Textbook of Practical Oral and Maxillofacial Surgery

Textbook of Practical Oral and Maxillofacial Surgery

DANIEL E. WAITE, D.D.S., M.S., F.A.C.D.
Professor and Chairman,
Department of Oral and Maxillofacial Surgery;
Assistant Dean for Hospital Affairs,
Baylor College of Dentistry
Dallas, Texas

THIRD EDITION

LEA & FEBIGER • 1987 • PHILADELPHIA

Lea & Febiger
600 South Washington Square
Philadelphia, Pa. 19106-4198
U.S.A.
(215) 922-1330

Library of Congress Cataloging-in-Publication Data
Main entry under title:

Textbook of practical oral and maxillofacial surgery.

   Includes bibliographies and index.
   1. Mouth—Surgery. I. Waite, Daniel E., 1926–
[DNLM: 1. Surgery, Oral. WU 600 T 3544]
RK529.T49 1986   617′.522   85-23973
ISBN 0-8121-1028-5

PRINTED IN THE UNITED STATES OF AMERICA
Print Number: 5 4 3 2 1

Preface

THE *Textbook of Practical Oral Surgery* was originally written with the belief that a need existed for an introductory textbook that dealt with basic concepts and selective clinical problems and was commensurate with the level of understanding of the dental student and the general practitioner of dentistry. This third edition continues to bear the same objective. With the passage of time and the exponential growth of knowledge in general dentistry, surgery, and medicine, it is easy and attractive to write about and propagate those interesting and expanding areas of information. However, it is the author's opinion that there is an important place for the emphasis of fundamentals and basic principles as outlined in the *Textbook of Practical Oral Surgery.* To this end, I have tried in my writings, and have extended the invitation to the contributing authors, to be clear in thought and basic in concepts that will be advantageous to those individuals desiring a basic understanding of what will be required of them throughout their practice of dentistry and their involvement in oral and maxillofacial surgery.

As in the previous editions, we are trying to introduce to the student the broad field of oral and maxillofacial surgery and some basic information a surgeon must possess to carry forth his responsibilities in a practice relating to this expanding field. The importance of taking an adequate history, interviewing the patient, conducting an appropriate oral examination, and using the laboratory aids for diagnosis is stressed. The sequential aspect of assessment, diagnosis, and treatment with appropriate postoperative management of patient care is established through individual chapters and their appropriate placement in the text.

Dentistry today is clearly a primary health care provider. Its role in the health professions increases daily with the ever expanding responsibilities that are part of patient health care needs. The increasing age of our population, with patients living longer as a result of advanced medical care, brings into focus patients with geriatric needs relating to complex medications, various implant prostheses, and the broadening parameters for maintenance of oral health. The ever changing delivery system relating to health care has placed continuing emphasis on the individual management of patients in the office, nursing homes, and hospices, as well as an emphasis on outpatient care. The reader will find the new chapters on anesthesia, pain control, management of chronic and craniofacial pain, and implants especially helpful in understanding the care of older persons.

The text of the third edition has been divided into four distinct sections. Each section builds upon the other, commencing with the basic principles of oral and maxillofacial surgery as taught to dental students, expanding into the necessary techniques of oral surgery as described in Section 2, and advancing to increased areas of surgical responsibility outlined in Section 3. Section 4 focuses on the ever increasing scope of oral and maxillofacial surgery as defined in the responsibility for the patient care in the hospital, new developments, and understanding of patients with temporomandibular joint disease and the ever increasing knowledge and technical skills to manage the closely related field of developmental jaw deformities, cleft lip, and cleft palate.

As often happens, work of this kind is of most value to those who have lived the closest to it. Such is the case for me and, therefore, I am the benefactor. During the course of laying out the project, stimulating the contributors and maintaining contact with them, and with final editing and the pressure of deadlines, I felt very much a part of the third edition of the *Textbook of Practical Oral and Maxillofacial Surgery*. It is my hope that each of the readers, over the years, will sense some of this feeling, and my desire is that, to some degree, it also becomes a part of them.

Dallas, Texas   DANIEL E. WAITE

Acknowledgments

Many persons have contributed their time, talent, knowledge, and illustrated material to the excellence of this textbook. In such an undertaking, the present authors and contributors owe a great deal to those who have gone before. Those who have developed the diagnoses, surgical procedures, and patient treatment plans are those who have laid a great foundation for the discipline of oral and maxillofacial surgery as practiced today. It is impossible to identify or express appropriate appreciation to all of the past educators and researchers in oral and maxillofacial surgery who have made such contributions.

Many new authors in this third edition bring significant contributions. The material that is presented, coupled with the background and experience of the authors, makes this particular edition the best. The completion of such a task encompassed in the pages of this textbook is the accumulated effort of many more persons than can be identified. Such an effort represents the skills of many besides the authors—secretaries, residents, colleagues, photographers, publisher, and, of course, patients. The secretaries who have been especially helpful in final typing and preparation of manuscripts have been Ellie Weigand and Darlene Amos. The kindly encouragement and confidence expressed to me by Christian C.F. Spahr, Jr. of Lea & Febiger is greatly appreciated. Raymond R. Kersey, executive editor for Lea & Febiger, has been especially helpful in guiding the overall plan and timing of the publication. Dr. Hak Joo Kwon has helped in coordination and organization of the chapters, and Dr. Robert Wardrop has contributed by proofreading and helping with editing. Dr. Donald Chiles, Director of the Undergraduate Oral Surgery Program at Baylor College of Dentistry, has been especially supportive and offered excellent guidance and personal support to me. He also contributed his own chapter.

In the first edition, I acknowledged that good residents make a good chief, as good residents make for a good training program. Their intellectual sharpness and their consistent cooperation have kept me alert and progressive in the surgical field. To them I express my deepest appreciation. The following pages carry a collage of photographs of these fine young people who gave me outstanding support over many years as Chairman of Oral and Maxillofacial Surgery at the University of Minnesota. Two other groups of residents, who do not appear in the photographs but who equally deserve mention, are those who were with me during their training at the Mayo Clinic in Rochester, Minnesota, and now at the Baylor College of Dentistry in Dallas, Texas. To these young people, as well as to the institutions I have served, I owe a debt of gratitude.

A special debt of gratitude is owed to my wife, Alice Waite. Throughout the preparation and laborious efforts of all three editions, she has been supportive, patient, encouraging, and truly my companion.

D.E.W.

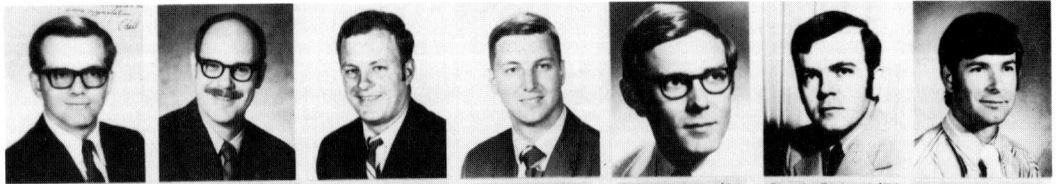

Anderson, Odell '69 Richter, Kenneth '69 Benson, David '70 Miller, John '71 Servine, John '71 Check, Richard '72 Grammer, Frank '72

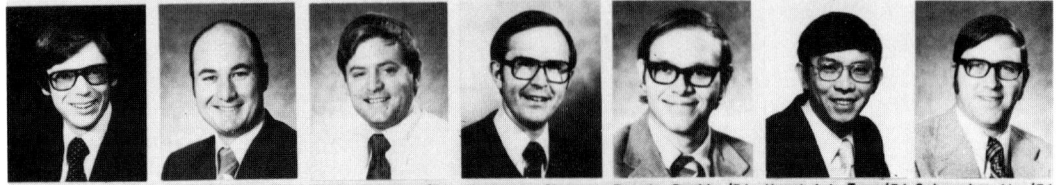

Boerger, William '72 Erickson, Gary '73 Coyle, Thomas '73 Anderson, Clennan '73 Broude, David '74 Huynh Anh, Tuan '74 Schmucker, Alan '74

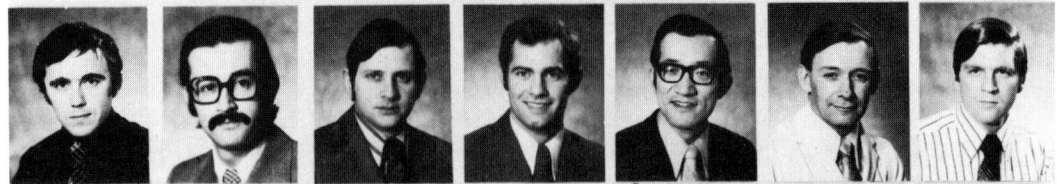

Piercell, Michael '74 Barrera, Alfonso '74 Freeman, Neal '75 Short, Sinclair '75 Wang, Joseph '76 Curran, John '76 Jensen, Guy '76

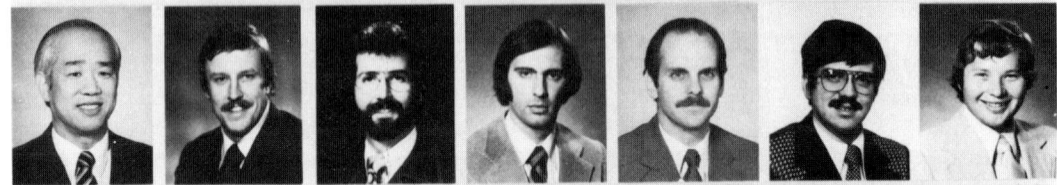

Kwon Hak, Joo '76 Olson, Dale '76 Hanson, Gerald '76 Ballin, Richard '77 Gatto, Daniel '77 Hebda, Thomas '77 Sokoloski, Peter '77

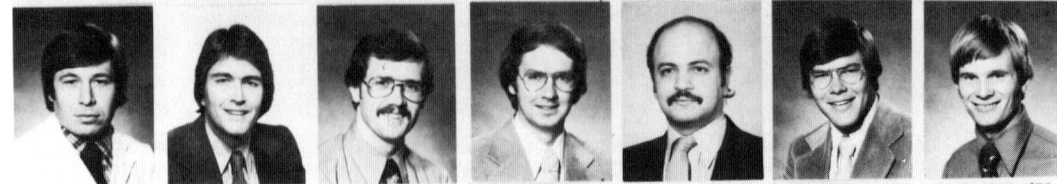

Block, James '78 Anderson, Stephen '78 Fleener, Michael '78 Amundson, Kevin '79 ElDeeb, Mohamed '79 Durtsche, Timothy '79 Omlie, Mark '79

NOT PICTURED: Heldridge, John '69; Wilkes, Clyde '69; Runck, Dennis '70; Nguyen Minh, Truong '72; Nelson, Robert '76

ORAL SURGERY GRADUATE PROGRAM 1969–1984
UNIVERSITY OF MINNESOTA SCHOOL OF DENTISTRY

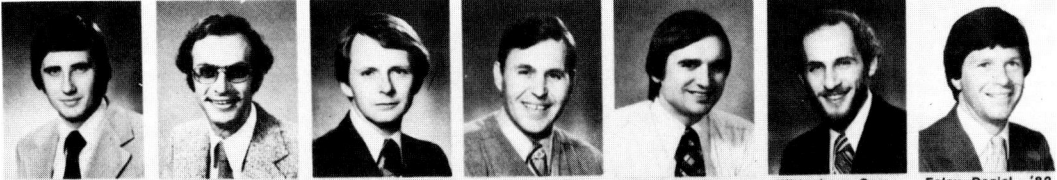

Babst, Charles '80   Nasser, Joseph '80   Sorochan, Robert '80   Cisler, Terry '81   Seidelmann, Thomas '81   Wittenberg, Gerry '81   Foley, Daniel '82

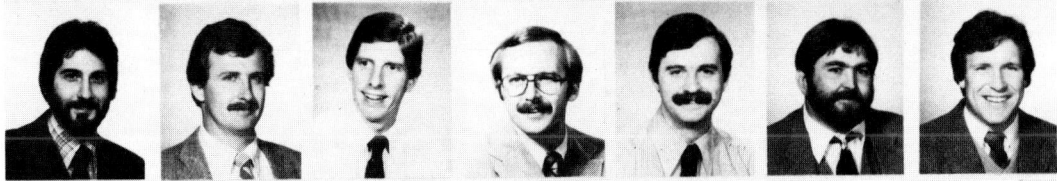

Fiola, Thomas '82   Whinery, John '82   Martin, Brent '83   Paulson, Eric '83   Tunis, Wayne '83   Deeter, William '84   Haas, Fred '84

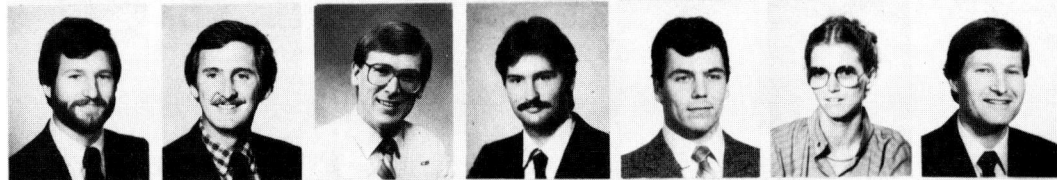

Weisbecker, Richard '84   Hoffmann, William '85   Horswell, Bruce '85   Roszkowski, Matthew '85   Bruksch, Kurt '86   Pinholt, Else '86   Templeton, Bruce '86

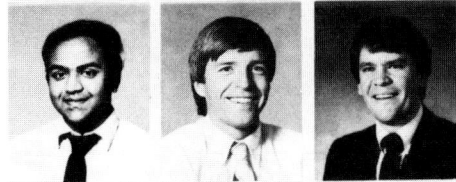

Cumarasamy, Thayalan '87   Florine, Brent '87   Wade, Marshall '87

Contributors

GRAEME A. BROWNE, B.D.S., M.Sc., F.R.C.D.
Clinical Assistant Professor, University of Minnesota
Staff Oral and Maxillofacial Surgeon, Veterans Administration Medical Center
Minneapolis, Minnesota

DONALD G. CHILES, D.D.S., F.A.C.D.
Associate Professor, Oral and Maxillofacial Surgery
Baylor College of Dentistry
Dallas, Texas

JOHN J. DELFINO, D.M.D., M.S.
Chairman, Division of Oral and Maxillofacial Surgery
Director of Residency Programs
St. John's Mercy Medical Center
St. Louis, Missouri

THOMAS R. FLYNN, D.M.D.
Assistant Professor of Oral and Maxillofacial Surgery
School of Dental Medicine; Assistant Professor of Surgery,
School of Medicine, University of Connecticut
Farmington, Connecticut

JAMES R. FRICTON, D.D.S., M.S.
Associate Professor, Department of Oral and Maxillofacial Surgery;
Co-director, TMJ and Craniofacial Pain Clinic
School of Dentistry, University of Minnesota
Minneapolis, Minnesota

JOSEPH A. GIOVANNITTI, JR., D.M.D.
Adjunct Assistant Professor
Baylor College of Dentistry; Consultant, Department of Dentistry,
Baylor University Medical Center
Dallas, Texas

JOHN F. HELFRICK, D.D.S., M.S.
Professor and Chairman, Department of Oral and Maxillofacial Surgery
Health Science Center, University of Texas
Houston, Texas

FRANK W. HILLIARD, D.D.S., M.S.
Orthodontist
Arlington, Texas

ROBERT A. JAMES, D.D.S., M.S.
Professor, Department of Restorative Dentistry;
Director, Postdoctoral Studies in Oral Implantology
School of Dentistry, Loma Linda University
Loma Linda, California

MARK T. JASPERS, D.D.S., M.S.
Associate Professor, Department of Oral and Maxillofacial Surgery
School of Dentistry, University of Minnesota
Minneapolis, Minnesota

KENNETH K. KEMPF, D.D.S.
Assistant Professor and Director, Department of Hospital Dentistry
Division of Oral and Maxillofacial Surgery
University of Iowa Hospitals and Clinics
Iowa City, Iowa

MICHAEL C. KINNEBREW, M.D., D.D.S.
Clinical Associate Professor, Oral and Maxillofacial Surgery;
Adjunct Clinical Associate Professor, Department of Communication Disorders, Louisiana State University
New Orleans, Louisiana

HAK JOO KWON, D.D.S., Ph.D.
Associate Professor (DEU), Department of Oral and Maxillofacial Surgery
School of Dentistry, University of Minnesota
Minneapolis, Minnesota

PAUL H. MCFARLAND, JR., D.D.S.
Associate Dean for Graduate Studies
Professor of Oral and Maxillofacial Surgery
Health Science Center, University of Texas
Houston, Texas

DONALD R. MEHLISCH, M.D., D.D.S.

Adjunct Associate Professor, Department of Oral and Maxillofacial Surgery, Baylor College of Dentistry, Dallas, Texas;
Clinical Professor, Department of Oral and Maxillofacial Surgery, University of Texas, Houston, Texas;
President, Biomedical Research Group, Inc.
Austin, Texas

ROGER A. MEYER, D.D.S., M.D.

Associate Professor, Department of Oral and Maxillofacial Surgery
School of Dentistry; Assistant Professor, Department of Surgery
School of Medicine, Emory University
Atlanta, Georgia

STEPHEN B. MILAM, B.A., M.A., D.D.S.

Assistant Professor, Coordinator of Pain and Anxiety Control Curriculum,
Department of Pharmacology
Baylor College of Dentistry
Dallas, Texas

EDWARD L. MOSBY, D.D.S.

Associate Professor and Vice Chairman, Department of Hospital Dentistry;
Associate Director, Oral and Maxillofacial Surgery Graduate Training
Truman Medical Center, University of Missouri
Kansas City, Missouri

JEFFREY L. RAJCHEL, D.D.S.

Assistant Professor, Department of Oral and Maxillofacial Surgery
Baylor College of Dentistry
Dallas, Texas

DONALD W. ROBERTSON, Ph.D.

Associate Professor
Department of Anatomy, School of Medicine
University of Minnesota
Minneapolis, Minnesota

RICHARD G. TOPAZIAN, D.D.S.

Professor and Chairman, Department of Oral and Maxillofacial Surgery
School of Dental Medicine; Professor of Surgery, School of Medicine
University of Connecticut
Farmington, Connecticut

DANIEL E. WAITE, D.D.S., M.S., F.A.C.D.

Professor and Chairman, Department of Oral and Maxillofacial Surgery;
Assistant Dean for Hospital Affairs, Baylor College of Dentistry
Dallas, Texas

PETER D. WAITE, M. Ph., D.D.S., M.D.

Assistant Professor, Department of Oral and Maxillofacial Surgery
School of Dentistry, University of Alabama
Birmingham, Alabama

ROBERT W. WARDROP

Research Fellow; Department of Oral and Maxillofacial Surgery
Baylor College of Dentistry
Dallas, Texas

LARRY M. WOLFORD, D.D.S.

Professor of Oral and Maxillofacial Surgery;
Baylor College of Dentistry
Dallas, Texas

Contents

CHAPTER 1

History, Scope, and Objectives: The Speciality of Oral and Maxillofacial Surgery

DANIEL E. WAITE

The direction in which education starts a man will determine his future life. PLATO

The origins of oral surgery are credited to Dr. S.P. Hulliehen, who practiced in Wheeling, West Virginia from 1835 until his death in 1857. He performed over 500 operations for cleft lip, cleft palate, and other abnormalities and diseases of the mouth and jaws. Dr. Hulliehen, honored as a pioneer in the field, is known as "the father of oral surgery." Dr. James Edmund Garretson, 1828–1895, Professor of Anatomy at the Philadelphia School of Anatomy, was the first person to envision oral surgery as a specialty that would develop only with special training. He named the field "oral surgery" and advised others who limited their practice to surgery of the mouth and surrounding tissues to call themselves "oral surgeons."

The first recognition of oral surgery as a specialty came in 1869 when Garretson was appointed oral surgeon to the University of Pennsylvania Hospital. At that time, he published the first book on surgery of the mouth known as Garretson's *System of Oral Surgery.*

Many other distinguished individuals helped establish oral surgery as a specialty. Truman W. Brophy, noted for his work on cleft lip and cleft palate; Matthew H. Cryer for his knowledge of the anatomy of the face and cranium; Thomas Fillebrown for his improved method in anesthesia; Thomas L. Gilmer for his outstanding work in fractures of the jaws; and John S. Marshall for his scholarly writings in oral surgery are but a few. Chalmer J. Lyons is noted for his remarkable teaching skills and his establishment of the first three-year postgraduate hospital internship in oral surgery. George B. Winter is equally

1

significant for his development of the principles involved in removal of impacted and unerupted teeth.[1]

Around 1912, physicians began to appreciate the important relationship of dentistry and oral disease to systemic disease. Hospital administrators became aware that to provide complete care for treatment of the sick, they had to include oral diagnosticians and dental surgeons as part of the health team. Dentists in general practice were soon to recognize the special qualifications of those who devoted their time to surgery of the mouth and the need for specialized care of hospital patients.

Developments and refinements in oral surgery techniques have been greatly influenced by experience gained in treating war injuries and by general advancements in medicine and dentistry. Such advancements include those in local and general anesthesia, and radiographic technology. A major advancement occurred in surgical technology with a new understanding of the principles of blood flow, bone grafting, wound healing, and pharmacology. This has promoted progress in the fields of orthognathic and cleft palate surgery.

The fact that people live longer has positively influenced oral surgery as new information has evolved from geriatric medicine and the need for specialized health care for older individuals. There has also been a resurgence of scientific information and research relating to the temporomandibular joint and preprosthetic surgery that has involved the dentist and specifically the oral and maxillofacial surgeon.

Organized Oral Surgery

The American Society of Exodontists was organized in August 1918, with 29 charter members of the society at the organization meeting in Chicago. At the society's second meeting, held in New Orleans, Dr. M.R. Howard circulated a petition regarding a name change. This change did not occur until the Milwaukee meeting in 1921, when the society's name became the American Society of Oral Surgeons and Exodontists. In 1943 Exodontists was dropped, and the present name, The American Society of Oral and Maxillofacial Surgeons, was adopted in 1977.

The American Board of Oral Surgery was established in 1946. In 1955, educational requirements for oral surgery were established as 3 years of advanced study and training. Although this has remained unchanged over many years, in 1983, the House of Delegates of the American Society of Oral and Maxillofacial Surgeons passed a resolution requesting the American Dental Association to look into the establishment of a fourth year of training. As of this writing, approximately half of the 116 training programs offer 4 years of training. Several also include the medical degree.

Although oral surgery training programs are sponsored by dental schools, and most certainly arise out of the dental profession, a major part of the training occurs in hospitals. A typical training program in oral and maxillofacial surgery requires a resident (graduate student) to spend a significant amount of time on a medicine service, anesthesia, and general surgery. Many programs may require shorter periods of time in such related areas of interest as neurosurgery, otolaryngology, and plastic surgery. The greater emphasis in training, however, is within the oral surgical discipline, treating patients with problems relating to the oral cavity and related head and neck structures. Oral surgery training encompasses basic research, leading to the acquisition of higher academic qualification. This emphasis on research has acted as a catalyst for the development of new ideas and their application in the clinical field of oral and maxillofacial surgery. The explosion of new knowledge and refinement of new techniques in the surgical treatment of cleft palate and jaw deformities is a direct result of research. The broad scope of oral and maxillofacial surgery is defined as that part of dental practice dealing with the diagnosis and surgical and adjunctive treatment of diseases, injuries, and defects of oral and maxillofacial regions.

The oral and maxillofacial surgeon as a dental specialist with advanced surgical and hospital training has a sound appreciation of the dental and surgical needs of the cleft palate patient. He provides a variety of surgical services at various stages in the growth and development of the cleft palate patient. The need for an oral and maxillo-

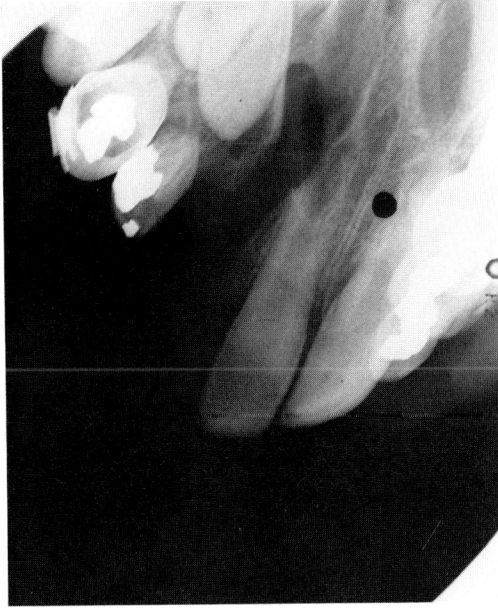

Fig. 1-1. *Alveolar cleft defect in a 6-year-old boy.*

facial surgeon's consultation regarding treatment occurs early in the patient's life. Jaw discrepancies, supernumerary teeth, impacted teeth, quality of the dentition, the cleft defect (Figs. 1-1 and 1-2), velopharyngeal insufficiency, and diet are but a few of the many problems that require participation from an oral and maxillofacial surgeon. It is not unusual for a patient to require multiple surgical procedures at different ages. These interrelated procedures have the common goal of providing a dentofacial configuration that is optimal relative to function and esthetics. Ideally, this goal is achieved as the patient reaches physical maturity.

The wide acceptance of the interdisciplinary team approach to the habilitation of the cleft palate patient has not eliminated

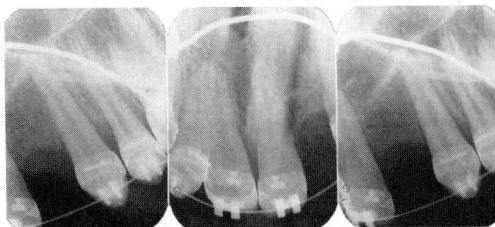

Fig. 1-2. *Defect has been grafted with bone from iliac crest. Canine tooth has erupted through the graft.*

controversy over treatment approaches. It has, however, encouraged the coming together of a group of professionals who, through their mutual concern for the patient, can establish realistic treatment goals. Such scientific curiosity, often stimulated by the inadequacies perceived in current treatment modalities, will bring about improvements in treatment for patients.

The scope of an oral surgery practice varies with the skills and training of the individual practitioner. This may also be affected by the locale in which he practices. Many related academic and clinical courses are necessary to provide an adequate foundation in oral surgery: some of these are oral diagnosis, oral pathology, oral medicine, radiology, anesthesia, and pharmacology. When carefully planned and integrated into the dental curriculum, such courses provide the basis for the experience in oral and maxillofacial surgery.

One must understand and appreciate that experience in providing oral surgery care comes slowly. At no one time can anyone know all there is to know about surgical management. After acquiring a strong foundation and experience in undergraduate oral surgery in dental school, the practitioner will gradually broaden his scope of surgical management. It is impossible for all undergraduate students or practitioners, for that matter, to receive exactly the same experience or to be exposed to all surgical problems. Some general practice surgical procedures may never be performed by a dentist in the early years of his experience. This does not imply that the dentist should never perform them. As a result of the understanding of the principles of surgery relating to anatomy, physiology and pathology, the student should have the confidence to select and manage patients with a high degree of skill. As one adheres to these basic principles and accumulates experience, his confidence should increase along with his grasp of the variety and complexity of oral surgery technique.

General Objectives

General objectives of the course in oral surgery include the following:

1. To provide a foundation of professional knowledge associated with surgical skills to enable the student to diagnose and

treat competently the various disorders related to his practice.

2. To stimulate the student to recall basic science information and to correlate it with the disease processes occurring in and about the oral cavity, particularly those lending themselves to surgical care.
3. To teach the student to examine his case findings critically and intelligently and to diagnose with competence.
4. To guide the student in developing a sense of confidence in his own skills and clinical judgment and to encourage the desire for continued professional study and self-improvement.
5. To help the student become familiar with and evaluate critically the scientific publications in oral surgery.
6. To filter out those students with a special interest in research. Students with either clinical or basic research interests should be given additional counselling and guidance in selecting special problems that would enhance their discovery of new information and contributions to the field of research.
7. To train the student to select cases that lie within the limits of his surgical ability and to exclude or refer those that he is not fully competent to handle.
8. To provide the student with a basis for continuing graduate or postgraduate study or for a teaching career.

Specific Objectives

Upon completion of his course in oral surgery, the student should be able to provide treatment for surgical patients accordingly:

1. To administer a local anesthetic effectively and safely.
2. To extract teeth in uncomplicated cases and recover root fragments effectively and efficiently.
3. To prepare the mouth for the reception of a prosthesis, which may entail bone and soft tissue surgery.
4. To care for infection of the oral cavity resulting from dental disease.
5. To perform root canal and apicoectomy procedures.
6. To recognize, treat, and prevent, whenever possible, syncope and shock that might result from surgery.

7. To treat and control hemorrhage from oral surgical procedures.
8. To perform a biopsy of suspected lesions or neoplasms and submit the properly prepared specimen to an oral pathologist.
9. To reduce and immobilize fractures of the teeth, alveolus, and uncomplicated fractures of the jaws.
10. To be familiar with the hospital operating room and capable of managing hospitalized dental patients.
11. To utilize sedatives, analgesics, and antibiotic medications, when necessary, with confidence.
12. To be aware of the relationship between oral and systemic disease pathophysiology, to request medical consultation when appropriate, and to refer for medical treatment when necessary.
13. To diagnose and refer, when appropriate, oral and facial deformities that may be amenable to oral surgical management.[2]

American Dental Association guidelines summarize the required experience for the graduate dentist. Graduates must be proficient to perform uncomplicated, minor oral surgical procedures. They must be competent in the surgical exposure of unerupted teeth and in uncomplicated alveoloplasty and preprosthetic surgery. Students should be exposed to the management of abscesses through intraoral procedures, the uncomplicated biopsy of hard and soft tissue lesions, and surgical extractions of impacted and erupted teeth.[3]

The dentist assumes an ethical as well as a legal responsibility when he accepts a patient for oral surgery. He must be qualified to diagnose and operate on patients presenting with surgical conditions; otherwise, it is his professional responsibility to refer the patient where he can be treated adequately. The health and welfare of the patient must always be the prime concern of the dentist. Good ethics and good surgical judgment based on his own surgical training and experience should clearly indicate to the dentist his responsibility for each surgical problem.

Since every oral surgeon is also a dentist, his background will make him sensitive to his patient's needs from a dental stand-point, and his hospital, anesthesia, and surgical experience will make him more aware of medical needs and medical counsel. The general dentist should rely upon the oral surgeon for assistance and guidance whenever complications arise as a result of surgically related diagnosis and treatment. At the same time, the oral surgeon should be sympathetic, alert, and willing to aid the general dentist in such instances. Difficult impaction procedures, roots, or foreign bodies lost in the maxillary sinus or tissue spaces are problems obviously within the experience of the oral surgeon. Fractures of the facial bones, skin grafts to the oral cavity for complicated prosthodontic cases, bone grafts, and problems relating to the temporomandibular joint will also have been a part of his training. The hospital management for the dental surgical treatment of patients with complicated systemic disease may become the joint responsibility of the general dental practitioner, the oral surgeon, and the physician. The salivary glands and their disease states often come to the attention of the dentist first. A detailed history and examination, which may include sialography or other special evaluations, may need to be done before a diagnosis can be made (Figs. 1-3 and 1-4). Only at that time can one decide on the best course of management, which may include a referral to the oral surgeon.

Oral surgery bears a close relationship to orthodontics. Jaw deformities and severe malocclusion may necessitate both surgical

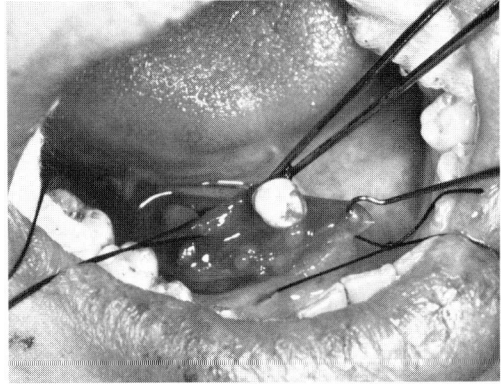

FIG. 1-4. *Salivary stone being removed from Wharton's duct.*

and orthodontic management. Prognathism, micrognathism, maxillary retrognathism, and unilateral condylar hyperplasia are only a few conditions that require the cooperation of these two specialists (Fig.1-5). Moreover, the general dentist must be able to recognize these deformities, obtain the appropriate records and history, and refer patients accordingly.

Oral pathology is another dental specialty requiring close cooperation with oral surgery. Tissue change through frozen section or conventional techniques can be identified only when adequate biopsy specimens and good case histories have been provided. Prosthodontics also requires close cooperation by the dentist in the surgical preparation of the denture base for a prosthesis. Alveoloplasty, immediate denture surgery, frenectomy, tuberosity reduction, and vestibuloplasty are a few situations in which this close cooperation must exist.

The educational program should provide the student with a basic understanding of hospital protocol, practice, and organization. The primary role of the hospital experience at the level of predoctoral dental education should be to reinforce the concept of treating the "total" patient and the application of the biomedical sciences. Sufficient experiences in clinical laboratory medicine should be presented to enable the student to order and interpret appropriate laboratory tests. Experience in applied pharmacology, physical evaluation, pain and anxiety control, and general anesthesia, which are part of the predoctoral

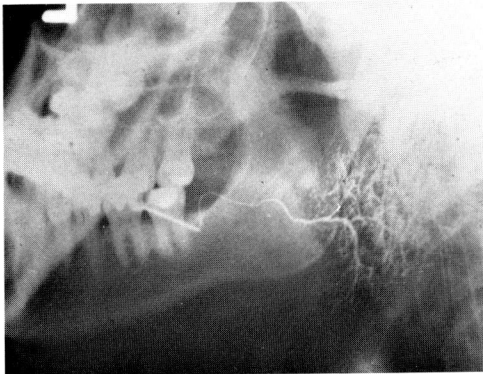

FIG. 1-3. *Sialography. The use of a contrast medium placed within the salivary duct of the parotid gland. Normal filling of the duct and gland.*

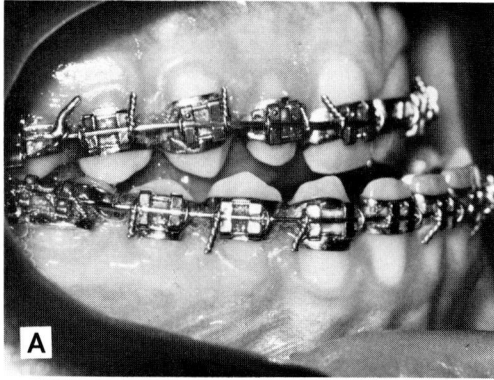

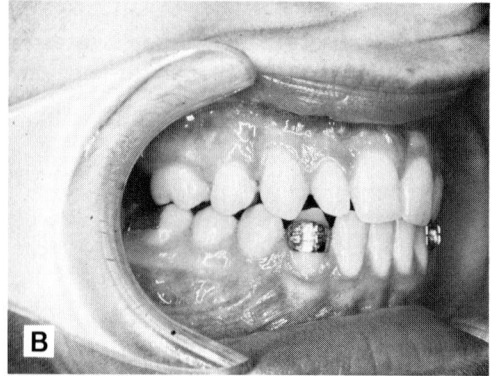

FIG. 1-5. *Treatment of prognathism by the orthodontist and oral surgeon. (A) Before surgery. (B) After surgery and removal of orthodontic appliances.*

student's education, should be reinforced in the hospital rotations. The student should gain familiarity with the hospital record and be able to enter and retrieve necessary information from the chart. The student should also receive general information about the organizational adminis-

FIG. 1-6. *Lateral chest x-ray of a patient with a heart valve prosthesis. Wire sutures are seen along the anterior chest wall.*

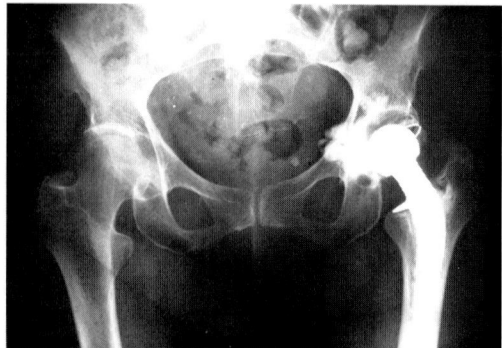

tration, financing, protocol, and governance of the hospital. Topics to be covered include the process of applying for hospital privileges, patient admission procedures, operating room protocol, and interprofessional patient management.

The relationship of oral surgery to the practice of medicine has become increasingly important. Even though preventive dentistry is making great advances, so is preventive medicine, and thus many patients outlive the life of their dentitions. Many surgical procedures have to be carried out on patients receiving anticoagulant medication, antihypertensive drugs, sedatives, or immunosuppressive agents. Many patients are unaware of the significant relationship between a variety of medical conditions and even minor surgical procedures. This serves to emphasize the

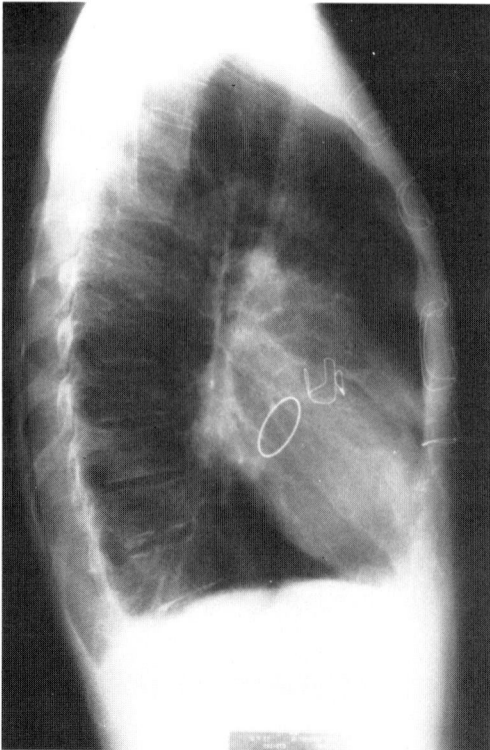

FIG. 1-7. *Total hip prosthesis. Because of potential foreign body response and infection, antibiotic coverage for dental surgery is indicated.*

great need for the dentist to be knowledgeable about general medical problems (Figs. 1-6 and 1-7). On occasion, patients have to be hospitalized for medical reasons in order to perform otherwise routine office procedures. Laboratory procedures such as urinalysis, bacterial culture, and hematologic evaluation may have to be done on many surgical patients. This immediately draws the dentist into medical-dental discussion with physicians, nurses, and paramedical personnel. It may necessitate the writing of medication orders, pre- and postanesthetic care, admission, progress, and discharge notes by the dentist when these patients are hospitalized. There is no substitute for experience and understanding when dental care is offered to the otherwise medically ill patient.

Finally, there is no substitute for the constant awareness of up-to-date literature, discussion with dental and medical colleagues and, of course, just plain clinical experience if the objectives of this text are to be realized. These pages are designed to be stimulating and to extend the invitation to learn more. An important concept is to do first things first. Thomas Henry Huxley aptly said, "perhaps the most valuable result of all education is the ability to make yourself do the thing you have to do when it ought to be done whether you like it or not; it is the first lesson that ought to be learned; and however early a man's training begins, it is probably the last lesson that he learns thoroughly."

References

1. The Bulletin, American Society of Oral Surgeons, June 1949.
2. American Society of Oral Surgeons: Principles of undergraduate education in oral surgery. J. Dent. Educ., *30*:403, 1966.
3. Accreditation Standards for Dental Education Programs, December 1984.

CHAPTER 2

Principles of Surgery

PETER D. WAITE

Medicine, to produce health, has to examine disease, and music, to create harmony, must investigate discord.

PLUTARCH

Approach to the Patient

No greater opportunity, responsibility, or obligation is afforded an individual than that of serving another person as a physician. In treating patients, a physician needs technical skill, scientific knowledge, and human understanding. One who uses these with honesty, humility, and wisdom will provide a unique service to all with whom he comes in contact.

We in the healing arts must possess many qualities, but most of all we must have genuine concern for those we serve. We must provide our patients with the care that we would expect and want. If we can avoid a superior air and a condescending attitude toward those who need the service we offer, we will maintain the respect of life: the basic principle of surgery. Disregard for the basic principles of surgery, human life, and personal ethics is the preliminary step to the collapse of the tenets of surgical care. Surgical care is based upon "doing unto others as you would have them do unto you."

Dr. T.R. Harrison once wrote:
Tact, sympathy, and understanding are expected of the physician, for the patient is no mere collection of symptoms, signs, disordered functions, damaged organs, and disturbed emotions. He is human, fearful, and hopeful, seeking relief, help, and reassurance. To the physician, as to the anthropologist, nothing human is strange or repulsive. The misanthrope may become a smart diagnostician of organic disease, but he can scarcely hope to succeed as a physician. The true physician has a Shakespearean breadth of interest in the wise and foolish, the proud and the humble, the stoic hero, and the whining rogue. He cares for people.[1]

Development and Scope

It has been said that "those who cannot remember the past are condemned to repeat it." Therefore, we should develop and retain basic principles that protect us from past mistakes and yield satisfactory results. The history of disease is as old as mankind, and the basic forms—trauma, infections, tumors, and congenital abnormalities—have not changed. Surgeons have responded to disease on the basis of compassion that the patient needs and deserves and have been influenced by their own sense of wholeness and good health. In many ways the concept of good health or lack of disease is being analyzed, evaluated, and changed. For example, we no longer accept arthritis, hypertension, angina pectoris, and periodontal disease as normal conditions associated with aging. Many of these diseases are not curable, but medical science can make them less severe and better tolerated. In reality, physicians rarely cure an illness but modify the annoying symptoms.

Oral and maxillofacial surgeons are involved not only with the cure of disease, but more importantly, with improving the quality of a person's life. Because of the aura and mystique that surround some surgeons and their procedures, society has imposed a disproportionate subjective value system for the treatment of disease. Some procedures are viewed as important and others less important for the wholeness and well-being of an individual. It is difficult to quantitate the value and significance that a surgical procedure has on improving the quality of life of any given individual. One cannot measure the value of a surgical correction of a person's deformity by the complexity of the anatomy, length of surgery, the stature of the surgeon, or the financial cost to the patient.

Since the development of medical insurance, an erroneous dichotomy of the human body has appeared to influence patients' and physicians' concepts of complete health care. Dental practices are not generally considered under medical insurance. Although dental surgery is certainly similar to any other subspecialty of surgery that improves a patient's quality of life, it is viewed differently by national and private insurance companies. It is unfortunate that health care has been fragmented. Dental health is no less important than any other aspect of individual health care.

Many technically simple procedures have resulted in greatly improving the quality of life for an individual. Perhaps only someone with a similar problem can fully empathize with the individual unable to perform simple daily routine functions such as eating, drinking, or speaking.

Since the prehistoric ages, medicine men have responded to the diseases of mankind and contributed to our present knowledge of patient care. Many physicians, such as the early Egyptians, Hippocrates, Celsus, Galen, and Theodoric, have influenced the present approach to the surgical patient. Originally, patient care was provided in a general manner, without distinction of a physician or dentist. During the fourteenth century, barbers and surgeons arose as the two major groups or guilds caring for the sick and diseased. The union guilds attempted to relieve human suffering but differed in their approach. Simple dental care, provided mainly by the barbers, met a large portion of the public's somatic complaints. While the barbers offered a significant service to people at that time, the surgeon's role was extremely limited.

Surgeons worked under many myths and misconceptions that influenced the knowledge of general patient care. Benefits from surgical care were very small because of factors such as pain, infection, hemorrhage, shock, and lack of anatomic knowledge. Dentistry, on the other hand, was of greater benefit because of its technical simplicity at that time. Basic conflicts of interest and theory must have led to an agreement in 1540 that the barbers would perform no surgery if the surgeons would perform no dentistry. Although the barber and surgery union guilds lasted only 200 years from their inception, the subtle limitation of practice continued much longer.

Pain, infection, hemorrhage, and shock were the most difficult obstacles for the surgeons to overcome, but as they did the scope of their practice grew substantially. The successful demonstration of ether anesthesia by William T. G. Morton (1819–1868), a Boston dentist, was a landmark event in the history of surgery. Joseph Lister (1827–1912), the originator of antiseptic surgery, and Louis Pasteur (1822–1895), the originator of the germ theory, greatly reduced the dangers of infection. Not until Sir Alexander Fleming discovered penicillin in 1945 did surgeons truly conquer the problem of infection. Only recently have great strides been made in treating hemorrhage and shock, because of increased knowledge in anatomy, physiology, and vascular surgery.

Oral and maxillofacial surgery is defined as the part of dental practice that deals with the diagnosis and the surgical and adjunctive treatment of the diseases, injuries, and defects of human jaws and associated structures. Viewed as a subspecialty of surgery, it is a blend of dentistry and surgery requiring strict adherence to surgical principles as well as intricate understanding of dental applications. It cannot function on the precepts of surgery or dentistry alone but requires both disciplines to avoid the failures of the past.[2]

Risk Assessment in Surgical Evaluation

Patient evaluation or "risk assessment" is very important for a surgeon. The dentist who provides surgical treatment must evaluate the total surgical trauma elicited in relation to the systemic status of the patient to arrive at the operative risk. The oral surgeon must understand the systemic nature of disease and how it influences the surgical therapy. He must recognize systemic disease states that contraindicate surgery and expeditiously refer to proper medical specialties. The oral and maxillofacial surgeon must be able to recognize very early pathologic states even if oral manifestations are not present.

The principles of evaluating a patient by history taking, physical examination, and laboratory data are designed to provide an assessment or diagnosis of the individual's state of health. A good history is the most important part of evaluating a patient prior to surgery. Time spent listening to the patient provides valuable clues that can lead the practitioner to the proper conclusions about a patient's health status. Although this data is subjective, it is the largest and most important portion of data to collect.

A patient may have no complaints of poor health, but when the surgeon reviews past medical history, he may realize that the risk involved with the patient may be much greater than normal. For example, a 50-year-old white male allergic to penicillin, taking antihypertensives, cardiac glycosides, and bronchodilators, is obviously a great risk for any surgery even if he "feels fine." Further questioning into the review of systems directed by the past medical history provides additional subjective data. One would specifically question the patient to determine the degree of residual reserve available in each related organ system. (Residual reserve is the functional capacity to perform beyond the basal level.) If no residual reserve exists, the risk of elective surgery must be evaluated for the good of the patient. In other words, in the above example one would closely evaluate the cardiovascular and pulmonary systems. Subjective data is the summation of the history and review of systems, while objective data is the physical examination.

In the preoperative evaluation the surgeon should take each organ system and ask himself "how will my surgery, anesthesia, position or duration of surgery, and convalescent period affect this aspect of my patient's disease state?" When the trauma of surgery increases risk to the patient, the benefit of surgery must be questioned.

The preoperative examination is not designed to discover occult disease but to establish whether a particular individual can successfully and safely undergo the psychologic and physiologic stresses of surgery. The surgeon should determine what minimizes those stresses and what increases the risk of a routine procedure in different and variable circumstances.

All aspects of systemic disease are important considerations for minor outpatient dental surgery and cannot be inclusively addressed at this time. No universal statements can be applied to all situations, but basic principles can be offered to the student.

In general, one should avoid elective surgery in a compromised patient until he reaches his optimal state of health. For example, postpone surgery if possible for individuals with transient neurologic deficits or recent cerebrovascular accidents until medically stable. It also is best to wait 6 months after a myocardial infarct for elective surgery because the cardiac risk is greatly reduced. Dyspena and/or chest pain at rest or with even mild activity represents "end stage" disease with minimal reserve in the pulmonary or cardiovascular systems. It also indicates probable micro-angiopathic disease in all organ systems and should signify caution to the surgeon.

Patients with congestive heart failure and orthopnea obviously cannot lie flat in a dental chair for long periods of time without developing pulmonary edema. The condition of individuals with chronic obstruction pulmonary disease generally improves in the afternoon after they have had time to clear pulmonary secretions. However, if they are hypercarbic, then respiration is stimulated by hypoxia, and nitrous oxide and oxygen analgesia may cause respiratory suppression. Well-controlled diabetics generally can be managed best in the morning without modifying their medical therapy, but if uncontrolled or brittle may require management by a physician.[3]

In conclusion, of the many principles of surgery, only two are accurate 100 percent of the time: "do no harm" and "know thy patient."

TABLE 2-1. *Factors influencing the stages of wound healing*

Accelerate Healing	Decelerate Healing	
Suturing	Foreign Body	Radiation
Grafting	Mobilization	Chemotherapy
Debriding	Pressure	Immune Suppression
Function	Hemorrhage	Diabetes
Halsted's Principles	Dehisence	Obesity
Gentleness	Chronic Disease	Age
Hemostasis	Starvation	Vitamin Deficiency
No Tension	Hypoxia	
Blood Supply	Sepsis	
Asepsis	Shock	
Approximation	Acidosis	
Obliteration of Dead Space	Uremia	
	Liver Disease	
	Steriods	

Wound Healing

Surgery has been defined as the art and science of wounding. Without the restoration of wound continuity, there would be no surgery. In other words, if wounds did not heal, surgery could not be performed. Since even the most minor delicate form of surgery produces tissue trauma, the surgeon must know what processes minimize, prevent, and eliminate factors that retard would healing (Table 2-1 and Fig. 2-1).

Normal healing follows an orderly sequence of cellular and biochemical steps that are initiated by injury. Damaged capillaries cause hemorrhage, platelet aggregation, and activation of coagulation. Tissue disruption activates complement and kinin cascades, initiating chemotaxis of inflammatory cells into the avascular wound. Macrophages appear and predominate in the direction of the tissue regeneration process. Fibroblasts are induced at the wound edge and produce a collagen matrix that supports angiogenesis. This process continues in the wound space until the wound edges fuse. The physiologic signals that initiate, propagate, and terminate the fibroblastic collagen process are poorly understood, but clearly many fragile and susceptible steps exist.

The healing process can be conceptualized in four biologic stages. The first is the coagulation stage, in which clot formation is crucial and fibrinogen is a key macromolecule. Hemorrhage hematoma, edema, or contamination retard this stage. The second stage occurs up to the seventh day, during which the neutrophils function to combat infection. Purulence, foreign body, fistula, or abscess delay progression to the third stage. The proliferative stage, which occurs during the second week, is characterized by the presence of fibroblasts and is controlled by the macrophage. Collagen and proteoglycans form a matrix that holds the wound together. Wound tension, mobility, decrease in vascularity, hypoxia, and metabolic factors influence this process. The fourth stage is that of restoration and continuity, which occurs by connective tissue remodeling. It produces normal mature tissue with 50 percent of the final tensile strength by the third or fourth week.

STAGES IN WOUND HEALING

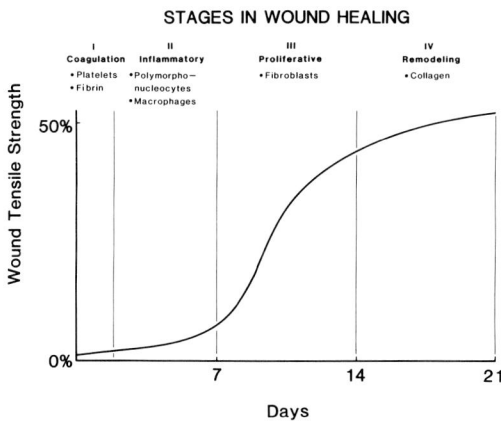

FIG. 2-1. *Wound strength during various stages of healing.*

The obviously complex physiology of wound healing is beyond the scope of this chapter. However, a thorough understanding is essential for the surgeon, who must be aware of basic principles that dictate current patient management and practice. For example, sutures are generally removed at 7 days because the wound has passed through the coagulation and inflammatory stages of healing. During the next 7 days the wound rapidly increases in tensile strength in what is referred to as the proliferative stage. Certain factors, such as increased vascularity, however, can accelerate this healing process. Therefore, sutures in the head and neck can be removed in 5 days when the tensile strength is similar to other wounds. This also decreases the inflammatory response to the suture material and less scar formation occurs.[4,5]

Nutrition

Trauma produces certain metabolic responses that increase energy and protein requirements. Surgery elicits trauma and requires wound healing, which in turn produces similar metabolic needs. Proper surgical technique can reduce these metabolic demands and encourage anabolism. The summation of metabolic needs is related to the degree of wound healing required. Although the metabolic and physiologic demands may be minimal in minor oral surgery, they are present and should be considered.

The goal of nutritional support is maintenance of calories (carbohydrate), nitrogen (protein), and vitamins. Nutritional requirements can be estimated from the basal metabolic rate (BMR). BMR is the metabolic rate of a fasting individual at *complete* rest. It is a function of age, sex, and body size that is reproducible and predictable. It is listed in standard tables in units of kilocalories per square meter of body surface per hour ($kcal/m^2/hr$). The basal caloric requirement per day is simply the body surface area multiplied by the basal metabolic rate. The total caloric requirement represents the total caloric need of the individual to heal wounds and provide routine daily functions. It is the product of the basal caloric requirement, the surgical stress factor, and an additional 25 percent metabolic need for a nonactive but incompletely resting convalescent patient.

$$\text{Total Caloric Requirement} = \text{Basal calories} \times \text{stress factor of surgery} \times 1.25$$

Nutritional support should provide at least 15 percent of the total calories as protein and at least 60 percent as carbohydrate. The remaining 25 percent can be either fat or carbohydrate. Most enteral feeding formulas reflect this balanced composition of carbohydrate, fat, and protein. Malnutrition is seldom a problem for the oral surgery patient but the principle of good nutrition is important. Obstacles to good nutrition may be obstruction, decreased function, or as described previously, increased metabolic needs. These can all be solved by blended or enteral formula feeding.

Example: 35-year-old male, 3rd molar patient.
10% increase in metabolic needs for surgery
Body surface area = $2m^2$
BMR = 36.5 kcal/m^2/hr.
Basal calories = (36.5) (2) (24) = 1752

(1752 Basal calories) (1.10 stress factor) (1.25 activity factor) = 2409 total caloric needs[6]

Management of Infections

Head and neck infections most often are odontogenic in origin. The offending organism usually has a low virulence and can be eliminated easily in the normal host after extraction of teeth, root canal therapy, and/or incision and drainage of abscesses. Because most odontogenic infections are caused by penicillin-sensitive microorganisms, however, antibiotics are of great assistance. Antibiotics must be viewed only as an aid in infectious disease management. They cannot take the place of definitive treatment. The cause of the odontogenic infection must be eliminated before the surgeon can assume the cure. Persisting infections after routine therapy may indicate the presence of one or more of the following: antibiotic resistance, poor defense mechanisms, foreign body, occult abscess, sequestration, complex microbial populations, and/or increased virulence.

Infectious disease control is a complex and extensive speciality, beyond the scope of this chapter; however, basic principles apply to oral surgery. Antibiotics cannot replace good surgical technique but only support it if it fails. Maxillofacial infections generally involve mixed populations of streptococcus and gram-negative anaerobes. Penicillin is the drug of choice because it is the least toxic, most effective, and cheapest, with the broadest spectrum and most specificity for maxillofacial infections.[7]

Operative Care

The care of the surgical patient involves three specific stages: preoperative, intraoperative, and postoperative. Preoperative care begins with the diagnostic work up, involving a thorough history and physical examination. Preoperative evaluation or risk assessment is an overall survey of the patient's general health status. Its purpose is to identify significant problems that may increase the risk of surgery or influence the convalescent stage.

In pure elective surgery no operation must begin unless every subsystem is optimal. The surgeon must weigh the benefits and risks of surgery in relation to various aspects of the patient. Some of these specifics are:

(1) Nutrition, hydration, and electrolyte balance
(2) Blood volume
(3) Status of coagulation
(4) Cardiovascular reserve
(5) Respiratory reserve
(6) Kidney function
(7) Association of concurrent disease

No universal statement can preclude or justify surgical intervention because compromise always exists between the lesser of evils.[8]

During the preoperative period discussing potential problems and expected results with the patient greatly allays anxiety and improves the patient-physician relationship. One about to undergo surgery must have confidence in his surgeon. A patient with a reasonable expectation and understanding of surgery is generally satisfied. A common complaint heard in many lawsuits is the lack of informed consent. With the medical legal system of today, it behooves surgeons to inform patients tactfully, but thoroughly, of potential problems and expected results of their particular surgery. Good patient rapport improves all aspects of a surgeon's practice.

Intraoperative care is primarily good surgical technique but also involves monitoring the patient's response to surgery. This stage of operative care is so critical and consuming that in major cases an anesthesiologist is required. The principles still apply, even in minor surgery. The surgeon must be aware of the patient's pain threshold, mental status, and vital function reserves. This requires monitoring vital signs and recording the data. Although the surgeon may not practice anesthesiology, he should know the effects and limitations of the drugs administered. This is particularly true in outpatient intravenous sedation. All medications have side effects and toxic levels; therefore, they should be used with caution.

Good intraoperative care is surgical technique that does not jeopardize a patient's health status. The patient must be rendered pain free to allow surgery, then be successfully restored to the presurgical state. The procedure must be performed in a manner that does not negatively alter the patient's health status. The technique should not impede vital functions. The oral surgeon must concentrate on the procedure as well as observe the patient's airway for regular respirations. One also must periodically ensure that the vascular state is normotensive. All surgery induces some degree of stress, and the patient's emotional response to this stress must be moderated if possible. Control of a patient's emotional response improves the perception of pain and stabilizes the vital signs. Good intraoperative care involves all aspects of the patient's well-being beyond the surgical field.

Postoperative patient care extends from the time of surgery through the convalescent stage to the restored presurgical health state. It varies for each individual and requires attention directly to wound healing and systemic function. No aspect of systemic function nor its relationship to the surgical procedure can be ignored because continuity of the surgical defect is so dependent upon it.

One must differentiate variable convalescence from true pathology, and have the discernment to intervene. Care must be directed to surgical complications, for which the surgeon must provide appropriate definitive treatment. Complications are to be expected with frequent surgical procedures and not be equated with negligence. Despite surgical problems, good patient care will result in a happy, well-satisfied patient.

References

1. Harrison, T.R.: Harrison's Principles of Internal Medicine. 9th Ed. Edited by K. J. Isselbacher, et al. New York, McGraw-Hill Book Co., 1980.
2. Sabiston, D.C.: Textbook of Surgery. 12th Ed. Philadelphia, W. B. Saunders Co., 1981.
3. Matukas, V. I.: Implications of systemic diseases in the surgical patient. *In* Oral and Maxillofacial Surgery. 1st Ed. Edited by D. Laskin. St. Louis, C.V. Mosby Co., 1980.
4. Hunt, T. K.: Studies on inflammation and wound healing: Angiogenesis and collagen synthesis stimulated in vivo by resident and activated wound macrophages. Surgery, *96*:1, 1984.
5. Schilling, J.: Wound healing. Surg. Rounds, 7:46, 1983.
6. Souba, W. W., and Bessey, P.O.: Nutritional support of the trauma patient. Infect. in Surg., *3*:727, 1984.
7. Topazian, R.G.: Management of Infections of the Oral and Maxillofacial Regions. Philadelphia, W.B. Saunders Co., 1981.
8. Waite, D.E.: Textbook of Practical Oral Surgery. 2nd Ed. Philadelphia, Lea & Febiger, 1978.

Selected Reading

Dunphy, J.E., and Way, L.W.: Current Surgical Diagnosis and Treatment. 5th Ed. Los Altos, CA, Lange Medical Publications, 1981.

CHAPTER 3 # Surgical Anatomy

DONALD ROBERTSON AND GRAEME BROWNE

The nature of the body is the beginning of medical science. HIPPOCRATES

A thoroughly integrated knowledge of gross anatomy, topographic anatomy, and pathophysiology forms the cornerstone of a sound clinical practice. Basic sciences provide insight into the mechanisms of disease processes. Applied anatomy reflects a comprehensive working knowledge of gross anatomy. It is as important to the family practitioner as it is to the surgeon for clinical diagnosis. The interpretation of physical signs is predicated upon a fundamental understanding of anatomy—essential for developing a differential diagnosis. A detailed knowledge of anatomic relations is important to the surgeon for preserving structures and reconstructing resected regional anatomy to minimize morbidity and loss of function and symmetry.

It is axiomatic that clinical skills are closely allied to a dynamic appreciation of gross anatomy. Periodic review is therefore encouraged. The following specific clinical oral surgery problems have been selected to highlight certain conditions that clinicians encounter:

1. Accessory innervation of the mandible
2. Regional lymphatics—concept of afferent and efferent limbs
3. Fascial planes, potential anatomic spaces, and the spread of odontogenic infection in the head and neck
4. The maxilla—its sinus, canine eminence, and exodontia/endodontia
5. Impacted mandibular third molar teeth and their neural and vascular relations
6. Mandibular fractures—muscle displacement of segments
7. The temporomandibular joint

Sensory Innervation of the Head and Neck

Pain is the most common symptom expressed by patients receiving dental or oral surgery. Symptomatic relief from presenting pain or pain that arises from surgical therapy is obtained effectively from regional nerve blocks or field blocks. Occasionally, patients appear to be immune to repeated attempts at providing conventional regional sensory blockade to the mandible. These patients indicate consistently that pain continues following successive attempts by their clinician to provide an effective nerve blockade. They conclude "that local anesthetic just doesn't work," thereby implying a biochemical basis for the persistent sensation. Accessory innervation to the mandible offers an anatomic explanation for the persistent sensation, following competent attempts at inferior alveolar nerve blockade.

Some individuals believe that the most frequent apparent source of accessory innervation arises from the cervical plexus; however, it is more likely to arise from the nerve to the mylohyoid. This sensory supply may be blocked by depositing a bolus of local anesthetic at approximately lingual and inferior to the apices of the first molar.

The other, less common, source of accessory innervation to the mandible derives from an aberrantly high origin of a dental branch of the inferior alveolar nerve. The subjective clinical ratio of occurrence of these two accessory sources of sensory innervation to the mandible is about 4:1. This suggests that when an accessory innervation is suspected, the clinician should

15

block the nerve to mylohyoid prior to attempting to block the less frequently occurring, high divergent origin of the sensory branch from the third division of the trigeminal nerve. The technique for blockade of this latter aberrant nerve involves entering the retromolar trigone in a cephalad direction ($+30°$) to the standard inferior dental nerve blockade and parallel to the medial surface of the ramus.

A later section deals fully with extraoral blockade of the second and third divisions of the trigeminal nerve. The reader should examine a skull and articulated mandible to review the geometry of these useful approaches to securing regional analgesia.

Anatomy

Two abnormal routes of innervation of mandibular teeth center about the third molar and the incisors. In the first case, the nerve to the third molar, which normally arises from the inferior alveolar after it has entered the mandibular canal, arises early and enters the mandible separately by way of a small foramen anterior to the mandibular foramen. In the second case, the most likely source of aberrant innervation is the nerve to the mylohyoid, which may contain sensory fibers that enter the mandible near the symphysis and hence supply incisors of that side of the jaw. Some controversy centers over the role of the cervical plexus in supplying mandibular teeth.

Lymphatics of the Head and Neck

The cardinal clinical signs of pathology associated with this auxiliary circulation for blood vessels are (1) palpable lymph nodes, (2) red streaks in the skin (lymphangitis), and (3) lymphedema. All head and neck examinations *must* include inspection and palpation for any of these cardinal signs. The method of examination is outlined in Chapter 4. Clinical examination alone cannot differentiate between inflammatory and metastatic lymphadenopathy. Lymph node biopsy is the only way these conditions may be identified. Note that lymphadenopathy may arise de novo and requires diagnosis. The clinician must know afferent lymphatics to regionally enlarged nodes to examine the area being drained by those nodes. An isolated neck mass must be examined to rule out organomegaly (e.g., thyroid), neoplasm, developmental

sinus tract (e.g., branchial cleft cyst), granulomatous disease (e.g., tuberculosis), and infection.

Firm and nontender lymph nodes suggest neoplastic involvement, and tender enlargement of regional nodes suggests inflammatory involvement. These two conditions are *not* mutually exclusive. A high index of suspicion is indicated when "lumps" are being investigated. Clinical staging of neoplasms employs the TMN classification (T = tumor, M = metastatic, N = nodes).

Neoplasms may be submucosal; therefore, inspection alone does not disclose their presence. Palpation is essential especially in the posterior third of the tongue. If no obvious cause exists at examination for the adenopathy, consultation with an otolaryngologist provides further clinical examination by panendoscopy or selective laryngoscopy.

Anatomy

In any consideration of the lymphatic drainage of the head and neck structures, several general features should be kept in mind. First, extremely diverse nomenclature is utilized. The text that follows includes various terms encountered relative to any node group. Second, the ultimate drainage of all head and neck structures is by way of a single chain of nodes and associated channels. All other drainage feeds this single channel. Third, frequently a given region or organ within the head and neck can drain through two or more routes. Thus, only general patterns of drainage can be described in many cases.

DEEP CERVICAL NODES

The *deep cervical chain* (Fig. 3-1) of nodes and associated lymph vessels is the ultimate channel for all lymph draining from the head and neck. For that reason, it is appropriate to describe it initially. It consists of 20 to 30 nodes related to the carotid sheath and the internal jugular vein. The chain extends from the base of the skull to the confluence of the internal jugular vein and the subclavian vein. For descriptive purposes, they are commonly subdivided into two groups:

1. *Superior deep cervical nodes*—extending from the base of the skull to the point where the omohyoid muscle crosses the

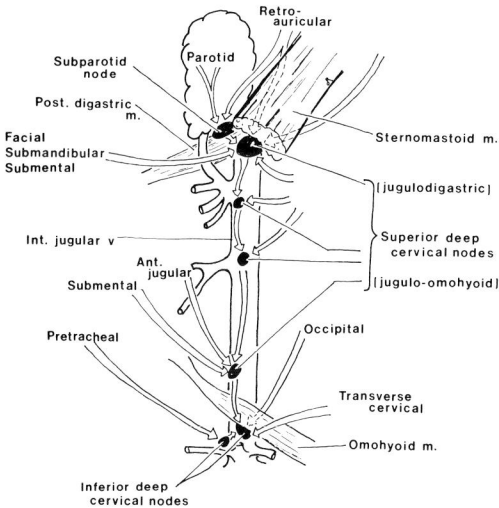

FIG. 3-1. *The deep cervical nodes and their afferent channels.*

internal jugular vein. One of the most superiorly located nodes in this subdivision, as well as one of the most functionally significant, is the *jugulodigastric* (tonsillar-subdigastric) node, located just below the posterior belly of the digastric muscle where it crosses the internal jugular vein.

2. *Inferior deep cervical* (supraclavicular) *nodes*—situated below the omohyoid muscle. The *jugulo-omohyoid node* is a relatively large and constant member of this group. The group receives efferent lymph channels from the superior deep cervical nodes, the tongue, the posterior neck and scalp, the superficial aspect of the pectoral region, and part of the arm. In addition, it may receive a part of the lymph drainage of the liver.

Considered by some to be a superiorlateral extension of the deep cervical chain are the *retropharyngeal* nodes, located within the buccopharyngeal fascia just posterior to the pharynx, at the base of the skull. These nodes, send their efferents to the superiorly situated nodes of the deep chain.

SATELLITE NODE GROUPS, SUPERFICIAL

The *occipital* (nuchal) nodes, a group of one to three nodes, are located near insertions of the semispinalis capitis and trapezius muscles (Fig. 3-2). They drain poste-

rior regions of the scalp, and for the most part, their efferent channels pass to the superior deep cervical nodes. Some efferents may drain into a small and variable group of nodes disposed along the length of the spinal accessory nerve (the *accessory* or *deep lateral* nodes), which ultimately drain into the inferior deep cervical nodes.

The *retroauricular* (postauricular, posterior auricular, mastoid) nodes consist of one or two small nodes located near the insertion of the sternomastoid muscle. They drain a portion of the auricle and the external auditory meatus. Efferents from these nodes drain into superior deep cervical nodes.

The *superficial parotid* (preauricular) nodes, varying in number, are located over the parotid gland and immediately anterior to the tragus of the ear. Some authors refer to a specific node of this group that is located immediately inferior to the apex of the gland as the *subparotid* node. These nodes receive lymph drainage from the auricle and the external auditory meatus, temporal, and lateral aspect of the front of the scalp, both upper and lower eyelids, and posterior portion of the cheek. Their efferents pass to the superior deep cervical nodes.

The *facial* nodes drain an extensive area that includes the medial portion of the forehead and scalp, the external nose and anterior third of the nasal cavity, the anterior portion of the cheek, the upper lip, and lateral portions of the lower lip. They

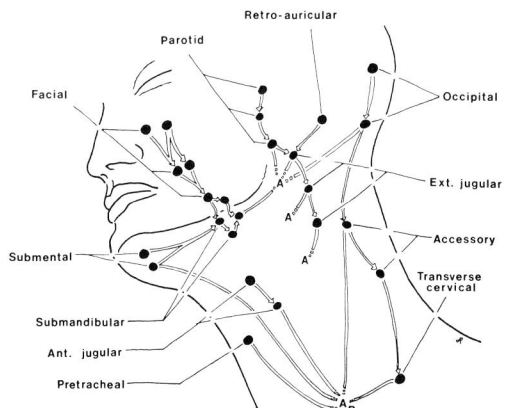

FIG. 3-2. *Superficial node groups of the head and neck and the course of their efferent channels. (A) Superior deep cervical nodes. (B) Inferior deep cervical nodes.*

are subdivided, rather arbitrarily, into a *maxillary* (infraorbital) group, a *buccal* group situated just lateral to the angle of the mouth, over the buccinator muscle, and a *mandibular* (supramandibular) group located over the inferior and lateral aspect of the mandible in close association with the facial vessels. All groups drain into the submandibular nodes.

The *submandibular* (submaxillary, dental) nodes, located in the submandibular triangle between the bellies of the digastric muscle and lower border of the mandible, are sometimes subdivided into anterior, middle, and posterior portions according to their relationship to the facial vessels. The largest and most constant of this group of three to six nodes is situated at the intersection of the facial artery and lower border of the mandible. In addition, some small nodes of this group may be situated deep to the gland. The more anterior nodes of the group may be situated in the angle between the medial surface of the mandible and the mylohyoid muscle, making them difficult to palpate.

The *submental* (suprahyoid) nodes are situated in the triangle between anterior bellies of the digastric muscles and the hyoid bone. Consisting of two to four nodes, they drain the medial portion of the lower lip and the floor of the mouth, the tip of the tongue, and skin over the chin. Their efferents project in part to the submandibular nodes, in part directly to the superior deep cervical nodes. In the latter instance, both cranial and caudal nodes of the deep chain are involved.

The *superficial cervical* nodes are located along the course of the external jugular vein, and hence on the surface of the sternomastoid muscle. This group, which is continuous with the inferior portion of the superficial parotid group, receives afferent lymph vessels from a portion of the external ear and the superficial parotid nodes. Their efferents terminate in the superior deep cervical chain.

The *anterior cervical* (anterior jugular) nodes, an irregular and variable group, has both superficial and deep components. The superficial nodes, when present, are related to the vein of the same name and drain skin of the neck below the level of the hyoid bone. Their efferents pass to lower nodes of the superior deep cervical chain.

SATELLITE NODE GROUPS, DEEP

The *deep parotid* nodes are located within the substance of the gland, for the most part, with some situated medial to the gland, along the lateral wall of the pharynx. This group drains to the superior deep cervical nodes.

The *deep facial* (internal maxillary) nodes lie deep to the ramus of the mandible, on the lateral surface of the lateral pterygoid muscle. They are related to the maxillary artery. Their efferents project to the superior deep cervical nodes.

The *lingual* nodes consist of two or three nodes between the hyoglossus and genioglossus muscles. They drain into the superior deep cervical nodes.

The *prelaryngeal* and *pretracheal* nodes are simply superior and inferior components of a variable group that drains the lower larynx, the thyroid gland, and upper trachea. Their efferents extend to the inferior deep cervical nodes.

SPECIFIC REGIONAL CONSIDERATIONS

Cheeks, lips, labial, and buccal gingiva. The anterior portion of the cheeks, the upper lip, and lateral portions of the lower lip drain via the facial and submandibular nodes, and hence to the superior deep cervical chain. The middle portion of the lower lip drains into the submental nodes and subsequently into both cranial and caudal portions of the superior deep cervical chain.

Drainage of the labial and buccal gingiva corresponds to that of the cheeks and lips.

Palate, floor of the mouth, lingual gingiva. The palate has two primary routes of lymphatic drainage. The anterior portion drains into the facial chain, and hence to the submandibular nodes. The posterior portion (including the soft palate) drains into the retropharyngeal and superior deep cervical nodes.

The anterior portion of the floor of the mouth drains either into the submental nodes or directly into nodes of the superior deep cervical chain, bypassing any regional nodes. The posterior portion of the floor of the mouth drains either to submandibular nodes or directly into superior deep cervical nodes.

Mandibular lingual gingiva has two routes of drainage. Anteriorly, the channels enter the submandibular nodes, while more posterior drainage is via channels into the superior cervical nodes (i.e., corresponding to drainage of the base of the tongue).

Teeth and periodontal membrane. Only a general pattern is applicable. As a rule, lymph drainage of all teeth, with the exception of the lower incisors, is into the submandibular nodes, although some molars of both jaws may extend directly into superior deep cervical nodes. The lower incisors drain into submental nodes, reflecting a pattern seen for the central part of the lower lip and the gingiva.

Tongue. The tongue (Fig. 3-3) has a particularly complex pattern of drainage. It is divided into four zones, each with a characteristic route of drainage.

The *apical* zone, or tip, drains along with the central portion of the lower lip into the submental nodes, or directly into the superior deep cervical nodes. The drainage of the apical portion of the tongue is to nodes of both sides.

The *marginal* (lateral) zones drain into the submandibular or superior deep cervical nodes of the corresponding side.

The *central* zone has a very extensive drainage into the submental, submandibular, and both superior and inferior portions of the deep cervical chain. Drainage is to both sides.

The *basilar* zone, or that part posterior to the vallate papillae, drains into the superior deep cervical nodes of both sides.

Palatine tonsil. The palatine tonsil drains directly into superior deep cervical nodes, especially the jugulodigastric node.

Fascial Planes and Spaces

Odontogenic infections may track into the deep cervical spaces and communicate with the thoracic cavity, to the base of the skull, or extend intracranially. The sequelae are major medical and surgical concerns. Odontogenic infections are discussed in Section 3; however, the general principles of surgical management of infections about the face and neck evolve from an understanding of gross anatomy.

Descriptions of the fascial layers and associated spaces within the head and neck lack consistency in terminology and agreement over what constitutes defined fascial layers. The following description considers only those fasciae and spaces germane to the discipline.

The Fascial Layers

The *prevertebral* and *alar* fascial layers (Figs. 3-4 through 3-8) are closely related to the cervical vertebral column. The prevertebral layer invests the column and associated musculature, including the scalene muscles. It creates the axillary sheath surrounding the brachial plexus and the axillary vessels. Between the transverse processes of the vertebrae, and anterior to the column, the prevertebral fascia splits into two layers separated by an area of loose connective tissue. The layer immediately opposed to the vertebral musculature is designated prevertebral fascia, and the more anterior layer is termed the alar fascia. The potential space between these two layers extends down from the base of the skull into the mediastinum.

The *superficial layer of deep cervical fascia* (investing fascia) forms an outer, tubelike fascial investment of the neck, enclosing the superficial muscles of the neck (trapezius, sternomastoid, the strap muscula-

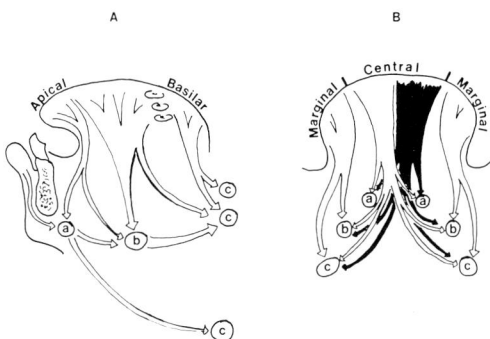

Fig. 3-3. *Lymphatic drainage of the tongue. (A) Submental nodes. (B) Submandibular nodes. (C) Deep cervical nodes.*

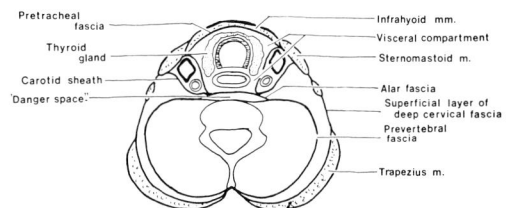

Fig. 3-4. *Cross-section through the neck at the level of the thyroid gland, showing the primary layers of deep cervical fascia.*

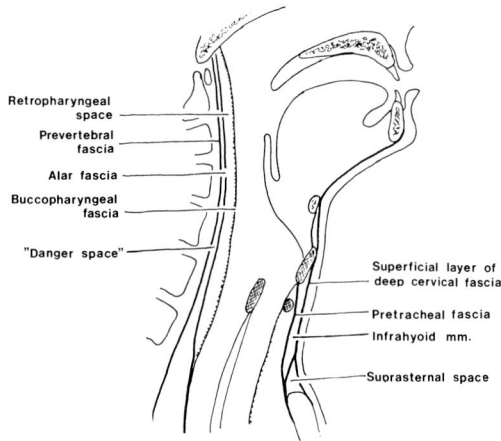

FIG. 3-5. *A sagittal section through the neck and the jaw. Both fascial layers and spaces are indicated.*

FIG. 3-7. *Cross-section through the left parotid region, showing the primary fascial layers and spaces at this level.*

ture). As it invests the infrahyoid musculature, its posterior leaf, which opposes the deep surface of the muscles, is designated the *pretracheal fascia*, or middle layer of deep cervical fascia. This layer should not be confused with the superficial fascia of the head and neck, which is the tela subcutanea.

Above the hyoid bone, the superficial layer of deep cervical fascia continues superiorly toward the mandible. Behind the ramus, it splits to enclose the parotid gland. Just below the border of the body of the mandible, it encloses the submandibular gland. Approaching the border of the body and posterior margin of the ramus, the fascia splits again. The superficial leaf continues onto the face; the deep leaf passes medial to the pterygoid musculature of the infratemporal region.

The *carotid sheath* invests the common carotid artery, the internal jugular vein,

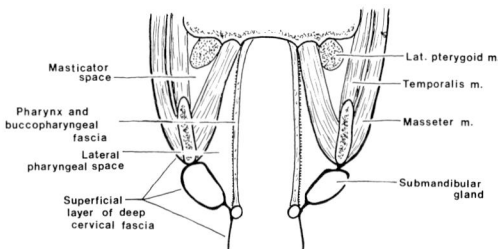

and the vagus nerve. It is formed by contributions from the superficial layer of deep cervical and pretracheal fasciae.

It should be remembered that the pharynx has associated with it a rather thin and filmy layer of fascia termed the *buccopharyngeal* fascia. This layer continues anteriorly and laterally over the buccinator muscle, inferiorly onto the esophagus.

The Fascial Spaces

The *suprasternal space* (of Burns) is formed by splitting of the superficial layer

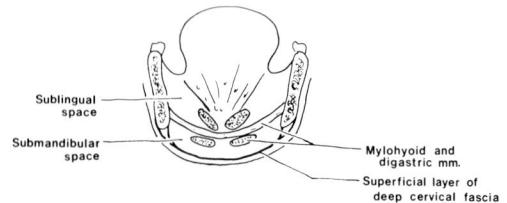

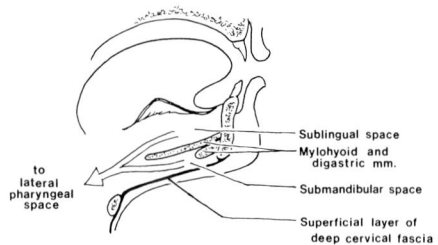

FIG. 3-8. *Diagrammatic coronal and sagittal sections through the mandible, showing the position and relationships of the sublingual and submandibular fascial spaces.*

FIG. 3-6. *A diagrammatic coronal section through the mandible and the muscles of mastication.*

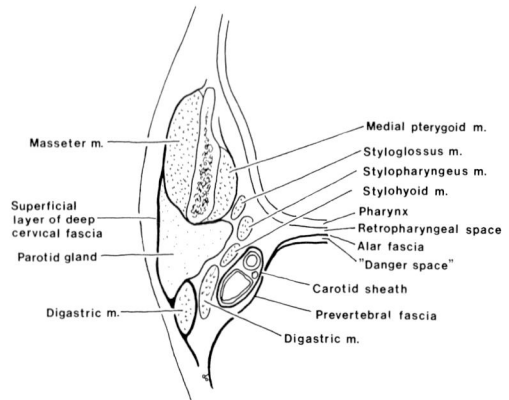

of deep cervical fascia just above the sternum. The posterior leaf attaches to the deep surface of the sternum, the anterior to the ventral surface of the sternum. The space, bounded laterally by the sternomastoid muscles, contains the terminal portion of the anterior jugular vein.

The *"danger space"* is the potential space between the prevertebral and alar fasciae.

The *visceral compartment* is bordered anteriorly by the pretracheal fascia, posteriorly by the prevertebral and alar fasciae, and laterally by the carotid sheath and the deep layer of fascia surrounding the sternomastoid muscle. This space encloses the trachea, the thyroid gland, and the esophagus. It can be subdivided into a pretracheal space and a retrovisceral space. The former space surrounds the trachea; the latter lies between the lower pharynx and esophagus and the pretracheal fascia. These two spaces, continuous with one another, extend down into the upper mediastinum. The retrovisceral space extends superiorly to the base of the skull.

The *carotid space,* or space of the carotid sheath, is simply that space within the sheath. Reports on the spread of infections via this space vary; some investigators report the extension of an infection from the upper neck to the lower neck and mediastinum via this route but others deny this possibility.

The *space of the body of the mandible* is a potential space or cleavage plane between the superficial layer of deep cervical fascia and the lower border of the mandible. Infections may either spread to the masticator space or be confined to the space itself.

The *space of the submandibular gland* is a misleading description since the superficial layer of deep cervical fascia, as it splits to envelop the gland, is adherent to the capsule of the gland. Hence, the "space" is totally filled with the gland itself.

The *space of the parotid gland,* like that of the submandibular gland, is a potential space occupied by the parotid gland. Very significantly, from a practical point of view, this space is closely related, medially, to the lateral pharyngeal space.

The *masticator space* is formed by splitting the superficial layer of deep cervical fascia at the ramus and body of the mandible.

The internal leaf continues superiorly, medial to the muscles of mastication, to attach to the base of the skull. Laterally, the external or superficial leaf continues up over the temporalis muscle. Posteriorly, the two leaves come together behind the posterior border of the ramus of the mandible. Anteriorly, the fascia attaches to the body and ramus of the mandible ahead of the masseter and temporalis muscles, respectively. An anterior extension of the external leaf to the maxilla and the fascia overlies the buccinator muscle.

The masticator space contains the muscles of mastication, the maxillary artery, and the mandibular nerve. It is closely related to the lower molar teeth.

The *retropharyngeal space* is the superior continuation of what has already been described in the neck as the retrovisceral space. Lying between the pharynx and associated buccopharyngeal fascia and the alar fascia, it continues up to the base of the skull. The *lateral pharyngeal space* is simply the lateral extension of the retropharyngeal space around the lateral aspect of the pharynx. It is bounded laterally by the internal fascia of the masticator space and the parotid gland. Medially, it is limited by the fascia of the pharynx. The lateral spaces communicate freely with the retropharyngeal space and are related closely to both the parotid gland and the masticator space.

The *submandibular space* is made up of two spaces that communicate with one another and with the lateral pharyngeal spaces. The two spaces are the *sublingual space,* which lies above the mylohyoid muscle, below the mucous lining of the floor of the mouth, and lateral to the musculature of the tongue, and the *submaxillary space,* which lies between the mylohyoid muscle, superiorly, and the superficial layer of deep cervical fascia that bridges the interval between borders of the body of the mandible, inferiorly. The two spaces communicate with one another at the posterior border of the mylohyoid muscle and lateral pharyngeal space posteriorly.

The *peritonsillar space* is the area of loose connective tissue lying in the tonsillar bed and connecting the capsule of the tonsil loosely to underlying pharyngeal musculature.

The Maxillary Sinus and Canine Eminence

Dental anlage, differentiation, maturation, and emergence of succedaneous dentition through the alveolar process contribute to the volume and conformation of the maxillary sinus. The development of the sinus is known as pneumatization. Exodontia may be iatrogenically associated with creation of an oroantral communication. Dental extractions apparently facilitate extension of the sinus into the alveolar process. However, this is most likely an illusion since the alveolar bone undergoes disuse, atrophies, and resorbs, creating the appearance that the volume of the sinus is increasing. Care must be exercised during exodontia of isolated posterior teeth that are in function, as the extraction may be complicated by a fracture of the alveolar process with a resultant opening into the maxillary sinus. The clinical management of a potentially complicated extraction and the maxillary sinus is discussed in Chapters 11 and 16.

Anatomy

The maxillary sinus, like the paranasal sinuses, displays considerable variations in size and shape. These variations are significant in relation to the maxillary teeth. Three salient features should be kept in mind when considering these relationships.

1. In the "normal" instance, the anterior wall of the sinus is relatively thick, helping to form the "canine pillar," one of the primary buttresses of the facial skeleton. Characteristically, this pillar widens at its base to extend some distance posteriorly and laterally—in effect, providing a plate of bone over the apices of the premolar teeth. As a rule, this covering of bone is considerably thicker over the first premolar, and may consist of nothing more than a thin layer of cortical bone over the apex of the second premolar.

2. The molars commonly bear a close relationship to the sinus, the apices of their roots frequently projecting up into the sinus and producing elevation of the floor. These protuberances usually have a thin bony wall, but it is not rare to have an imperfection in the bone, leaving the tooth separated from the lumen of the sinus by the mucosal lining.

3. The posterior extremity of the maxillary alveolar process forms the maxillary tuber. Normally, the maxillary wall thickens at this region. This thickening, in conjunction with the pterygoid processes of the sphenoid bone, assists in forming the posterior buttress of the visceral skeleton. When the maxillary sinus is very large, the wall of the maxilla can become very thin, rendering the tuber susceptible to fracture with the application of stress.

Impacted Mandibular Third Molar

Removal of mandibular impacted third molar teeth is a technically demanding procedure. It is attended by potential trauma to the lingual nerve, the inferior alveolar nerve, the buccal artery, and reversible but obvious motor paralysis to the facial nerve that may cause ipsilateral peripheral palsy (Bell's palsy).

Interpretation of existing preoperative radiographs provides a two-dimensional appreciation of the relationship of the apex of no. 17 or no. 32 with respect to the inferior alveolar neurovascular bundle. The patient should be advised of the potential for nerve injury during dissection. Close examination of the radiograph may disclose evidence of proximity between tooth and neurovascular canal.

The close relationship between the third molar and the lingual nerve, as it passes immediately medial to the third molar region, necessitates a need for cautious instrumentation in this area. A misdirected long buccal nerve blockade or excessive volume of local anesthetic may cause lateral extension by clysis of the anesthetic to encroach on the motor nerve to the muscles of facial expression. An ipsilateral, peripheral seventh nerve palsy results. Its duration is related to pharmacodynamics of the drug used.

Buccal artery trauma is likely when a distobuccal releasing flap is used. This vessel may be of considerable size and may be a source of postoperative reactionary hemorrhage that requires definitive management. The reader is referred to Chapter 10 for further discussion of the preoperative assessment of impacted third molar teeth.

Anatomy

THE LINGUAL NERVE

The lingual nerve, in its course through the infratemporal fossa, descends along the lateral surface of the medial pterygoid muscle, anterior and slightly medial to the inferior alveolar nerve. As it approaches the upper end of the mylohyoid line on the inner surface of the mandible, it starts to swing forward to gain the upper surface of the mylohyoid muscle. At this point, it is rather superficially located just below the mucous membrane of the sublingual sulcus, close to the alveolus of the third molar.

THE SEVENTH CRANIAL (FACIAL) NERVE

The seventh nerve, after emerging from the stylomastoid foramen, swings forward, at about the level of the neck of the mandible, to enter the face. Commonly, the nerve is embedded within the substance of the parotid gland. However, because of wide variation in extent of nerve/gland relationships, the facial nerve or one of its primary branches may be relatively exposed medial to the gland. The auriculotemporal branch of V3 is also closely related to this area.

THE INFERIOR ALVEOLAR NERVE

The inferior alveolar nerve descends through the infratemporal region along the lateral surface of the medial pterygoid muscle. As it descends, it lies posterior and slightly lateral to the lingual nerve. It becomes closely related to the inner surface of the ramus only as it attains the mandibular foramen. At some point prior to its entrance into the mandible, it gives off the nerve to the mylohyoid. Once within the substance of the mandible, the nerve, with its accompanying vascular elements, runs through the mandibular canal to be distributed to the teeth. In premolar and molar areas, the relationship of the nerve to the teeth varies considerably.

As a rule, the apices of the third molar roots are closely related to the canal, and the distance separating the roots and canal gradually increases with anterior progression. This is subject to considerable variation, depending upon the conformation of the mandibular body, age, stage of dental development, and positioning of the molars.

THE BUCCAL NERVE

The buccal nerve descends forward through the infratemporal fossa to pass between the anterior portion of the masseter muscle and the buccinator muscle. As it runs forward on the lateral surface of the buccinator, giving off sensory branches that pierce the muscle to supply the cheek, it lies medial to elements of the facial nerve. Throughout most of its course, the nerve is accompanied by the buccal artery, which supplies the underlying muscle and the mucosa of the cheek, and participates in formation of anastomotic connections with the underlying transverse facial and facial arteries.

Mandibular Fractures and Segment Displacement Resulting From Muscle Contraction: Selected Fractures

Displacement of mandibular fractures is influenced by the *direction* of the line of osseous fracture and the *resultant vectors* imposed on the bony segments by the attached musculature. Relatively little displacement results from the direction and magnitude of force precipitating the injury to the mandible when compared to injuries sustained to the maxilla, nasal bone, and zygomatic complex exclusive of high velocity missile avulsive injuries. A notable exception to this occurs with LeFort I and II midface fractures, in which displacement occurs under the influence of myospasm from the palatopharyngeus, palatoglossus, buccinator, and the superior and middle constrictor muscles. Distinction should be made between this and a telescoping that frequently occurs in maxillary fractures as a result of the architecture of the bone with its maxillary sinus.

The principles of management of facial bone trauma are based on mechanical effects that muscle attachments and the direction of the lines of fracture have on the *stability* of the component bones of the injury. Section 4 deals with specific injuries to the maxillofacial complex. It is appropriate, therefore, to review the significant features of myology and the mandible.

Anatomy

SUPERFICIAL MUSCLES OF MASTICATION

The *masseter* muscle consists of two components. The superficial, which makes up the largest part of the muscle, arises from the anterior two thirds of the zygomatic arch. The fibers of this component run down and back to insert upon the lateral surface of the ramus of the mandible. The deep component arises from the posterior third of the zygomatic arch. Its fibers run down and forward to insert on the upper part of the ramus.

The masseter, acting as a unit, elevates the jaws.

The *temporalis* muscle has an extensive origin from the temporal fossa on the lateral aspect of the skull and from the overlying temporal fascia. The fibers converge to insert upon both lateral and medial surfaces of the coronoid process of the mandible. The medial attachment extends down for some distance onto the medial surface of the ramus, some fibers forming a tendon that inserts into the anterior border of the ramus and some by a tendon inserting more medially and distally. The two tendons lie in the lateral and medial margins of the retromolar fossa.

By virtue of its origin, the muscle has two actions. The anterior and intermediate fibers, situated more vertically from origin to insertion, act as powerful elevators of the mandible. The more posterior fibers, situated more horizontally, act to retract the jaw.

DEEP MUSCLES OF MASTICATION

The *medial pterygoid* muscle arises from the medial surface of the lateral pterygoid plate, extending onto the lateral surface, and from the tuberosity of the maxilla. Its fibers run down, laterally, and back to insert upon the medial surface of the ramus of the mandible, opposite the masseter. The medial pterygoids function as elevators of the mandible.

The lateral pterygoid muscles arise from the undersurface of the greater wing of the sphenoid bone (superficial head) and from

the lateral surface of the pterygoid plate (inferior head). Both heads converge to insert in the pterygoid fovea of the mandibular neck, with some components of the superior head attaching to the anterior surface of the articular capsule of the temporomandibular joint and articular disc.

The lateral pterygoid muscle acts primarily as a protractor of the jaw. The portion of the superior head attaching to the articular capsule and disc has classically been ascribed the function of pulling the articular disc forward to keep it opposed to the condyle during protraction of the jaw. Whether this is the case, or whether the disc moves passively with the condyle, has yet to be resolved.

THE SUPRAHYOID MUSCLES

The suprahyoid musculature considered in displacement of fragments following mandibular fracture are the digastric, mylohyoid, geniohyoid, and genioglossus muscles. Although these muscles can function in fragment displacement, the degree to which they do is affected by the activity of the infrahyoid musculature.

The *digastric* muscle arises from the mastoid process, posteriorly, and inserts in the digastric fossae of the mandible, anteriorly. It consists of two bellies and an intermediate tendon, the latter being bound to the hyoid bone.

The *mylohyoid* muscle arises from the body and greater horns of the hyoid bone. Its fibers course superiorly to insert upon the prominent mylohyoid line on the inner surface of the body of the mandible. The more medial fibers insert with those from the opposite side in the mylohyoid raphe.

The *geniohyoid* muscle, as implied by its name, extends between the genial tubercle of the mandible and the hyoid bone.

The *genioglossus* muscle, the largest muscle of the tongue, forms the bulk of that organ. Its bony attachment is to the genial tubercle on the inner aspect of the symphysis region of the mandible.

Condylar Fractures

With a unilateral condylar fracture (Fig. 3-9A), the lateral pterygoid muscle pulls the condylar neck medially and forward while the temporalis, masseter, and medial pterygoid muscles elevate the ramus. The medial pterygoid also pulls the ramus slightly forward. Clinical findings include premature ipsilateral occlusion, ipsilateral deviation with opening of the mouth, hemotympanum, and preauricular depression.

In a bilateral condylar fracture (Fig. 3-9B), the actions of the muscles are similar to those described previously, the difference being that the forces acting are applied to both sides. In such instances, a bilateral premature occlusion is accompanied by an anterior open bite. Hemotympanum and preauricular depression obtain, as before.

Fractures of the Angle

With an unfavorable fracture of the angle (Fig. 3-10), the combined actions of the masseter, medial pterygoid, and temporalis muscles rotate the proximal segment forward and medially. The symptoms accompanying this fracture may include swelling, submucosal ecchymosis, decreased range of movement, and sialorrhea.

Fractures of the Body—Unfavorable

In a unilateral fracture of this type (Fig. 3-11A), the pterygomasseteric sling and the temporalis muscle act to rotate the proximal segment up and medially, thereby producing premature occlusion of the teeth associated with that fragment. The teeth of the distal fragment remain in normal occlusion. Other symptoms may include swelling, submucosal ecchymosis, decreased range of movement, intraoral hemorrhage, mobility of the tooth in the line of fracture, and fetor oris. There may be neuropraxia or axonotmeses of the ipsilateral inferior alveolar nerve.

With bilateral unfavorable fracture of the body (Fig. 3-11B), the pull of the su-

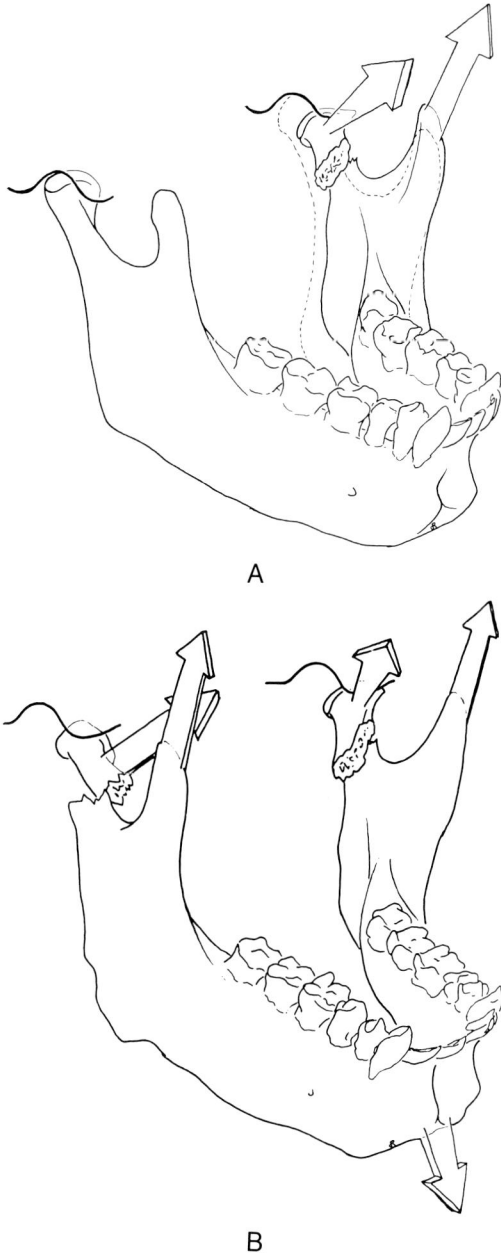

A

B

FIG. 3-9. (A) Unilateral condylar fracture. (B) Bilateral condylar fractures.

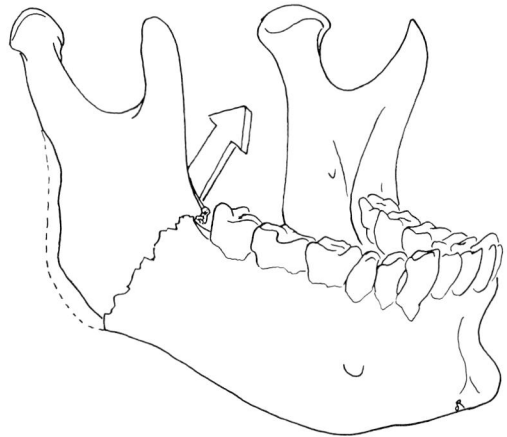

FIG. 3-10. Unfavorable fracture of the angle of the mandible.

A

B

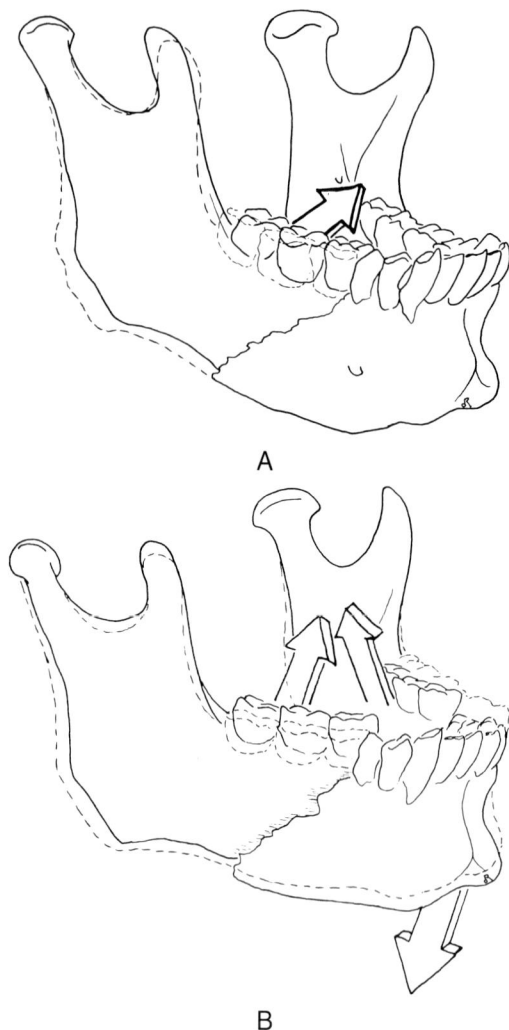

FIG. 3-11. *(A) Unfavorable unilateral fracture of the body. (B) Bilateral fracture of the body.*

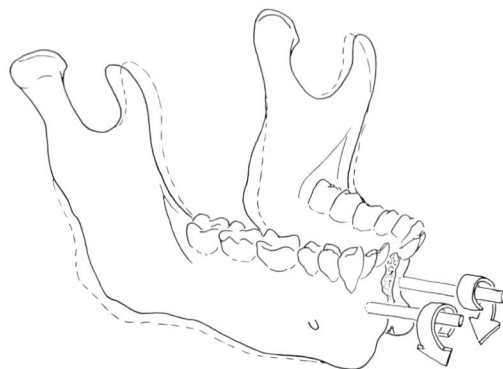

FIG. 3-12. *Fracture of the symphyses of the mandible.*

prahyoid musculature tends to depress and retract the distal segment, producing an anterior open bite. Other symptoms are similar to those of a unilateral fracture.

Fractures of the Symphysis

In this case (Fig. 3-12), the mylohyoid muscle has the effect of pulling down the mandibular halves while rotating them slightly, producing a lateral tilt of the transverse occlusal table. The geniohyoid and digastric muscle go into spasm, retracting and depressing the jaw. In addition to a diastema, submucosal ecchymosis, a decreased range of motion, malocclusion, sialorrhea, fetor oris, and intraoral hemorrhage occur.

The Temporomandibular Joint

The temporomandibular (TM) joint, both architecturally and functionally one of the most complex and sophisticated joints of the human body, remains one of the most poorly understood. (For a further discussion of the temporomandibular joint, refer to Chapter 21.) While it is classified as a simple, synovial, ellipsoid joint, its structure and function are complicated by its being a composite of four joints that function differently with different movements of the mandible. Similarly, movement in the joint on one side of the body always involves movement on the opposite side.

Joint Morphology

The osseous elements of the joint consist of the mandibular (glenoid) fossa of the temporal bone and the condyle of the mandible. The concave mandibular fossa is situated on the inferior surface of the squamous portion of the temporal bone, just anterior to the bony external auditory meatus of the ear. The sloping anterior wall of the fossa, which is its primary articular plane, is formed by the *articular eminence.* (Note: the term *articular tubercle* is commonly and erroneously used in reference to the eminence. The articular tubercle is located on the lateral extremity of the anterior zygomatic root of the temporal bone. It is a point of attachment for ligaments of the temporomandibular joint, and is nonarticular.)

Extending forward from the apex of the eminence is the horizontal *preglenoid plane*. The posterior wall of the fossa, a nonarticular surface, is formed by the bony tympanic portion of the temporal bone, together with a variably sized ridge of bone extending down from the squamous temporal bone. The latter is the posterior articular ridge, which becomes prominent laterally, forming the cone-shaped *postglenoid process*. The ridge and the bony portion of the external meatus are separated by the *tympanosquamosal suture*, which, when followed medially, is continuous with the *petrotympanic suture*. The fossa, somewhat constricted medially, possesses a bony wall formed by the lateral surface of the spine of the sphenoid. Although there is no real bony lateral wall, a slight elevation extends from the lateral end of the articular tubercle to the postglenoid process. The thickness of the roof of the fossa varies, but characteristically it is quite thin, indicating a lack of pressure-bearing function. Importantly, the roof of the glenoid fossa forms the floor of the middle cranial fossa.

The mandibular component of the joint is the ovoid condyle, which sits asymmetrically atop the neck, its pointed lateral pole projecting only slightly from the plane of the ramus of the mandible and its rounded medial pole lying considerably medial to the ramal plane. The medial pole is braced from below by the *mandibular crest* (dental trajectory), which extends up the posteromedial length of the neck.

The condyles measure from 15 to 20 mm in their long axes and are 8 to 10 mm from anteriorly to posteriorly. They are situated with their axes at right angles to the rami of their respective sides, but together form an angle of 145 to 160° with respect to the sagittal plane of the skull. They are strongly convex in an anterior-posterior plane; only slightly convex in a mediolateral plane, with the convexity increasing at the medial pole. The *articular surface* of each condyle occupies the anterior and superior aspects, and continues medially down and around the medial pole that faces the bony medial wall of the fossa when the jaw is in the occluded position.

The temporomandibular joint is unique in that the articular surfaces of the participating bones are *not covered with hyaline cartilage*, as is characteristic of other synovial joints, but with *fibrocartilage* plates that may contain cartilage cells. The cartilaginous elements are said to decrease with age and abnormal pressure.

The *articular disc* separates the two articular surfaces and divides the joint cavity into superior and inferior compartments. This is an oval fibrous plate of great firmness. Characteristically, its central part is considerably thinner than the periphery with the posterior border being especially thick. The variation in thickness appears to be correlated with the prominence of the articular eminence; the more prominent the eminence, the thicker the disc. Occasionally, the disc is perforated in the center. Posteriorly, the disc continues into a thick layer of loose and vascularized connective tissue that reaches to and fuses with the posterior wall of the articular capsule. This is the *retrodiscal pad*. The disc lacks blood vessels in its thinner central portion.

The articular capsule surrounding and limiting the synovial cavity of the temporomandibular joint attaches to the border of the temporal articulating surface and to the neck of the mandible. The relationships of the capsule to the disc and of the disc to the condyle are highly significant. Anteriorly, the disc and capsule are fused. Posteriorly, they are connected by a pad of loose, vascularized, and innervated connective tissue, giving the disc freedom of anterior movement. Laterally and medially, the disc and the capsule are attached independently to the lateral and medial poles of the condyle. The capsule between the neck of the mandible and the disc is thicker, and the nature of its relationship to the disc allows only rotation between disc and condyle. The capsule between the disc and the attachments to the base of the skull is thinner, allowing the sliding, or translational, movement between the disc and upper articular surfaces.

The articular capsule is strengthened by the *lateral* (temporomandibular) *ligament*. This ligament has two components: a wide superficial (lateral) layer, and a deep or medial band. The former arises from the outer surface of the articular tubercle at the root of the zygomatic arch and extends obliquely down and back to insert on the mandibular neck behind and below the lateral pole of the condyle. The deep layer arises from the articular tubercle. Its fibers pass backward and horizontally to attach with the disc to the lateral pole of the condyle and to the back of the disc.

The synovial capsule of the temporomandibular joint lines the fibrous capsule, attaching to the periphery of the articulating facets and to the neck of the condylar process.

In addition to the articular capsule, two accessory ligaments are classically described with the temporomandibular joint. They are the *sphenomandibular* ligament, extending from the spine of the sphenoid to the lingula and adjacent surface of the ramus, and the *stylomandibular* ligament, running between the styloid process and the mandibular angle.

The function of these ligaments is not clear. Although some investigators have ascribed no functional significance to them, others regard them as having a role in normal mandibular movements. Clinically, they are significant because they can influence the spread of anesthetic (the sphenomandibular ligament) and serve as a landmark for the localization of other structures. With respect to the latter function, the *pterygomandibular raphe* should also be mentioned. This tendinous intersection of the superior constrictor and buccinator muscles extends from the hamulus of the medial pterygoid plate to the posterior end of the mylohyoid line of the mandible. Although it is not a true ligament, it is significant as an observable landmark within the oral cavity. Some investigators believe it has a stabilizing function in mandibular fractures.

The vascular supply of the temporomandibular joint is via the superficial temporal and maxillary arteries posteriorly and the masseteric artery anteriorly. The maxillary artery, as it runs forward, is closely related to the temporomandibular joint, passing between the neck of the mandible and the sphenomandibular ligament. Slightly anterior and medial to the neck of the mandible and the joint, the middle meningeal artery arises from the maxillary to ascend to the base of the skull. Venous drainage of the joint is through a plexus surrounding the joint (collectively forming the temporomandibular vein) that drains into either the maxillary or retromandibular veins.

Innervation of the temporomandibular joint is by the auriculotemporal nerve, closely related to the joint and passing adjacent to the lower part of the medial surface of the capsule. In addition to the auriculotemporal nerve, there are regular contributions by the masseteric nerve and occasionally by the posterior deep temporal nerve.

CHAPTER 4 # History and Examination

GRAEME BROWNE

Never treat a stranger.

The skillful garnering of symptoms or events described by a patient and placing them in chronologic sequence enable a clinician to develop a basis for preliminary conclusions about the causes of the patient's complaints. The subjective statements (symptoms) are then evaluated against objective findings (signs) obtained through a physical examination. The clinician may find it necessary to isolate emotional gain from facts to judge the value of specific symptoms and signs. Subsequently, he arrives at a differential diagnosis. The importance of an orderly sequential analysis obtained from the patient's history is clearly as relevant to safe and effective oral surgery as it is to medical practice. Finally, he confirms the preliminary diagnosis from laboratory data consistent with the clinical signs and symptoms. Such laboratory tests may include radiographs, blood smears, serum analysis, tissue microscopy, immunology, and cytochemistry.

The accumulation of facts requires skill that is acquired from learning. It reflects the integration of basic science with the art of performing a thorough clinical examination, and it represents the essence of communication in providing the patient with confidence and guidance, while preserving his dignity.

The History

A patient's dental and medical histories are carefully assembled narratives that reflect, chronologically, his background and problems. The facts are secured from reliable informants, and their scope is influenced by the nature of the presenting problem. For example, a middle-aged white male complains of unilateral mandibular pain following the loss of a dental restoration, while a middle-aged black male reports intermittent left-sided mandibular pain occurring during meals, as well as while washing his car. For the first individual, the relationship between the lost restoration and the pain on a prima facie basis is plausible and could be quickly corroborated with evidence found upon direct examination. The diagnostician would require a broader perspective of the second individual to provide a basis for a diagnosis. Since odontalgia is among the most frequent causes of jaw pain, this tentative diagnosis would be a primary one. It is also widely accepted that pain with meals may result from salivary gland obstruction. He would include this source of pain in the differential diagnosis. Exertional factors enter the history as the course of the jaw pain progresses, suggesting that the pain may be due to cardiac pathology. Considering age, sex, and ethnic origin, the diagnostician would need to rule out the myocardium as the underlying cause of the jaw pain. Consequently, the scope of the interview becomes closely governed by information provided by the patient.

The astute clinician provides an environment of receptiveness for his patients. They should feel that they are in a non-threatening and nonjudgmental situation as they relate their problems. The clinician's interested, sympathetic and leisurely manner greatly improves rapport. With gentle guidance, he keeps the interview from stalling on peripheral and irrelevant material. He should establish a common understanding of language and idioms by interjecting queries like "do you mean . . . ?" "is it like . . . ?" etc. He should write sparingly during the interview and endeavor to maintain eye contact with the patient. If the patient's reliability as a historian is assessed early in the interview, time and effort will be conserved.

Format of the Recorded History

The formal history is a standardized sequence of sections in which the emphasis may vary to reflect subspecialty interest. The format is the following:

CC	Chief complaint
HPI	History of present illness
MEDS	Current or recent medications
All	Allergies
PMH	Past medical history
PSH	Past surgical history
ROS	Review of symptoms
FH	Family history
SH	Social history

Because a formal medical history is often not necessary or perhaps not relevant to a current dental problem (but occasionally the two are intimately related), an alternative format, the problem-oriented record, succinctly provides dental practice with a satisfactory record. This alternative format is SOAP:

S = subjective (symptoms)
O = objective (signs)
A = assessment
P = plan

The clinician decides when to apply these formats on the basis of the four general categories of patients whom he is likely to manage.

(F) 1. New patient with a specific oral surgery problem
(S) 2. New patient for routine maintenance and supervision
(S) 3. Regular follow-up for routine maintenance
(F) 4. Hospital patient primarily for dental treatment.

(F refers to formal history and S refers to simplified history.)

With the passage of time, medical histories require updating. Intercurrent illnesses may require special management as the dental practitioner plans his therapy. Prior to implementing the treatment plan, he should review the medical history with the patient. This is important if he has not seen the patient recently, and particularly as patients become older. For each decade of life beyond 30 years, one major medical diagnosis may be added to the existing list. A corollary to successful medical care is that more geriatric patients are ambulatory, self sufficient, and living longer, causing the family dentist to provide continuing supervision and treatment.

THE CHIEF COMPLAINT (CC)

This list contains the symptoms that caused the patient to seek professional advice or management. The chief complaint may be in the patient's own words; however, that is not essential. What is essential is that no diagnosis be made at this point as it may later emerge as an erroneous assumption and delay an appropriate course of therapy.

HISTORY OF THE PRESENT ILLNESS (HPI)

This is the cornerstone of the formal history. An accurate description prepared by the clinician relates precipitating or exacerbating factors (e.g., motion, thermal stimuli), alleviating factors (e.g., three ASA tablets every four hours), duration, frequency, intensity, and time of onset to the chief complaint. If previous records exist, they should be reviewed when they are considered germane to the current problem.

CURRENT OR RECENT MEDICATIONS (MEDS)

Listing all current, recently prescribed, or self-medicated drugs is useful at this early stage in writing the history. This information provides the clinician with additional insights into previous diagnoses, and may suggest a contraindication or additional medications to the dental management.

ALLERGIES AND HYPERSENSITIVITIES (ALL)

Knowledge of any medications, adhesive tape, surgical skin preparations, specific metals, or rubber that may precipitate an anaphylactic response or hypersensitivity must be documented. Medication hypersensitivities should be recorded. The patient's statements about drug reactions should be respected. Alternative forms of therapy are commonly available. Consultations with an allergist may be indicated to investigate reported adverse drug reactions.

PAST MEDICAL HISTORY (PMH)

Relevant to a safe dental and oral surgery practice is a thorough comprehension of the pathophysiology and complications of certain medical conditions. These conditions may present a significant risk to the patient if specific safeguards are not undertaken prior to rendering dental or oral surgery services. A history of rheumatic fever, evidence of heart murmur, hypertension, previous myocardial infarction, cerebrovascular accidents, diabetes mellitus, thyroid dysfunction, renal disease, hepatic disease, or blood dyscrasias that include hemorrhagic diatheses and leukocyte dysfunction require thorough evaluation. The reader should refer to a standard text on these organ system diseases for a review of the pathophysiology, distilling areas of particular relevance to oral surgery or general dental practice from the review.

PAST SURGICAL HISTORY (PSH)

This section of the history itemizes the procedures, dates, hospitals, and previous transfusion and general anesthetic records. Complications related to previous surgical procedures should also be recorded. In addition, radiotherapy is noted and the region treated specified.

REVIEW OF SYSTEMS (ROS)

This comprehensive inventory of each anatomic or physiologic system seeks to augment the information in the HPI. Inquiring into the functional health of the patient uncovers clues of subclinical disease or finds corroborative evidence that would aid in coupling symptoms with the diagnosis. For example, difficulty with micturition in an elderly male patient who presents for multiple dental extractions requires that these facts be integrated into the dental or oral surgery treatment plan.

In addition to medical follow-up of the dysuria, the clinician providing oral surgery management would avoid the use of diazepam or belladonna alkaloids for premedication of intravenous sedation. These medications exacerbate urinary outflow difficulties.

FAMILY HISTORY (FH)

This section may not always be of value for general dental disease but may be important in recording the incidence of cleft lip and palate, orthognathic dysplasias, or inherited neuromuscular diseases. A family history of diabetes, hypertension, cancer, cardiac and renal disease, or hematologic disorders may highlight programs designed to supervise patients at known risk in some of the foregoing categories.

SOCIAL HISTORY (SH)

This social history provides background on the patient's emotional stability and socioeconomic level, as it relates to his occupation, hobbies, and habits (e.g., the consumption of tobacco, alcohol, or "recreational," nonprescribed, scheduled drugs). Interactions between anesthetic agents, analgesics, or drug history are best avoided by planning. Similarly, pulmonary complications caused by chronic bronchitis and smoking can be addressed preoperatively.

The Office Health History Review Form

A brief, easy-to-understand series of questions that the patient completes prior to the clinical interview provides a useful source of health-related information (Figs. 4-1 and 4-2). Although the questions do not encompass a vast range, they pertain to the majority of office patients and permit them to reflect on their general health and to prepare for the forthcoming interview with the clinician. The questionnaire serves only as a guide for the clinical staff who *should* take time to review the responses with the patient to ensure that his responses have been recorded accurately and that he has the opportunity to question the clinician to obtain clarification or relevance of the condition(s) to dental practice.

Occasionally a few clinicians ignore the questionnaire entirely and leave the interpretation to auxiliary staff who may be

General Health History   Name _____ Ht _____ Wt _____ DOB _____
MD/DO _____ Location _____ Telephone _____
Date of Recent Physical Examination _____
                                    LMP _____

1. Current medications _____
2. List any drug-related allergies: _____
3. Have you ever been treated for:

	No	Yes	When:
asthma	____	____	_____
anemia	____	____	_____
bleeding disorders	____	____	_____
bone marrow disorder	____	____	_____
diabetes	____	____	_____
heart disease	____	____	_____
angina/pain	____	____	_____
murmurs	____	____	_____
rheumatic fever	____	____	_____
infarcts	____	____	_____
surgical correction ___ valve	____	____	_____
___ bypass	____	____	_____
hepatitis/jaundice	____	____	_____
hypertension/strokes	____	____	_____
kidney disease	____	____	_____
nervousness	____	____	_____
seizure disorder/tics/fainting episodes	____	____	_____
tuberculosis/pneumonia	____	____	_____
sudden weight change	____	____	_____

4. Previous operations:

	Date	Place
_____	_____	_____
_____	_____	_____

	No	Yes
5. Have you ever had radiation treatment to the head, face, or neck?	____	____
6. Have you experienced any of these symptoms:		
palpitations/skipped heart beats	____	____
swollen ankles/feet	____	____
shortness of breath at rest	____	____
shortness of breath with exercise	____	____
need to urinate throughout night or day	____	____
frequent thirst	____	____
change in bowel habits:	____	____
frequently		
consistently	____	____
shape	____	____
color	____	____
rectal bleeding	____	____
7. Are there some foods that you cannot eat?	____	____
8. Have you had changes of 8-10 pounds of weight recently?	____	____
9. Do you bruise readily, have nosebleeds, blood in urine?	____	____
10. Headaches	____	____
11. Visual disturbances	____	____
12. Changed sensation	____	____
13. Frequent colds and sore throat	____	____
14. Skin rashes/discoloration/brittle nails/hair	____	____

FIG. 4-1. *General health history questionnaire.*

General Dental History

DDS _____ Location _____ Telephone _____

Date of recent dental examination/treatment _____

1. Do you have ulcers or lumps in your mouth?
2. Do you have pain in or around your jaws?
3. Do your gums bleed or burn?
4. Do you have persistent bad breath?
5. Do you get frequent headaches/earaches?
6. Have you had orthodontics?
   endodontics?
   periodontics?
7. Do you get jaw stiffness or cramps?
8. Do hot/cold/sweet foods cause pain?
9. Do you want to maintain your teeth?
10. Do you wear dentures?
11. Do you get cold sores/fever blisters?
12. Have you previously had complicated/difficult extractions?

FIG. 4-2. *General dental history questionnaire.*

unfamiliar with medical screening techniques. This practice is inconsistent with safe and approved clinical conduct and must not be condoned.

A potential disadvantage of the questionnaire is the perfunctory response necessary to answer the questions. Telling patients beforehand that dental care is often related to specific medical conditions will avoid having the patient ask "why do you need to know this?" Priming the patient in this way should quickly dispel his notions of irrelevance. Consequently, the dental practitioner is able to provide rational and timely care. In summary, the health questionnaire is a valuable adjunct and a likely time saver, when used with its limitations in mind.

Mental Status Examination (MSE)

The patient's reliability should be established while obtaining his history. Although less than 15 percent of the elderly population suffers from different degrees of dementia that arise without evidence of etiology, a number of organic brain syndromes are iatrogenically induced by the chronic use of psychotropic medications. The subtle emergence of altered thought patterns and increasing lapses in memory may not be apparent to the patient or his close family; therefore, a screening MSE should be unobtrusively woven into the interview.

This examination surveys nonlocalizable cerebral functions such as thought content, affect, judgment, and insight. It requires few specific questions, but close observation and attentive listening by the clinician. The practitioner must generate his own subjective norms during his daily practice.

The MSE requires observation of the level of consciousness of the patient. Since the majority of patients who visit the office are self-sufficient, they will be alert. A few may be lethargic as a result of the effects of medications or the effects of self-prescribed drugs. Stuporous and obtunded patients may reflect metabolically compromised conditions. Any impaired level of consciousness must be considered a potential emergency and one that requires intensive monitoring and management by trained personnel.

General appearance and affect are easily noted. Affect reflects the mood and its appropriateness to the clinical situation. Judgment and insight are assessed by asking the patient about his appreciation of his situation and its accompanying problems. The refinement and localization of focal cerebral disease is the realm of the neurologist.

Essential areas of patient evaluation for those facing dental or oral surgery include the following:
1. General status
2. Cardiovascular function

3. Pulmonary function
4. Neurologic status
5. Renal and hepatic function
6. Endocrine function
7. Hematopoietic function

These are discussed in the following section.

The Examination

The physical examination of the patient begins during the interview. Clinical examination classically consists of inspection, palpation, percussion, and auscultation. The clinician may detect such odors as ketones on the breath of diabetic patients in ketoacidosis, the sweet smell of pseudomonas, or the fetid odor of fusospirochetal organisms and anaerobes such as Bacteroides in infections.

Meaningful examinations emerge only with practice. Systematic observations and their integration with facts that are known to be consistent with the suspected pathophysiology require skill. It is essential to finally refine one's routine for conducting regional or complete physical examinations, to avoid missing important but perhaps subtle evidence that would support a provisional diagnosis. However, examinations may be classified broadly into (1) routine, (2) specific complaint, and (3) emergency.

The time expended in establishing a history may be minimal in comparison to what is spent on evaluating multiple systems during the course of the patient's care.

Vital Signs (VSS)

Obtaining the vital signs—blood pressure, pulse, respirations, and temperature—should be the first step in patient contact. It should be performed in a manner that does not arouse anxiety or fear of exacerbating already present pain or of impending loss of dignity.

While recording blood pressure, the clinician should ensure the correct positioning of the patient's arm and the blood pressure cuff with respect to the heart level. Systolic and diastolic pressures must be recorded. The symmetry of pulses is checked, and the rate, rhythm, and volume of the peripheral vasculature are noted. Care must be taken in palpating carotid pulses of elderly patients to avoid mobilizing atheromatous plaques and potentiating a vascular occlusion. The stimulation of the carotid sinus while examining pulses may yield profound vagal bradycardia. Both events may lead to serious cerebrovascular insufficiency. Ventilatory rate should be noted without the patient's knowledge. Alterations in volume and rhythm are indicative of pulmonary, metabolic or brainstem diseases, e.g., chronic obstructive disease, Kussmaul's, and Cheyne-Stokes respirations. Temperature is conveniently recorded sublingually, but reflects approximately a difference of 1° C less than the higher rectal temperature. Axillary temperatures are variable and therefore unreliable. Diurnal variations and ovulation by fertile women will be noticeable on recorded temperatures.

General Impression of Patient Status

Normally, the clinician enters the examining room to a seated patient. The opportunity to obtain unobtrusive impressions on the patient's station, gait, posture, general vitality, and agility is forfeited. Apparent age, degree of agitation, facial appearance, shape and size of hands, fingernails, grooming, speech (content and cadence) in addition to the use of aids such as a cane, eye glasses, or hearing aid may be inventoried quickly (Fig. 4-3). For example, hands may reflect occupation, smoking habits, emotional distress, metabolic disturbances, and arthritis (Fig. 4-4 A-C). Nailbeds may have stigmata of hematopoietic, cardiovascular, or pulmonary pathology by alterations of their color and shape (Fig. 4-4D). In addition, the quality of nails may reflect chronic fungal infections (suggesting T cell depression) or brittleness associated with a fine finger tremor of hyperthyroidism. Close inspection of the hands may reveal splinter hemorrhages associated with subacute infective endocarditis or palmar erythema and Dupuytren's contracture, frequently associated with chronic alcoholism. Alteration of hand size bilaterally suggests acromegaly, or if unilaterally present in a young patient, it suggests a vascular anomaly such as an arteriovenous shunt or hemangioma. (Cyanosis is not a reliable sign of hypoperfusion or hypoxia because it is

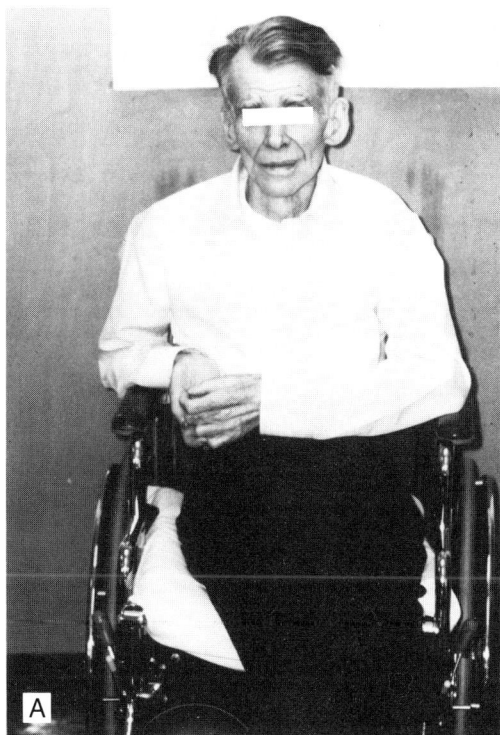

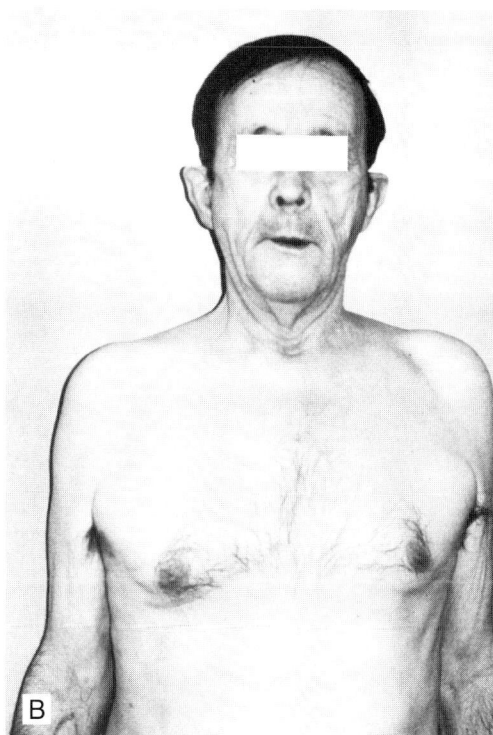

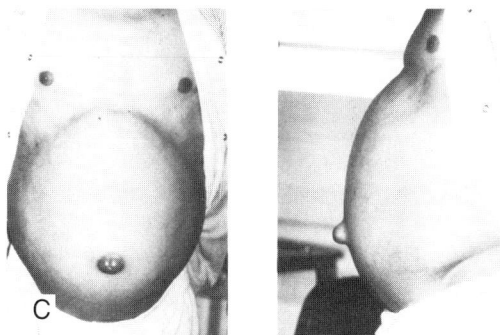

FIG. 4-3. *General physical appearance. (A) Advanced neurologic disease. (B) Chronic obstructive lung disease. (C) Massive ascites with caput medusae from portal venous hypertension.*

inversely related to the degree of anemia present.)

Head and Neck Examination

All dental patients must receive a complete head and neck examination. The frequency of re-examination is determined by occupational risks (e.g., glass blower, bootmaker) or by personal habits (e.g., tobacco and alcohol consumption). Patients not at known risk for oral cancers should receive examinations at regular but less frequent intervals.

The patient should be seated comfortably with his head and neck in an upright and normal position (Fig. 4-5). This attitude avoids patient fatigue and permits soft tissue contour to be evaluated for symmetry. Frontal, profile, tangential, and posterior views are undertaken prior to focusing attention on the cervical triangles, thoracic inlet, face, and calvarium (the clinician should remove the patient's eye glasses and inspect the areas covered by the frames). Palpation is conveniently accomplished from behind the patient for most areas of the anterior cervical triangle, including the submandibular and submental regions (Fig. 4-6). The posterior cervical triangle, external auditory meati, and calvarium are conveniently palpated while standing in front of the patient. Regional lymphatic drainage is carefully examined, and the presence of lymphadenopathy noted. When such a condition exists, the primary and secondary nodal station afferent sites must be explored thoroughly to exclude the possibility of a malignant proc-

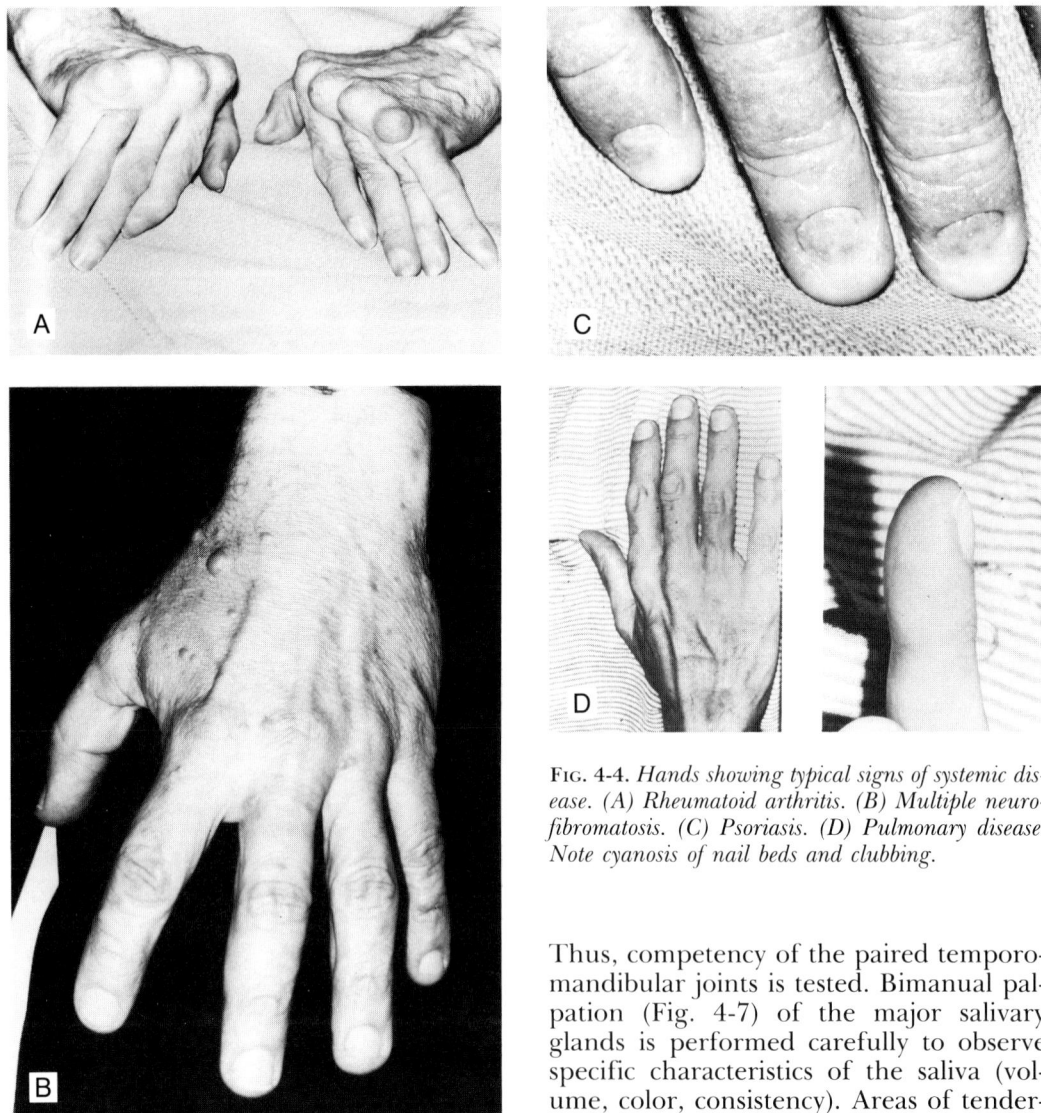

FIG. 4-4. *Hands showing typical signs of systemic disease. (A) Rheumatoid arthritis. (B) Multiple neurofibromatosis. (C) Psoriasis. (D) Pulmonary disease. Note cyanosis of nail beds and clubbing.*

ess. Fiberoptic inspection is often the sequel to finding an oral cancer, since second synchronous tumors may exist. Panendoscopy is therefore an appropriate procedure to complete the examination. Tissue biopsies may be required if the initial examination fails to find why the efferent nodes are enlarged. Careful palpation of the thyroid gland must be performed.

The maxillofacial examination includes a functional anatomy review, noting nasal patency, facial symmetry, adequacy of dental occlusion, and demonstration of a full range of active motion of the mandible.

Thus, competency of the paired temporomandibular joints is tested. Bimanual palpation (Fig. 4-7) of the major salivary glands is performed carefully to observe specific characteristics of the saliva (volume, color, consistency). Areas of tenderness or firmness along the body or ducts of these glands must be noted and their cause sought. Sympathetic autonomic facilitation may substantially reduce salivary gland function; therefore, residual saliva in the collecting ducts and stroma of the gland will be quickly evacuated by preparatory "milking" of the gland. Major tranquilizers, anxiolytics, and diuretics reduce salivary flow. Permanent alteration of serous acinal function follows radiation therapy to these structures. This is an expected complication that accompanies such tumor therapy. Note also that secretory IgA (S-IgA) is also depressed following radiotherapy. Depression of S-IgA titer parallels an observable increased incidence of dental

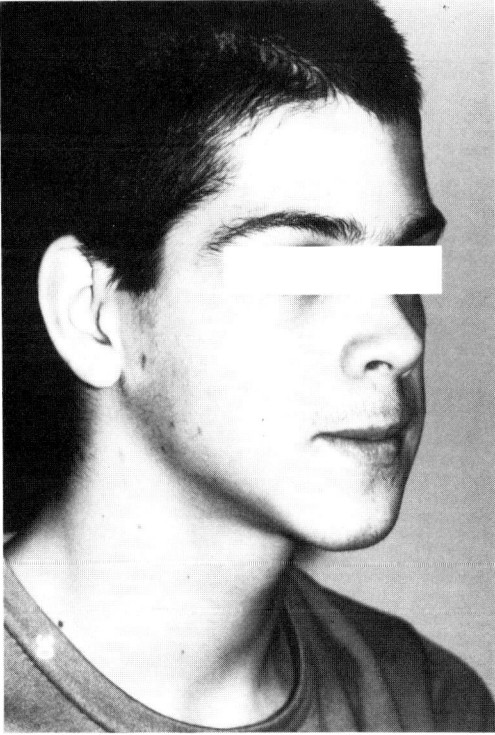

FIG. 4-5. *Patient position for a routine head and neck examination.*

caries and periodontal disease that is a common sequel to radiotherapy of the oral cavity.

Prior to examining the oral cavity and its related structures, the clinician should carefully inspect the lips and perioral region for evidence of herpetic lesions. Examination gloves are routinely recommended. He should inspect the lips for abnormalities of contour, consistency, color, and mucosal continuity. He then inspects and palpates the oral vestibule and oral cavity. Drying the mucosa facilitates detection of early mucosal changes commonly associated with erythroplasia. A high proportion of erythroplastic lesions are dyskeratotic and may proceed to carcinoma in situ or invasive squamous cell carcinoma. The hard and soft palates are inspected for soft tissue pathology and bony abnormalities such as clefts, tori, or exostoses.

The tongue is inspected for shape, color, papillae distribution, and mobility. It is best examined by applying gauze to the tip

FIG. 4-6. *(A) Palpation of the neck from behind the patient. (B) Palpation of the submandibular region from behind the patient.*

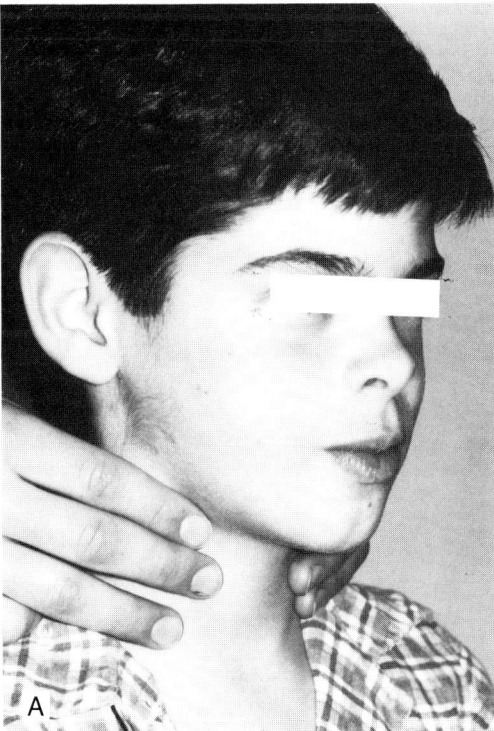

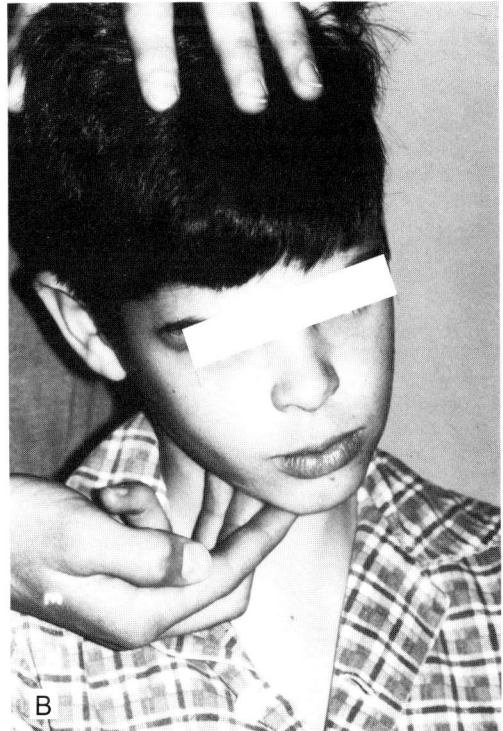

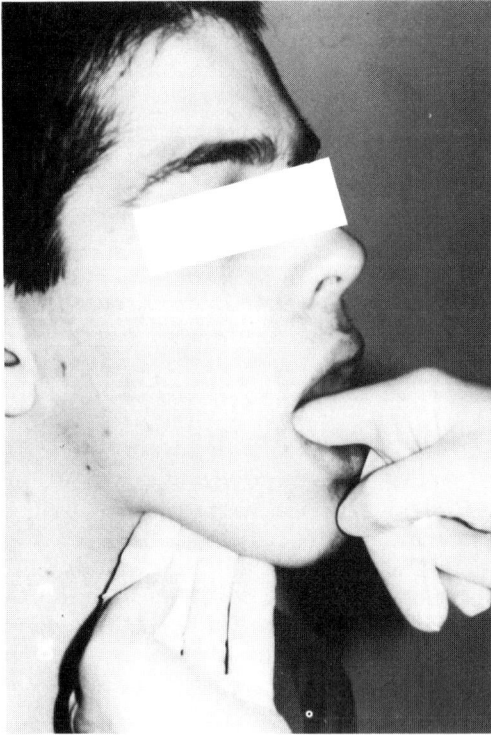

FIG. 4-7. *Bimanual palpation of the floor of the mouth and, in particular, the submandibular gland.*

and the periodontal condition with special reference to exudate, contour, and degree of abnormal dental mobility. Finally, the muscles of mastication are palpated to note the existence of altered tone, bulk, and tenderness in conjunction with the envelope of mandibular motion.

Pulmonary Examination

While obtaining the history, the clinician can make key observations. Ventilatory effort is apparent by the prominence of the accessory muscles of respiration, color of the facial skin, lips and earlobes, clubbing and cyanosis of the fingernails and their beds, cadence of speech, and the patient's facial expression which may reflect anxiety. Specific notation is made of the labored phase of the ventilatory cycle (inspiration or expiration). Normally, the ratio of inspiration to expiration is:

1. Vesicular—3:1
2. Bronchovesicular—1:1
3. Bronchial—1:3
4. Asthmatic—1:5 accompanied by sibilant or sonorous rales

Symmetry of excursion of the chest wall and diaphragm is inspected. Tactile and

(Fig. 4-8) and extending it with gentle traction. Lateral displacement permits glossofaucial inspection and palpation, while elevation of the tongue provides for ventral surface examination. The posterior one third is depressed by palpation. Inspection of the oro- and hypopharynx is performed by direct and indirect means using small dental or laryngoscopy mirrors (Fig. 4-9). Careful placement of the mirror enables the posterior nasopharynx to be inspected. Because this part of the examination requires a cooperative patient, considerable practice is necessary to achieve competency. Digital palpation of the soft palate should be performed to detect low level masses in this region. Nasopharyngeal neoplasms frequently metastasize to the posterior pharyngeal wall where lymphadenopathy may be appreciated during palpation. This may be the *only* presenting sign of remote pathology.

The alveolar processes and dentition are examined, noting erupted and missing teeth, the location of bridges and crowns,

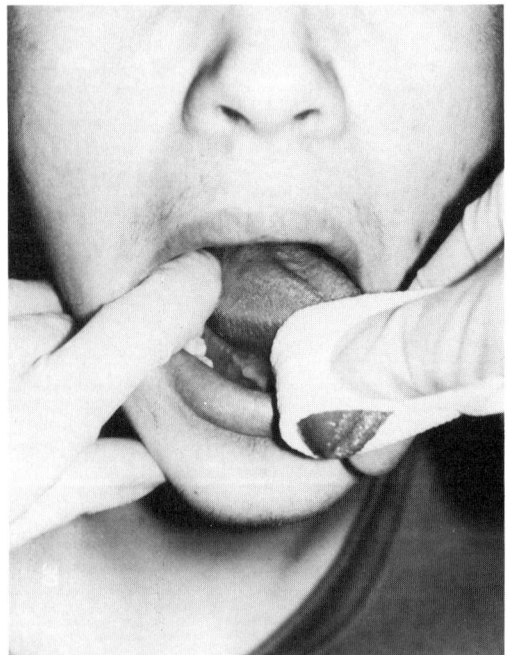

FIG. 4-8. *Examination of the tongue demonstrating traction, visualization, and palpation.*

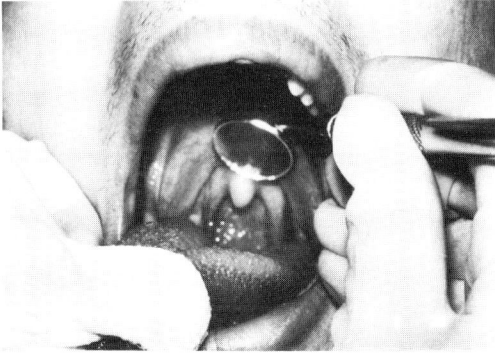

FIG. 4-9. *Inspection of the hypopharynx by direct visualization. The mirror permits indirect laryngoscopy.*

vocal fremitus provide clues to the modification of patency of the conducting airways and the degree of pulmonary consolidation with intervening pleural effusion. Percussion dullness, decreased breath sounds, and altered voice sounds (e.g., whispered pectoriloquy or egophony and adventitious sounds) strongly suggest active pulmonary disease.

Formal pulmonary function tests (PFTs) provide excellent information about existing lung pathology. Useful clinical testing of ventilatory capacity is assessed by the match test or with conversation fluency, following a leisurely ascent up two flights of stairs.

Cardiovascular Examination (COR)

Pallor, cyanosis, peripheral edema, dyspnea, chest pain, and altered arterial pulsations may indicate cardiovascular disease. Distended neck veins reflect increased venous pressure and can be readily assessed with the patient seated in the dental chair. The vertical height of the venous pulse wave from a level at the right atrium provides the clinician with venous pressure measured in centimeters of blood to the right side of the heart. Thus, if the jugular venous pulse waves (a, c, v) are noted in the upright patient, there is reasonable evidence of congestive heart failure or of local venous obstruction by a space occupying mass. Venous pulsations exclude causes of jugular venous distention (JVD) due to increased intrathoracic pressure or of obstruction to the right atrium.

The point of maximum impulse (PMI) should be visualized or palpated. This is usually located in the midclavicular line and the fourth intercostal space. Left ventricular hypertrophy causes the PMI to shift to the left toward the axilla. Right ventricular hypertrophy will cause the heart to rotate to the right, moving the PMI sagitally and resulting in a precordial heave. Percussion of the area of cardiac dullness will confirm the shifts in PMI associated with cardiomegaly or pericardial effusion. Auscultation of heart sounds for rate, rhythm, valve closure (S1, S2) and flow murmurs requires substantial practice to identify the pathophysiology of this system. Consultation with a physician is indicated should aberrations become evident. Finally, the peripheral vasculature is assessed for pulsation symmetry, collateral flow (Allen's test) and strength, noting integumental changes that accompany altered flow states.

Neuromuscular Examination

The clinician should test all the cranial nerves systematically during the head and neck examination. (Table 4-1 lists the cranial nerves and some common disorders.)

Muscle tone, bulk, power, and symmetry can be quickly assessed. Fasciculations, tremors, or clonus must be noted as they may be signs of metabolic, localized peripheral, or central disorders of the nervous system. The glabellar, snout, or sucking reflexes indicate frontal disinhibition and are correlated with the dementias and cerebrovascular insufficiency. Biceps, triceps, brachioradialis, knee, and ankle reflexes in addition to the Babinski, Romberg, and peripheral primary sensory testing should be performed as the minimum neurological exam for patients who are to receive a general anesthetic. The reader should refer to a standard text on physical assessment for details on this facet of the examination.

Hepatorenal Examination

Percussion of the right upper abdominal quadrant discloses the caudal extent of the liver. Palpation of the dependent border may reveal a smooth, nontender liver. Tenderness, nodularity, and hepatomegaly should alert the clinician to consult a physician. Viral, parasitic, or chemical induction of hepatitis is potentially dangerous when

TABLE 4-1. *Cranial nerves and some disorders*

Cranial Nerves	Disorders	Cranial Nerves	Disorders
I. Olfactory	Trauma, dementias, depression, nasal obstruction	VII. Facial	Bell's palsy, trauma, CVA, middle ear disease
II. Optic	Retinal detachment cataracts, cerebrovascular insufficency, multiple sclerosis	VIII. Vestibulo-cochlear	Acoustic neuroma, CVA
III. Oculomotor	CVA, tumor, cavernous sinus disease	IX. Glossopharyngeal	Basalar artery insufficiency, myasthenia gravis
IV. Trochlear	Same as III	X. Vagus	CVA
V. Trigeminal	MS, trauma, cavernous thrombosis, demyelinating disease	XI. Accessory	Brain stem disease
VI. Abducens	Trauma, MS, CVA	XII. Hypoglossal	CVA, demyelinating diseases myasthenia gravis

associated with anesthesia and surgical treatment. Full disclosure of the nature of the pathology should be obtained prior to proceeding with definitive oral surgical management. All patients over the age of 35 should have a fecal occult blood test and rectal examination to screen for colorectal cancer. Renal function tests provide dynamic information on the physiologic status of the urinary system.

Assessment and Plan

Upon completion of the history and physical examination, integration of the patient's chief complaint and supporting clinical evidence may suggest one or more clinical diagnoses. Since statistical probability dictates the most likely diagnosis to be the one that occurs most often in a given population, the clinician is able to plan a cost-effective series of laboratory tests supporting or nullifying the working diagnosis. The clinician commonly chooses from among the tests listed in Table 4-2.

TABLE 4-2. *Common laboratory tests*

Radiographs	Biopsy
Microbiological	Complete Blood Count
Coagulation Parameters	Blood Chemistry
Electrocardiogram	Urinalysis
Serum Electrolytes	Pulmonary Function

Radiographs

Radiography is an integral part of the majority of dental and oral surgery patient evaluations. The *radiogram* is the resultant image recorded on electromagnetically sensitive emulsion following exposure to a controlled source of medical radiation. This process, termed radiography, provides a permanent record.

Interpretation of radiographs presupposes an understanding of the regional anatomy, a tacit appreciation of the diverse range of normal radiographic appearances, including developmental changes, and a concise knowledge of pathophysiology likely to occur in the region under examination. The recently trained clinician should know the following modalities employed in radiography: intraoral, extraoral, panoramic views; CT scans; tomograms and arthrograms; sialography; bone scans; chest films (PA and lateral). (See Figs. 4-10 through 4-13.)

Appropriate selection of radiograms is based upon the working diagnosis obtained from the history and physical examination. Exodontia *must* be prefaced by a review of recent radiographs of diagnostic quality that fully disclose the anatomy being investigated. (This point will be developed further in the sections on exodontia.) Special techniques assist in localizing the spatial relationship of retained roots, impacted teeth, or foreign bodies (Clark's technique, triple exposure of Bosworth). Fracture injuries of the facial skeleton require a minimum of two views, each at right angles to the other, to provide sufficient information for a diagnosis and to determine the best method of treatment. The clinician should *defer* definitive treatment until he has secured adequately pre-

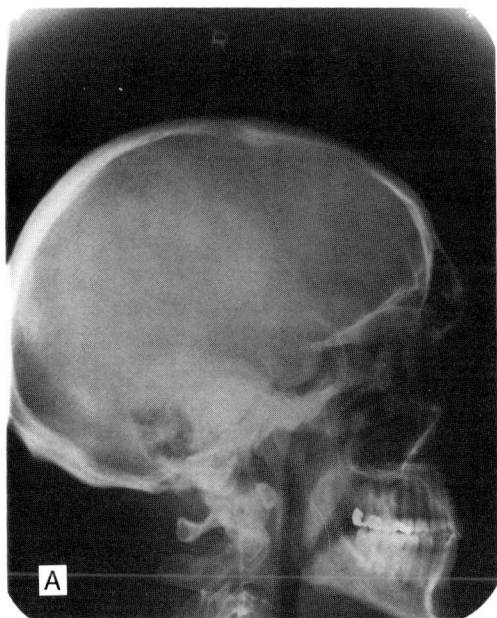

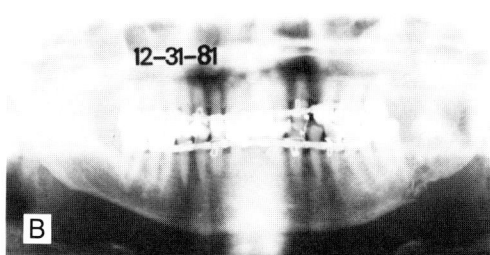

FIG. 4-10. *Extraoral radiographs. (A) Lateral head view showing enlarged sella turcica. (B) Panorex showing osteomyelitis.*

8. Internal architecture (unilocular, multi-locular, variegated density)

A diagram in the record is an invaluable aid in providing a reference for long-term follow-up of a radiographic lesion.

Complete Blood Count: CBC

A complete blood count provides a general survey of the erythrocyte and leukocyte series (Table 4-3). Number, shape, size, and the presence of inclusions, particularly in the red cell cytoplasm, reflect the status of the bone marrow, or the presence of heavy metals (e.g., lead).

pared radiograms and has reviewed the differential diagnosis in conjunction with selected and relevant laboratory tests.

Radiographic findings should be recorded noting:
1. Anatomic location
2. View (type)
3. Shape
4. Size
5. Radiopenetrance (opaque, lucent)
6. Type of periphery (irregular, lytic, sclerotic)
7. Related structures (tooth, neurovascular bundle, sinus)

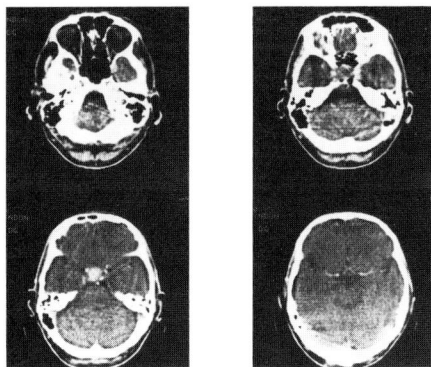

FIG. 4-11. *Computerized axial tomogram of patient shown in Figure 4-10.*

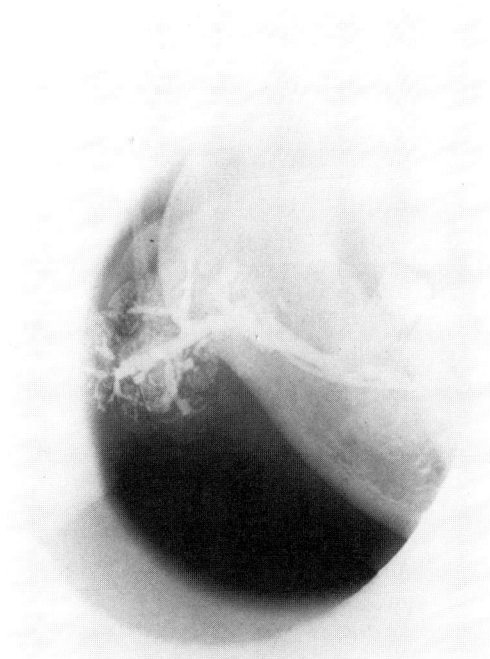

FIG. 4-12. *Sialogram of chronic obstructive salivary gland disease.*

Diagnoses are made from a CBC, e.g., anemias, bone marrow activity, oxygen transport, and heavy metal poisoning. The erythrocyte sedimentation rate (ESR) is a nonspecific index of rouleau formation. This may be increased during pregnancy, infection, rheumatic fever, immune disorders (e.g., rheumatoid arthritis), or medication induced.

TABLE 4-3. *Normal values for erythrocyte series*

Parameter	Male	Female
RBC $\times 10^6$	4.6 - 6.0	4.3 - 5.5
RETICS %	0.5 -	1.5% RBC
Hb mg %	14 - 17	12 - 16
HCT %	40 - 50	37 - 45
MCV μ^3	82 -	92
MCH $\mu\mu$g		
ESR min/hr (Westergren)	15	20

The white cell count (WBC) reflects the patient's immune competency, presence of parasitic conditions, or the existence of malignant granular cell lines, such as leukemias (Table 4-4).

TABLE 4-4. *Normal values for leukocyte series*

Parameter	Proportion
WBC $\times 10^3$ mm^3	5 - 10
Differential %	
Neutrophils	60 - 70
Lymphocytes	20 - 30
Monocytes	2 - 3
Eosinophils	1.6 - 3
Basophils	0.1 - 1

Coagulation Tests

Coagulation study is warranted when a history reflects unusual bruising, bleeding to minor trauma, or when a patient is con-

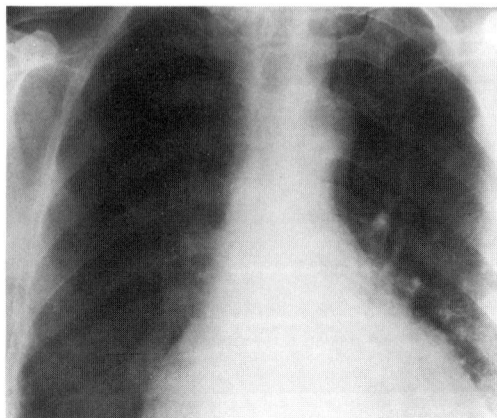

FIG. 4-13. *Chest x-ray of cardiomegaly and congestive failure. Note cephalization.*

suming anticoagulant medications (Table 4-5). Liver disease and certain bowel resections increase the risk of hemorrhage.

TABLE 4-5. *Laboratory tests for coagulation disorders*

Test	Normal Values
Tourniquet test (capillary fragility)	
Bleeding time (IVY) min	1 - 6
Platelets $\times 10^3$	200 - 400
Prothrombin time (PT) sec (extrinsic)	11.0 - 12.5
Partial thromboplastin time (PTT) sec (intrinsic)	32 - 35
Factors	

A hematologist should be consulted if the history or laboratory tests identify abnormal values (Table 4-6).

A common clinical dilemma occurs when a patient who is taking anticoagulants presents for exodontia. In general, it is reasonably safe to proceed with surgery if the PT value does not exceed 1½ to 2 times the control.

Blood Chemistry

Blood chemistry includes a diverse range of tests to identify the presence of en-

TABLE 4-6. *Hemorrhagic diathesis and coagulation tests*

CONDITION	TESTS					
	Platelets	Bleeding Time	Clot Retraction	Coag. Time	PT	PTT
Thrombocytopenia	⤓*	⤒*	Poor	N	N	N
vonWillebrand's Disease	N	⤒*	N	⇅	N	⇅
AHA (VIII)v	N	N	N	↑	N	↑
Christmas Disease	N	N	N	↑*	N	↑
Heparinization	N	N-↑	N	↑		
Hypoprothrom-binemia		N-↑	N	↑	↑*	↑

↓ =low; ↑ =high; ⇅ =variable
N = normal; ◯=very reliable tests

zymes, proteins, cations, anions, glucose, nitrogen products, lipids, and osmolality. Abnormalities identified within this examination may indicate important underlying metabolic disorders. Follow-up by a physician is indicated for diagnosis and treatment of the underlying disorders.

Blood chemistry, therefore, seeks to locate abnormal biochemical processes. It presupposes a tacit understanding of which tests must be obtained as a systemic screening tool and the correct interpretation of the laboratory data generated.

Serum Electrolytes

The principal cations and anions in the extracellular compartment are Na^+, K^+, and Cl^-. Additional cations present in plasma include Mg^{++}, Ca^{++}, and p^{+++}. These are referred to as the electrolytes. Table 4-7 gives normal values of electrolytes and associated disease.

TABLE 4-7. *Normal values of electrolytes and associated disease*

Electrolyte	Amt MEQ/L	Elevated	Lowered
Na	135 - 145	Dehydration	Aldosterone
K	3.5 - 4.5	Renal Disease	Diuretics
Ca	8.5 - 10.5	Adenoma	Hypothyroidism Cystic fibrosis Malabsorption
Mg	1.5 - 2.5	Renal Hypothyroid	Malabsorption Hyperthyroid
Cl	100 - 106	ASA toxicity Ketosis (diuretics)	Adrenal cortical insufficiency
HCO^3	24 - 28	Acidosis (metabolic or respiratory)	Chronic renal failure Acute renal failure Alkalosis

TABLE 4-8. *Normal values of urinalysis and condition*

Parameter	Normal	Condition
Color	Straw	Hematuria
pH	4.5 - 8.0	↑ Infection, ↓ drugs (ASA, barbiturates), COPD
SG	1.010	↑ Infection, tumor; ↓ trauma CNS
RBC	<10PHF	↑ Trauma, tumor, infection, parasites
WBC	<5PHF	↑ Infection, 2° obstruction
Casts	Few	Hypertension, nephron disease
Bacteria	0	↑ Infection, ♂ contamination
Glucose	0	Diabetes mellitus, renal disease, pregnancy
Ketones	0	Starvation, keto acidosis (D.M.)
Proteins	2 - 8 mg/ml	↑ Nephrotic syndrome, Waldenstrom's macroglob-inemia, lymphomas (Bence-Jones), amyloidosis
Bil	0	↑ Obstructive liver disease, hemolytic disease

Urinalysis

Urinalysis is a simple screening test for renal disease. In addition, metabolic and endocrine disorders may be identified and monitored during therapy of these diseases by detecting and quantifying specific parameters, e.g., sugars, ketones, products of epinephrine, etc. The diagnosis of pregnancy and its progress can be followed by determining progesterone levels.

Collection of the specimen requires midstream, first void samples, to be carefully obtained. To avoid bacterial contamination, patients must be instructed in the mechanics of obtaining the specimen. Note that erythrocytes are not unusual findings in the urine of menstruating women. When red cells appear in urine of male patients, the coexistence of pathology in the renal-urinary tract system is likely, and further evaluation by appropriate clinicians is required. Color, specific gravity, and odor are noted. Biochemical tests for protein, sugar, and ketones are routinely performed (Table 4-8). Microscopic examination of the specimen identifies casts, white cells, red cells, crystals, and bacteria.

Electrocardiogram (ECG)

The electrocardiogram (Fig. 4-14) records the electrical events that control the cardiac cycle. It notes rate, rhythm electrical axis, R wave progression, PR interval, QRS complex, ST depression, and T wave inversion. Electrical junction between the atria and ventricles is identified, and U and Q waves are noted. Reference to serum

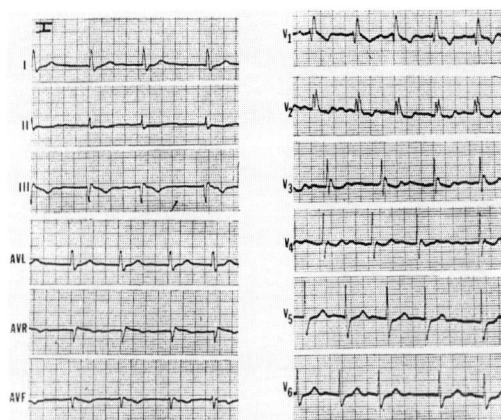

FIG. 4-14. *Lead electrocardiogram.*

TABLE 4-9. *Pathology and related laboratory values*

System Disorder	Laboratory Test
Hepatic	↑ SGOT, ↑ LDH, ° Bil(T), ↑ alk phos ↓ BUN, ↓ glucose, ↓ total protein
Cholecystitis	↑ 5′N, ↑ WBC, ↑ ESR, ↑ alk phos, ↑SGOT
Renal • prerenal • postrenal	↑ BUN, ↑ P, ↑ creat, ↑ K, ↓ Na, ↓ Ca, ↑ Mg BUN:creat > 10:1
Cardiac	↑ SGOT, ↑ LDH, ↑ CPK (isoenzymes)
Skeletal	Ca, P, alk phos, acid phos

electrolytes and the intercurrent use of cardioactive drugs is made with respect to the ECG. Evidence of arrhythmia, ischemia, and infarcts should alert the clinician to obtain a cardiology opinion or preoperative management of an unstable cardiac condition, when dental and oral surgery therapy is pending. Anesthesia work-up may require an ECG if the patient is male and over age 35, or if a lengthy surgical procedure is planned.

Other Laboratory Tests

The history and physical examination in conjunction with the results of previously obtained screening tests may direct the clinician to obtain additional specific tests to further characterize the patient's condition. Suggested screening tests for patients scheduled for oral surgery may include those indicated in Table 4-9.

Prior to interpreting the laboratory values derived from any investigation, the clinician should refer to a table of normal values prepared by the laboratory providing the service and then compare specific test results.

Interpretation of Laboratory Tests

A range of normal values exists for laboratory tests. This variability accommodates about 95 percent of the population and considers age, race, gender, circadian rhythm, and eating patterns. Experimental variability imposes additional bias to the range of "normal" laboratory values, e.g., shaking a hemovac tube will cause hemolysis of the red cells yielding an apparently high plasma concentration of K^+. Consequently, the interpretation of laboratory values must be undertaken with common sense and clinical acumen. Reflect on *known sources* of error. The clinician should ask "do these data obtained by examination fit the profile of the patient and are the data consistent with known pathophysiologic criteria that ultimately form the basis of a definitive diagnosis?"

If the clinician is satisfied with the results of the tests as representative of the patient's condition, he should integrate and synthesize the facts to formulate a therapeutic plan. An alternative, or "plan B," should be available for implementation if "plan A" no longer fits the facts. Finally, consultation with a physician may be appropriate for many circumstances; in others, it is *essential*.

CHAPTER 5

Medical Emergencies

Jeffrey L. Rajchel and Robert W. Wardrop

The only complete catastrophe is the catastrophe from which we learn nothing. W. E. HOCKING

The incidence of medical emergencies in the dental office is low. However, they are likely to increase as a result of medical advances that allow compromised patients a more normal lifestyle. Surveys demonstrate that approximately 35 percent of patients undergoing ambulatory anesthesia have a significant medical history that may lead to complications.

Effective management of a medical emergency depends upon prevention, recognition, and treatment. The clinician must obtain a complete medical history, carefully observe the patient, and recognize predisposing or precipitating factors to prevent an impending emergency. Although this chapter focuses on recognition and treatment of certain medical emergencies, prevention is of primary importance.

Vital Signs

The vital signs are important for baseline information on the status of a patient. They are often the primary guides to accurate diagnosis of an emergency and subsequent therapy. The cardinal physical signs include pulse, blood pressure, respiration, and skin color.

Pulse

The average pulse rate for normal adults is 60 to 80 beats per minute, and 80 to 110 per minute for children. It should be both strong and of regular rhythm. A heart rate of less than 60 beats per minute for an adult and 70 for a child is termed *bradycardia,* whereas a rate above 100 in the adult is called *tachycardia.* The American Heart Association suggests that "the carotid pulse is the most accessible, most reliable, and the most easily learned position." Abnormal rates or rhythm may indicate cardiac or pulmonary disease. Lower heart rates with a normal blood pressure are frequently seen in athletic individuals.

Blood Pressure

Blood pressure is a function of heart action and vascular resistance. Blood pressure equals stroke volume times heart rate times total peripheral resistance (BP = S.V. × H.R. × T.P.R.). Thus, any effect on the heart or the vascular compartment is manifested by comparable change in the blood pressure.

Normal average blood pressures include: 90/60 at 5 years of age, 100/65 at 10 years, 120/75 for a young adult, and 140/90 for middle-aged and elderly individuals. (Normal adult systolic pressure is often estimated to be 100 mm Hg plus the age of the patient. If the diastolic pressure is greater than 100 mm Hg, treatment should be delayed until medical consultation is obtained.) Because excitement or exertion may alter readings by 20 to 30 mm, it is suggested that a reading be repeated after the patient has relaxed for a short time. Hypertension encountered in an emergency in the dental office commonly results from patient anxiety. This can usually be controlled with discontinuing the procedure and placing the patient in a comfortable position. If signs and symptoms persist, nitroglycerin can be administered sublingually to produce vaso-dilation and subsequent decrease in blood pressure.

Hypotension, a reduction in arterial blood pressure, is generally a more immediate life-threatening emergency than a hypertensive episode. Adult systolic readings less than 80 mm Hg are significant. (A reduction in blood pressure to 80/60 is more significant in a patient with a starting pressure of 130/95 than in one with a pre-operative reading of 100/75.) Initial treatment for a patient who feels faint or loses consciousness is to place the legs in an elevated position with the head reclined. If this is unsuccessful in restoring normal blood pressure and the patient is bradycardic (heart rate less than 60), atropine 0.4 mg IM should be administered. If, however, the patient remains hypotensive with a normal or elevated heart rate, mephentermine 15 to 30 mg IM is injected.

Respirations

The depth, rhythm, rate, and effort of breathing should be observed. The respiratory rate ranges between 20 and 40 per minute during early childhood and 15 and 25 during late childhood, reaching adult levels of 14 to 18 per minute at age 15. The depth and rhythm should be regular. Evidence of respiratory distress suggests obstruction, acute allergic reactions, asthmatic attack, or heart disease. For each 1° F temperature elevation, the heart rate increases ten beats per minute and the respiratory rate increases four per minute.

Breath odors can also be of value. An acetone odor is often associated with hyperglycemia and a potential diabetic coma. Alcohol on a patient's breath can demonstrate anxiety or an alcohol problem. This could alert the dentist to appropriate alteration of the treatment plan.

Skin

A brief examination of the skin gives the practitioner valuable information regarding the state of oxygenation and status of the cardiovascular system. Pallor (lack of normal color) is often seen in states of anxiety, a tendency towards syncope, and in hypotensive episodes. Cyanosis (dusky or bluish appearance) of the lips and nail beds is due to inadequate oxygenation of blood and may be associated with cardiac or respiratory arrest and airway obstruction. The skin is usually moist during a hypoglycemic reaction, whereas it is often dry during hyperglycemic crisis.

Syncope

Syncope (fainting, vasodepressive syncope, vasovagal syncope) is the most common cause of loss of consciousness in the dental office. Predisposing or contributing factors may include fear and anxiety, pain, sight of blood, hot environment, fasting, and exhaustion.

Early signs and symptoms of syncope include a feeling of warmth, nausea, and weakness. The patient may complain of "feeling faint" and lose facial color, giving rise to a pale, ashen gray complexion with beads of perspiration on the forehead. Initially, the heart rate may rise with little change in blood pressure.

As the process continues, the patient develops coldness of the extremities, dizziness, pupillary dilation, and acute depression of the heart rate and blood pressure. Without appropriate intervention, loss of consciousness ensues, with shallow irregular breathing, convulsive movements of limbs, and twitching of facial muscles. The period of unconsciousness is usually brief (lasting seconds to minutes), and recovery follows quickly once the patient is placed in the supine position.

The pathophysiology of syncope follows release of catecholamines in response to stress. This leads to a decrease in peripheral resistance and a pooling of blood into the muscles. A relative decrease in circulatory blood volume and falling arterial blood pressure initiates compensatory mechanisms that attempt to maintain cerebral blood flow. Fatigue of these mechanisms leads to a reflex bradycardia and fall in blood pressure, resulting in cerebral ischemia and loss of consciousness.

Early recognition of signs and symptoms of syncope and placement of the patient in the supine position improve venous return and usually prevent the progression of the episode. Tight clothing should be loosened and the airway cleared and maintained. Oxygen may be administered and vital signs should be carefully monitored. A respiratory stimulant, such as aromatic spirits of ammonia, can be crushed between the fingers and waved 4 to 6 inches beneath the patient's nose. If unconsciousness persists for longer than five minutes after initiating treatment, or if complete recovery does not occur in 15 to 20 minutes, another cause for the "fainting" should be sought.

SUMMARY OF TREATMENT
1. Early recognition
2. Place patient in supine position, elevate feet
3. Administer oxygen
4. Give respiratory stimulant (aromatic spirits of ammonia)

Hyperventilation

Hyperventilation is one of the most common causes of collapse seen in a dental surgery. It can be defined as ventilation in excess of that required to maintain normal oxygen and carbon dioxide blood levels. Commonly observed in overly anxious patients, hyperventilation may be precipitated by stressful procedures resulting in an increase in respiratory rate and depth.

Blood carbon dioxide levels following hyperventilation become depleted from normal values of around 40 mm Hg to as low as 15 mm Hg (hypocapnia). A reduction in the partial pressure of carbon dioxide shifts the oxyhemoglobin dissociation curve upward and to the left, allowing hemoglobin to be more saturated in oxygen and less readily available to the tissues (Bohr effect). Hypocapnia produces cerebral vasoconstriction (carbon dioxide is a powerful cerebral vasodilator). The change in oxyhemoglobin dissociation curve combines with cerebral vasoconstriction to decrease oxygen availability to the brain tissues, resulting in neurologic symptoms of dizziness and giddiness. Hypocapnia also results in an increase in pH of the blood (respiratory alkalosis). As the pH of the blood rises, calcium metabolism becomes altered and the level of ionized calcium in the blood decreases. Decreases in blood-ionized calcium may lead to symptoms of tingling and paresthesia of the extremities and perioral region, cramps, and possible convulsions.

Treatment of hyperventilation is aimed at reducing the anxiety level of the patient and correcting the respiratory problem. The patient should be reassured, seated in an upright position with the airway cleared, and told to decrease and regulate breathing to about four to six breaths per minute. Most cases of hyperventilation revert to normal at this stage.

If these steps are not effective, the patient should rebreathe exhaled air that contains increased amounts of carbon dioxide. This can be accomplished by placing a bag over the patient's mouth and nose and instructing the patient to breathe into the bag slowly (six to ten breaths per minute). The dentist may avoid potential hyperventilation by being alerted to the patient's anxiety and increased breathing rates and taking appropriate preventive measures at that time.

SUMMARY OF TREATMENT
1. Early recognition
2. Reassure patient and reduce anxiety
3. Reposition patient in upright position
4. Clear airway and control breathing rate and depth
5. Rebreathe exhaled air through paper bag

Heart Disease

Although a wide variety of diseases affect the cardiovascular system, the general practitioner should be acutely aware of coronary heart disease and hypertensive heart disease. If overlooked or taken lightly, either of these conditions may result in a medical emergency. Groups at potential risk include: middle-aged to older males, cigarette smokers, and persons with a family history of heart disease.

Coronary heart disease results from decreased blood supply to the myocardium through the coronary arteries. A mild imbalance between the myocardial oxygen supply and demand results in angina pectoris, whereas a myocardial infarction or "heart attack" is precipitated from partial or complete cessation of coronary arterial perfusion.

Angina Pectoris

Angina pectoris is the primary symptom of ischemic heart disease. No consistent

relationship exists between the severity of angina pectoris and extent of coronary artery disease. Typically, the pain is described as a sensation of pressure, tightness, or heaviness. It is generally mild to moderate in intensity and less commonly sharp or burning. The location of chest pain varies widely among different individuals. The presenting symptom may be substernal pain that spreads across the chest and radiates to any area above the diaphragm including the neck, mandible, teeth, shoulders, arms, back, and epigastrium. Radiation to the left shoulder is especially common. An anginal attack is often precipitated by physical exertion, emotional upset, cold weather, and eating a heavy meal. The pain usually lasts for 2 to 10 minutes after the patient has rested. The cause of the pain is unknown, but is thought to result from release of lactic acid, histamine, and related kinins by ischemic cardiac muscle.

Initial treatment is directed toward increasing oxygen delivery to the myocardium while reducing oxygen demand. This is achieved by administration of 0.3-0.6 mg nitroglycerin placed under the patient's tongue. The drug is absorbed rapidly, bringing relief within 1 to 3 minutes. For many years, it was thought that this and similar drugs produced their effect by dilation of the coronary arteries. However, it is now believed that these calcified and atherosclerotic vessels are incapable of this. The present theory is that the drug produces a generalized systemic arterial dilation (reduces total peripheral resistance and decreases myocardial afterload—the net effect is a decrease in myocardial oxygen demand), thus lowering blood pressure, venous return, and cardiac output. This effect may be responsible for headaches, flushing, and occasional reflex tachycardia.

Myocardial Infarction

Myocardial infarction results from a sudden, severe arterial insufficiency to the heart. It is an acute medical emergency in which over 60 percent of deaths occur within 60 minutes of the onset of symptoms. A heart attack most commonly occurs from partial or complete occlusion of one or more of the coronary arteries by atherosclerosis, thrombosis, or embolis.

The anterior descending branch of the left coronary artery, which supplies the anterior left ventricle, is the most common site of involvement.

Signs and symptoms of angina pectoris may closely mimic myocardial infarction. In an acute myocardial infarction, the pain is typically described as crushing, squeezing, pressing, burning or vice-like in quality. It presents substernally with radiation to the mandible, shoulders, neck and arms. In 15 to 20 percent of individuals there is no presentation of pain, although nausea, vomiting, cold sweats, and weakness are accompanying symptoms. An anginal attack can potentially be excluded with greater suspicion of a myocardial infarction if:

1. The pain can be localized with one finger
2. The pain lasts for less than 30 seconds or more than 30 minutes
3. The intensity of the pain is severe
4. The pain is not relieved by rest
5. The pain is not relieved by nitroglycerin
6. The pain is accompanied with hypotension (Arterial hypotension has been identified in 80 percent of all patients with myocardial infarction.)

Primary management of myocardial infarction is focused towards prevention of further necrosis of muscle cells. The ischemic area in the heart is surrounded by a zone of compromised cells. If oxygen demand continues to be greater than the supply, these cells will also die, thus increasing the amount of damage to the heart wall. An oxygen debt can result from pain and anxiety that usually accompanies a heart attack. The practitioner should quickly attempt to alleviate these symptoms with morphine (10-15 mg IM) and nitrous oxide/oxygen. Oxygen deficiency can also result from inadequate myocardial perfusion in hypotension and/or bradycardia. These specific problems should be treated as they arise. The importance of continuous monitoring of vital signs cannot be overemphasized.

SUMMARY OF TREATMENT—CHEST PAIN
1. Terminate surgery and all stimulation
2. Keep the patient at rest in a comfortable position (A semi-sitting position with

slight elevation of the head and feet is preferred to maximize cardiac perfusion.)

3. Administer 100% oxygen by face mask
4. Administer one tablet (0.3-0.6 mg) nitroglycerin sublingually. Repeat dose in 5 to 10 minutes if pain persists (to a maximum of three tablets)
5. Monitor vital signs (heart rate, blood pressure, respirations). Failure to relieve anginal symptoms by appropriate agents is suggestive of myocardial infarction
6. Summon medical assistance
7. Administer morphine 10-15 mg IM for relief of pain
8. Administer nitrous oxide/oxygen for relief of anxiety
9. Treat specific problems as they arise: Hypotension—The systolic pressure should be maintained above 80 mm Hg Bradycardia—Heart rate should be maintained above 60 beats per minute

Respiratory Obstruction

The dental patient is frequently at risk from aspirating foreign bodies that fall into the posterior pharynx. Most objects such as root canal reamers, teeth, inlays, or crowns are small enough to pass through the larynx into the trachea without causing obstruction. However, an object may enter the trachea and obstruct the airway. Therefore, the dentist should be familiar with management of such problems.

If airway obstruction is not complete and the patient is capable of forceful coughing and adequate respiration, he should be left alone. If air exchange subsequently deteriorates (as in the case of complete obstruction), prompt management is necessary in order to avoid loss of consciousness and possible death.

The abdominal thrust, or Heimlich maneuver, should be used to rapidly increase intrathoracic pressure and dislodge the foreign body (Fig. 5-1). During the Heimlich maneuver, the patient is held from behind with the operator's hands firmly clasped below the patient's xiphoid process. Six to ten thrusts are then made into the abdomen of the adult and usually succeed in dislodging the object. It may be possible in the unconscious patient to insert the fingers into the oral cavity and remove foreign objects located above the epiglottis. A laryngoscope can be used for direct visualization by trained personnel.

If the above measures are ineffective, an airway must be established below the obstruction. Tracheotomy can be a hazardous procedure, and is not recommended for use in the dental office. Cricothyroid membrane puncture (cricothyrotomy) can be carried out more simply.

1. With the chin elevated and neck extended, locate the thyroid cartilage and cricoid cartilage. Stabilize the trachea and identify the cricothyroid membrane

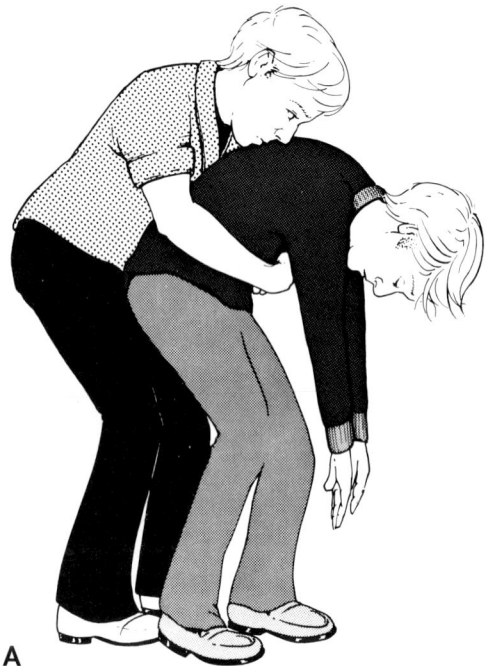

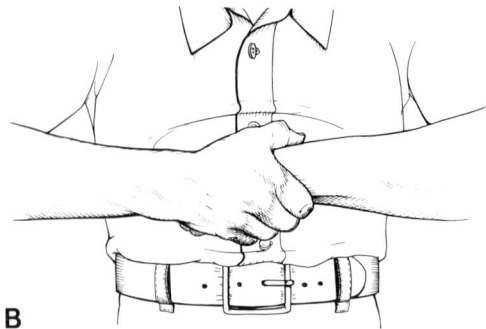

FIG. 5-1. *Heimlich maneuver. (A) Positions of patient and person performing maneuver. (B) Position of hands on patient.*

2. Insert a 12-13 gauge needle through the cricothyroid membrane entering the tracheal lumen

3. Ensure adequate oxygenation via the cricothyrotomy

Following establishment of an airway, oxygen should be administered and the patient transferred to an emergency center for follow-up management and removal of the foreign object.

SUMMARY OF TREATMENT

1. Recognize complete obstruction
2. Abdominal thrust (Heimlich maneuver)
3. Check mouth for foreign objects
4. Attempt to ventilate
5. Cricothyrotomy if necessary

Cardiopulmonary Arrest

Cardiopulmonary arrest in the dental office is a serious event. The dentist and his staff should be prepared to recognize and treat it with efficiency and effectiveness. Although cardiovascular collapse usually occurs in patients with preexisting cardiovascular disease, additional causes may include: drug overdose, airway obstruction, anaphylaxis, seizure disorders, and acute adrenal insufficiency. Prevention of a cardiopulmonary arrest requires full knowledge of the patient's medical history, vital signs, and presurgical consultations where appropriate.

Diagnosis of cardiopulmonary arrest is based on the absence of both ventilation and circulation. Clinical findings include lack of chest or abdominal movement, no breath sounds, and a lack of carotid pulse. The patient is unconscious with dilated pupils and an ashen gray appearance. Cardiopulmonary resuscitation (CPR) must begin immediately since anoxia may produce irreversible brain damage after 3 to 4 minutes.

Although an individual can perform CPR effectively, a team approach is more efficient. Therefore, dental office personnel should be trained together. The following description is based on the American Heart Association recommendations.

Recognition of unconsciousness can be based on a lack of response to sensory stimulation, and basic life support should be initiated immediately. Assistance should be called for and the patient placed in a supine position. The airway should be cleared and opened by head tilt combined with either neck or chin lift. If this maneuver is unsuccessful in opening the airway, the fingers should be placed behind the angles of the jaw, forcefully displacing the mandible forward, tilting the head backward.

If spontaneous breathing does not occur, artificial ventilation should be commenced. Ideally, this is accomplished with an anesthetic machine or positive pressure device (i.e., bag valve mask or demand valve system); however, if these are not available, then mouth-to-mouth or mouth-to-nose ventilation can be used. Use of an oropharyngeal airway in an unconscious patient helps maintain an adequate airway during artificial ventilation. Four quick, full breaths are given initially without allowing time for lung deflation between breaths. Subsequent ventilation should be continued at a rate of one every 5 seconds (12 per minute) for the adult victim, one every 4 seconds (15 per minute) for small children, and one every 3 seconds (20 per minute) for infants. Immediately following the first ventilatory cycle of four quick breaths, the circulation should be assessed.

The presence or absence of effective circulation can be determined by palpation of a carotid pulse. In the absence of a pulse, external chest compression must be initiated immediately, and the emergency medical service (EMS) should be summoned.

With the patient placed in a supine position on a hard surface, the emergency personnel should be close to the patient's side. The heel of one hand is placed over the lower half of the sternum, 1 to 1.5 inches superior to the xiphoid process, with the other hand placed immediately above the first one. The fingers must be kept off the chest wall, with the axis of the heel of the hand placed on the long axis of the sternum to maintain the compression force over the sternum (Fig. 5-2). With arms straight and shoulders positioned directly over the hands, pressure is exerted to depress the lower sternum 1.5 to 2 inches for a normal-sized adult (Fig. 5-3). External chest compression is effective in providing cerebral and systemic circulation by in-

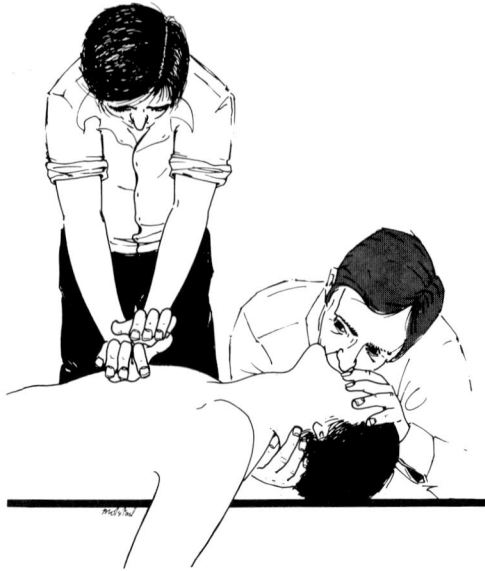

Fig. 5-2. *Positions of the patient and those administering resuscitation.*

creasing intrathoracic pressure. This pressure is transmitted into the extrathoracic arteries to a greater extent than the veins, creating a pressure gradient and, therefore, a systemic blood flow. The compression rate for two-person CPR is 60 per minute. When performed without interruption, this rate will allow cardiac refilling. With two rescuers, one long inflation should be quickly interposed after each five chest compressions (ratio of 5:1) without any pause in compression. In children, only the heel of one hand is used for cardiac compression, and with infants, only the tips of the middle and index fingers are used at a higher rate around 80 to 100 per minute.

The effectiveness of CPR can be assessed by evaluating the response of the patient. Four indicators can be observed:
1. The color of the skin and mucous membranes
2. The carotid pulse
3. Respiratory movements
4. Pupils of the eye

Upon transferring a victim of cardiopulmonary arrest to an emergency room, advanced life support becomes available and includes electrocardiography, defibrilla-

tion, and additional drugs to control acidosis and/or arrhythmias.

SUMMARY OF TREATMENT
1. Establish unresponsiveness, tap or gently shake and shout
2. Call out for help
3. Position the patient (supine); proceed with the ABCs of CPR
4. Airway
   a. Open the airway (head tilt)
   b. Establish apnea (look, listen, feel)
5. Breathing
   a. Perform rescue breathing (mouth to mouth)
   b. Manage foreign body airway obstruction, if present
6. Circulation
   a. Establish presence or absence of pulse
   b. Activate EMS system
   c. Begin chest compression (if pulse absent)

Anaphylaxis

One of the most severe and potentially life-threatening emergencies that occur in the dental office is an anaphylactic-type allergic reaction. It can occur during or after administration of a drug. The incidence of such a reaction is uncommon, but the dental practitioner should be familiar with its

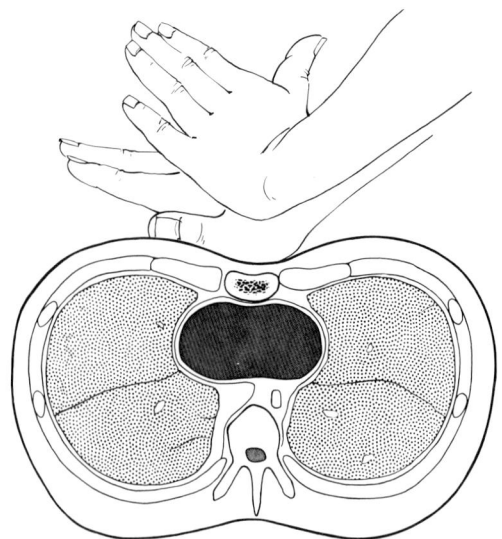

Fig. 5-3. *Cardiac compression.*

recognition and treatment. (Although the incidence of developing an anaphylactic reaction in the dental office is unknown, it has been estimated that the risk in a hospital is 1 to 4 percent.)

Allergic reactions following administration of a drug can occur unpredictably in any patient. Anaphylaxis generally requires previous exposure to the drug and production of antibodies. The drug responsible for eliciting a reaction is called an antigen. The initial exposure of the body to this antigen stimulates the patient's lymphocytes to produce antibodies specific to the drug. These antibodies attach to receptor sites on cell membranes of both mast cells present in the tissues and basophils circulating in plasma.

Sensitized mast cells and basophils bound with antibodies are capable of initiating an anaphylactic reaction when stimulated by reexposure to the drug. This severe reaction is the result of degranulation of mast cells and basophils and release of chemical mediators. Histamine is the most important substance released and is responsible for increased capillary permeability and contraction of bronchial smooth muscle. Other chemical mediators include SRS (slow reacting substance of anaphylaxis) and prostaglandins.

The amount of drug and route of administration are important factors influencing severity of the allergic reaction. (Drugs administered intravenously have a greater potential of resulting in an anaphylactic reaction than those administered orally.)

Signs and symptoms of an acute drug-induced anaphylactic reaction may occur within seconds to minutes. The patient should be observed for 30 minutes following administration of an unfamiliar medication.

The reactions may be grouped as follows:

Eye: Lacrimation, ocular itching, conjunctivitis

Nose: Sneezing, rhinorrhea, nasal congestion

Respiration: Laryngeal edema, dyspnea, stridor, wheezing (asthma), bronchospasm, suprasternal retraction

Cardiovascular: Weakness, thready low volume pulse, tachycardia, hypotension, syncope, cardiac arrest

Gastrointestinal: Nausea, vomiting, diarrhea

Skin: Erythema of upper body, edema (angioneurotic edema), wheal formation (transudation of fluid secondary to increased vascular permeability)

Central Nervous System: Convulsions, coma

A life-threatening allergic reaction is characterized by hypotension, cardiac dysrhythmias, and bronchospasm. The goals of treatment are to inhibit further release of chemical mediators, restore intravascular fluid volume, and relieve bronchospasm. The treatment includes maintenance of a patent airway and administration of oxygen. The patient should be placed in a horizontal position with the legs slightly elevated (Trendelenburg position). Intramuscular or sublingual injection of 0.3 to 0.5 cc of epinephrine 1:1000 is administered immediately. The ability of epinephrine to decrease the release of chemical mediators from mast cells and basophils is the most likely explanation for its rapid lifesaving effect. Additionally, alpha and beta adrenergic effects relax bronchial smooth muscle and supply peripheral vasoconstriction.

After administration of epinephrine, an antihistamine should be injected intramuscularly. Diphenhydramine (Benadryl) 25 to 50 mg helps reduce the attachment of circulating histamine to unoccupied histamine receptors.

Steroids are no longer commonly recommended for the treatment of anaphylaxis because their beneficial effects are delayed for 30 to 90 minutes following administration. They do not block the interaction between antigen and antibodies or prevent release of chemical mediators. Nevertheless, hydrocortisone is used and does not appear to have an adverse effect.

Mild allergic reactions are not life-threatening and are often alleviated by discontinuation of the responsible agent. If signs and symptoms such as urticaria (rash), pruritis (itching), or ocular reactions occur, antihistamines are generally effective. Initially, diphenhydramine (Benadryl) 25 to 50 mg is given IM or orally, followed by oral administration every 6 hours for 24 hours.

SUMMARY OF TREATMENT

1. Maintain a patent airway. Administer oxygen
2. Place patient in Trendelenburg position if hypotensive and in shock. If the patient has difficulty breathing, a semi-reclined position may be more helpful
3. Inject epinephrine 0.3 to 0.5 cc 1:1000 IM or sublingual. Repeat in 10 to 15 minutes as needed
4. Administer diphenhydramine (Benadryl) 25 to 50 mg IM
5. Monitor vital signs
6. Initiate CPR if necessary
7. Summon medical assistance

Hypoglycemia

Glucose is essentially the only source of energy available to maintain normal intracellular metabolism in the brain. The brain is particularly vulnerable since it has no way to store glucose in contrast to almost every other tissue in the body. This condition is caused by the brain's inability to utilize circulating free fatty acids as an energy source.

Regulation of plasma glucose levels is primarily a function of the alpha and beta cells in the pancreatic islets of Langerhans. These cells produce glucagon and insulin, respectively. Their effects are exactly opposite. Insulin decreases plasma glucose levels whereas glucagon increases them. (Epinephrine, corticosteroids, and growth hormone also increase plasma glucose levels.) Although hyperglycemia has numerous causes, diabetes is the most common endocrine disease that results in hyposecretion of insulin and an inability to maintain glucose concentrations within the relatively narrow bounds of normal. Normal blood sugar levels are 80 to 120 mg%.

A full medical history of a diabetic patient must include consideration of onset, duration, severity, and present medications. (Treatment may include: diet control, oral hypoglycemic agents, or insulin injections.) If insulin-dependent, the patient usually receives an injection each morning. In this way, high postprandial blood glucose levels will be prevented. If, however, the patient takes his normal insulin dose but omits a meal, he can depress the glucose level precipitously.

An attack of hypoglycemia generally gives the practitioner sufficient warning so that an unconscious state should seldom occur in the dental office. Signs and symptoms may include: twitching of the limbs, headache, visual disturbances, confusion, hunger, faintness, nausea, weakness, and moist skin and tongue. If the patient is conscious and able to swallow, glucose should be given orally. Orange juice, two or three tablespoons of granulated sugar dissolved in water, or a candy bar may be given. The response is usually rapid. If the patient has lost consciousness, 20 to 50 ml of 50 percent dextrose solution should be given intravenously over a period of 2 to 3 minutes. An alternate therapy is the administration of 1.0 to 2.0 mg of glucagon IM.

The possibility of a hyperglycemic reaction, or diabetic coma, occurring in an ambulatory patient is quite small. Generally, such a patient has been ill for several days prior to collapse. Additionally, the signs and symptoms are different. They include dry skin, dry tongue, hypotension, and acetone breath.

SUMMARY OF TREATMENT

1. Recognize characteristic signs and symptoms
2. Administer oral glucose if patient is conscious
3. Administer 1.0-2.0 mg glucagon IM if unconscious—repeat dosage if necessary
4. Summon medical assistance if necessary

Asthma

Bronchial asthma is a respiratory disease of hyperreactivity characterized by dyspnea and wheezing, due to a narrowing of bronchi by smooth muscle spasm, mucosal edema and congestion and mucous hypersecretions. Airway obstruction occurs particularly during expiration. Asthma, a common condition affecting more than 2 percent of the population, begins in childhood or early adult life. Extrinsic asthma typically occurs in children with an allergic predisposition. An attack in these patients may be precipitated by exposure to specific allergens such as house dust, foods, or drugs. Intrinsic asthma usually develops in

adults, is not allergic in nature, and may be precipitated by infection, irritating inhalants, and emotional stress.

Prevention of an acute asthmatic attack requires a detailed medical history, along with a knowledge of those factors that may precipitate an attack. Any known allergens should be eliminated from the surgery. An asthmatic patient who reports respiratory symptoms of a cold or flu should have his elective procedures rescheduled. Stress and anxiety should be minimized, and use of conscious sedation with nitrous oxide-oxygen may be helpful.

The clinical presentation of an asthmatic attack may vary depending on severity of the condition. Commonly, a patient is wheezing during inspiration and expiration. The patient often coughs to clear excess mucous from the respiratory tract. Breathing soon becomes labored with use of accessory muscles (sternocleidomastoid, trapezius, scalenus). The patient may be anxious and become panic-stricken.

Management of an acute asthmatic attack in the dental office should begin with use of bronchodilators supplemented with oxygen. Usually a patient feels more comfortable sitting upright. He should be allowed to take his own tablets or inhalant. If these are unavailable, the dentist should provide a suitable bronchodilator inhalant such as Alupent. If little change follows administration of the inhalant, epinephrine (0.3 to 0.5 mg) is given subcutaneously and may be repeated as necessary in 5 to 15 minutes. If the above measures have not terminated the attack, the patient should be transported to an emergency room for further management.

SUMMARY OF TREATMENT
1. Place patient in comfortable position
2. Administer bronchodilator (Alupent inhaler)
3. Administer oxygen
4. Parenteral medication—epinephrine 0.3 to 0.5 mg subcutaneously, repeated 5 to 15 minutes if necessary
5. Summon medical assistance

Adrenal Insufficiency

Over 50 steroids have been isolated from the human adrenal cortex, but only a few provide significant biologic activity. The most abundantly secreted steroid is commonly known as cortisol or hydrocortisone. This glucocorticoid functions to maintain electrolyte and water homeostasis, sustain the blood pressure, and promote metabolism of carbohydrate, fat, and proteins. It also reduces inflammatory tissue swelling by lessening fluid formation, and maintains life in situations of stress or shock.

Production of cortisol by the adrenal cortex is regulated directly by the anterior pituitary gland and indirectly by the hypothalamus. Although plasma cortisol levels are subject to minute-to-minute variation, the concentration is much higher in the early morning than through the afternoon and evening. The normal adult secretes approximately 20 mg of cortisol per day. Under maximal stress, adrenal glands secrete 200 to 300 mg per day.

Adrenocortical insufficiency, or Addison's disease, has an incidence of three to four persons per 100,000 population. It may be a result of primary adrenal insufficiency or secondary adrenal insufficiency. Over 90 percent of primary adrenal insufficiency is caused by an autoimmune mechanism or bilateral tuberculosis of the adrenal glands. Additional causes include amyloidosis, blastomycosis, coccidiomycosis, histoplasmosis, lymphomas, and leukemia. Over 80 percent of both glands must be atrophied before signs and symptoms of insufficiency develop. Secondary insufficiency may be caused by disease of the pituitary gland and hypothalamus or commonly by ACTH suppression due to exogenous glucocorticoid administration.

Consequences of adrenal insufficiency are inability of the body to manage the challenge of stresses, such as infection, trauma, surgery, pain, or apprehension. When the adrenal gland is unable to supply necessary cortisol, an Addisonian crisis ensues. It is generally manifested by weakness, syncope, hypotension, rapidly progressing with hyperpyrexia to vascular collapse, shock, and death.

A patient with inadequate adrenal cortex function, therefore, needs supplemental steroids prior to dental treatment. This is usually reserved for appointments of anticipated stress such as exodontia or periodontal surgery. Although recent investigations have seriously questioned the general principles of corticosteroid therapy, adrenocortical suppression should be suspected if a patient has received the equivalent of 20 mg of hydrocortisone per day for a continuous period of 2 weeks or longer within the last 2 years (Rule of Two's).

The choice of prophylactic regimen depends upon the physician's recommendation, patient's physical status, and potential stress involved in the planned dental procedure. In general, a two- to threefold increase in glucocorticoid treatment on the day of the appointment is adequate to prepare a patient. Some authorities advocate a single presurgical bolus, whereas others suggest tapering the dose to original levels over the next 24 to 48 hours.

An Addisonian crisis is not easy to diagnose and can be circumvented by taking a good medical history. Treatment includes 100 mg hydrocortisone intramuscularly (preferably intravenously) and transferring the patient to a hospital. There is no contraindication to such a clinical trial in an ill patient if an incorrect diagnosis of adrenal insufficiency has been made.

SUMMARY OF TREATMENT
1. Recognize signs and symptoms
2. Place patient in supine position, elevate feet
3. Basic life support
4. Administer hydrocortisone 100 mg IM
5. Summon medical assistance

Epilepsy

Epilepsy is a recurrent disturbance of the central nervous system manifested by loss of consciousness and convulsions. It affects over 1 percent of the general population, and usually has no identifiable etiology, although in a few patients it may be secondary to factors such as local or generalized brain disease.

Epilepsy has a variety of clinical manifestations. A major concern in treating these patients in the dental office is the occurrence of a convulsion or epileptic seizure. In patients with a past history of epilepsy, the degree of control should be ascertained and elective procedures delayed if the patients are not well controlled. It is also im-

portant that patients take their prescribed medication (e.g., Dilantin).

A grand mal epileptic seizure typically begins with a warning (aura) followed by loss of consciousness, tonic and then clonic convulsions, and finally a variable prolonged recovery. Fecal and urinary incontinence may occur, and patients may injure themselves by falling.

Management of a seizure includes maintaining the airway and protecting the patient. The patient should be laid on his side and any oral appliances removed. Tight, restrictive clothing should be loosened. A towel or padded tongue blade may be placed between the teeth to prevent tongue biting (although this maneuver may be impractical), and the patient should be placed away from equipment or furniture so that he cannot injure himself.

Usually a convulsion is brief; however, should it continue after several minutes, the patient may require transfer to an emergency room and administration of intravenous sedation. Following a seizure, the patient may have significant CNS depression and/or airway obstruction requiring basic life support.

SUMMARY OF TREATMENT
1. Position patient on his side
2. Prevent injury to patient
3. Maintain airway
4. Monitor vital signs
5. Basic life support
6. Summon medical assistance if necessary

Emergency Kit

Every dentist has a moral responsibility to maintain an emergency kit in his office. The kit should be well planned and contain appropriate drugs and equipment with which the practitioner is familiar. Although specialty training in intravenous injections and advanced cardiac life support would be most ideal, these techniques are beyond the scope of this chapter.

Recognition and management of a medical emergency is dependent upon an office staff that is well trained and coordinated in a team approach. This can best be maintained with regular practice sessions. All emergency materials should be checked regularly and stored in an accessible area known to all office personnel (Fig. 5-4).

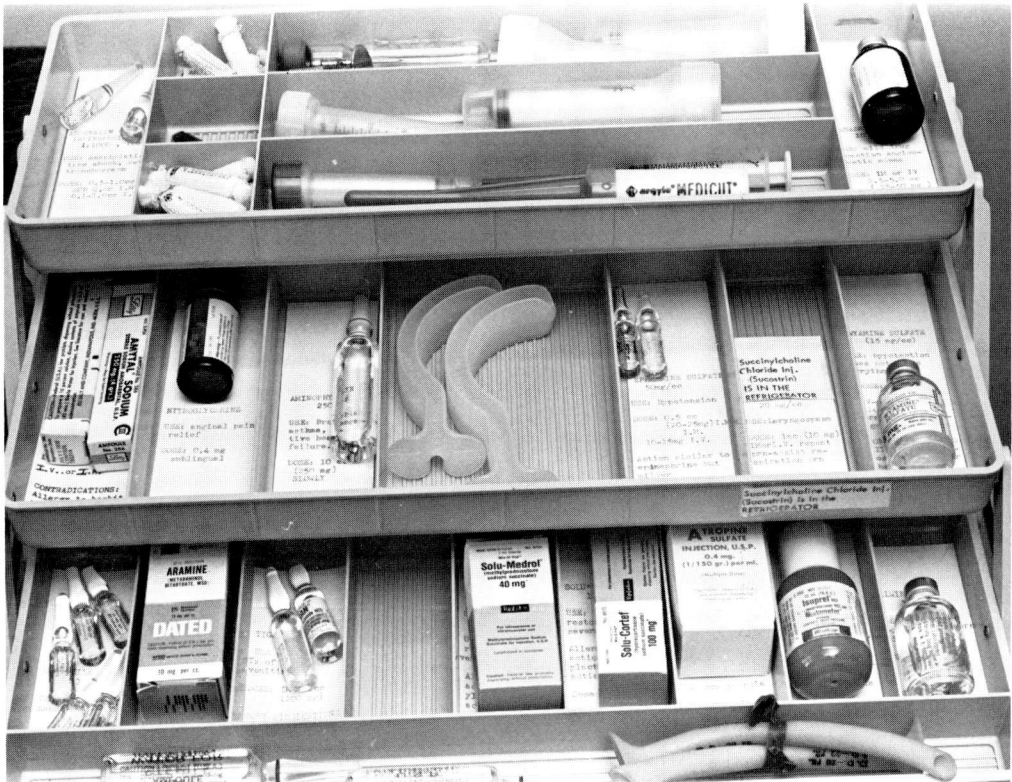

FIG. 5-4. *An emergency kit should always be available in the dental office.*

Most emergencies do not require drug administration; however, it may be a necessary part of life support. The following recommended drugs do not require proficiency in intravenous injections. All dosages are based on average-sized adults. Because recommended drugs and their dosages often change with the passage of time, the clinician must be aware of these changes.

AMMONIA INHALANTS
Indications: Syncope
Actions: Stimulates the medullary respiratory and vasomotor centers through irritation of the sensory endings of the trigeminal nerve
Administration and dosage: Break ampule between fingers and hold 4-6 inches away from patient's nose

METAPROTERONOL (ALUPENT)
Indications: Asthma, Bronchospasm
Actions: Potent beta adrenergic stimulator that results in bronchodilation
Administration and dosage: 2-3 inhalations with patient in an upright position

ATROPINE
Indications: Bradycardia
Actions: Parasympatholytic action that blocks post ganglionic nerve endings. It also has an anticholinergic (drying) effect
Administration and dosage: 0.4 mg/ml 0.4 mg IM (Repeat if necessary.) Maximum dose 2.0 mg

DIPHENHYDRAMINE (BENADRYL)
Indications: Allergic reactions
Actions: Antihistamine that competes for receptor sites on the smooth muscle of lungs, skin, and intestine
Administration and dosage: 50 mg/ml 50 mg IM

EPINEPHRINE (ADRENALIN)

Indications: Anaphylactic reactions, Cardiac arrest

Actions: Stimulates both alpha and beta receptors resulting in: (1) an increase in the force of contraction and heart rate, (2) bronchodilation, (3) increased blood pressure, and (4) blockage of histamine release

Administration and dosage: 0.2-0.5 ml 1:1000 IM or subcutaneously (Repeat every 5-15 minutes as needed.)

GLUCAGON

Indications: Hypoglycemia in an unconscious patient

Actions: Increases blood glucose concentrations

Administration and dosage: 1.0 mg/ml 1.0 mg IM (Repeat if not conscious in 5-10 minutes.)

MORPHINE

Indications: Analgesia in myocardial infarction

Actions: Potent analgesia that acts as a central nervous system and respiratory depressant

Administration and dosage: 10-15 mg IM (Demerol may be used as an optional choice—50-100 mg IM.)

NITROGLYCERIN

Indications: Chest pain, Angina pectoris, Hypertension

Actions: Coronary and peripheral vasodilator

Administration and dosage: 0.3 mg tablet sublingual every 5 minutes for a maximum of three tablets

HYDROCORTISONE

Indications: Acute adrenocortical insufficiency

Actions: Anti-inflammatory, supportive of all organ systems

Administration and dosage: 50 mg/ml 100 mg IM (IV if possible.)

MEPHENTERMINE (WYAMINE)

Indications: Hypotension

Actions: Increases blood pressure by increasing the force of myocardial contraction with little or no peripheral vasoconstriction

Administration and dosage: 15-30 mg IM (Response is evident 5-15 minutes after injection.)

Although intravenous injections are most ideal in an emergency situation because of their rapid onset of action, intramuscular administration is the route of choice for one with limited experience. In general, the point of injection should avoid major nerves and vessels, and available muscle sites should be capable of holding a large volume of injected fluids. Suitable areas for injection include the buttocks and the deltoid.

The upper outer quadrant of the gluteal area is preferred when the buttock is chosen. Vessels and nerves of the sacral plexus are abundant in the upper inner quadrant, and the lower quadrants contain the sciatic nerve. The deltoid may be used in both adults and children. (In children, the gluteal area is small and composed primarily of fat.)

Administration of an intramuscular injection is as follows:

1. Cleanse the injection site and allow to dry
2. Secure the skin with the thumb and index finger of one hand
3. Hold the syringe as though it were a dart in the other hand
4. Insert the needle in one quick flick of the wrist perpendicular to the skin surface. The needle should be advanced only three fourths of its length
5. Aspirate the syringe
6. If no blood return, inject slowly and smoothly
7. Withdraw the needle while holding the skin in position
8. Massage the site vigorously to encourage rapid absorption

Additional emergency equipment should be available and arranged systematically. These items include:

1. Oxygen delivery system
2. Sphygmomanometer (blood pressure cuff)
3. Stethoscope
4. Syringes (sterile, prepackaged)
   a. 3 ml complete with 21-gauge needles, 1 inch

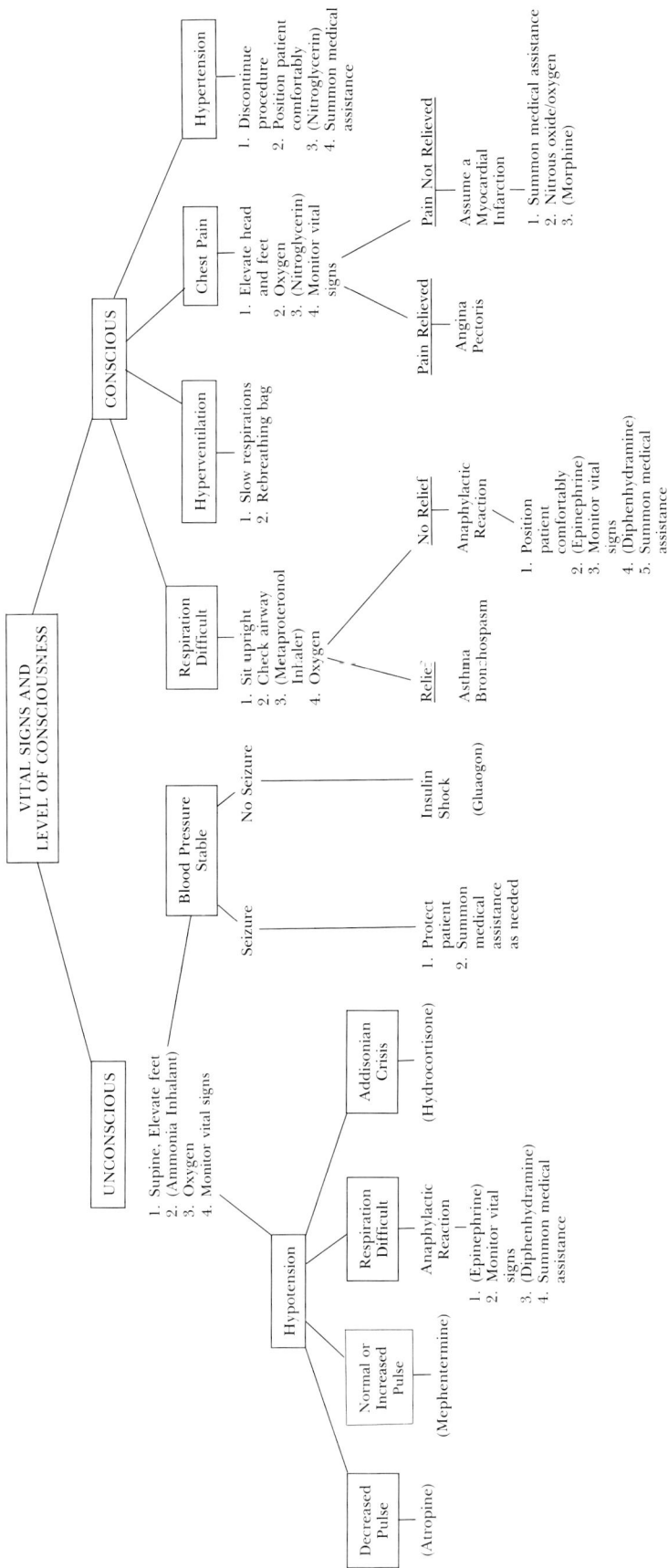

Fig. 5-5. *An organized approach to the recognition and treatment of medical emergencies.*

59

b. 1 ml complete with 21-gauge needles, 1 inch
5. Suction and tonsil suction tips
6. Alcohol sponges
7. Paper bag
8. Oropharyngeal airways
9. Cricothyrotomy needle
10. Sweetened orange juice/packets of sugar

Obtaining a complete medical history is paramount if emergency situations in the dental office are to be avoided. This, however, does not preclude the necessity for an awareness of potentially fatal signs, symptoms, and treatment modalities.

Figure 5-5 schematically illustrates an organized approach to the recognition and treatment of medical emergencies.

Selected Reading

Basic Life Support for Physicians. Dallas, American Heart Association, 1981-1983.

Bethune, J. E.: The Adrenal Cortex. Kalamazoo, Upjohn Co., 1975.

Braun, R. J.: Dentists' Manual of Emergency Medical Treatment. Reston, VA, Reston Publishing Co., 1979.

Elbadrawy, H. E.: Aspiration of foreign bodies during dental procedures. J. Canad. Dent. Assn., 51(2):145, 1985.

Harrison, T. R., et al.: Principles of Internal Medicine. 9th Ed. New York, McGraw-Hill Book Co., 1982.

Heimlich, H. J.: A life-saving maneuver to prevent food choking. JAMA, 234:398, 1975.

Irby, W. B.: Current Advances in Oral Surgery. Vol. 2. St. Louis, C. V. Mosby Co., 1982.

Laws, I. M.: The health of patients attending for dental anaesthesia. Br. Dent. J., 132:136, 1972.

Malamed, S. F.: Handbook of Medical Emergencies in the Dental Office. 2nd Ed. St. Louis, C. V. Mosby Co., 1982.

McCarthy, F. M.: Emergencies in Dental Practice. 3rd Ed. Philadelphia, W. B. Saunders Co., 1979.

Office Anesthesia Evaluation Manual. Chicago, American Association of Oral and Maxillofacial Surgeons, 1978.

Smith, B. H.: The unconscious patient. J. Oral Surg., 27: 709, 1969.

SECTION 2. *This section is basic to understanding and performing good oral surgery technique. Principles of oral surgery, treatment planning, and the management of complications are discussed.*

CHAPTER 6 # Anesthesia and Pain Control

JOSEPH A. GIOVANNITTI and STEPHEN B. MILAM

The beginning is the most important part of the work.

PLATO

Anticipation of pain is the most common cause of anxiety associated with a dental visit and accounts for the avoidance behavior of 6 to 9 percent of the U.S. population who neglect needed dental care.[1] Ironically, modern dentistry is virtually painless as a result of the development of new techniques to control pain and anxiety. These include behavioral management strategies, improved regional analgesia techniques, and conscious-sedation techniques. To be successful in modern dental practice, every practitioner should understand the psychology and physiology of pain and be familiar with methods of pain and anxiety control. Without this foundation, the stigmatic relationship between pain and dentistry will continue to impede dental health care delivery in our society.

Psychology and Physiology of Pain

Pain can be defined simply as the perception of and reaction to a noxious stimulus. *Pain is a subjective experience influenced by numerous cognitive activities such as attention, anxiety, and previous experiences.* In addition, factors such as age, sex, certain environmental conditions, and disease states affect the pain experience. These factors may explain why some patients remain overtly calm during a painful dental procedure, while others are noticeably affected by mild stimuli.

The pain experience begins with an environmental change (i.e., noxious stimulus) of sufficient magnitude to depolarize high threshold receptors called nociceptors. Generated nerve impulses travel along neural pathways composed of type A-delta and C nerve fibers to central nervous system structures responsible for processing spatial, temporal, and magnitudinal properties of the input (neospinothalamic tract, spinocervical tract, and the dorsal column system), for producing motivational drive and unpleasantness (reticular formation and limbic system), and for regulating the final response to the stimulus (cerebral cortex).

Techniques to control pain in dentistry interrupt these processes at various levels. For example, a local anesthetic deposited in close proximity to stimulated nerve fibers interrupts pain perception by interfering with depolarization and impulse propagation. Conscious-sedation and general anesthesia techniques interfere with both the pain perception and reaction process by depressing higher central nervous system functions. Behavioral management strategies (i.e. progressive relaxation, hypnosis, biofeedback, systematic desensitization) affect pain response presumably by altering the regulatory function of the cerebral cortex. The effectiveness of any technique depends upon patient charac-

61

teristics, operative requirements, and the clinician's skills. Each clinician should be aware of his skill limitations, as well as the effective limits of the technique selected. These limitations must be respected at all times, for if the clinical situation supersedes them, serious injury and even death may result.

Regional Anesthesia in Dentistry

According to National Institutes of Health statistics, dentists perform more than one-half million local anesthetic injections each day in the United States.[2] This figure accounts for 95 percent of all local anesthetic administrations.[3] Clearly, regional analgesia techniques provide the foundation for all other methods of pain and anxiety control in dentistry.

Pharmacology of Local Anesthetics

Local anesthetics are lipid-soluble organic compounds capable of producing reversible blockade of nerve impulses. They act on all excitable tissues including the central and peripheral nervous systems and the heart. Local anesthetics constitute the major drug class for pain control in dentistry.

CLASSIFICATION

In 1859, Albert Niemann extracted an alkaloid from the leaves of *Erythroxylon coca*, which he named cocaine. This is the first and only naturally occurring local anesthetic drug; the rest are synthetic compounds. Local anesthetics may be classified on the basis of common chemical configurations. Stuctural features common to all local anesthetics are a cyclic (aryl-), lipophilic group linked to a secondary or terti-

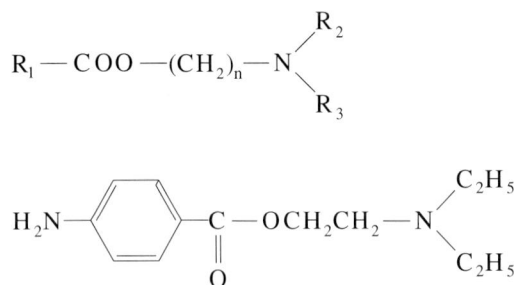

FIG. 6-2. *General formula for the amide-linked local anesthetics and the prototype, lidocaine.*

ary hydrophilic amine group by an intermediate alkyl linkage. The clinically useful local anesthetics are classified into two groups on the basis of the structure of the intermediate linkage: the amino-ester and the amino-amide local anesthetics. Ester-linked local anesthetics have the general formula shown in Figure 6-1, and are represented by the prototype procaine. Amide-linked local anesthetics have the general formula shown in Figure 6-2, and are represented by the prototype lidocaine. Other examples of local anesthetics are listed in Table 6-1. Variations in the structure of these drugs modify their potency, toxicity, pharmacokinetic properties, and duration of action.

MODE OF ACTION

Local anesthetics are weak bases, and as such they have low water solubility, low tissue diffusibility, and are unstable in solution. Manufacturers combine the local anesthetic base with a strong acid, such as hydrochloric, to improve its water solubility and thus enhance its tissue diffusibility. Combination with a strong acid stabilizes not only the local anesthetic drug in solution, but also stabilizes the vasoconstrictor, if present. When a cartridge of local anes-

FIG. 6-1. *General formula for the ester-linked local anesthetics and the prototype, procaine.*

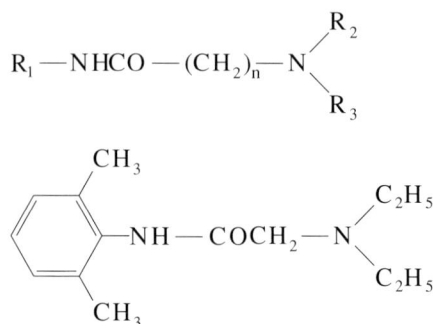

TABLE 6-1. *Commonly used local anesthetics*

Ester-linked	Amide-linked
procaine (Novocain)	lidocaine (Xylocaine)
tetracaine (Pontocaine)	mepivacaine (Carbocaine)
	prilocaine (Citanest)
	bupivacaine (Marcaine)
	etidocaine (Duranest)

thetic is injected into the tissue, it interacts with tissue buffers in the following manner:

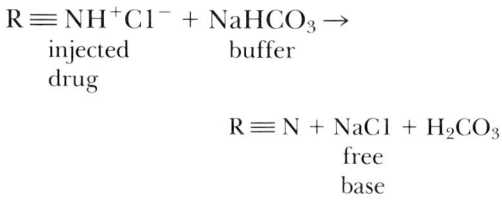

$$R \equiv NH^+Cl^- + NaHCO_3 \rightarrow$$

injected   buffer
drug

$$R \equiv N + NaCl + H_2CO_3$$
free
base

The free base, or un-ionized form of the local anesthetic, is capable of diffusion across the nerve membrane. Once the local anesthetic is within the axoplasm, it is presumed to dissociate into a charged, or ionized, form:

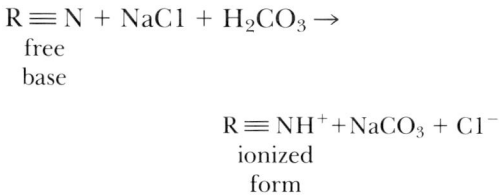

$$R \equiv N + NaCl + H_2CO_3 \rightarrow$$
free
base

$$R \equiv NH^+ + NaCO_3 + Cl^-$$
ionized
form

It is believed that the charged form of the local anesthetic molecule binds at a receptor site in the sodium channel and inhibits the influx of sodium, which is responsible for the production of the action potential. As the concentration of local anesthetic molecules at the active site is reduced by redistribution and metabolism of the drug, recovery from the nerve block follows.

Techniques of Administration

TERMINOLOGY

The sequence of disappearance of sensations following the administration of a local anesthetic agent is related to the size of nerve fibers exposed to the drug and the presence of myelination. In 1929, Gasser and Erlanger[4] demonstrated that small diameter nerve fibers could be blocked with lower concentrations of cocaine than large diameter nerve fibers. Additionally, the myelin sheath surrounding larger nerve fibers acts as a barrier to the diffusion of local anesthetic molecules intracellularly. Thus, small, unmyelinated nerve fibers are blocked before the larger myelinated nerve fibers. Since neurons carrying pain sensation are generally of small diam-

eter, the sequence of disappearance of sensations following a local anesthetic injection is: pain, temperature, touch, proprioception, and motor function.

Analgesia is a reduced sensitivity to pain without the loss of consciousness. When local anesthetics are administered, a loss of pain sensation over a specific portion of the anatomy occurs without the loss of consciousness. This is known as *regional analgesia*. The terms *regional anesthesia* and *local anesthesia* are commonly used interchangeably with regard to the production of regional analgesia. This can be semantically misleading since *anesthesia* means the loss of all sensation.

A *nerve block* is produced when a local anesthetic solution is deposited in close proximity to a nerve trunk (Fig. 6-3). The entire area distal to the site of the block supplied by that particular nerve trunk is rendered insensible to pain. The deposition of an anesthetic solution in proximity to larger terminal nerve branches is termed an *infiltration* (Fig. 6-4). Analgesia is produced in a limited circumscribed area supplied by these nerve branches. Deposition of anesthetic solution at the level of the apex of a tooth is an example of an **infil-**

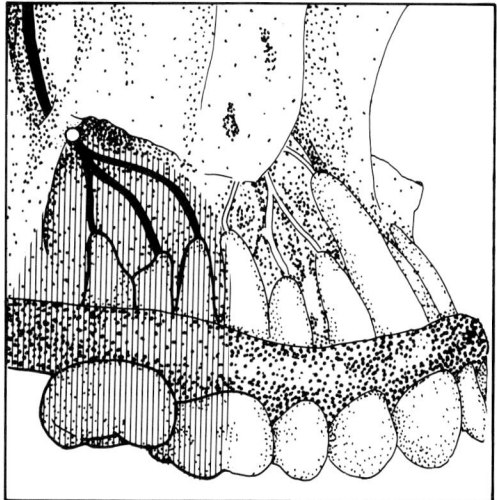

FIG. 6-3. *Nerve block. The entire distribution (shaded area) of the posterior superior alveolar nerve is rendered insensible to pain when the injection is made in proximity to the nerve trunk (white dot). (From: Manual of Local Anesthesia in Dentistry. 3rd ed. New York, Cook-Waite Laboratories, Inc., 1980.)*

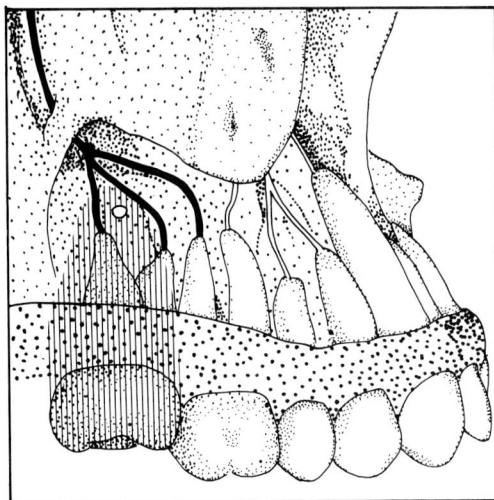

FIG. 6-4. *Infiltration. The circumscribed area (shaded) supplied by this branch of the posterior superior alveolar nerve is rendered insensible to pain when the injection is made in proximity to the nerve branch (white dot). (From: Manual of Local Anesthesia in Dentistry. 3rd ed. New York, Cook-Waite Laboratories, Inc., 1980.)*

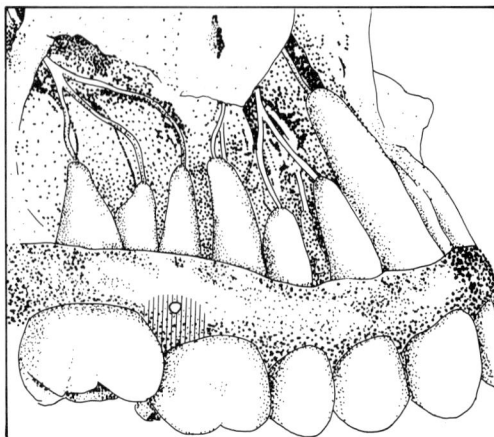

FIG. 6-5. *Local infiltration. The distribution of small terminal nerve endings is rendered insensible to pain when the injection is made into the interdental tissue (white dot, shaded area). (From: Manual of Local Anesthesia in Dentistry. 3rd ed. New York, Cook-Waite Laboratories, Inc., 1980.)*

tration. A *local infiltration* occurs when the anesthetic solution is deposited in proximity to small terminal nerve endings (Fig. 6-5). Instrumentation is performed in the same tissue into which the anesthetic has been injected. An example of a local infiltration is an intrapapillary injection.

Trigeminal Nerve

The fifth cranial (trigeminal) nerve is the major sensory nerve of the face, mouth, and nasal cavity. It also provides motor and proprioceptive innervation to the muscles of mastication. Its sensory origins are from nuclei in the upper part of the pons, while its motor origins are located separately in the inferior surface of the pons. Neurons from these nuclei coalesce in the semilunar ganglion located on the anterior surface of the petrous portion of the temporal bone. From here the trigeminal nerve diverges into three divisions: ophthalmic, maxillary, and mandibular. Discussion is limited to the second and third divisions, since the successful practice of dentistry is based upon blockade of the various branches of these nerves.

Maxillary Division

The maxillary division exits the cranium via the foramen rotundum and courses through the pterygopalatine fossa and intraorbital canal before exiting to the face via the infraorbital foramen. It supplies sensory innervation to the maxillary teeth and gingiva, maxillary sinus, hard and soft palate, lower eyelid, side of the nose, upper lip, mucous membrane of the nasopharynx, and skin over the anterior temporal region. It may be necessary to block one or more of the nerves or nerve branches listed in Table 6-2 to perform successful surgery in the maxilla.

POSTERIOR SUPERIOR ALVEOLAR NERVE

The posterior superior alveolar nerve (Fig. 6-6) leaves the maxillary nerve before it enters the infraorbital groove, crosses the tuberosity, and enters the maxilla through a foramen or group of foramina on its infratemporal surface. Branches supply the maxillary molars, with the exception of the mesiobuccal root of the first molar, the lining of the maxillary sinus corresponding to the molar teeth, and the buccal alveolar bone and soft tissue in the molar region. This nerve, or its terminal branches, must be blocked prior to surgical procedures involving the molars and supporting structures. In surgical procedures involving the first molar, a separate infiltration injection must be performed over the mesiobuccal root, because it is not supplied by the posterior superior alveolar nerve.

TABLE 6-2. *Regional analgesia of the maxilla*

Nerves Anesthetized	Areas Anesthetized
Posterior superior alveolar nerve	Maxillary molars (except mesiobuccal root of first molar); buccal alveolar bone and soft tissues; lining of maxillary sinus corresponding to the molar teeth
Middle superior alveolar nerve	Mesiobuccal root of first molar; premolars; corresponding buccal alveolar bone and soft tissues; lining of maxillary sinus
Anterior superior alveolar nerve	Canines, lateral incisors, central incisors; corresponding buccal alveolar bone and soft tissues
Greater palatine nerve	Hard palate and overlying mucosa from molars to first bicuspids
Nasopalatine nerve	Hard and soft tissues of the entire anterior hard palate to the canines bilaterally
Infraorbital nerve	Lower eyelid, side of nose, upper lip; areas supplied by the middle and anterior superior alveolar nerves

Technique. Prior to any local anesthetic injection, the tissue must be prepared properly by drying the target area with a gauze square, applying a topical anesthetic ointment, and again drying the site. An antiseptic solution may be applied at the practitioner's discretion, but the puncture site should always be dried prior to needle penetration.

The palpating index finger should be inserted into the mucobuccal fold of the maxilla until it contacts the zygomatic arch at its juncture with the maxillary bone. The cheek is gently retracted laterally to permit visualization. The mouth should be opened only partially, because excessive opening may cause the coronoid process of the mandible to impinge upon the target area and/or impair visualization. A long dental needle (1⅝ inches) should be inserted into the mucosa slightly posterior to the zygomatic arch at a 45° angle to all three planes of orientation (Fig. 6-7A). The needle should be advanced slowly in this orientation so that the path of insertion conforms to the medial curvature of the maxilla in this area (Fig. 6-7B). This ensures deposition of anesthetic solution in close proximity to the nerve as it enters its foramina, and avoids contact with the pterygoid plexus of veins, thus preventing possible hematoma formation. The needle should be advanced to a depth of one half to two thirds the length of the dental nee-

dle (Fig. 6-7C). Following negative aspiration, approximately two thirds of a cartridge (1.2 ml) of local anesthetic should be slowly injected and the needle withdrawn.

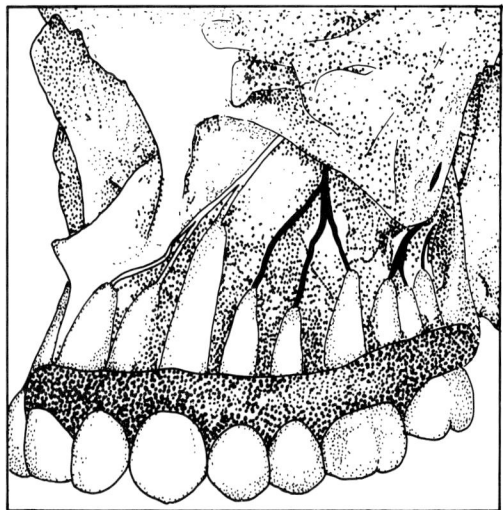

FIG. 6-6. *Representation of the three branches of the maxillary nerve that innervate the maxillary teeth. Posterior superior alveolar (shown in black): nerve supply to the molar teeth (except the mesiobuccal root of the first molar). Middle superior alveolar (shown in black): nerve supply to the mesiobuccal root of the first molar and the two bicuspids. Anterior superior alveolar (shown in white): nerve supply to the canine, lateral, and central incisors. (From: Manual of Local Anesthesia in Dentistry. 3rd ed. New York, Cook-Waite Laboratories, Inc., 1980.)*

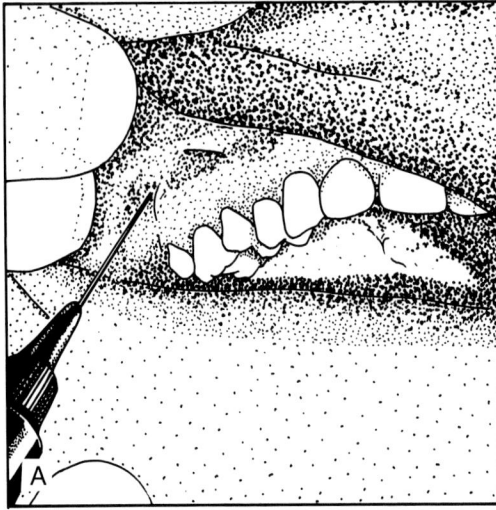

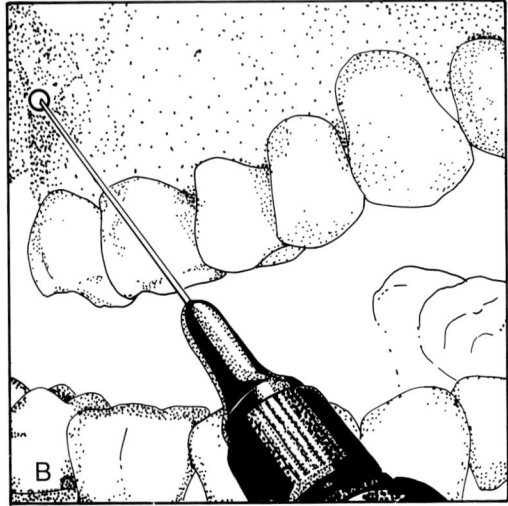

FIG. 6-7. (A) Proper orientation of the needle and syringe for the posterior superior alveolar nerve block. (B) The needle is advanced in close proximity to the curvature of the maxillary tuberosity to a depth approximating the posterior alveolar foramina. (C) Deposition of local anesthetic solution in this area blocks the posterior alveolar nerve along its entire distribution. (From: Manual of Local Anesthesia in Dentistry. 3rd ed. New York, Cook-Waite Laboratories, Inc., 1980.)

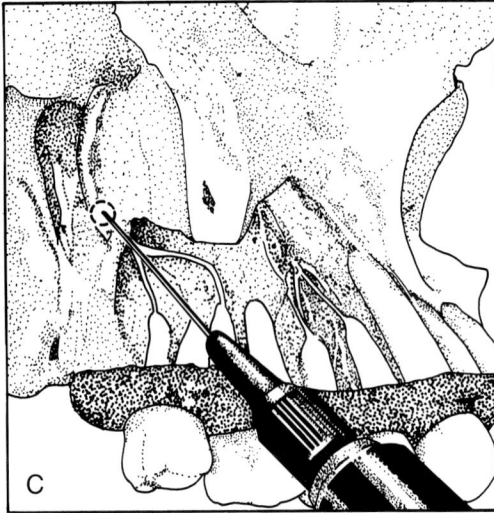

The remaining one third (0.6 ml) may be used to block the mesiobuccal root of the first molar or the palatal tissue as needed. The patient should not experience subjective signs of anesthesia, such as numbness or tingling, following this injection. Adequacy of the nerve block must be ascertained by instrumentation of the involved area without pain.

MIDDLE SUPERIOR ALVEOLAR NERVE(S)

This small group of nerves (Fig. 6-6) branches from the maxillary nerve as it courses through the infraorbital canal, and thus, is located within the maxilla. The middle superior alveolar nerve branches innervate the mesiobuccal root of the first molar, the premolars, the antral lining corresponding to these teeth, and the buccal alveolar bone and soft tissue in this area. These nerve branches must be blocked to perform surgical procedures involving the mesiobuccal root of the first molar, the premolars, and related structures.

Technique. After properly preparing the injection site as previously described, the practitioner should retract the cheek to expose the mucogingival junction in the premolar area. A 1⅝-inch or 1-inch needle should be inserted at the level of the mucogingival junction between the first and second premolars, and just a few millimeters buccally to the alveolar bone (Fig. 6-8A). The needle should be oriented so that it conforms to the curvature of the maxilla in this area, and advanced slowly to a depth whereby its tip approximates the level of the apices of the premolar teeth (Fig. 6-8B). Following negative aspiration, one cartridge (1.8 ml) of local anesthetic solution should be injected slowly and the needle withdrawn. The local anesthetic solution diffuses through the porous maxillary

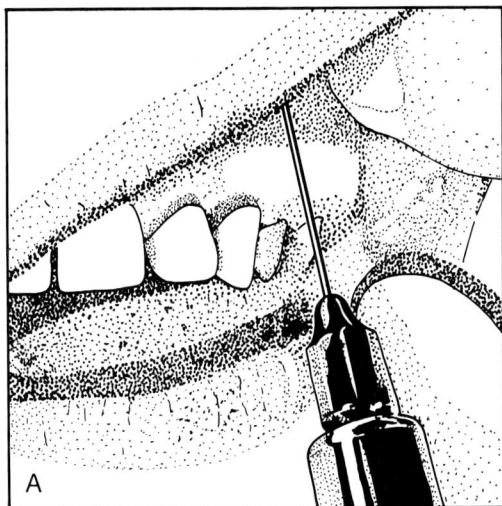

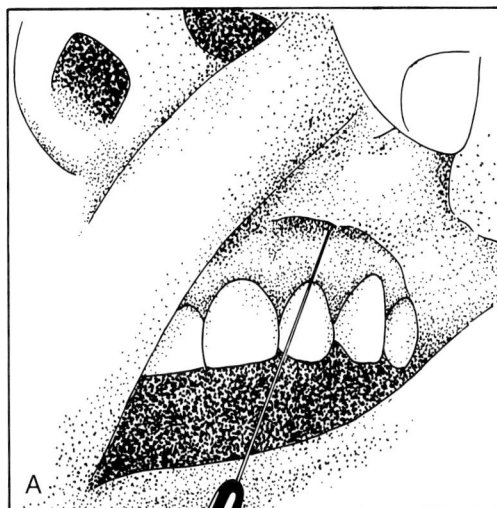

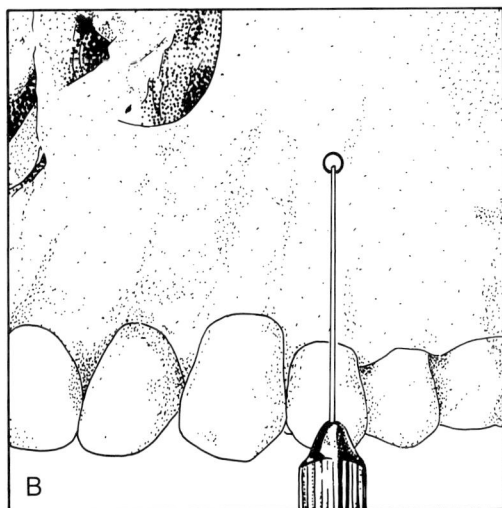

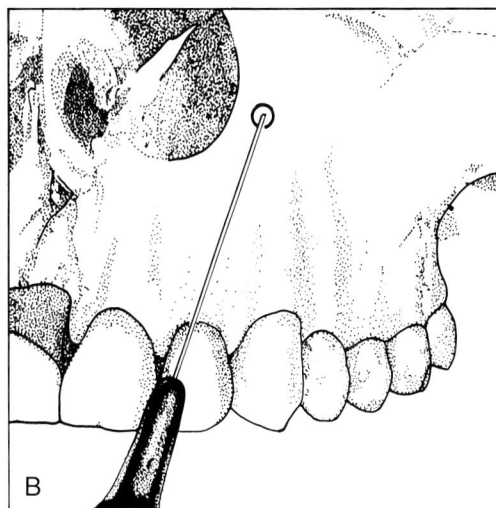

FIG. 6-8. (A) Proper intraoral orientation of the needle and syringe for the middle superior alveolar nerve block. (B) Local anesthetic solution deposited in this area diffuses through the buccal plate and blocks the middle superior alveolar nerve and its associated structures. (From: Manual of Local Anesthesia in Dentistry. 3rd ed. New York, Cook-Waite Laboratories, Inc., 1980.)

FIG. 6-9. (A) Proper intraoral orientation of the needle and syringe for the anterior superior alveolar nerve block. (B) Deposition of local anesthetic solution at the apex of the canine tooth produces loss of sensation over the distribution of the anterior superior alveolar nerve. (From: Manual of Local Anesthesia in Dentistry. 3rd ed. New York, Cook-Waite Laboratories, Inc., 1980.)

bone thereby blocking the middle superior alveolar branches. If these teeth are to be extracted, the palatal tissue must be anesthetized separately. The patient may experience subjective signs of numbness and tingling in the upper lip, but adequacy of the block is best determined by instrumentation without pain.

ANTERIOR SUPERIOR ALVEOLAR NERVE(S)

This small group of nerves (Fig. 6-6) leaves the maxillary nerve in the infraorbital canal anteriorly to the middle superior alveolar nerve, and just prior to the exit of the infraorbital nerve to the face. Terminal branches of the anterior superior

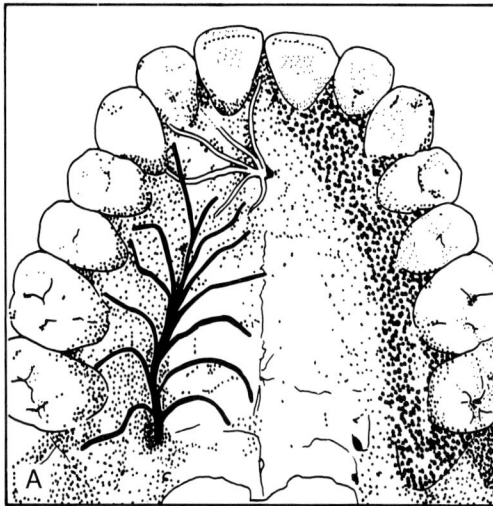

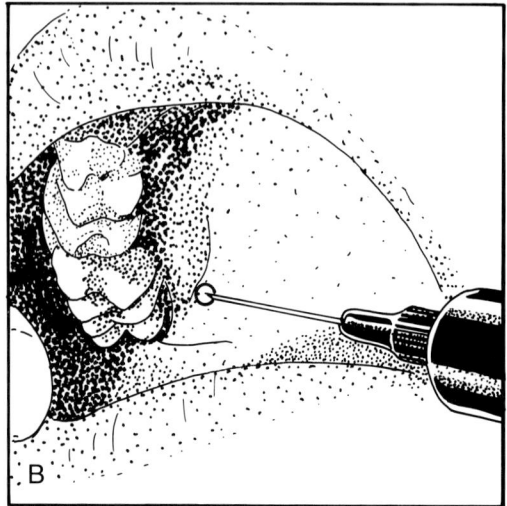

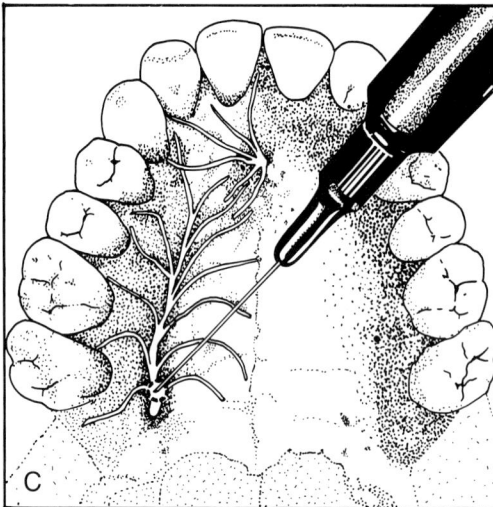

FIG. 6-10. *(A) The greater palatine nerve (shown in black) exits onto the hard palate from the greater palatine foramen and travels anteriorly to the bicuspid-canine area. (B) Proper orientation of the needle and syringe for the greater palatine nerve block. Note that the needle is perpendicular to the hard palate, and anterior to the greater palatine foramen. (C) Local anesthetic solution deposited slightly anteriorly to the greater palatine foramen will produce conduction blockade distal to the injection site. (From: Manual of Local Anesthesia in Dentistry. 3rd ed. New York, Cook-Waite Laboratories, Inc., 1980.)*

alveolar nerve supply the canine, lateral, and central incisors, and buccal alveolar bone and soft tissue in this region. The anterior superior alveolar nerves must be blocked to perform surgery involving the three anterior teeth and their supporting structures.

Technique. Following tissue preparation, the lip should be retracted and a 1 ⅝-inch or 1-inch needle inserted at the mucogingival junction adjacent and parallel to the long axis of the canine tooth (Fig. 6-9A). The needle should be advanced slowly along the canine eminence until its tip approximates the level of the apex of the canine tooth (Fig. 6-9B). After negative aspiration, one cartridge of local anesthetic

solution should be injected slowly and the needle withdrawn. Again, diffusion of the local anesthetic solution occurs through the maxillary bone and blocks the anterior superior alveolar branches. Extraction of any of the three anterior teeth warrants separate blockade of the palatal tissue corresponding to these teeth. The patient experiences the subjective signs of upper lip tingling or numbness, but the adequacy of the block must still be objectively ascertained by instrumentation without pain.

GREATER (ANTERIOR) PALATINE NERVE
The greater palatine nerve (Fig. 6-10A) is a continuation of the short pterygopalatine nerve, which branches from the maxillary nerve in the pterygopalatine fossa. Somatic afferent fibers pass through the pterygopalatine ganglion without synapse and become the greater palatine nerve as it courses through the greater palatine canal. The nerve exits onto the hard palate by way of the greater palatine foramen, travels anteriorly along the hard palate to the

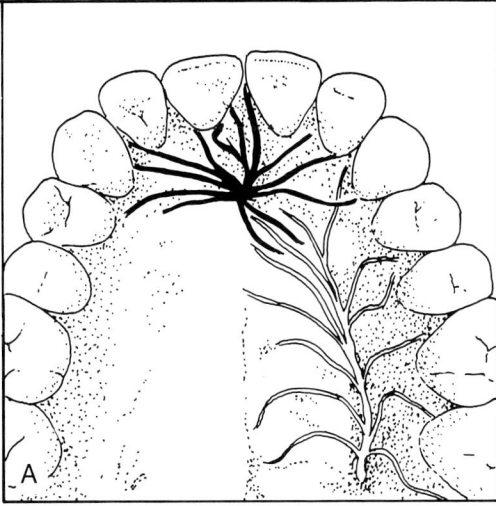

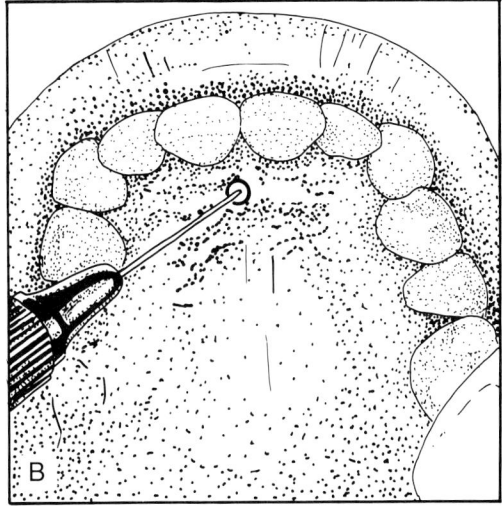

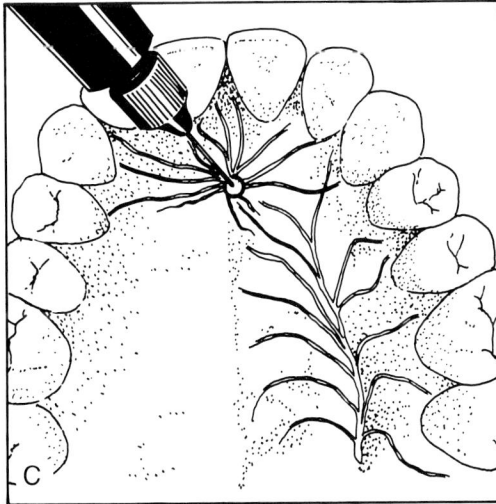

FIG. 6-11. (A) The nasopalatine nerve (shown in black) exits via the nasopalatine foramen and branches bilaterally over the premaxilla. (B) Proper orientation of the needle and syringe for the nasopalatine nerve block. Note that the needle enters the incisive papilla at an angle to the midline. (C) Deposition of local anesthetic solution at the rim of the nasopalatine foramen produces numbness bilaterally in the anterior hard palate. This injection is very painful, and the patient should be forewarned prior to administration. (From: Manual of Local Anesthesia in Dentistry. 3rd ed. New York, Cook-Waite Laboratories, Inc., 1980.)

first bicuspid area, and innervates the hard palate and overlying mucosa from the molars to the first bicuspid tooth. Occasionally, its innervation extends as far anteriorly as the canine. This nerve must be blocked to provide anesthesia for surgical procedures that may involve the palatal hard or soft tissue.

Technique. The greater palatine foramen is visualized intraorally as a depression on the hard palate located between the second and third molars. After preparing the tissue, the practitioner should insert the needle slightly anteriorly to the greater palatine foramen, and perpendicularly to the hard palate (Fig. 6-10B, C). The needle should be advanced to contact

bone, withdrawn 2 mm, and approximately one fourth (0.5 ml) of a dental cartridge should be injected. The patient experiences numbness of the hard palate and perhaps difficulty in swallowing, especially if the block is performed bilaterally.

NASOPALATINE NERVE

The nasopalatine nerve (Fig. 6-11A), one of the posterior superior nasal nerves, branches from the maxillary nerve in the pterygopalatine fossa and enters the nasal cavity. It enters the oral cavity via the nasopalatine foramen, located in the midline of the anterior hard palate directly between the two central incisors. From this point, the nasopalatine nerve sends branches bilaterally and posteriorly along the hard palate as far as the canine region. This nerve must be blocked for surgical procedures involving the anterior hard palate.

Technique. The nasopalatine foramen lies directly beneath the incisive papilla,

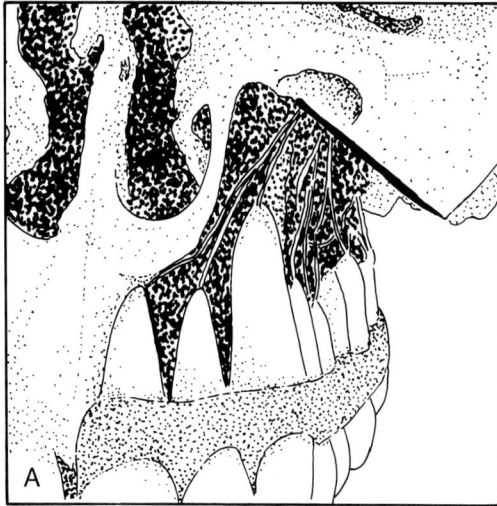

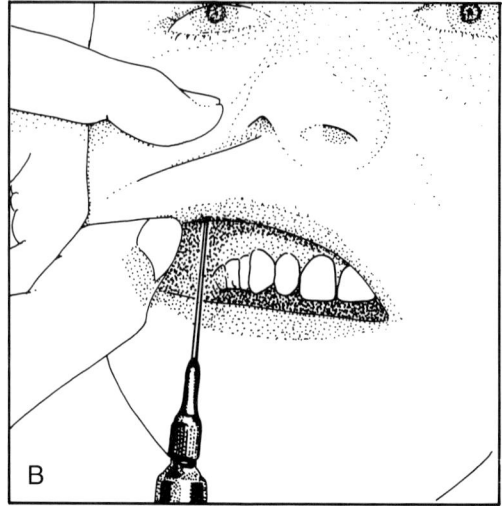

FIG. 6-12. *(A) Cutaway showing the branches of the infraorbital nerve (anterior superior and middle superior alveolar nerves), which are anesthetized following the infraorbital nerve block injection. (B) Proper orientation of the needle and syringe for the infraorbital nerve block. Note that the palpating finger remains over the infraorbital foramen. (C) It is not necessary to enter the infraorbital foramen with the needle. Following the injection, the patient's cheek should be massaged to ensure the spread of the anesthetic solution into the infraorbital canal. This action produces blockade of the anterior superior and middle superior alveolar nerves. (From: Manual of Local Anesthesia in Dentistry. 3rd ed. New York, Cook-Waite Laboratories, Inc., 1980.)*

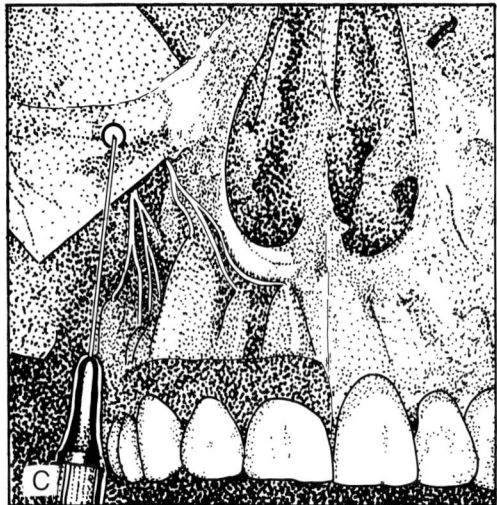

which is located directly between, and palatal to, the two central incisors. After the tissue is prepared, the needle should be inserted into the incisive papilla at an angle (not parallel) to the midline, and advanced until the rim of the foramen is contacted (Fig. 6-11B). The needle should be withdrawn 1 or 2 mm, and one fourth (0.5 ml) of a dental cartridge should be injected following negative aspiration. As with the greater palatine nerve block, it is not necessary to enter the foramen with the needle (Fig. 6-11C). The patient experiences numbness in the anterior hard palate bilaterally to signify onset of the block. As an added word of caution, a painful experience often occurs with needle insertion.

Occasionally, it may be desirable to perform a nerve block, resulting in a much more extensive area of regional analgesia than the more routine injections just described. A major nerve block may be indicated when extensive maxillary surgery is contemplated, when local infection precludes a more conventional block, or when extensive anesthesia acts as a diagnostic aid for certain chronic pain syndromes. The following nerves may be blocked for these purposes.

INFRAORBITAL NERVE

The infraorbital nerve (Fig. 6-12A) is the continuation of the maxillary nerve as it courses through the infraorbital canal and exits via the infraorbital foramen. As we have seen, branches from the infraorbital nerve are the middle superior and anterior superior alveolar nerves, and the inferior palpebral, lateral nasal, and superior labial nerves. With a single injection, it is possible to produce unilateral regional analgesia of the incisors, canine, bicuspids, mesiobuccal root of the first molar, the antral lining corresponding to these teeth, the buccal hard and soft tissues, the lower eyelid, the side of the nose, and the upper lip.

Technique. The infraorbital foramen must first be located. This is done by imagining a vertical line drawn through the patient's pupil as he looks straight ahead. The infraorbital foramen lies on this line just below the inferior rim of the orbit. After locating this depression, the palpating finger should remain over the foramen. Another finger or thumb should then retract the cheek to expose the buccal vestibule adjacent to the bicuspid teeth. Following tissue preparation, a 1⅝-inch needle should be inserted into the buccal vestibule between the bicuspids and parallel to their long axis (Fig. 6-12B). The penetration should be made far enough buccally to ensure that the needle passes to the infraorbital foramen without interference from the canine eminence. The path of insertion should be at an angle conforming to the curvature of the maxilla in this area, and the tip of the needle should pass as closely to the bone as possible. The needle should be advanced slowly toward the foramen until it is felt to drop into the infraorbital rim (Fig. 6-12C). Following negative aspiration, one cartridge (1.8 ml) of local anesthetic solution should be slowly injected and the needle withdrawn. The skin over the infraorbital foramen should be massaged to promote the spread of the anesthetic solution into the foramen. It is not necessary to enter the foramen with the needle during this injection. Spread of the solution into the infraorbital canal is necessary to produce a block of the anterior and middle superior alveolar nerves. The patient experiences the subjective signs of numbness and tingling of the lower eyelid, side of the nose, and upper lip. If surgery extends to the palatal tissue, a separate palatal injection must be performed.

MAXILLARY NERVE

In addition to the areas blocked by the infraorbital nerve block, a maxillary or second division nerve block results in unilateral regional analgesia of the molar teeth, the corresponding antral lining and buccal hard and soft tissues, and the hard and soft palates.

Technique. The target area for this nerve block is the main trunk of the maxillary nerve as it passes through the pterygopalatine fossa. The three techniques for blockade of this nerve are beyond the scope of this book. Generally speaking, the first technique is called the high tuberosity approach. This injection is similar to the posterior superior alveolar nerve block, but the needle is advanced beyond the posterior alveolar foramina to the pterygopalatine fossa. The second technique is approached through the greater palatine canal. This injection is similar to the greater palatine nerve block, but the needle is actually advanced up through the foramen and canal and into the pterygopalatine fossa. The third technique involves an extraoral approach. The needle is inserted into the side of the face, through the sigmoid notch of the mandible, and into the pterygopalatine fossa. The second division block also requires a greater volume of local anesthetic solution (approximately 5 ml) for success.

Mandibular Division

The third and largest division of the trigeminal nerve is composed of a motor and sensory root that exit the cranium by way of the foramen ovale. It provides motor innervation to the muscles of mastication, the anterior belly of the digastric muscle, the mylohyoid muscle, the tensor tympani, and tensor veli palatine. It is sensory to the mandibular teeth and gingiva, lower lip, cheek, anterior two thirds of the tongue, auricle, and skin over the temporal region. It may be necessary to block one or more of the nerves listed in Table 6-3 in order to perform surgery successfully in the mandible.

Although infiltration anesthesia is commonly used in the maxilla (by injecting at the apex of the involved tooth), it is usually unsuccessful in the mandible due to the density of the bone. Infiltration anesthesia of the mandible may be of value in children, since the mandibular bone may still be porous enough to allow diffusion of the anesthetic solution. Infiltrations may also

TABLE 6-3. *Regional analgesia of the mandible*

Nerves Anesthetized	Areas Anesthetized
Inferior alveolar nerve	Mandibular teeth; surrounding hard and soft tissues unilaterally to the midline (does not innervate buccal soft tissue in the molar area)
Lingual nerve	Mucosa of floor of mouth, anterior ⅔ of tongue; lingual gingiva
Long buccal nerve	Mucosa of cheek; buccal mucosa and mucoperiosteum of molar region
Mental nerve	Buccal gingiva; mucoperiosteum from bicuspids to midline; skin of chin and lower lip (does not innervate teeth)
Incisive nerve	First bicuspid, canine, incisor unilaterally to the midline; areas innervated by the mental nerve

be effective as an adjunct to nerve block in surgery involving mandibular anterior teeth.

INFERIOR ALVEOLAR AND LINGUAL NERVES

These two nerves (Fig. 6-13A) are commonly anesthetized with the same injection technique, so they will be considered together. The inferior alveolar nerve innervates the mandibular teeth and surrounding hard and soft tissues unilaterally to the midline. It does not, however, supply the buccal soft tissue in the molar area. It enters the mandible on the medial surface of the ramus through the mandibular foramen, courses through the inferior alveolar canal within the mandible, and exits as the mental nerve through the mental foramen. Incisive branches of the inferior alveolar nerve remain within the mandibular canal and travel anteriorly to supply the anterior teeth.

The lingual nerve separates from the mandibular nerve before the inferior alveolar nerve enters the mandibular foramen. It supplies the mucosa of the floor of the mouth, the anterior two thirds of the tongue, and the lingual gingiva. Therefore, blockade of the inferior alveolar and lingual nerves results in regional analgesia of the body of the mandible, the mandibular teeth, the mucosa and underlying tissues anterior to the first molar, the floor of the mouth, the anterior two thirds of the tongue, and the mucosa and periosteum on the lingual surface of the mandible.

Technique. Anatomic landmarks for this injection include the anterior border of the ramus, the external and internal oblique ridges, the coronoid notch, the retromolar triangle, and the pterygomandibular ligament. The target area for the inferior alveolar nerve block is the mandibular foramen, located in the midportion of the medial surface of the ramus about one centimeter above the occlusal plane (Fig. 6-13B).

After the tissue is properly prepared, the palpating thumb is placed in the mucobuccal fold. Once the external and internal oblique ridges and the coronoid notch (deepest concavity of the anterior border of the ramus) are identified, the thumb should be placed on the coronoid notch and oriented so that it is parallel to the occlusal plane when the mouth is opened maximally. The remaining fingers of the palpating hand should be placed on the face at the angle of the mandible. This gives an approximation of the width of the ramus (remember that the mandibular foramen is located in the mid-ramus). While maintaining this hand position, a 1⅝-inch needle should be inserted from the opposite canine or bicuspid area.

The orientation of the needle should be medial to the internal oblique ridge, lateral to the pterygomandibular ligament, parallel and 1 cm above the occlusal plane, and directed toward the mandibular foramen (Fig. 6-13C). The needle should be advanced slowly to a depth approximating one half to two thirds the width of the ramus, at which point bone should be contacted (Fig. 6-13D). The tip of the needle

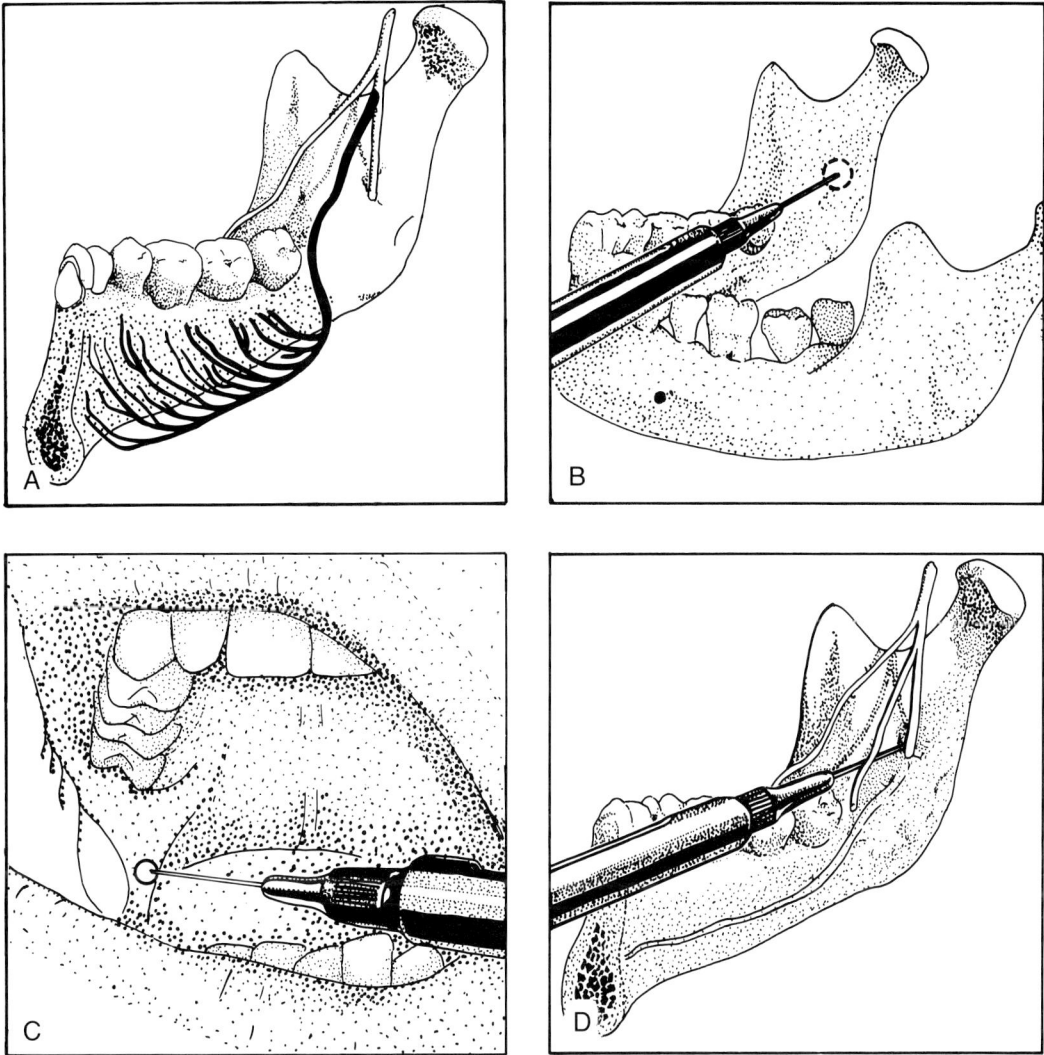

FIG. 6-13. *(A) The inferior alveolar nerve, shown entering the mandibular foramen on the lingual surface of the ramus, and the lingual nerve, shown in black, are commonly blocked during the same injection. (B) Target area for the inferior alveolar nerve block. The mandibular foramen is located in the midportion of the ramus, about 1 cm above the occlusal plane and on line with the coronoid notch. (C) Proper orientation of the needle and syringe for the inferior alveolar and lingual nerve blocks. (D) Proper orientation of the needle and syringe for the inferior alveolar nerve block. The needle tip is in contact with the target area. Withdrawing the needle along the same plane to half its original depth enables the practitioner to perform the lingual nerve block. (From: Manual of Local Anesthesia in Dentistry. 3rd ed. New York, Cook-Waite Laboratories, Inc., 1980.)*

should now be slightly above the mandibular foramen. After withdrawing the needle 1 to 2 mm, and obtaining a negative aspiration, two thirds (1.2 ml) of a dental cartridge should be injected. The needle should then be withdrawn to half its original depth, aspiration performed again, and the remaining anesthetic solution deposited effectively blocking the lingual nerve. The patient experiences numbness and tingling of the chin and lower lip to the midline, and the anterior two thirds of the tongue. It should be noted that the inferior alveolar nerve block does not anesthetize the buccal mucosa in the molar area. For surgical procedures involving the mandib-

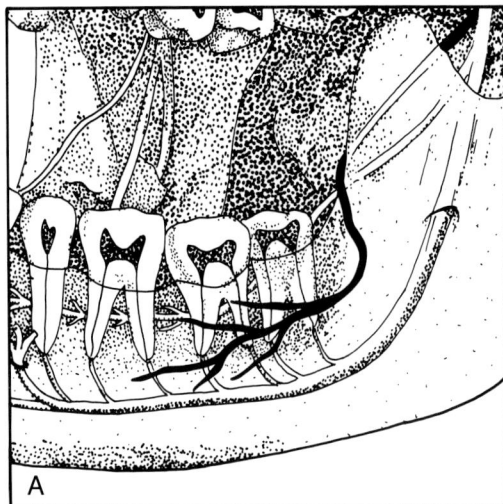

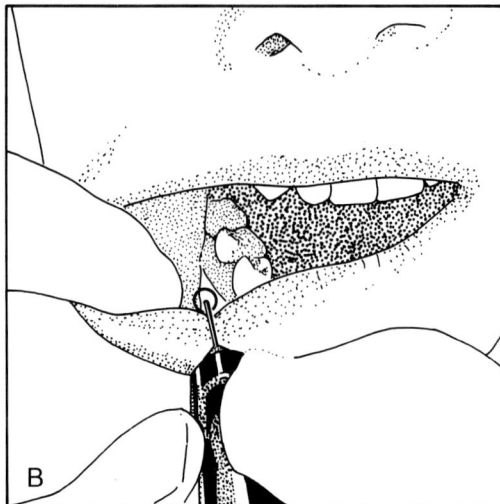

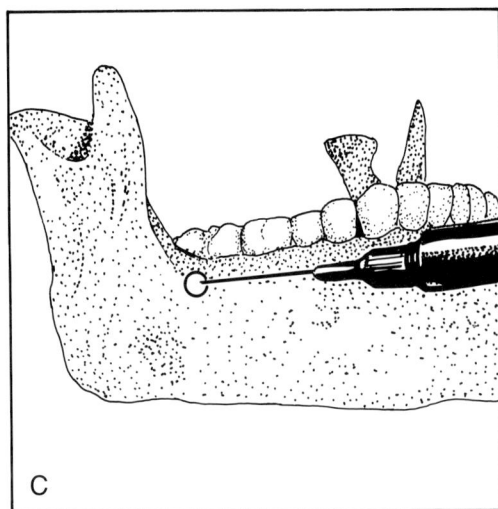

FIG. 6-14. *(A) The long buccal nerve (shown in black) crosses the external oblique ridge to innervate the buccal mucosa in the molar region. (B) Proper orientation of the needle and syringe for the long buccal nerve block. (C) The needle is in contact with the external oblique ridge. Deposition of local anesthetic solution in this area blocks the long buccal nerve as it crosses the external oblique ridge. (From: Manual of Local Anesthesia in Dentistry. 3rd ed. New York, Cook-Waite Laboratories, Inc., 1980.)*

ular molars, the long buccal nerve must also be blocked.

LONG BUCCAL NERVE

The long buccal nerve (Fig. 6-14A) provides sensory innervation to the mucosa of the cheek, and the buccal mucosa and mucoperiosteum of the mandibular molar region. It passes through the retromolar triangle and crosses over the external oblique ridge as its branches enter the cheek and buccal mucosa.

Technique. After preparing the tissue, the clinician should place the palpating finger on the external oblique ridge adjacent to the retromolar triangle. He inserts the needle into the mucobuccal fold just me-

dial to the fingertip until it contacts the external oblique ridge (Fig. 6-14B). The depth of penetration may be only a few millimeters. The needle should be withdrawn slightly, aspiration performed, and one fourth (0.5 ml) of a dental cartridge injected prior to removing the needle (Fig. 6-14C). The patient experiences numbness and tingling in the cheek when this block has been performed properly. The long buccal nerve block does **not** produce lip numbness to the midline.

MENTAL NERVE

The mental nerve branches from the inferior alveolar nerve and exits the mandibular canal via the mental foramen. It provides sensory innervation to the buccal gingiva and mucoperiosteum from the bicuspids anteriorly to the midline, and also supplies the skin of the chin and lower lip to the midline. The mental nerve does not innervate the teeth. A mental nerve block is useful in surgical procedures involving the lower lip and the mucolabial fold anterior to the first bicuspid.

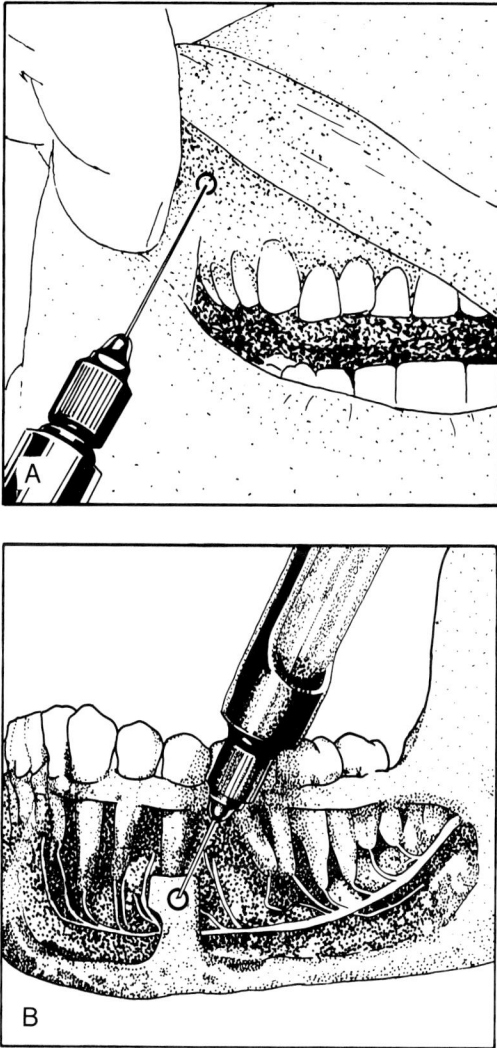

FIG. 6-15. (A) Proper orientation of the needle and syringe for the mental and incisive nerve block. Note that the needle is directed from posterior to anterior to ensure smooth entry into the mental foramen during the incisive nerve block. (B) Deposition of local anesthetic solution in proximity to the mental foramen produces blockade of the mental nerve only. Entry into the foramen produces blockade of incisive and mental nerves. Note again the posterior to anterior direction of the needle. (From: Manual of Local Anesthesia in Dentistry. 3rd ed. New York, Cook-Waite Laboratories, Inc., 1980.)

Technique. After preparing the tissue, the clinician should retract the cheek to expose the mucogingival junction adjacent to the bicuspid teeth. The mental foramen, located in the body of the mandible between and slightly inferior to the apices of the first and second bicuspids, should be palpated. The needle should be inserted into the mucogingival junction between the bicuspids and parallel to their long axis (Fig. 6-15A). The needle is advanced slowly to the level of the mental foramen, aspiration performed, and one half (0.9 ml) of a local anesthetic cartridge should be injected before withdrawal (Fig. 6-15B). It is not necessary to enter the mental foramen with the needle tip. Subjective signs of anesthesia include numbness and tingling of the chin and lower lip to the midline.

INCISIVE NERVE

The incisive nerve is a continuation of the inferior alveolar nerve within the mandibular canal after the mental nerve has exited. This nerve provides sensory innervation to the first bicuspid, canine, and incisors unilaterally. The incisive nerve block is performed infrequently since these same structures are routinely anesthetized by the inferior alveolar nerve block.

Technique. The incisive nerve block is best performed in two stages. First, the mental nerve should be blocked as above. Second, after mental nerve anesthesia has been obtained, the needle should again be inserted through the mucogingival junction adjacent to the bicuspid teeth. Since the mental foramen opens posteriorly, the path of insertion should be from posterior to anterior, as the intent is to enter the mental foramen with the needle tip. It may be necessary to probe the area gently with the needle to locate the opening of the foramen. This is why the mental nerve block should be performed prior to incisive block. After the needle drops into the foramen and aspiration is performed, approximately one third (0.6 ml) of a dental cartridge should be injected slowly. The subjective signs of anesthesia will be the same as for the mental nerve block. Anesthesia of the teeth must be ascertained by instrumentation without pain. If surgery extends to the lingual tissue, this must be injected separately.

Failure of Regional Analgesia

Although the success rate for obtaining profound regional analgesia is extremely high, at times a less than desirable result is achieved. There are many reasons for the

TABLE 6-4. *Failure of regional analgesia*

Poor technique
Improper needle selection
Improper selection of local anesthetic solution
Intravascular injection
Presence of tissue inflammation
Alternative innervation

failure to achieve adequate regional analgesia (Table 6-4). Foremost among these is poor injection technique. Poor technique is common among beginners unfamiliar with the oral anatomy and/or tentative in their approach to the patient. Poor technique is also not uncommon in the seasoned practitioner who may become complacent about proper injection procedures. The most common cause of a failed injection is improper identification of appropriate anatomic landmarks. This usually results in improper needle orientation or placement, which then leads to misdirection away from the target area.

Inappropriate needle selection may also contribute to failure. A needle that is too long or too short, coupled with uncertainty about the required depth of penetration, will lead to failure. The selection of a thin needle for certain injections may result in deflection away from the desired path of insertion. For this reason, a 25-gauge, $1\frac{5}{8}$-inch needle is preferred over a 27- or 30-gauge needle for the inferior alveolar nerve block injection.

The proper selection of the local anesthetic solution contributes to the success of regional analgesia. For example, local anesthetic drugs have vasodilator properties. When they are injected, this property actually enhances their uptake into the systemic circulation and thereby limits their duration of action. Local anesthetics are commonly combined with vasoconstrictors such as epinephrine or levonordephrin, in part, to delay the systemic absorption of the anesthetic drug and prolong the duration of action. In the case of the highly vascular maxilla, when infiltration injections are performed, it is advisable to use a local anesthetic solution containing a vasoconstrictor to ensure adequate working time.

Occasionally, patients may experience some subjective signs of anesthesia but may not be able to withstand instrumentation without pain. This may be due in part to the injection of an inadequate volume of anesthetic solution. This is especially common among students, who tend to resist injecting the contents of a dental cartridge into their patients. In this situation, usually all that is necessary is the administration of a greater volume of solution. This may also be of benefit in patients with anatomic variations.

A final cause of poor injection technique is the intravascular injection of anesthetic solution. It is to be avoided, since it will rapidly remove the local anesthetic solution from the target area and prevent interaction with the nervous tissue. More important, however, is that intravascular injection will undoubtedly lead to local anesthetic and/or vasoconstrictor toxicity reactions which can be life threatening. Negative aspiration must always be performed prior to primary injection, and each time the needle is repositioned.

Another possible cause of failed regional analgesia is the presence of tissue inflammation. Since inflammation increases tissue blood flow, the systemic absorption of local anesthetic solutions is usually increased. Inflammation may also modify the activity of peripheral nerves by lowering the response threshold, changing the protein structure of the nerve, or enhancing conduction. Most significantly, inflammation lowers the tissue pH and creates an acidic environment in which the anesthetic solution must work. Lowered tissue pH significantly reduces the ability of local anesthetic drugs to block nervous tissue, and may render them ineffective.

Finally, when all the above causes for failed regional analgesia have been ruled out, the possibility of alternative innervation should be considered. Variant nerves may exist that supply structures not usually associated with them. This can occur in patients with an extremely high palate and long alveolar process. The nasopalatine nerve may exchange fibers with the anterior superior alveolar nerve and contribute to the innervation of the incisor teeth. The long buccal nerve, although a branch of the third division of the trigeminal nerve, may innervate the buccal soft tissue in the maxillary molar area.

In the mandible, variant branches of the

inferior alveolar nerve may leave the nerve before it enters the mandibular foramen. These branches are not blocked by the conventional inferior alveolar nerve block. The mylohyoid nerve, which supplies sensory and motor function to the mylohyoid muscle and anterior belly of the digastric, may enter the mandible on the lingual side via a foramen in the bicuspid region. This occurs in about 10 percent of patients and may provide sensory innervation to the incisor teeth. A conventional inferior alveolar nerve block will not affect this nerve. The long buccal nerve, in most patients, assists in the supply of the mandibular molar and bicuspid teeth. The lingual nerve may assist in the supply of the mandibular bicuspids and first molar. Occasionally, the pharyngeal plexus of nerves, which normally supply the pharynx, may supply impacted mandibular third molars. Very rarely the cutaneous coli nerve, a branch of the cervical plexus in the neck, may enter the mandible on the inner surface of the lingual cortical plate and innervate the mandibular teeth. Finally, crossover innervation may exist in the mandible, whereby the incisors on one side are supplied in part by the opposite inferior alveolar nerve.

Complications of Regional Analgesia

Complications associated with regional analgesia may be either localized or systemic in nature. Although localized reactions are more frequent in everyday practice, systemic reactions can have more far-reaching consequences (Table 6-5).

Local Effects

Perhaps the most disconcerting localized anesthetic complication is the production

TABLE 6-5. *Complications of regional analgesia*

Local Effects	Systemic Effects
Paresthesia	Psychogenic
Trismus	Drug toxicity
Hematoma	Allergy
Mucosal irritation	
Infection	
Needle breakage	
Undesired nerve block	

of *paresthesia* in the trigeminal system. Paresthesia is described as an abnormal sensation such as burning or tingling, which manifests along the distribution of a particular nerve or nerve pathway. It results from direct mechanical needle trauma to the nerve or by injection of a contaminated anesthetic solution in close proximity to the nerve. Although relatively uncommon, paresthesia is most likely to occur following an inferior alveolar nerve block injection. The altered sensation is usually transient and may resolve spontaneously within days, weeks, or months. In rare instances, the damage can be permanent. No treatment is available for this condition, but patient rapport and reassurance may prove to be effective therapeutic tools.

Muscle *trismus* is another complication that may occur following an inferior alveolar nerve block. The internal, or medial, pterygoid muscle is most often affected. Limitation of muscular function after an intraoral injection may be caused by hematoma formation, direct muscle injury secondary to needle trauma, localized muscle necrosis secondary to the anesthetic drug or vasoconstrictor, infection in a fascial space, or the introduction of a foreign body. The treatment for trismus may include analgesics, saline mouth rinses, antibiotics, and physical therapy.

Hematoma formation is the result of direct needle trauma to a blood vessel, and is most likely to occur following a posterior superior alveolar nerve block injection. Signs and symptoms of hematoma include rapid swelling, a sensation of fullness in the area, facial asymmetry, and mild trismus. Management of a hematoma includes patient reassurance and ice on the day of injury, followed in 24 hours by the application of heat. Post-treatment antibiotics may also be necessary.

Mucosal irritation may be produced by a number of different causes. Topical anesthetics, when applied to the mucosa for longer than one minute, may diminish the capillary integrity of the underlying tissue and produce irritation. Additionally, the injection of excessive amounts of local anesthetics with vasoconstrictors into tightly attached tissue may produce localized tissue ischemia and ulceration. The tissue overlying the hard palate is most frequently damaged in this manner. High pressure injection techniques, such as the periodontal ligament injection, have been reported to produce irritation and even necrosis of the interdental papilla with exposure of the underlying bone. Self-inflicted injuries, such as cheek, lip, and tongue biting, are common causes of mucosal irritation following regional analgesia in children and occasionally in adults.

Infection is a rare complication of regional analgesia. It may result from injecting into or through an infected area, the use of the same cartridge or needle in more than one patient, and multiple injections of the same needle in the same patient. Preparing the injection site with an antiseptic agent prior to injection may reduce the amount of bacteria at the site, but it is inconclusive as to whether this action helps prevent infection.

Needle breakage is also very uncommon following local anesthetic administration. Single-use, disposable needles resulting from high-quality manufacturing techniques have minimized this problem. However, unexpected patient movement, excessive lateral force by the dentist, manufacturing defects, and intentional bending of the needle by the dentist may result in needle breakage. The needle is most susceptible to breakage at the hub. It is therefore recommended that the needle never be inserted to this depth, because breakage at this point would result in loss of the needle into the tissue.

Finally, inadvertent *undesirable nerve block* may result from local anesthetic administration. This may result from gross misdirection of the needle, or an unusual pattern of anesthetic distribution. Undesirable nerves that may be affected include the facial nerve, with resultant transient hemifacial paralysis of the sympathetic plexus and the recurrent laryngeal nerve. Blockage of the latter may produce hoarseness and difficulty with speech.

Systemic Effects

Perhaps the most common adverse reactions associated with regional analgesia are *psychogenic* in nature. A comprehensive pretreatment medical evaluation, with regard to prior adverse experiences, needle phobia, or emotional instability, is essential to the identification of potentially reactive patients. The most common psychogenic reaction is syncope, characterized by prodromal signs such as diaphoresis, pallor, nausea, dizziness, mental confusion, and hypotension. The most susceptible patients to syncope are young, healthy males in their early twenties. Another common psychogenic reaction is hyperventilation syndrome. This is precipitated by excessive anxiety and characterized by rapid, shallow breathing, which can progress to unconsciousness. Hyperventilation syndrome is most common in young female patients.

Drug toxicity reactions are an extension of the pharmacologic effects of either the local anesthetic or the vasoconstrictor. These reactions are positively correlated with the attainment of toxic blood levels of each drug as a function of the total dose administered and the time course of administration.

The central nervous and cardiovascular systems are the most sensitive to the actions of local anesthetic agents. As blood levels rise in the brain, the initial signs of toxicity are evident as excitatory activity. Patients may experience auditory and visual disturbances, dizziness, mental confusion, increased anxiety, muscle tremors, and finally generalized seizures. Central nervous system depression follows the excitatory phase and is manifested as lethargy, coma, and respiratory depression or arrest. The effect of local anesthetics on the cardiovascular system is also one of depression. Cardiovascular toxicity commonly occurs at approximately twice the dose required to produce the central nervous system effects. Cardiovascular toxicity is marked by profound hypotension and possibly circulatory collapse.

Toxicity reactions produced by vasoconstrictors also affect the central nervous system and the cardiovascular system. Central nervous system effects include restlessness, agitation, anxiety, and hysteria. Cardiovascular effects include tachycardia, hypertension, and ventricular arrhythmias.

Prevention is the best way to avoid undesirable side effects. This may be accomplished by strict adherence to proper injection techniques, maximal dose calculations for both local anesthetics and vasoconstrictors, and attention to the patient's medical history.

The least common systemic adverse reaction to local anesthetics is *allergy*. True allergy to local anesthetic drugs constitutes less than 1 percent of all adverse reactions to these agents. The clinical manifestations of allergy include erythema, urticaria, pruritus, edema, and respiratory embarrassment. Allergy should be suspected if any of these signs appear following the local anesthetic administration. However, allergic reaction seems unlikely in their absence. An extensive history of any previous reactions should be obtained in patients with suspected allergic responses to local anesthetics. Patients with complicated or confusing histories may be referred for additional testing.

Conscious Sedation

Most dental patients can be managed successfully with regional analgesia alone. However, some patients are excessively anxious and may react to the sounds, pressures, and vibrations of a dental procedure. When either anxiety or the stimuli become excessive, the patient may become uncooperative, making completion of the procedure difficult or even impossible. A variety of pharmacologic techniques have evolved in dentistry that are designed to reduce anxiety and/or alter the patient's level of awareness, thus enhancing his cooperation and facilitating treatment. Collectively, these techniques are referred to as conscious sedation techniques. The term "conscious sedation" emphasizes preservation of the conscious state in addition to the other goals of mood alteration and patient cooperation.

Pain Reaction Threshold

As previously mentioned, the pain experience is a complex psychophysical process affected by several factors. In particular, the patient's response to the perception of an unpleasant experience (i.e., pain reaction) can be greatly influenced by the situational factors, attention and anxiety. *Pain reaction threshold* is used to describe an individual's reactivity to a noxious stimulus. A person who is tolerant of a noxious stimu-

lus and appears relatively unaffected by it is said to have a high pain reaction threshold. Conversely, an individual who is hyperreactive to unpleasant stimuli has a low pain reaction threshold. The pain reaction threshold varies for each individual and is influenced by social learning, sex, age, attention, and anxiety. *Attention and anxiety are situational factors that can be affected by drugs used in conscious sedation techniques.*

The objectives of conscious sedation are to reduce the patient's awareness of his environment and allay anxiety while preserving the conscious state. In doing so, the patient becomes more tolerant of the dental procedure. Numerous conscious sedation techniques employ inhalation (nitrous oxide), enteral (oral), and parenteral routes (i.m., i.v., submucosal).

The safety of these techniques is directly related to maintenance of consciousness. A conscious patient is one capable of a rational response to command, with all protective reflexes intact, including the ability to clear and maintain an open airway. Consciousness is clinically assessed by continuously evaluating a patient's response to command. The elicited response must be a *rational* one. A response that is inappropriate or does not follow the command within a reasonable period of time may or may not be indicative of the conscious state.

Preservation of the conscious state during conscious sedation is important since loss of consciousness is frequently associated with significant changes in vital physiologic function. Most notable is the obtundation of protective reflexes, including airway maintenance. These changes can be extremely dangerous if not recognized and properly managed. Nonetheless, conscious sedation is remarkably safe when administered by properly trained clinicians and can be utilized to manage up to 95 percent of dental patients who are unsuccessfully managed with regional analgesia alone. The remaining patients are best managed with general anesthesia.

General Anesthesia

General anesthesia is defined as a reversible, drug-induced depression of the central nervous system, heralded by the production of unconsciousness and accompanied by a loss of all sensations including an insensibility to pain. It is a method of pain control that has been employed in dentistry for over 125 years. Although safer conscious sedation techniques frequently are preferable substitutes, some dental patients cannot be properly managed in a conscious state. Uncooperative children, mentally handicapped, excessively anxious, or medically compromised patients frequently require general anesthesia to facilitate dental treatment. The objectives of general anesthesia include the production of unconsciousness, inhibition of autonomic responses to noxious stimuli, production of amnesia, and relaxation of skeletal muscles.

Numerous drugs are available for inducing and maintaining general anesthesia. Barbiturates, psychosedatives, narcotics, dissociative agents, and inhalation anesthetics have been used singularly or in combination to produce general anesthesia. Selection of a suitable agent is based upon the physiologic status of the patient, operative requirements, and the physiologic effects the agent produces (i.e. pharmacodynamics). Because many dental procedures are performed in outpatient facilities, a rapid recovery to a mentally alert state is also desirable.

General anesthesia is unique to other methods of pain and anxiety control utilized in dentistry because unconsciousness is produced. The general anesthetic state is frequently compared euphemistically to natural sleep: "we are going to put you to sleep." However, general anesthesia is not sleep. Many vital physiologic functions including protective reflexes may be obtunded during general anesthesia. Airway obstruction and excessive cardiorespiratory depression are frequently observed during general anesthesia. Occasionally, publicized catastrophes involving dental patients result from inattentive and/or inexperienced clinicians who fail to recognize or effectively manage the dangerous sequelae that may accompany the unconscious state. With properly trained personnel in adequately equipped facilities, general anesthesia for dentistry has a remarkably safe record and is invaluable for managing selected patients.

References

1. Scott, D. S., and Hirschman, R.: Psychological aspects of dental anxiety in adults. JADA, *104:* 27, 1982.
2. U.S. Department of Health, Education, and Welfare: Oral Disease: Target for the 70's. Five-year Plan of the National Institute of Dental Research for Optimum Development of the Nation's Dental Research Effort. Bethesda, MD, National Institutes of Health, 1970.
3. Bennett, C. R.: The role of the dentist in anesthesiology. *In* Clinical Anesthesia: Public Health Aspects of Critical Care Medicine in Anesthesiology. Edited by P. Safar. Philadelphia, F. A. Davis Co., 1974.
4. Gasser, H. S., and Erlanger, J.: Role of fiber size in the establishment of nerve block by pressure or cocaine. Am. J. Physiol., *88:* 581, 1929.

CHAPTER 7 # Principles of Exodontia

Daniel E. Waite

Too far East is West. Dutch proverb

General Considerations

Halstead stated: "the surgeon should use his head as well as his hands." This statement is especially true in operating in and around the oral cavity. The removal of teeth has a remarkable psychologic influence on the patient. Women, particularly, view the loss of teeth as a serious disfigurement. Teeth reflect personality and individuality. Their removal, regardless of the reason, often inflicts embarrassment and produces varying degrees of psychologic adjustment. The removal of teeth can be ominous to the patient.

Cleanliness and sterilization are essential principles in any type of surgery. While a sterile drape across the chest with a clean head towel may be adequate for outpatient procedures, a far more detailed preparation and draping are necessary for hospital procedures (see Chapter 18). All instruments need to be sterilized, and all clinicians should have previous experience and training in microbiology and sterilization principles. As a general rule, steam autoclaving is the most common and efficient method for the control of microorganisms, including spores. Dry heat and gas are two additional very acceptable methods for sterilization. Although they take more time to accomplish similar results, they produce less corrosion on some instruments and are better suited for instruments with moving parts (such as the dental handpiece).

Prepping of the oral cavity reduces the potential for infection following surgery and is commonly done by intraoral lavage of saline-diluted hydrogen peroxide as a mouth wash. The hands, prior to surgery, are appropriately scrubbed; however, with the reduced cost of gloves and the increased need for the operator's and patient's protection many clinicians wear gloves for all surgical procedures.

Another basic principle involved in the removal of teeth is to know the indications for extraction. Occasionally, a patient feels that a particular tooth—or perhaps all of his teeth—should be removed. It is important to try to discover the reasons behind the patient's opinion. They may include: he wants beautiful white teeth or a better smile or he is tired of going to the dentist or can't afford to have his teeth repaired. These are not considered good indications for tooth removal. One may have to be very diplomatic in talking to such a patient.

As a general principle, a tooth that is not contributing to function in the dental arch may be considered for extraction. The more common indications would be teeth that are carious and present with nonvital pulps and where root canal treatment is not possible, severe periodontal conditions (Fig. 7-1), teeth that are not restorable, impacted or unerupted teeth, retained primary teeth (Fig. 7-2), teeth in malposition, and retained roots or tooth fragments.

Another indication for the extraction of teeth occurs when the teeth are directly in the line of treatment of a malignancy (as in a jaw tumor). Opinions vary about the amount and type of radiation to be used and the quality of the teeth and general health of the patient (Fig. 7-3). Such situations should be evaluated on an individual basis. In instances of trauma, when the blood supply may be sufficiently embar-

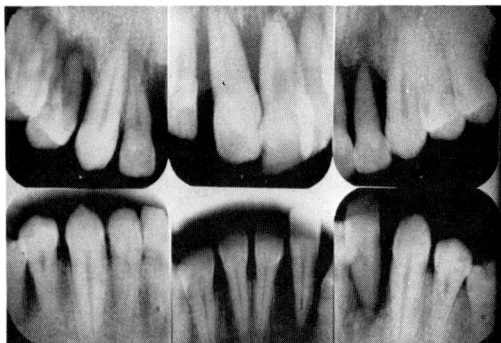

FIG. 7-1. *Periodontal condition necessitating extractions of teeth. (Courtesy of Dr. W. Hurt)*

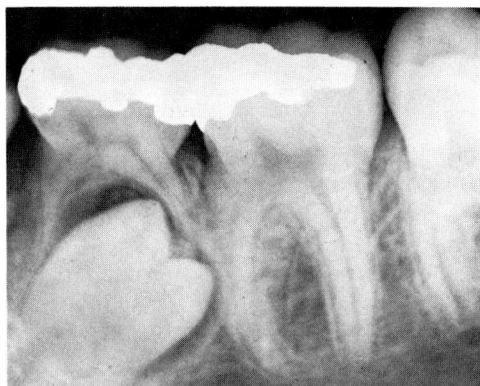

FIG. 7-2. *Impacted mandibular second biscuspid and retained deciduous molar.*

rassed or the supporting structures sufficiently injured, extraction may also be indicated (Fig. 7-4). Occasionally, a need occurs for extraction of permanent teeth for orthodontic reasons and, in some instances, at the time of orthognathic surgery. These unique and difficult decisions are generally arrived at in collaboration with the specialist managing the patient's care.

Contraindications

There are certainly some contraindications to the extraction of teeth. The patient's general health may be such that he cannot tolerate the injection of a local anesthetic or the removal of a tooth. Certain blood dyscrasias negate the extraction of teeth without very special preparation, particularly for those patients on anticoagulant therapy. Coronary artery diseases—

including hypertension and diabetes—require close cooperation with the patient's physician prior to treatment. Malignant conditions and patients receiving radiation therapy or various medications may contraindicate extraction. With certain infectious problems, both acute and chronic, a tooth extraction would be inadvisable. In such instances, the infection would need to be brought under control prior to the removal of the tooth.

The surgeon should take a history of the patient and perform a preoperative evaluation before proceeding with extraction (review Chapter 3). Moreover, he should carefully prepare a surgical plan, including any difficulties or complications that might occur during surgery. It is important to review the anatomy pertaining to the individual procedure. For example, knowing the distal curvature of the root of the maxillary lateral incisors would aid in their extraction, as would knowing that the central incisors have a conical root. The habit of sterile technique, and experience with infections both pre- and postoperatively, gives the clinician confidence in the management of these surgical cases.

The selection of the appropriate anesthetic in terms of its beneficial vasoconstricting action and its duration, and the skill with which it is administered, makes the patient comfortable over a longer period of time during the surgical procedure. In addition, the vasoconstriction action minimizes bleeding, creating a clear field for the surgeon. Appropriate sedative and

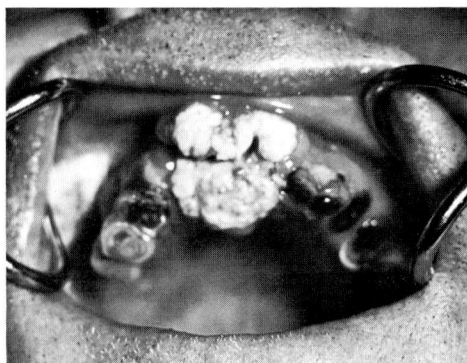

FIG. 7-3. *Advanced squamous cell carcinoma of anterior maxillary ridge treated by radiation. Teeth in and near the tumor were extracted.*

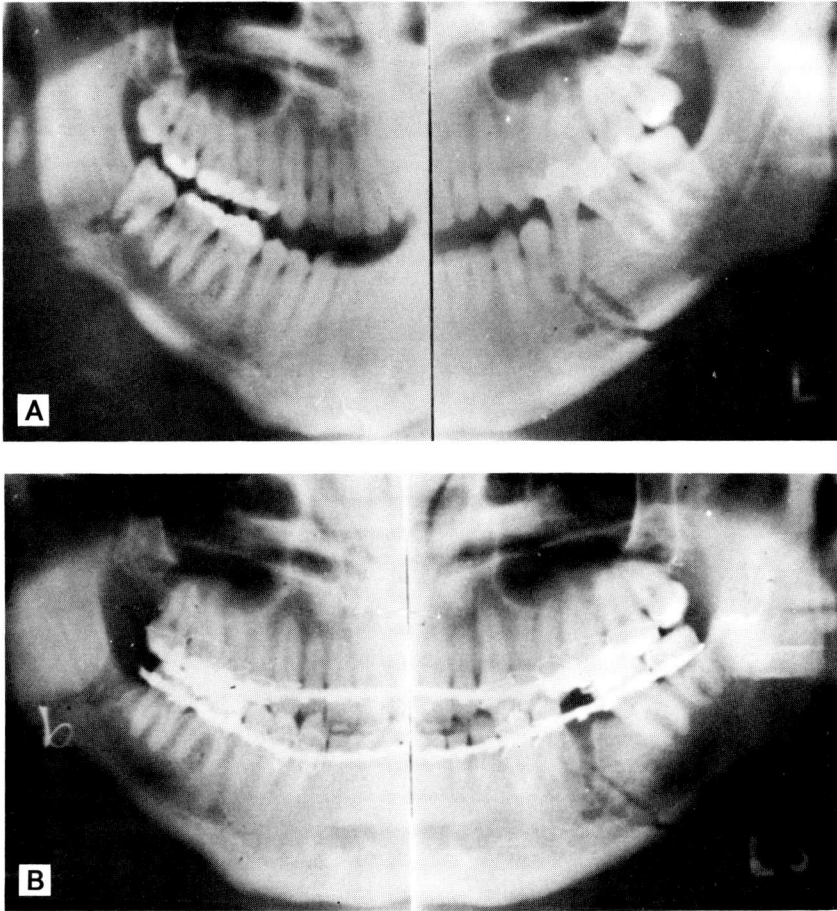

FIG. 7-4. *(A and B) Bilateral fracture of mandible. Bicuspid and third molar teeth were removed at time of treatment of the fracture. Note intraosseous wire at mandibular angle for immobilization of the proximal segment.*

analgesic medication also increases the efficiency of the procedure and allows a smooth postoperative recovery period. All these matters must be considered before undertaking the actual procedure.

When teeth are indicated for removal, it is of the utmost importance that the clinician know how to proceed. Every patient presents different problems and requires specific management. A patient who is to undergo a surgical procedure should have at least one preoperative visit to permit careful planning and thoughtful consideration of all facts. Laboratory reports should be available and radiographs mounted for proper study. The operator is then able to form a deliberate judgment that represents the best preparation for his patient's needs (Fig. 7-5).

After the diagnosis has been made, the treatment plan should be outlined. Important questions to consider initially include: "Does the patient need treatment?" "Is it within my scope of training?" "Am I capable of fulfilling this patient's needs?" If these questions can be answered affirmatively, a decision to proceed should be made. The proposed treatment should be reviewed carefully with the patient, or in the case of minors, with the parent or guardian. Such considerations as loss of work, postoperative pain, edema, and cost should be discussed. In this type of case presentation, several situations may become apparent.

1. An apprehensive patient
2. Evidence of lack of confidence in the dentist

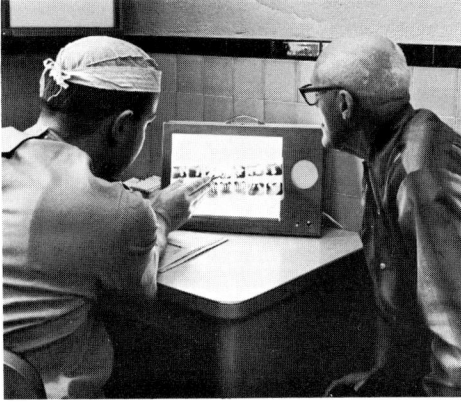

FIG. 7-5. *Interview with patient in the office, rather than in the dental chair, provides a relaxed doctor-patient relationship.*

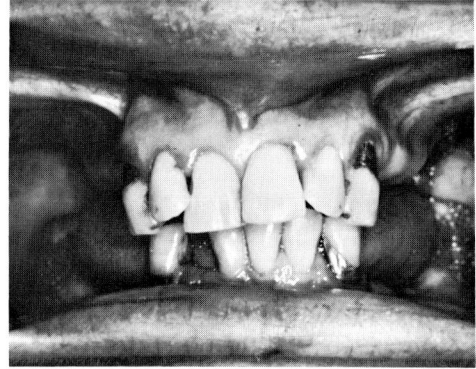

FIG. 7-6. *A case for immediate maxillary denture. Posterior teeth have been removed, retaining anterior teeth for final surgical appointment.*

3. A personality conflict or an attitude which may indicate lack of understanding of the operation or may prevent adequate communication during and after the procedure
4. Medical-legal complications
5. Consideration of hospitalization instead of outpatient care
6. Need for general anesthesia instead of local anesthesia

Any number of problems may come to light during the treatment planning appointment, and they must be appropriately answered before proceeding.

At this time also, instruments must be selected. From x-ray studies and the clinical examination, one can often ascertain whether the extraction can be made with or without a flap, bone removal, possible antral involvement, and so forth. A careful examination of the mouth may reveal mobile teeth, deep caries, areas of acute inflammation, or other situations that may dictate the order of the surgery. Depending on these findings, appropriate advice can be given to the assistant about such details as the selection of instruments, the time allotted for the surgery, and whether someone should accompany the patient.

Surgical Plan

In cases of a full mouth extraction, it is best to maintain the anterior teeth for aesthetic purposes, if possible, until the last

surgical appointment (Fig. 7-6). One should maintain vertical dimension when possible by leaving a bicuspid tooth in occlusion until the last surgical procedure. It is usually best to perform surgery in opposing quadrants to allow the patient to maintain a good vertical relation and comfortable chewing on one side during a portion of the surgical and healing process (Fig. 7-7). The removal of two teeth does not necessarily involve twice as much surgery as the removal of one. In fact, the removal of several teeth in one procedure is usually much less traumatic than their removal during individual surgical appointments.

When working in opposing quadrants,

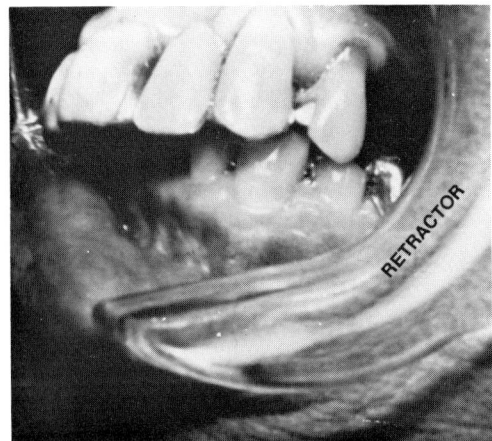

FIG. 7-7. *Note retained maxillary bicuspid tooth serving as vertical stop to maintain the natural vertical dimension.*

the surgeon must decide in which quadrant to start the surgery. One consideration is the duration of anesthesia. In the maxillary quadrant, where infiltration anesthesia is used, the anesthetic will dissipate early and should be administered just prior to commencing the surgery. If the maxillary quadrant is completed first, hemorrhage from it interferes with vision while working on the lower quadrant. If the lower quadrant is completed first, pieces of filling material or other foreign bodies may drop into the open mandibular sockets during the maxillary surgery. Since maxillary teeth are extracted by significant buccal and labial movement, the presence of mandibular teeth does not limit access. Because extraction forces of mandibular teeth are significantly more vertical, there is increased access for mandibular extraction when maxillary teeth have been removed first. In general, the decision about the first quadrant to be worked on must be made on an individual basis, keeping in mind these related problems.

Extraction usually begins with the most posterior tooth in the quadrant. When several teeth are removed, it is often necessary to consider a ridge trim or alveolectomy. When teeth from opposing quadrants are removed, attention must be directed toward providing adequate vertical dimension. To leave a pendulous or bulbous tuberosity after the molar complement has been removed creates inadequate space or vertical dimension and buccal undercut

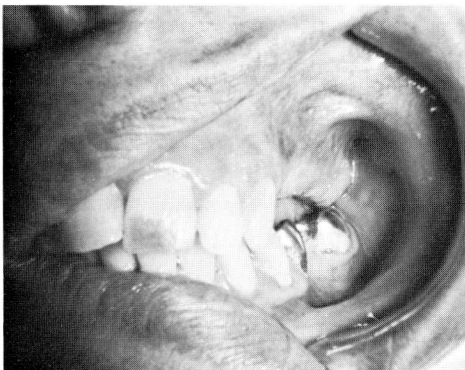

(Fig. 7-8). If other conditions, such as periapical granulomas, cysts, tori, or enlarged tuberosities are present, they may be considered for removal at the same time, depending on the operator's skill, the time required, and the patient's cooperation.

The removal of teeth need not be a totally frightful experience. Quiet, controlled, planned movements assure the patient of a good extraction procedure. If a tooth resists the general exodontic movements, a flap should be reflected and appropriate bone reduced, and/or planned tooth sectioning instituted (Fig. 7-9). At this time no detailed discussion should have to be made about the decision to proceed with the flap procedure or tooth sectioning. If the patient has been prepared properly and shows confidence in the dentist, a shift in the surgical plan should be managed in a calm, reassuring manner.

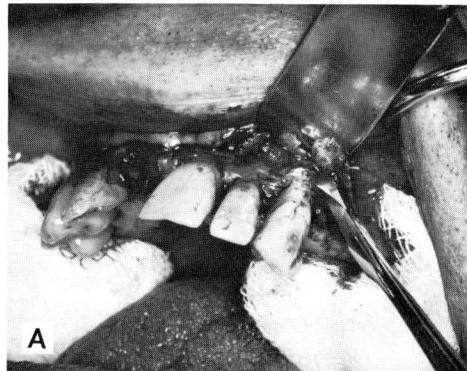

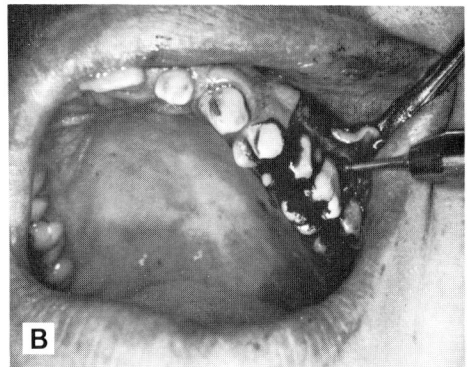

Fig. 7-8. *Posterior quadrant of maxillary teeth previously removed without adequately gaining vertical dimension in tuberosity region.*

Fig. 7-9. *(A) Cuspid tooth to be extracted showing collar of bone reduced with mono-angle chisel. (B) Difficult maxillary first molar extraction showing flap and tooth being sectioned with dental surgical bur.*

Flap Operation

Certain basic principles are to be followed in the planning, design, and manipulation of mucoperiosteal flaps. The indications for a flap operation are (1) to increase vision, (2) to gain surgical access, (3) to remove bone, and (4) to avoid injury to soft tissue that might occur from the contemplated work. The surgical principles underlying the design of the flap are (1) that it has a broad base that will ensure a good blood supply, (2) that it is large enough to allow good access without stretching, (3) that the flap is full-thickness and includes the periosteum when it is reflected, and (4) that when the flap is returned to its original site, the flap margins rest on a good bone table to minimize shrinkage, scarring, and contraction.

The healing time for a short flap is comparable to that for a long one; therefore, the incision length is not critical, and the necessary length of the incision should not be compromised. One should first mentally review the nerve and blood supply of the tissue to be included in the flap. Insofar as possible, incision line should parallel the nerve and blood supply. This obviously creates the least injury to the nerve and provides the best blood supply to the flap. The incision of the flap should begin in the interdental papillae to allow easier repositioning and suturing and provide a better blood supply at the termination of the incision.

Some have recommended a vertical incision at one end of the flap, and others, two vertical incisions (Fig. 7-10). If vertical incisions are used, they should be made in the interproximal area at least one tooth away from the margin of the bony wound, so that a plateau of bone will support the flap margin when it is sutured in position. Vertical incisions are not indicated in certain areas. The lingual tissues of the mandible are thin and reflect easily. Any flap reflected from the lingual is on an inside curve, and the relaxation of the flap is easily managed by increasing the length of the incision rather than making a vertical incision.

Several complications may arise if vertical incisions are made. They heal slowly due to retraction at the incision site, and are hard to suture. A vertical incision may

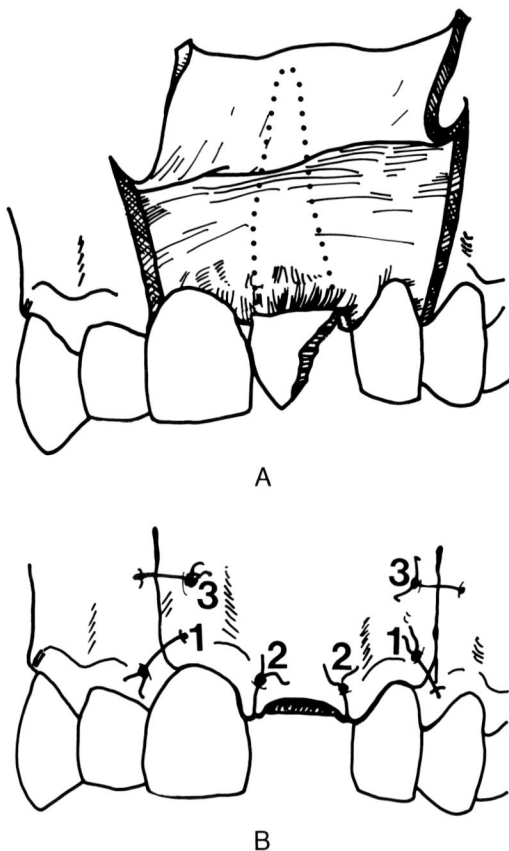

A

B

FIG. 7-10. (A) Mucoperiosteal flap reflection. Note vertical-type incision. (B) Flap returned, sutured. Note corner sutures placed first (1).

open the sublingual space if it extends beyond the mylohyoid muscle attachment. If the vertical incision were to be made in the second or third molar region, heavy bleeding, severing the lingual nerve, or extending into the lateral pharyngeal space are possible complications. The palate also is an example where the inside curve makes vertical incisions unnecessary. Complications that might occur include cutting the palatal artery, or the vessels and nerves of the nasopalatine region. The incision line should be so designed that the free corner of the flap does not have an acute angle (Fig. 7-11). This is important to avoid compromising the blood supply of the flap while obtaining adequate access without stretching or tearing. The base of the flap should always be wider than the free margin. The envelope flap often best serves these goals (Fig. 7-12).

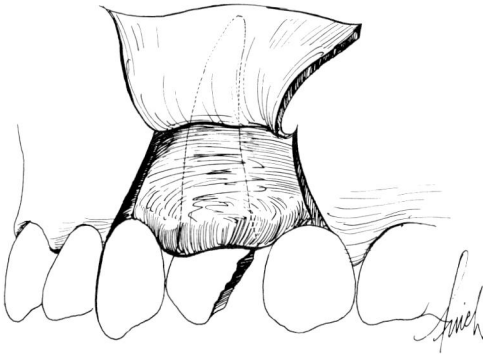

FIG. 7-11. *Incorrect flap design showing narrow base limiting blood supply and narrow neck of tissue on tip of flap.*

An important consideration of flap design is to ensure appropriate reattachment. This is true whenever repositioning tissue to gain a good tissue base on the ridge for a prosthesis and to avoid periodontal pocket formation around teeth, particularly when third molars are being removed. Applying the appropriate bevel to the incision is helpful, because it basically decapitates the rolled epithelial-lined papillae and gingival crevice tissue permitting new epithelialization and attachment (Fig. 7-13). This is particularly true in the case of the flap designed for the removal of third molars. When repositioning the flap, the sutures should be placed in a way that brings adequate tension and firmness to repositioning the flap around the second molar. This repositioning technique prevents a loosening of the flap and early pocket formation.

All tissue must be handled gently. Sharp scissors and needles, fine suture, and tissue forceps without teeth are part of the good surgeon's armamentarium.

Technique

1. Review the "seven minimum essentials" as originally described by Clark (see Chapter 9).
2. Appropriate anesthesia for the operation is, of course, indicated. There is some advantage to injecting small amounts of the anesthesia directly under the periosteum wherein the flap is to be reflected. This aids in the reflection of the flap as the fluid disperses itself beneath the periosteum, elevating it slightly. If additional anesthesia would

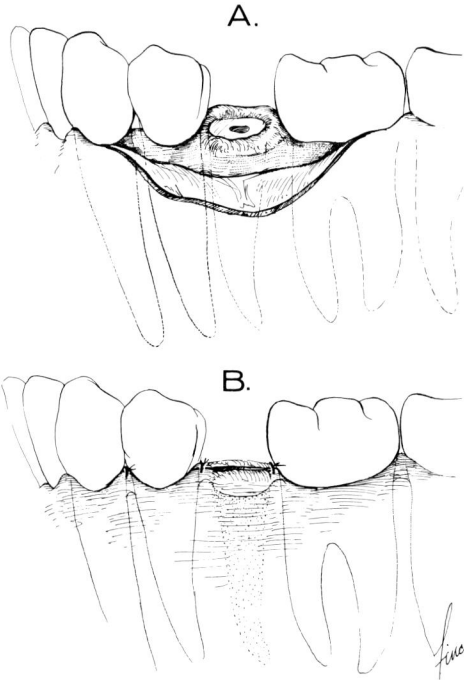

FIG. 7-12. *The envelope flap is best for most surgical procedures. It provides the broadest base and fully covers the bone cavity.*

be contraindicated, an injection of saline solution would accomplish the same thing. This is particularly helpful when reflecting the flap over a maxillary or mandibular torus. However, when a Z-plasty flap or a sliding soft tissue flap

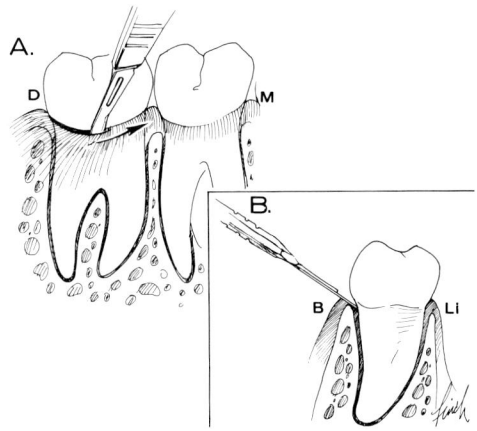

FIG. 7-13. *The no. 15 blade is shown incising at a 45° angle, thinning the mucosa to create an internal bevel.*

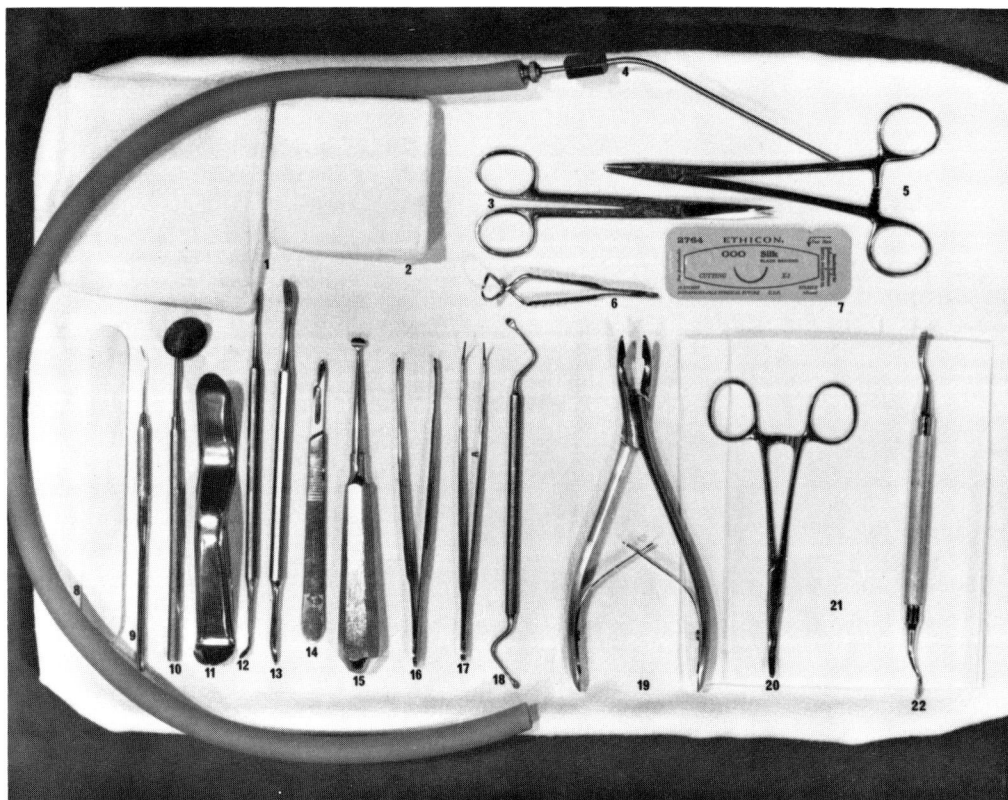

FIG. 7-14. *The flap tray should always be readily available. It should include 4" × 4" sponges (1); 3" × 3" sponges (2); scissors (3); suction (4); needle holder (5); towel clip (6); 3-0 silk (7); tongue blade (8); Gilmore probe (9); mirror (10); retractor (11); no. 1 Woodson elevator (12); no. 9 periosteal elevator (13); no. 15 blade and Bard Parker handle (14); no. 4 molt elevator (15); pick-up forceps (16); cotton pliers (17); small double-ended curette (18); rongeur (19); Kelly hemostat (20); pads to adjust light (21); bone file (22); and appropriate forceps and elevators.*

is planned, too much fluid injected near the surgical site could distort the soft tissue architecture, making flap design and planning difficult. For such cases, deposition of the anesthetic at appropriate innervation sites is better.

3. Prepare a flap tray (Fig. 7-14).
4. Make the incision with a sharp scalpel, keeping in mind the principles of flap design.
5. Reflect the flap with a periosteal elevator. Recommended instruments include the no. 7 wax spatula, the no. 1 Woodson, the no. 9 periosteal elevator, and the no. 4 molt curette (Fig. 7-15). To start the flap reflection, use the sharp portion of the elevator and immediately turn the instrument over so that the convexity of the elevator is against the

flap (Fig. 7-16). Use the largest instrument appropriate to the situation, and less tearing of the tissue will occur. Avoid overreflection of the flap, as well as heavy-handed retraction. Periodic relaxation of the flap by letting up on the retractor permits a return of the blood flow and general nourishment of the tissues. This is especially necessary during a long procedure.

6. After completing the surgery, smooth the bony margins with rongeurs and files and perform a complete toilet of the wound. Curettement, debridement, and irrigation are performed just prior to flap closure. Return the flap over the solid bone table and adequately suture into place. The edge of the flap (interdental margin) is trimmed to permit

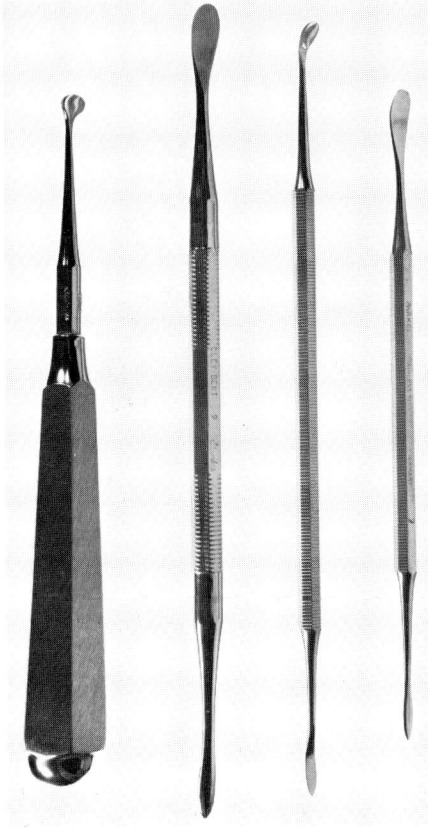

FIG. 7-15. *The instruments recommended for initiating and carrying out flap reflection are the nos. 7, 1, and 9 periosteal elevators or the no. 4 molt curette.*

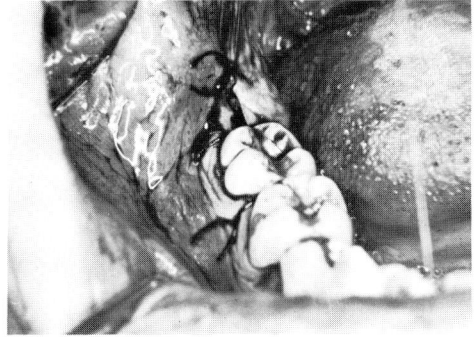

FIG. 7-17. *Flap returned after third molar removal, showing three interrupted sutures.*

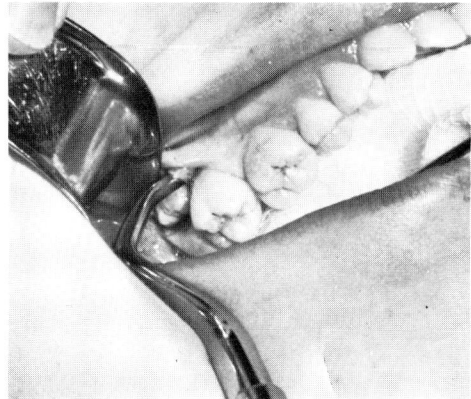

FIG. 7-18. *Flap reflected and third molar exposed for elevation.*

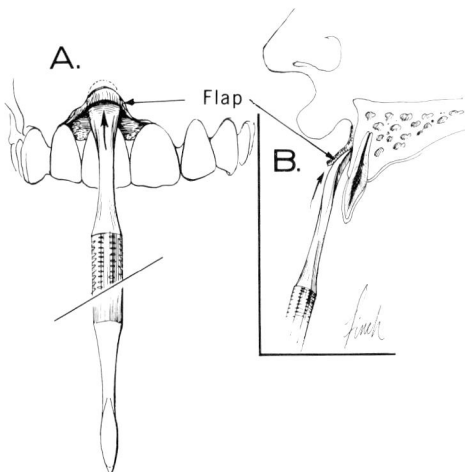

FIG. 7-16. *Use of the no. 9 periosteal elevator during flap reflection. The curved portion of the instrument should be against the soft tissue.*

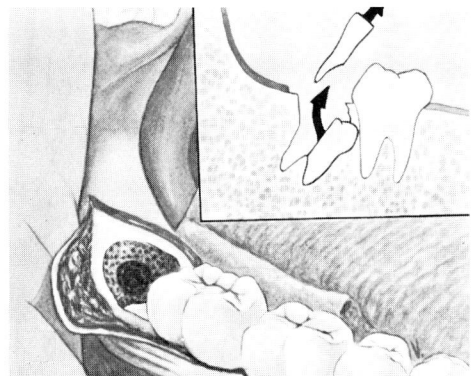

FIG. 7-19. *Distal one-half of tooth removed.*

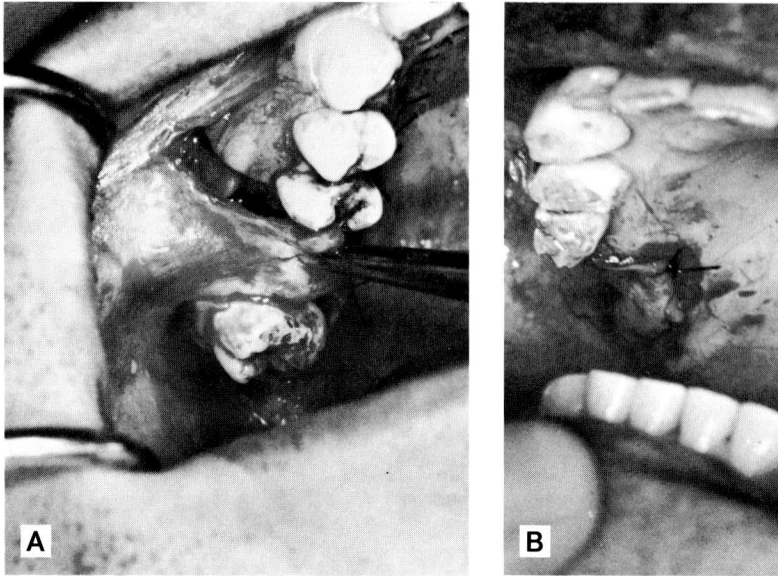

FIG. 7-20. (A) Buccal flap technique. Note relaxation of tissue and broad base of the flap. (B) Flap advanced and sutured to the de-epithelialized surface of palate.

appropriate proximation of the tissues but not allowing an overlap of the tissue margins. Either the running continuous lock stitch or the interrupted suture technique may be used (Fig. 7-17). Deep portions of the flap should then be milked toward the incised surface to ensure good adaptation with the appropriate pressure packs placed.

On occasion, the operator may wish to place a drain of gauze wick or rubber in a wound under a flap. For such instances, use only one piece of a given material, so that when it is removed, nothing is left behind as a foreign body and source of irritation.

7. Discuss with the patient the expected sequelae (e.g., pain, edema, ecchymosis), giving appropriate explanations, prescribing medication, and arranging the return appointment.

8. In general, remove sutures in 3 to 5 days, often coinciding with the next surgical appointment, if such is necessary. Patients often view the removal of sutures with undue apprehension. With good vision, light, suction, and assistance, the operator can make this procedure comparable to the examination.

There are many types of flaps other than envelope flaps (Figs. 7-18 and 7-19). Other examples include the advancement flap (Fig. 7-20), the rotation flap (Fig. 7-21), and transposition flaps (Fig. 7-22). Additional information on the mucoperiosteal flap operation for oral surgery appears in Chapters 9 and 10.

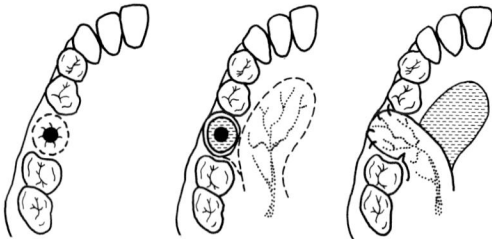

FIG. 7-21. Oroantral fistula closed by pedicle flap from palate.

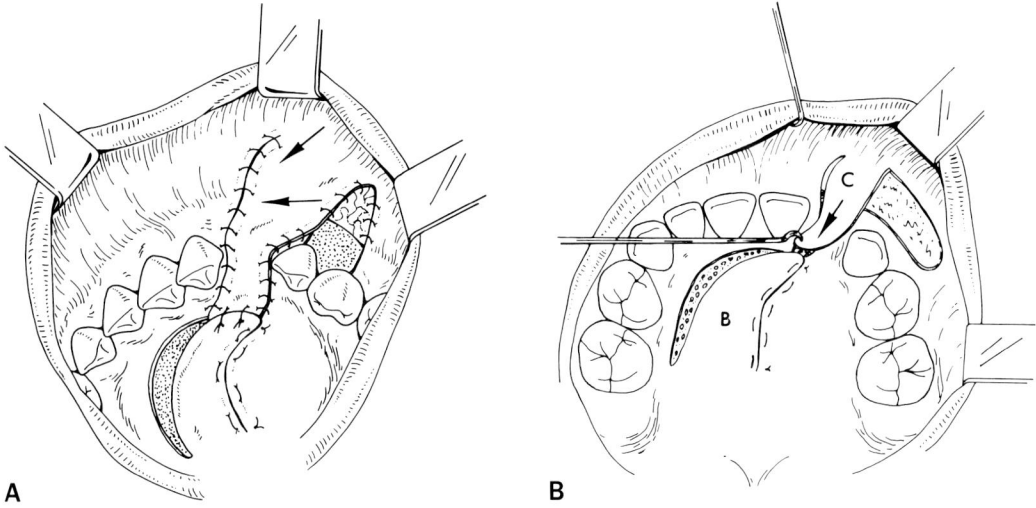

FIG. 7-22. (A) Partial mucoperiosteal sliding flap for closure of defect. Extension is from the lip. (B) A reversal pedicle flap is an alternative method for closure, best used for large defects. (From: Bell, W.H., et al., Surgical Correction of Dentofacial Deformities, Philadelphia, W.B. Saunders Co., 1980.)

CHAPTER 8

Instruments of Oral Surgery and Forceps Extraction

Daniel E. Waite

Don't throw away the old bucket until you know the new one holds water.
SWEDISH PROVERB

The instruments for oral surgical procedures are varied and many. As a general rule, the fewer instruments needed to complete a task, the more efficient the operation becomes. Every time an instrument is picked up, the task for which it was intended should be completed. Wasted movements indicate disorganization and lack of self-confidence or knowledge of how to proceed. Before one can expect to use instruments correctly, one must have a fundamental knowledge of them and their use.

Anesthesia Syringe

The obvious use of local anesthesia is for rendering the tissues pain free during the surgical procedures. In addition to anesthetization of nerves in the area of surgery, the vasoconstricting action of the local anesthetic reduces bleeding, greatly improving vision and making the surgical technique considerably easier. A more complete discussion on anesthesia and pain control appears in Chapter 6.

Two basic syringe mechanisms are available to deliver the anesthesia. Both should be of the aspirating type. The more commonly used syringe is the breach-loading metal syringe which receives a presterilized 1.8 ml of anesthetic solution in the glass cartridge. If more than one cartridge is needed, one simply changes the capsule and proceeds with the injection. The other type of syringe is either glass or a disposable type that is filled with anesthetic solution by withdrawing whatever amount is desired from a larger vial of solution. Disposable needles, usually 25- or 27-gauge, are used (Fig. 8-1).

Scalpel

Three blades and two knife handles are in general use. The blades are Bard Parker nos. 11, 12, and 15, and the handles are nos. 7 and 3 (Fig. 8-2). The no. 11 blade is used primarily for incision and drainage when a puncture-type incision is preferred and when blind cutting of deep tissue is necessary. The no. 12 blade is especially good for incision of the marginal gingivae and adapts well for following the cervical lines of the teeth (Fig. 8-3). The no. 15 blade, for general use, is used most frequently. It is excellent for most skin and mucosal incisions. Personal preference determines the choice of handles.

When using the scalpel, the pen grasp is utilized (Fig. 8-4). The fourth and fifth fingertips rest on a solid base. Tissue should be placed under tension while the curved portion of the blade is placed on the tissue surface. Firm pressure is directed downward and the blade drawn with a steady stroke for the desired distance. Even pressure on the blade should be applied and when the stroke is completed, the handle is raised, finishing with the tip of the blade.

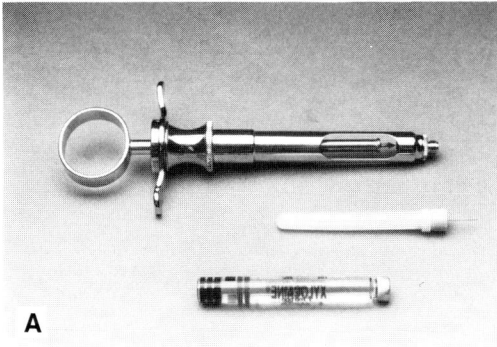

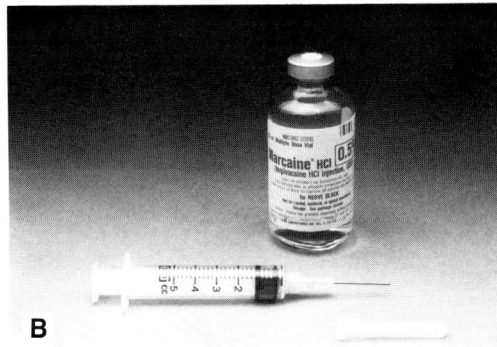

FIG. 8-1. *(A) Aspirating type of dental syringe with disposable needle and anesthetic carpule. (Walter Lorenz Surgical Instruments, Inc.) (B) Disposable-type syringe and needle with vial of anesthetic from which desired amount of solution can be withdrawn. (Sterling Drug, Inc.)*

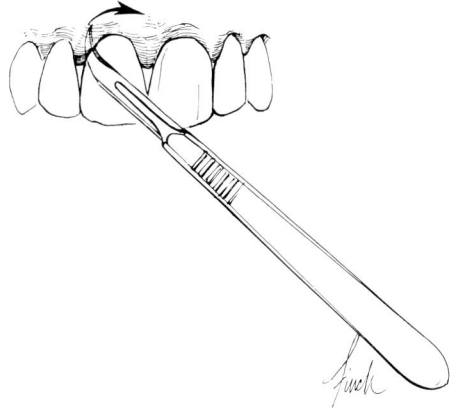

FIG. 8-3. *Knife blade no. 12 being used to incise gingival attachment.*

When incising mucoperiosteum, the surgeon should make the incision direct to bone with one movement. Whenever possible, always make complete incisions. Stopping midway through an incision is unnecessary, even if bleeding is evident. Hemorrhage can be controlled as soon as the incision has been completed.

When incising an abscess, the no. 11 blade is most useful. Place the point of the blade at the dependent point of the swelling, usually near its lower edge, and direct it toward the center with the cutting edge up (Fig. 8-5). Again, one stroke is made, and the incision should extend well into the center of the abscess. If necessary, a curved hemostat can then be placed in the point of the incision to improve the drainage. Incision and drainage frequently can be done without anesthesia because the pain is brief and may not be significant until after the incision has been made. In addition, local anesthesia at the site of infection is often ineffective and may further distend the painful tissues and spread the infection.

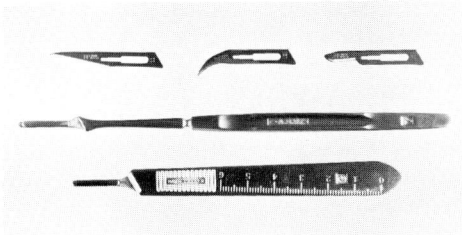

FIG. 8-2. *Knife blades nos. 11, 12, and 15; handles nos. 7 and 3.*

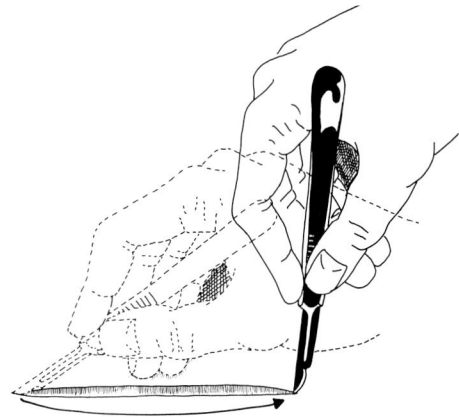

FIG. 8-4. *No. 15 blade with no. 3 handle, showing pen grasp. (From: Clark, Practical Oral Surgery, Lea & Febiger, 1965)*

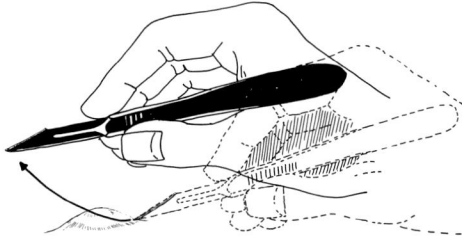

FIG. 8-5. *Incising an abscess with no. 11 blade. (From: Clark, Practical Oral Surgery, Lea & Febiger, 1965)*

Periosteal Elevators

The no. 1 Woodson and the no. 9 periosteal elevators are excellent (Fig. 8-6). They are used primarily for the reflection of mucoperiosteum. The ease of flap reflection varies considerably. The mucoperiosteum of the anterior palate is attached tightly to bone and difficult to reflect throughout its entirety because of the heavy, thickened tissue and the roughness of the palatal bone. In contrast to this, the tissue overlying the palatal torus is extremely thin and tears easily. The mandibular lingual mucoperiosteum is also thin and must be raised with care, although it reflects rapidly and easily.

When handling mucoperiosteal flaps, use the largest portion of the instrument that works well with its convexity toward the flap; less tearing and puncturing of the flap occur. Three major strokes are used in developing a periosteal flap; the push stroke, the pry stroke, and the pull stroke. In each instance, the instrument is held at an approximate 45° angle to the surface. Again, the pen grasp is best, with the fourth and fifth fingers resting on a solid base, usually the teeth. In initiating the pry stroke, the flap is developed first in the interdental papilla area with the small end of

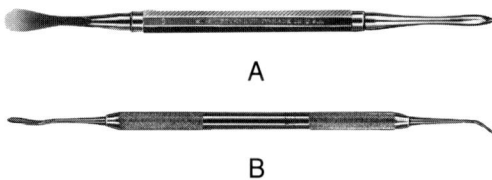

FIG. 8-6. *(A) Periosteal elevator no. 9. (Walter Lorenz Surgical Instruments, Inc.) (B) Woodson no. 1. (Hu-Friedy)*

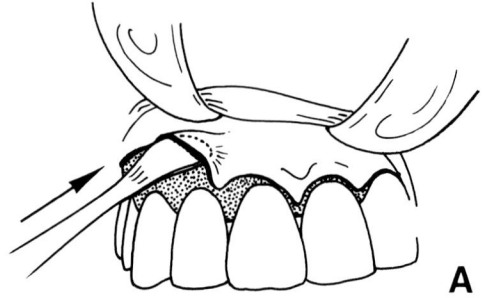

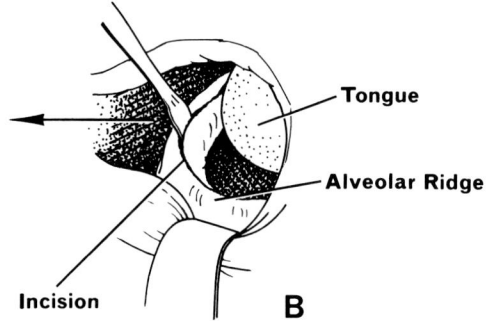

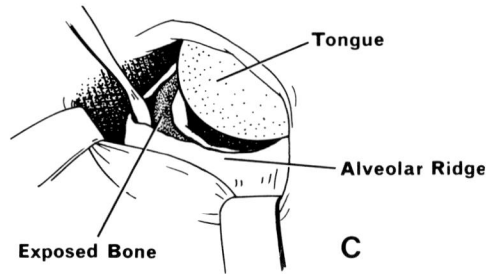

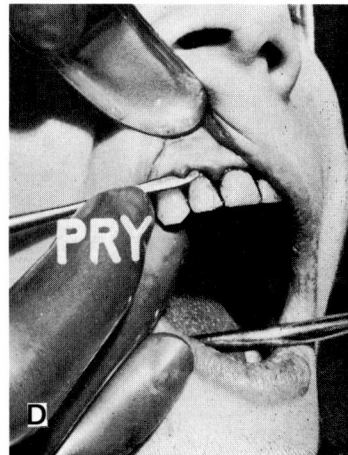

FIG. 8-7. *Flap reflection with a periosteal elevator. (A) Push stroke. (B and C) Pull stroke. (D) Pry stroke.*

the instrument (Fig. 8-7). The point is inserted firmly under the papilla and the adjacent tooth is used as a fulcrum. It is wise not to reflect the mucoperiosteal flap beyond the area of tissue to be exposed, because a certain degree of bone resorption takes place whenever a flap is reflected. If the reflection of the flap extends too far into the sulcus, edema accumulates in this area, thus retarding the healing process and shortening the overall depth of the mucobuccal fold.

Another broad periosteal bladed elevator described as the Seldin no. 23 is a helpful instrument (Fig. 8-8). The broad blades of this elevator and the curvature are helpful in reflection of some larger flaps and can be used as a retractor to protect tissues from other instrumentation. This is particularly true of the lingual soft tissues during the surgical removal of the lower third molar.

Retractor

A number of excellent retractors are available. The Minnesota retractor is a most common cheek retractor used in oral surgery. A ribbon retractor, commonly used for extraoral surgical procedures, has

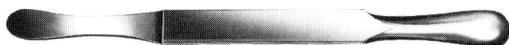

FIG. 8-8. *Seldin type periosteal elevator. (Walter Lorenz Surgical Instruments, Inc.)*

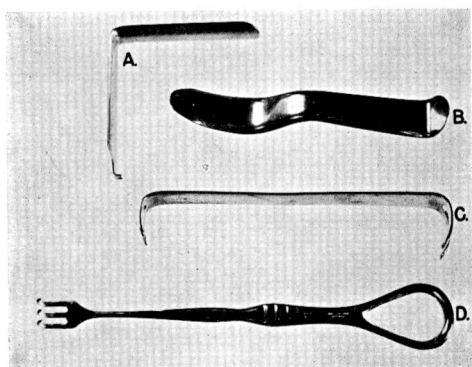

FIG. 8-9. *Retractors useful in oral surgery. (A) Austin. (B) University of Minnesota type. (C) Ribbon. (D) Catspaw. (From: Clark, Practical Oral Surgery, Lea & Febiger, 1965)*

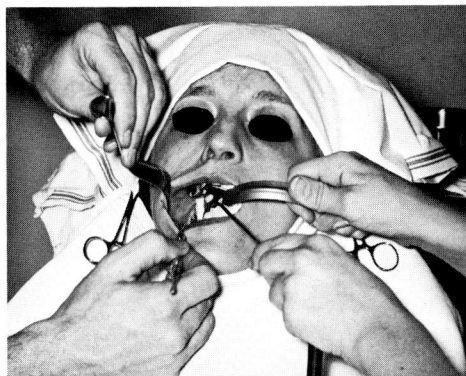

FIG. 8-10. *Tongue retractor in place over gauze, depressing the tongue and protecting the pharynx.*

several advantages (Fig. 8-9). The tongue retractor is most serviceable when a gauze sponge is placed as a curtain in the pharynx and partially under the retractor.

The retractors are used primarily by the assistant, and should be in the right hand to leave the left hand free for handling the suction, malleting, and cutting the sutures (Fig. 8-10). The assistant must be aware of what he is doing with the retractor. His main purpose is to retract the tissues gently but firmly and steadily so that the surgeon has the area under direct vision. The assistant must be careful not to pinch the lip or other tissues; moreover, it is easy to concentrate on the surgical procedure so much that the retractor may gag the patient or otherwise hinder the operator. Remember that constant retraction of tissues minimizes the blood flow through them. Therefore, whenever possible and when retraction is not needed, one should relax the tissues to let the blood supply return. A heavy-handed assistant can greatly increase the trauma to the retracted tissues.

Handpiece and Bur

The surgical bur is often used in the removal of bone and the sectioning of teeth. Carbide burs are much preferred over steel burs for cutting tooth structures and bone. High-speed instrumentation has greatly advantaged the surgeon and patient for surgical needs in reducing bone and sectioning teeth. A variety of surgical burs are available but generally can be categorized as cross-cut fissure burs, tapered, or round. All burs should be sharp and of the carbide or diamond type. Sterile water irrigation or saline should always be used to reduce the generation of heat, to keep the area clean, and to improve the efficiency of the cutting instrument. Several shapes and sizes of bone burs and bone wheels are available for the rapid reduction of exostosis or other large amounts of bone.

The handpiece and burs should be available at all times. The time lost in setting up the equipment is considerable, and when equipment is needed, it is needed immediately (Fig. 8-11).

General Principles

Because mandibular bone is much more dense than maxillary bone, the bur can be used to much advantage. Use a pen grasp with the straight handpiece, providing a steady, firm base with the fourth and fifth fingers to assure secure handling. The as-

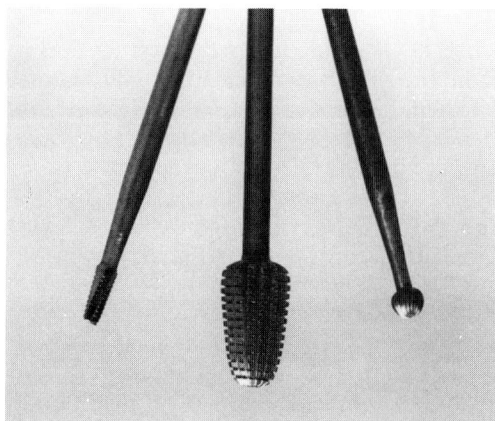

FIG. 8-11. *Surgical burs. (Brasseler USA, Inc.)*

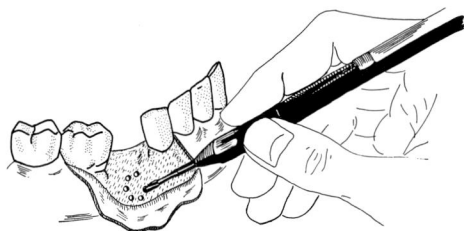

FIG. 8-12. *Method of gaining entry to mandible for removal of root fragment. Circle of drill holes being made. (From: Clark, Practical Oral Surgery, Lea & Febiger, 1965)*

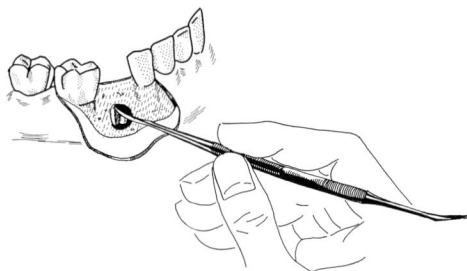

FIG. 8-13. *Root revealed after circle of drill holes has been completed and disc of bone pried up. (From: Clark, Practical Oral Surgery, Lea & Febiger, 1965)*

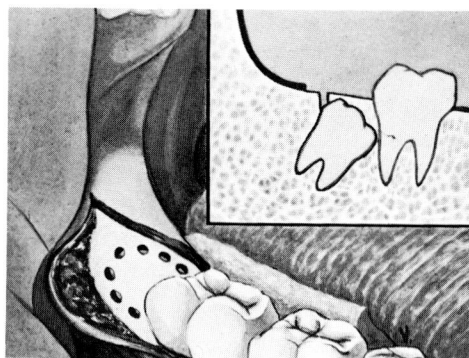

FIG. 8-14. *Necklace of drill holes with surgical bur to gain access for surgical removal of impacted tooth. (Courtesy of M.L. Hale)*

sistant directs an intermittent stream of water at the area and regularly uses the suction tip to evacuate the waste water and debris. The periosteum must be carefully retracted away from the revolving bur, for it is quickly mutilated if it becomes entangled in the instrument. Lingual reduction of bone with the handpiece should be done cautiously. Bony correction of lingual anomalies often are best managed with chisels and smoothed with a bone file.

To recover a root with the bur, the overlying bone can best be removed by creating a necklace of holes above the area where the root tip is anticipated (Figs. 8-12 and 8-13). These holes are then connected and the disc of bone is removed, permitting entry into the area of the root tip and making an easy removal. The bone overlying a third molar impaction can be similarly removed (Fig. 8-14).

When the bur is used for the sectioning of teeth, irrigation may be even more necessary (Fig. 8-15). Considerable heat can be

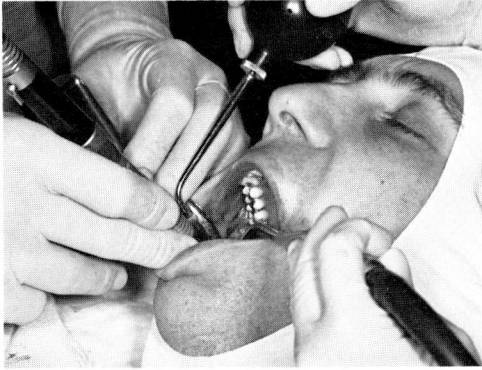

FIG. 8-15. *Irrigation is necessary when bur is used for the sectioning of teeth.*

generated, and the tooth structure clogs the bur blades quickly. (The sectioning of teeth is discussed in detail in Chapter 10.) The bur can also be used to make a purchase point for elevation (Fig. 8-16).

Mallet and Chisel

The chisel is another fine instrument for the removal of bone. Maxillary bone, much more porous than mandibular bone, is reduced easily with the chisel by using either hand pressure or the mallet (Fig. 8-17). The entire cranium acts as a countermass to receive the mallet blows, causing much less irritation than when the mallet is used on the mandible.

The chisel—especially the bi-level chisel—is also used for splitting teeth (Fig. 8-18). The monoangle chisel is preferable for bone reduction. The chisel must be razor sharp and should be honed after each use. When splitting teeth, give a single sharp bouncing blow with the mallet with no follow-through. When reducing bone with the chisel, the mallet should follow with a sequence of taps appropriate to the job being done. The chisel and/or osteotome has the advantage of always being sterile because of the ease of autoclaving them and having several instruments always available. In addition, irrigation is not necessary and less assistance is usually required.

Elevator

The elevator or exolever is one of the most valuable instruments to aid in the extraction of teeth. Whenever possible, it should be used to luxate all teeth before

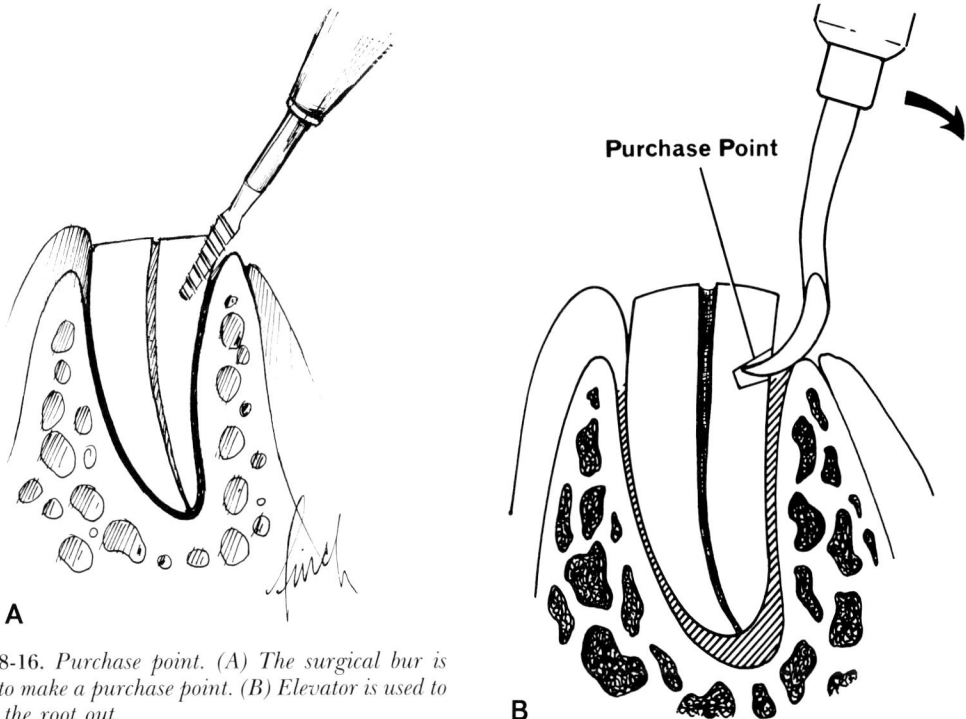

Purchase Point

A

B

FIG. 8-16. *Purchase point. (A) The surgical bur is used to make a purchase point. (B) Elevator is used to lever the root out.*

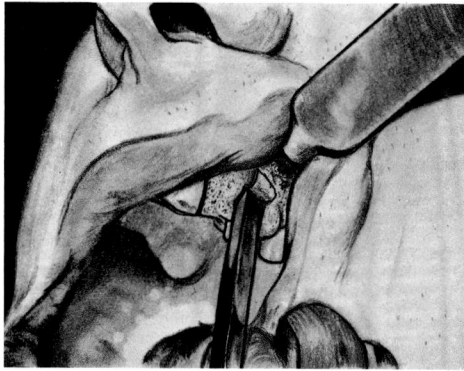

FIG. 8-17. *Use of chisel to shave bone from root of upper tooth. (From: Clark, Practical Oral Surgery, Lea & Febiger, 1965)*

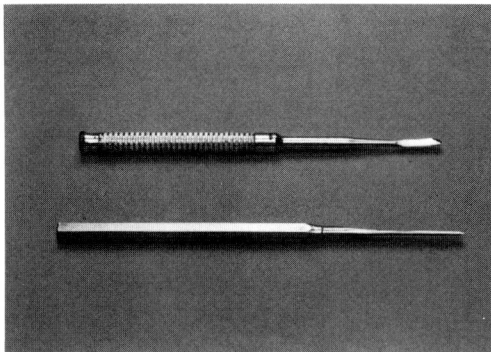

FIG. 8-18. *(Top) Chisel for removing bone. (Walter Lorenz Surgical Instruments, Inc.) (Bottom) Bi-level chisel for splitting teeth. (Hu-Friedy)*

applying the forceps. This facilitates the removal of the tooth; it minimizes the breakage of the tooth; it facilitates the removal of broken root tips if the tooth has been luxated prior to breakage; and it reduces the forceps pressure felt by the patient.

The elevator consists of three basic parts: the handle, shank, and blade. The concave blade of the straight elevator is used with the concave surface toward the tooth to be luxated. The occlusal edge of the blade engages the interseptal bone, which is the fulcrum (Fig. 8-19). The determination of the occlusal edge and the gingival edge varies according to the arch quadrant. Some elevator designs vary from the straight elevator in that the blade is set at an angle to the shank and handle; this

allows a better application of the elevator in certain areas of the mouth.

As used in the extraction of teeth, the elevator is a lever of the first class; that is, a lever with the fulcrum (which is the alveolar bone) between the resistance (which is the tooth) and the force (which is the hand of the operator) (Fig. 8-20). The function of a lever is to gain a mechanical advantage, calculated by dividing the input length by the output length. For example, 4 inches divided by 1 inch equals the mechanical advantage of 4 (Fig. 8-21). Thus, tremendous force is generated with this instrument.

Another type of lever application is that of the wedge. The force is supplied by the hand of the operator, and the resistance is supplied by the tooth or root tip. The size

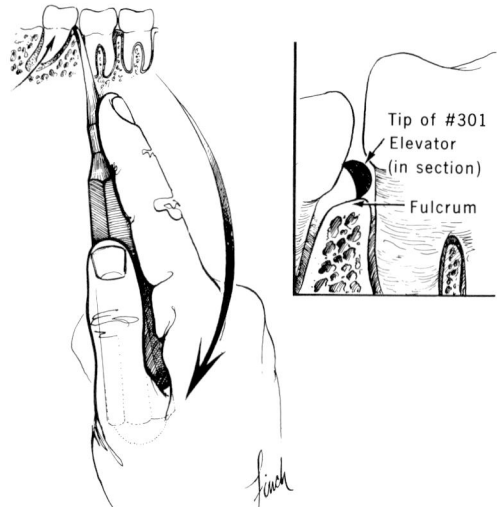

FIG. 8-19. *Correct application of the elevator for the luxation of teeth.*

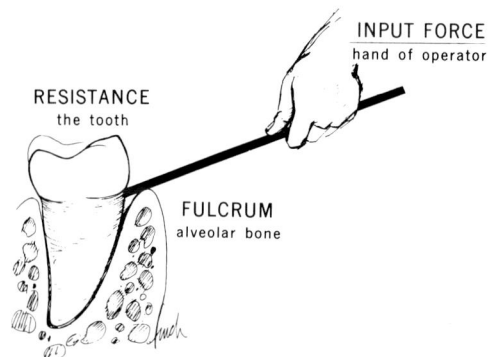

FIG. 8-20. *Illustration of the lever principle.*

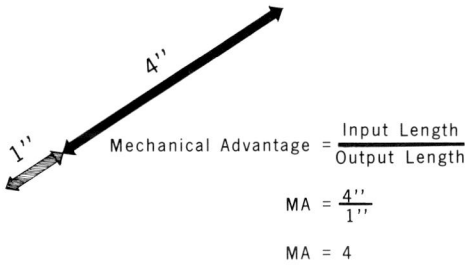

$$\text{Mechanical Advantage} = \frac{\text{Input Length}}{\text{Output Length}}$$

$$MA = \frac{4''}{1''}$$

$$MA = 4$$

FIG. 8-21. *Formula demonstrating increased force using the lever principle.*

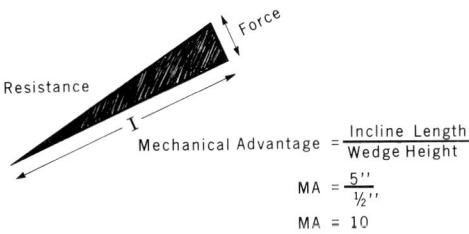

$$\text{Mechanical Advantage} = \frac{\text{Incline Length}}{\text{Wedge Height}}$$

$$MA = \frac{5''}{\frac{1}{2}''}$$

$$MA = 10$$

FIG. 8-22. *Formula using the principle of the inclined plane as a wedge.*

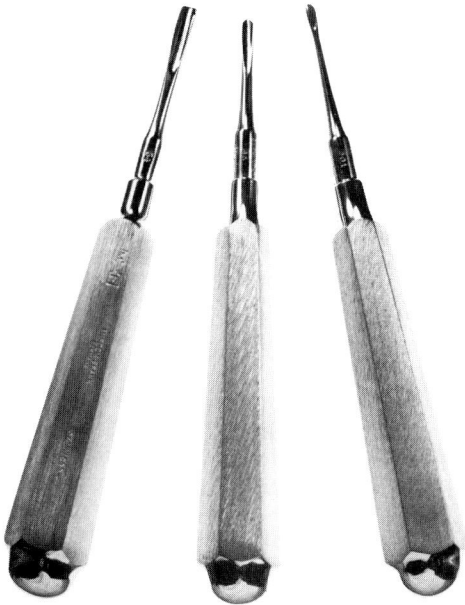

FIG. 8-23. *Straight elevators are often used as a wedge for displacement of the root or tooth.*

and shape of the wedge determine the force and the mechanical advantage. The mechanical advantage is the inclined length divided by the wedge height (Fig. 8-22). The wedge action of the elevator

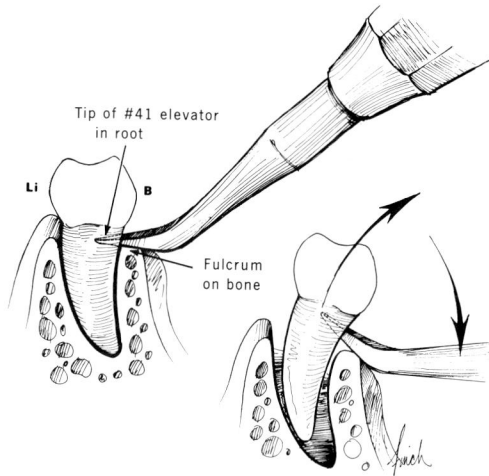

FIG. 8-24. *Demonstration of the lever principle using the no. 41 elevator.*

may be used to advantage in the delivery of fractured root tips.

Elevators may be grouped according to their primary use. The 301, 46, and 34 elevators vary only in size and are used to luxate teeth and root tips (Fig. 8-23). The no. 41 elevator is designed to be used in the bifurcation of lower molars or on teeth with a prepared purchase point (Fig. 8-24). The root apex instruments 1, 2, and 3 are designed primarily for the recovery of upper molar root tips (Fig. 8-25).

For the luxation of the anterior teeth, the 301 elevator is the instrument of choice. The blade is inserted into the interproximal space, with the concave surface toward the tooth to be extracted and with the fulcrum edge of the blade well engaged on the alveolar process adjacent to the tooth. The blade is then rotated toward the tooth and is engaged on its surface below the greatest point of convexity or at the cementoenamel junction. The elevator is then rotated until engaged, and the handle is moved inferiorly so that the tooth is elevated vertically as well as slightly horizontally (Fig. 8-26). In the upper arch, the elevator handle would be moved superiorly after it has been rotated to engage the tooth. The 301 may also be used to advantage as a wedge-type lever for the recovery of root tips in some areas of the mouth, such as the anterior maxillary area. The blade is inserted between the root tip and

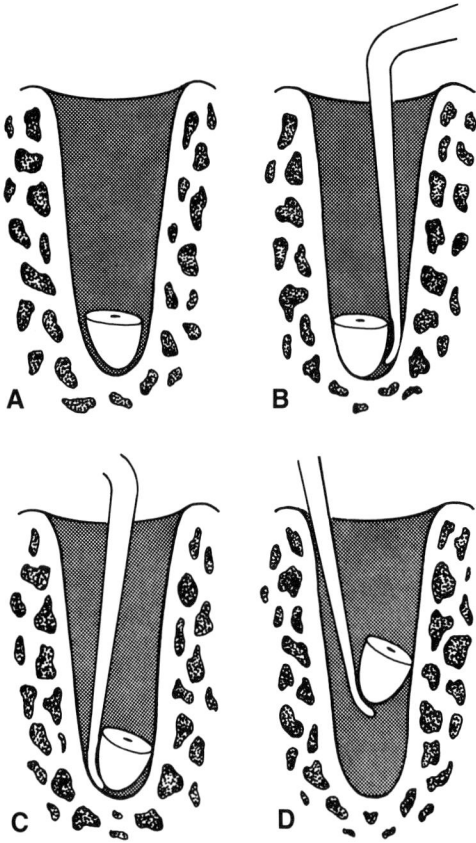

FIG. 8-25. *Curved root pick is used to displace a retained root in the process of recovery.*

FIG. 8-27. *Use of straight inclined plane elevator on upper cuspid root. (From: Clark, Practical Oral Surgery, Lea & Febiger, 1965)*

edge is engaged into the tooth. A slow, steady, upward distal and arc-like movement of the handle elevates the tooth in a distal and occlusal direction (Fig. 8-28B).

The Potts elevators are also available for use in the delivery of maxillary third molars. The application is entirely opposite to

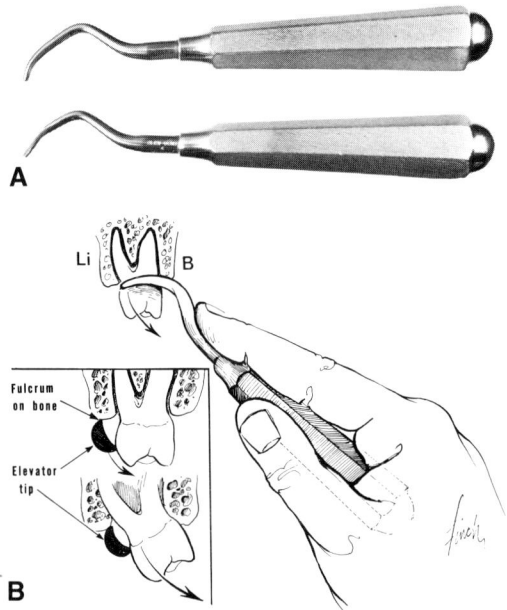

the alveolar bone, displacing the root tip by wedge action (Fig. 8-27). The larger size and strength of the 46 and 34 elevators make them more useful for the posterior teeth.

The 3 and 4 elevators are designed specifically for the luxation of the upper third molars (Fig. 8-28A). The blade is placed between the alveolar crest and the mesial surface of the third molar. The gingival

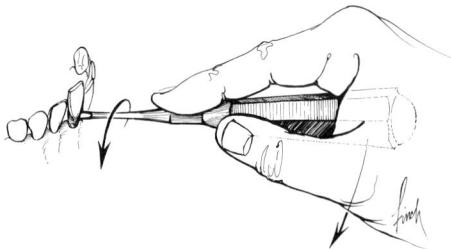

A

B

FIG. 8-28. *(A) No. 3 (top) and no. 4 (bottom) displacement elevators for removal of maxillary third molars. (B) Nos. 3 and 4 displacement elevators are used in an arc-like movement to elevate maxillary third molars.*

FIG. 8-26. *The 301 elevator used to luxate an anterior tooth.*

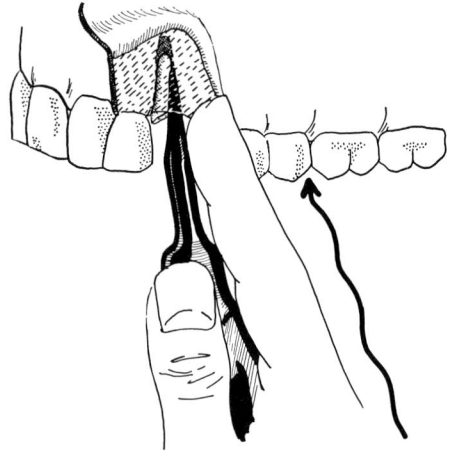

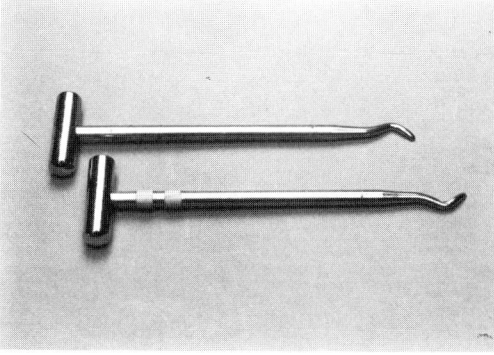

FIG. 8-29. *Potts elevators, right and left. (Walter Lorenz Surgical Instruments, Inc.)*

3 and 4, displacement elevators, in that the superior edge of the instrument is engaged into the tooth for removal. This particular instrument has limited use in that the short working surface of the elevator does not lend itself for good application when the impacted tooth is quite high (Fig. 8-29).

The 190 and 191 elevators have an offset shank to facilitate access to the lower molar roots (Fig. 8-30). These elevators are designed primarily for the recovery of lower molar root tips that have been fractured during the extraction of the tooth. For example, if the crown and distal root of a lower right molar are delivered, and the mesial root remains in the socket, the blade of the 190 elevator is inserted into the distal socket and rotated so that the point moves toward the apex of the mesial root and occlusally brings the root with it (Fig. 8-31A). The Cryer elevator is a similarly designed instrument, but to be effective, must be sharp (Fig. 8-31B and C).

The oral surgeon must adhere to certain basic precautions when using elevators.

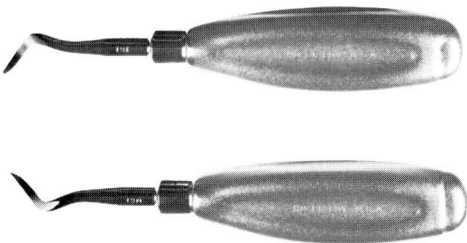

A

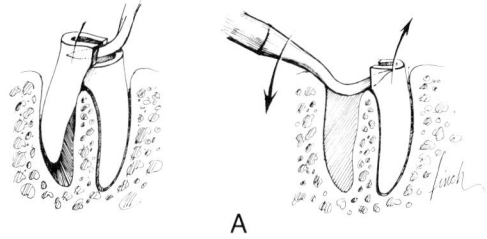

B

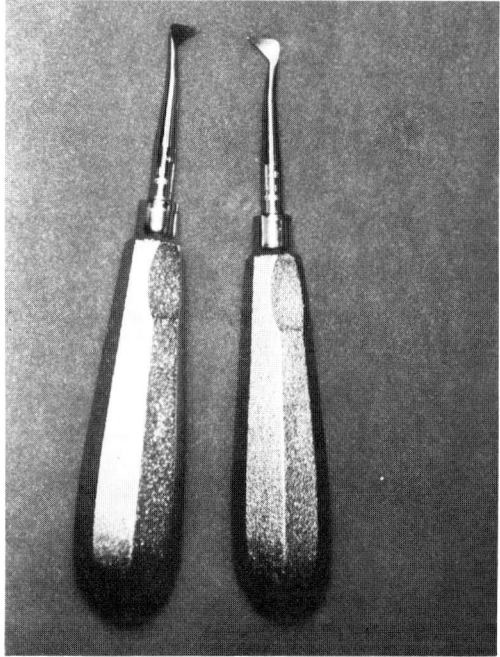

C

FIG. 8-31. *(A) Using 190 and 191 elevators to remove molar roots. (B) Cryer root elevators. (Hu-Friedy) (C) Cryer elevator—close-up view of the working blade. (Hu-Friedy)*

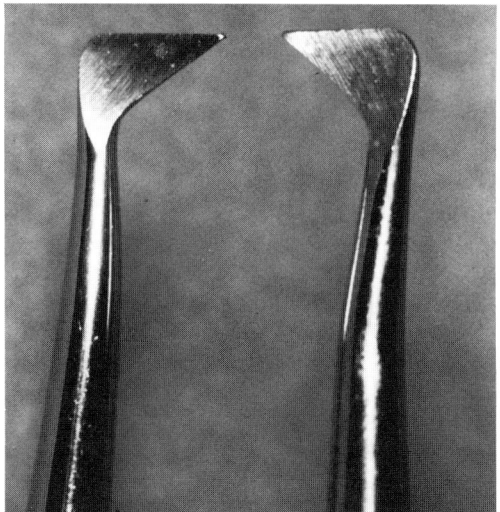

FIG. 8-30. *No. 190 (bottom) and no. 191 (top) elevators.*

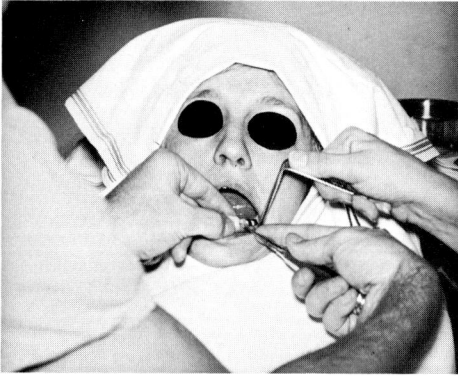

FIG. 8-32. *Use of the straight elevator, showing finger protection on lingual and elevator grasp.*

Proper application of elevator position, direction, and force is essential to prevent damage to the adjacent teeth, the alveolar process, and the mandible or maxilla. The danger of damage to adjacent tissues may be minimized by placing a finger along the shaft of the elevator and another on the lingual to act as stops in the event of a slip (Fig. 8-32).

Rongeur Forceps

The rongeur is a forceps-like instrument used to remove bone by shearing on a planing action. There are basically two types; the side-cutting rongeur and the end-biting rongeur (Figs. 8-33 and 8-34).

The end-biting rongeur is good for enlarging the bony wall of a cyst or the antrum, removing the peripheral bone by its biting action. It is also helpful in performing an alveolectomy. Occasionally, it can be used to remove heavy fibrous tissue attachments, such as a pericoronal sac or scar tissue masses posterior to the third molar area. Finally, this instrument may be used to extract a portion of a tooth when the specific biting action of the rongeur is needed.

The side-cutting rongeur is ideal for alveolectomy procedures. It should be used in a horizontal position with one of the biting edges of the forceps locked high on the alveolus while the other blade is brought to it in a planing action. This provides a controlled reduction of the excessive bone and creates less fracture or breakage of large amounts of bone. It is especially useful for

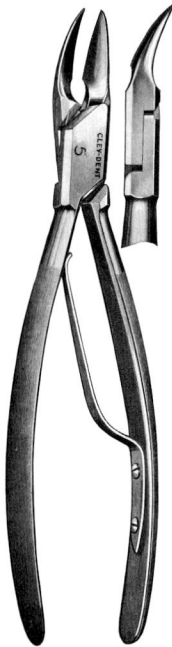

FIG. 8-33. *Side-cutting rongeur. (Cleveland Dental Mfg. Co.)*

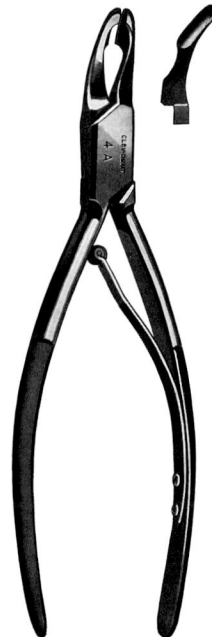

FIG. 8-34. *End-biting blunt-nosed rongeur. (Cleveland Dental Mfg. Co.)*

approaching a root by inserting its spear-pointed blade into a socket to remove a portion of the socket wall.

Whenever the rongeur is used, a constant cleaning of the blades is necessary. The operator holds the instrument with open beaks toward the assistant after each rongeuring action, and the assistant wipes them clean with a gauze sponge. The rongeur is a radical instrument that reduces large amounts of bone rapidly. However, when used carefully with good judgment, it serves the surgeon well.

Bone File or Rasp

The bone file or rasp (Fig. 8-35) is used for final trimming of the bony ridge after gross removal with the rongeur. Filing should follow use of the rongeur. The file should be placed high on the interseptal crest and, using the pull stroke, drawn toward the crest. Cross filing should be avoided because it tends to fracture the small and unsupported interseptal bone. Careful cleansing of the instrument is necessary; the assistant wipes the grooved ends with a sponge. Bone dust or chips may easily remain in the wound if careful cleansing is not done after each stroke or when filing is completed.

Gilmore Probe

The Gilmore probe is a surgical explorer. A slender instrument, it can be broken easily. No leverage should be applied to it. It explores and teases out small root tips near such structures as the inferior alveolar canal and the lining membrane of the antrum (Fig. 8-36). Remember that this is a sharp and dangerous instrument and can penetrate and injure these same structures.

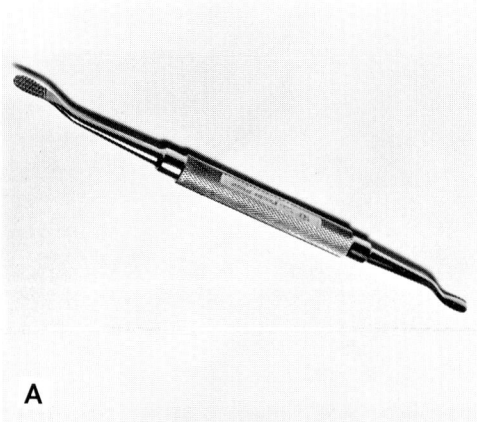

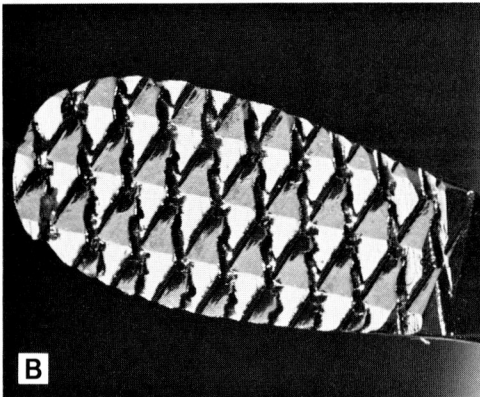

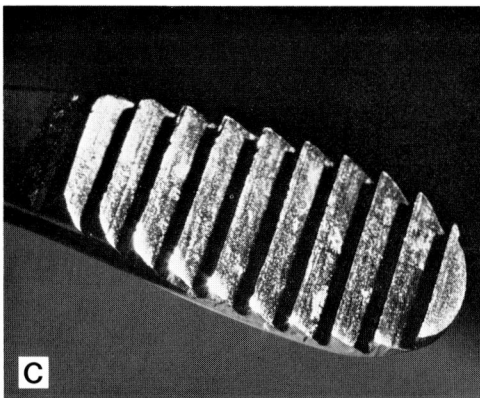

FIG. 8-35. (A, B, and C) Bone file or rasp.

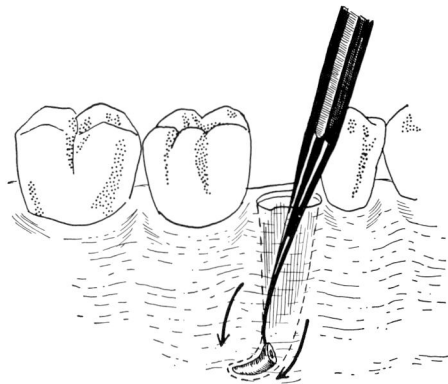

FIG. 8-36. Method of teasing out loosened root tip with Gilmore probe. (From: Clark, Practical Oral Surgery, Lea & Febiger, 1965)

Double-Ended Curette

The double-ended curette is available in small, medium, and large sizes. It explores the apices of sockets and enucleates granulomas, soft tissue tumors, cysts, and the like. The curette is a sensitive instrument designed to reveal to the surgeon the quality of the structures with which it comes in contact. When one becomes skilled in using this instrument, he can differentiate bone tissue from tooth structure and, of course, soft tissue.

When curetting the apices of a tooth socket, place the concave aspect of the curette near the superior edge of the socket wall and push the contents apically, following around the entire socket wall with this same movement. The total apical contents can then be drawn toward the surface in a scooping fashion until the socket is clean (Fig. 8-37).

Scissors

Although a great variety of scissors are available to the surgeon, two main types—

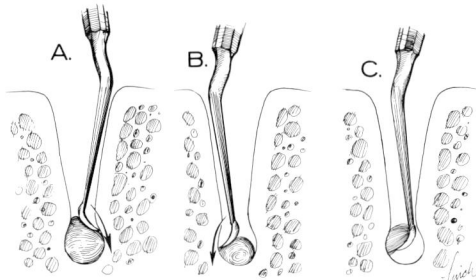

FIG. 8-37. *Proper use of the curette.*

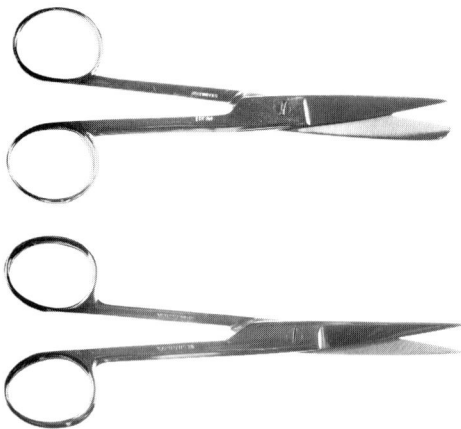

FIG. 8-38. *Curved and straight 6-inch scissors.*

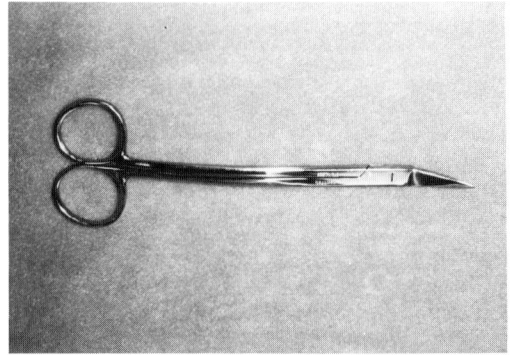

FIG. 8-39. *Dean scissors. Note angle of the blade. (Hu-Friedy)*

referred to as the suture scissors and the tissue scissors—are in general use (Fig. 8-38). The curved Mayo 6-inch scissors with two sharp points works well for dissecting and trimming wound margins. When trimming tissue margins, it is best to immobilize the tissue by means of the tissue forceps, permitting accurate and careful trimming.

The Dean scissors is another common scissors used for oral surgery techniques. It is a little longer-handled instrument, and the cutting surface is at an angle from the body of the instrument to permit easy access to the tissues in the oral cavity (Fig. 8-39).

When dissecting or undermining with the scissors, the incised margins are again immobilized with the skin hook or forceps and the scissors are inserted in the closed position and forcibly spread apart (Fig. 8-40). The purpose of this technique is to bluntly dissect the tissues with minimal hemorrhage or risk of cutting significant anatomic structures. Undermining is often done to permit advancement of tissue to a new location, and to lessen tension as a flap is sutured into its new position.

Although tissue scissors can also be used for sutures in many instances, the specific suture scissors is a straight-bladed instrument with a Mayo 6-inch blunt surface and one sharp point that permits the assistant to slide the blade down the suture strand until it stops on the knot, at which point the suture is cut. This is especially important for sutures that are to remain deep in the wound without a long tail.

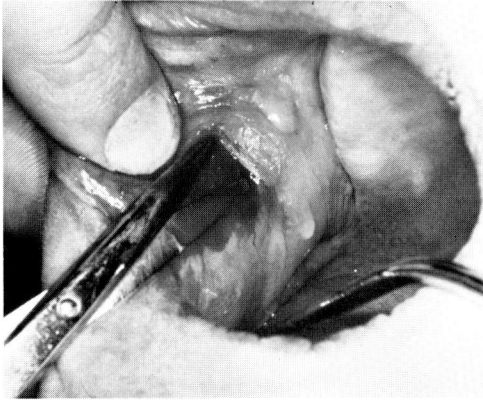

FIG. 8-40. *After excisional biopsy of the left paries, scissors is used to undermine the tissue flaps for closure.*

Tissue or Sponge Forceps

The forceps is a versatile instrument, and the operator should have the thumb forceps in hand at all times during suturing. Tissue forceps are used to immobilize the tissue when the needle is passed through it. Several types are available; however, the Rochester oral tissue forceps is a good general one for oral surgical use. In addition, there are small O'Brien tissue forceps without teeth, the nasal dressing forceps (a bayonet-type instrument), the cotton pliers for the placement of dressings in sockets, and the tissue forceps with sharp teeth. The Allis clamp is also used for handling tissue (Fig. 8-41).

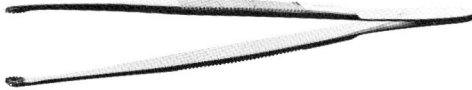

A

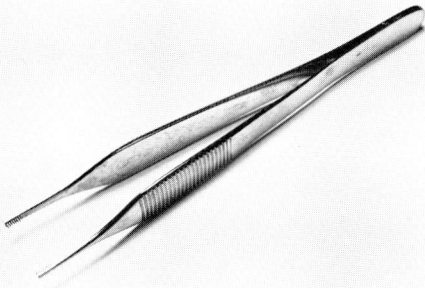

B

Suture, Needle, and Needle Holder

Specifications

For suturing oral mucosae, use 3-0 or 4-0 black silk. This material is treated to be serum proof and braided to resist coiling and snarling. Nonabsorbable suture mate-

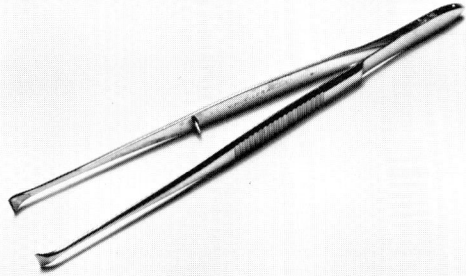

C

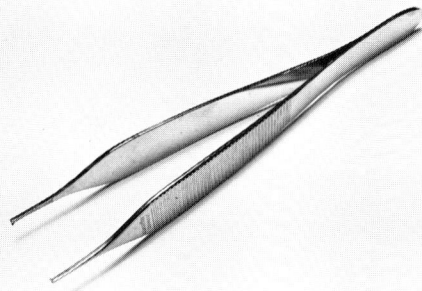

D

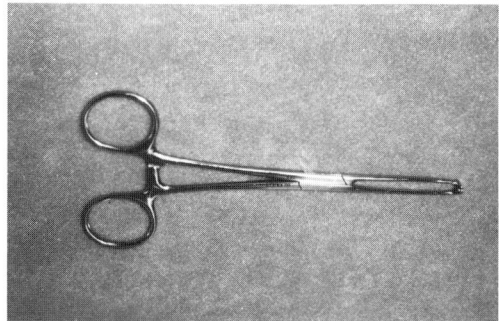

E

FIG. 8-41. *(A) Rochester Russian tissue forceps, 6 inches. (B) Brown-Adson side-grasping forceps. (C) O'Brien fixation forceps. (D) Adson forceps with mouth tooth. (E) Allis tissue forceps. (Walter Lorenz Surgical Instruments, Inc.)*

rial has uniform tensile strength whether wet or dry, lending itself well to the time-saving technique of instrument tying of knots. The stitches are easily seen when the patient returns for their removal. One reason for using nonabsorbable material is to bring the patient back for the all-important postoperative "look." For tying bleeders or closing muscles or fascia, use Pycktanin catgut, plain type A, 000, or chromic or plain catgut, size 000.

The needle should have a cutting edge for suturing mucosae; use Anchor brand 1822-18 (large) or 1822-20 (small), or Hu-Friedy three-eighths circle, size 18 or 20. Use a round (noncutting) needle for stitch tying or closing muscle or fascia: Anchor brand 1833, no. 2 or 3.

For all purposes, use the Hegar-Mayo needle holder, 6 inches long.

The needle is always grapsed just ahead of the eye to give maximal length of the needle for passing through tissue. Needles are readily broken when grasped on the eye (Fig. 8-42).

The needle holder is grasped the same way, with just the tip of the thumb through one ring, one phalanx of the fourth finger through the other ring, and the index finger braced against the shaft, halfway down. The other fingers close on the instrument in a natural position, giving a secure grasp, but one that permits instant dropping of the instrument when all fingers are straightened (Fig. 8-43). (The same grasp is used for hemostatic forceps.) The palm grasp for suturing is also used and, in the experienced hand, provides more rapid manipulation.

Technique for Suturing Oral Mucosae

The tissue is immobilized with a tissue forceps and the needle thrust through at

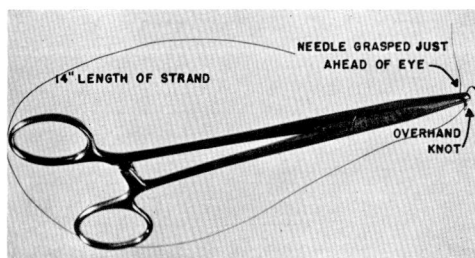

FIG. 8-42. *Needle, suture, and needle holder. (From: Clark, Practical Oral Surgery, Lea & Febiger, 1965)*

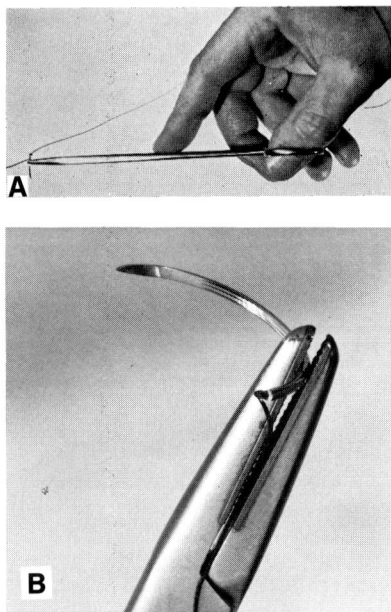

FIG. 8-43. *(A) Proper grasp of needle holder. (From: Clark, Practical Oral Surgery, Lea & Febiger, 1965) (B) Needle is grasped with the needle holder at the junction of the middle posterior third of the needle.*

right angles to the surface, ¼ inch from the edge of the incised wound. The motion then becomes curved, since the needle is curved. The stitch should be arranged so that it crosses at right angles to the line of closure. When first learning to suture, it is best to go through each side of the wound with separate bites of tissue. With more experience, opportunities will be found to pass through both sides with one stroke.

After the first thrust of the needle, the shaft should emerge enough so that the beaks of the needle holder can grasp it back of the point. The delicate tip of the needle is easily broken or bent by rough handling. The needle is drawn through the tissue with a curved motion. With the second side of the wound immobilized, this same procedure is repeated. The knot is then completed as a square knot or surgeon's tie (Fig. 8-44).

Figure 8 Stitch to Control Bleeding (Stitch Tie)

Direct clamping of a bleeding vessel with a hemostat is preferred, but if this cannot be done due to inadequate facilities in an emergency, this method is acceptable and effective: the probable location of the

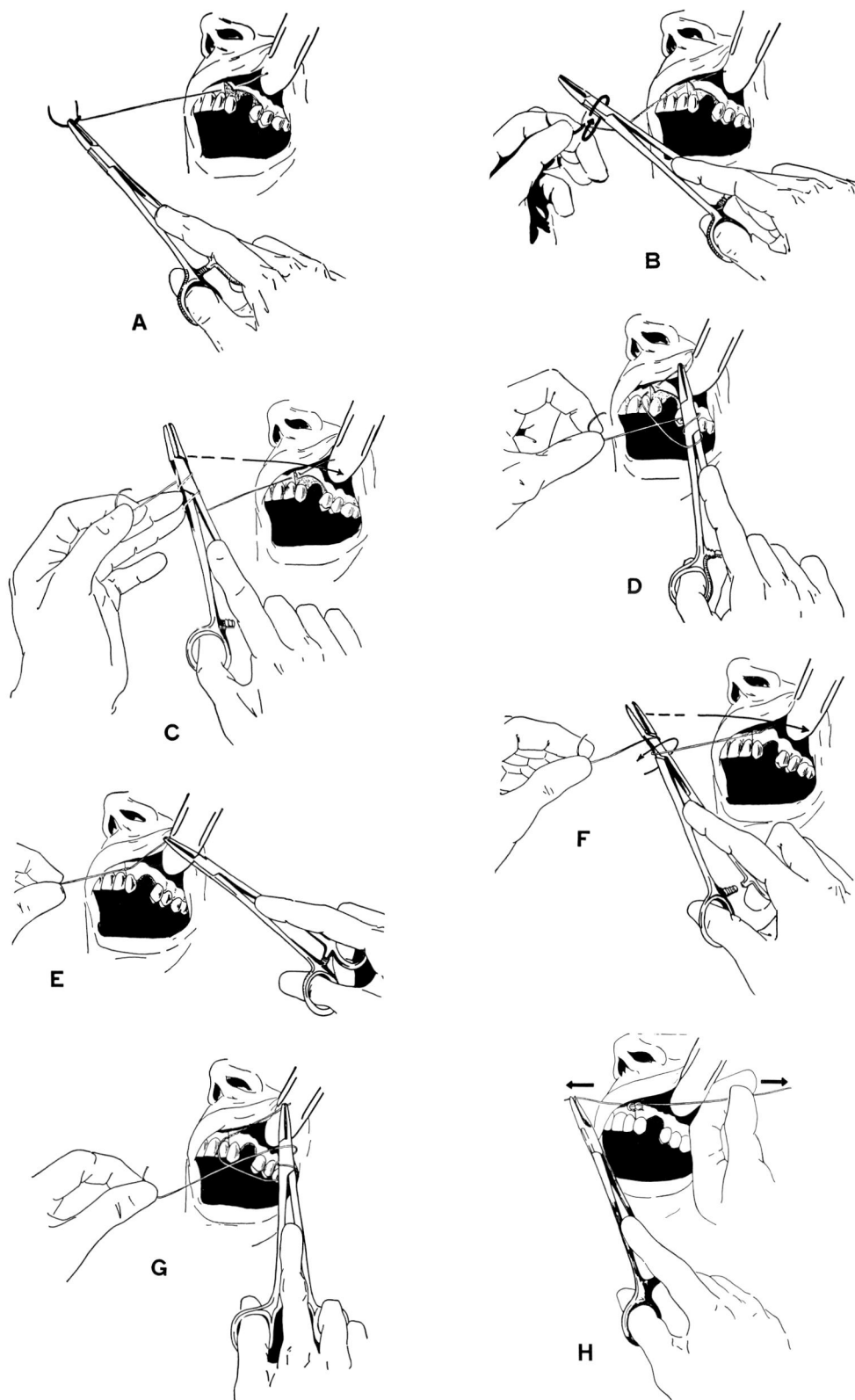

FIG. 8-44. *Instrument tie of the surgeon's knot. (A) Ready to tie the knot. Assistant retracts and holds back lip or cheek. Unlock needle holder, grasp needle between left thumb and forefinger (where it remains for the entire knot tie), pull forward until only 1 inch of suture remains. (B) Place needle holder on top of the long strand of suture (Legend continues on Page 108.)*

FIG. 8-44 Continued.
and pointed up, toward the left shoulder. *Wrap needle holder around the long strand two complete turns (clockwise—to the right). (C) With the left middle finger, stroke coils toward ring handles to keep suture away from box lock. Steady needle holder on left middle finger, carry open jaws of needle holder to the very tip of the short end. (D) Grasp the tip of the short end and lock needle holder. (Grasping short strand in the middle will produce a bow knot.) (E) Draw coils off of needle holder by pulling on the long strand. Keep short end 1 inch long. Direct short end toward the throat and pull long strand toward you, adjusting knot to desired tightness. Release suture from needle holder. From here on, if both strands are kept slack at all times, the double wrap will prevent knot from loosening. (F) The second half of the tie is much like the first, but this time place the needle holder under the long strand, point it toward the left shoulder, wrap it around only once (counterclockwise—to the left). (G) Repeat steps C and D as before. (H) Draw coils off the needle holder by pulling on the long strand. Now you have a choice: (1) To form the surgeon's knot shown in the picture, draw the short end forward and the long end to the rear, or (2) again direct the short end toward the throat and draw the long end toward you. Opinions differ on the best technique for finishing the knot. Some prefer to draw the short end forward and the long end to the rear; this will produce the neat surgeon's knot shown in H. However I prefer to direct the short end to the rear both times. The great convenience of avoiding finger manipulation of suture material inside the mouth, especially in posterior areas, more than compensates for the altered appearance of the knot. In our experience knots made in the manner described fulfill the essential requirement of remaining tied for five to seven days. In either event, now give one or two tugs on the strands, pulling in opposite directions, away from the knot, to set it firmly. Gather everything into the left palm—equal tension on both strands, then cut both ¼ inch from the knot. Remove short piece from jaws of needle holder. Lock it on the needle just ahead of the eye in preparation for the next stitch. (From: Clark, Practical Oral Surgery, Lea & Febiger, 1965)*

bleeding vessel is estimated and the needle passed deeply through both edges of the wound slightly ahead of the bleeder. Another generous "bite" is taken through both sides of the wound slightly behind the bleeder (Fig. 8-45). The suture is pulled up snugly and tied with a surgeon's knot, somewhat tighter than for an ordinary interrupted stitch.

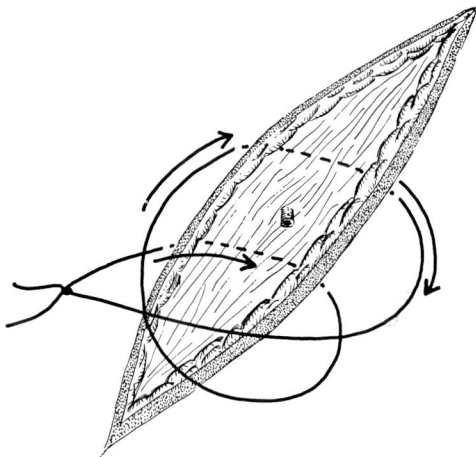

FIG. 8-45. *Figure 8 stitch tie. (From: Clark, Practical Oral Surgery, Lea & Febiger, 1965)*

Mattress Stitch

There are two types of mattress stitch: the horizontal and the vertical (Fig. 8-46).

The mattress stitch is used to produce slight eversion of wound edges or to provide more absolute apposition of two raw surfaces, as in closure of an oroantral fistula. The wound margins are considered as near and far edges. The needle is passed through the margins in the following sequence; near, far, far, near. The vertical mattress suture usually is used when more tension is needed. The suture is tied with a surgeon's knot.

Traction Suture

Occasionally, when the steel retractor cannot be used, this atraumatic, nonslipping method of securing retraction can be used to good effect. The cutting edge needle is passed through the flap margin, ¼ inch from the edge. The double strand of suture material is grasped with a hemostat attached (Fig. 8-47).

Use of Absorbable Suture Material

For Tying Bleeders. Refer to the section describing the hemostat. The catgut is held in the two hands and passed completely around the clamped vessel. The first half

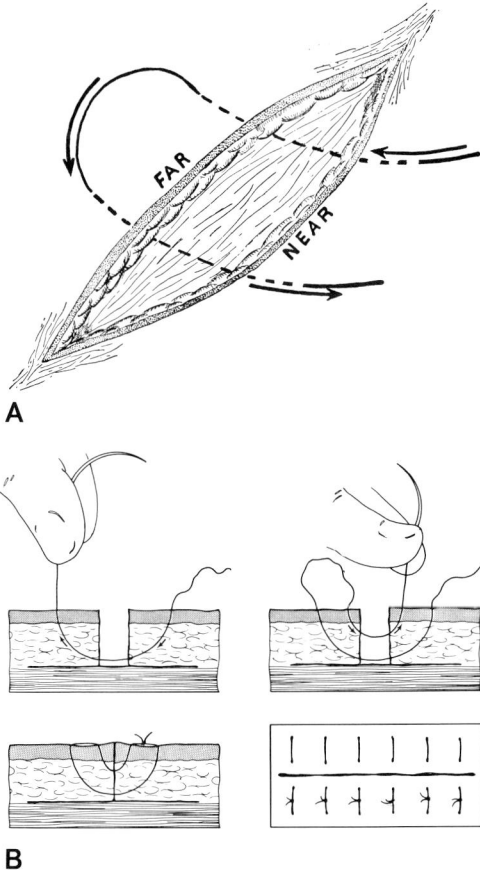

A

B

FIG. 8-46. *(A) Mattress stitch. (From: Clark, Practical Oral Surgery, Lea & Febiger, 1965) (B) Vertical mattress stitch.*

of the surgeon's knot is tied and tension maintained while the assistant carefully opens and removes the hemostat. This step seats the knot on the stalk of the vessel where it has been crushed. With care not to jerk the strands and thus loosen the knot, the second half is tied tightly and the ends cut approximately ⅛ inch long.

The instrument tie may be used, but well-soaked catgut will often cut through when grasped with the needle holder or hemostat. If the bleeding vessel is difficult to clamp and tie, the figure 8 stitch tie, using a round (noncutting) needle, may be employed.

For Closing Muscle or Fascia. The catgut is threaded on a round (noncutting) needle, leaving one long and one somewhat shorter strand. Because of the greater friability of catgut, it is usually not practicable to secure it to the needle with an overhand knot. The fascial or muscle margin is immobilized with a traction hook or tissue forceps. Ample bites of tissue, at least ¼ inch from the wound margin, are taken. The catgut is tied by hand, with the surgeon's knot.

If the initial passage of the needle is made from beneath upward and the second passage from superficial to deep surface of the tissue, the resulting knot will come to rest in the depth of the wound so that there will be no projecting ends of suture material (Fig. 8-48).

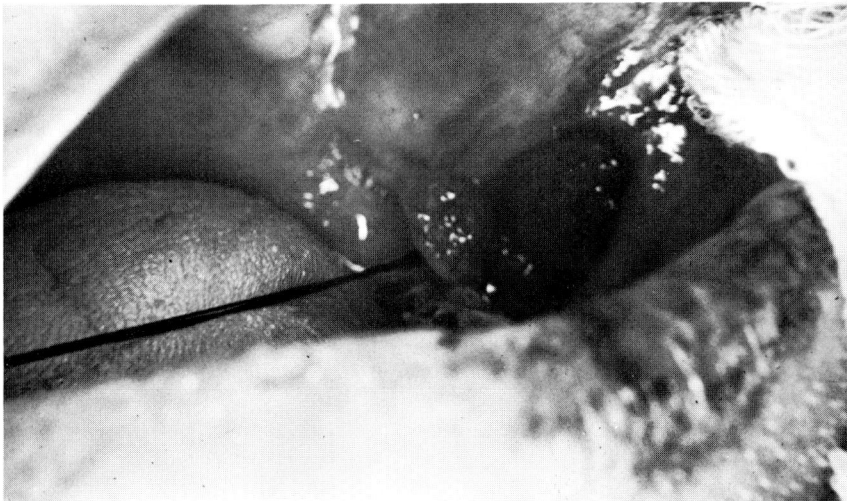

FIG. 8-47. *Traction suture.*

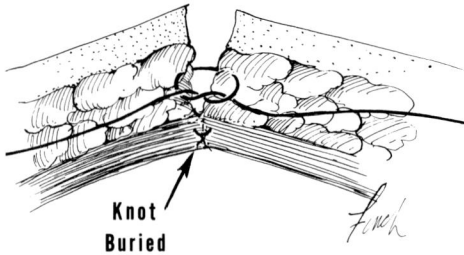

FIG. 8-48. *Method of keeping the knot near the depth of the wound.*

quickly into position while the tissue is still blanched to grasp the bit of the tissue that appears to be bleeding. The bleeding vessel can then be tied beneath the hemostat or, in many instances, the hemostat can be left in position during the operative procedure and the hemorrhage controlled at the tissues as they are sutured into position. The hemostat is also used to remove tooth fragments and root tips, and to grasp and hold tissues such as follicles or cyst membranes.

Hemostat

Although a large variety of hemostats are available for general hospital operating room procedures, the mosquito forceps and the Kelly forceps are generally used for intraoral use (Fig. 8-49). These come in both straight and curved designs. The Allis forceps is good for grasping tissue margins during dissection, and in some cases, retraction of the tissue segment that is to be removed.

When a hemostat is used to control bleeding, the area is first compressed with a gauze sponge and, as the assistant retracts the sponge from the previously bleeding site, the hemostat is moved

Aspirator

The aspirator is a necessary piece of equipment in oral surgery. The Frazier suction tip and the Hu-Friedy suction tip are excellent.

The assistant holds the aspirator in his left hand, freeing his right hand for retraction of tongue or lip as necessary (Fig. 8-50). Effective suctioning means keeping several areas of the oral cavity free of blood, saliva, and debris at all times. Saliva quickly pools in the floor of the mouth and near the tongue and soft palate. This area must be suctioned carefully without gagging the patient. The operative field is paramount, and it too must be kept clean with-

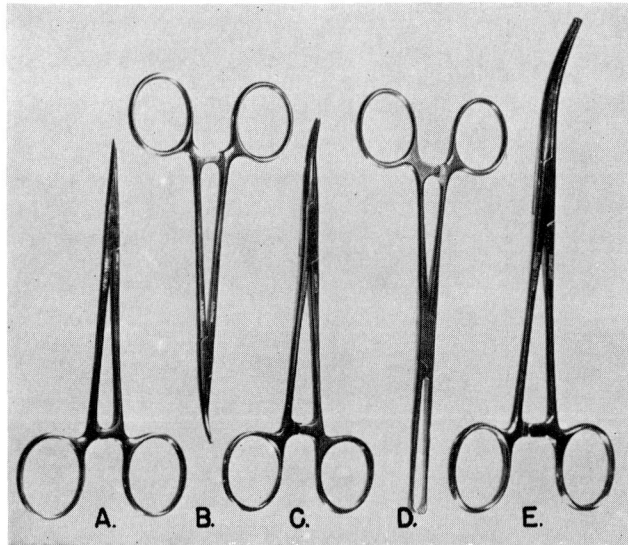

FIG. 8-49. *Various types of hemostats. (A) Straight mosquito. (B) Curved mosquito. (C) Curved Kelly. (D) Allis. (E) Carmault. (From: Clark, Practical Oral Surgery, Lea & Febiger, 1965)*

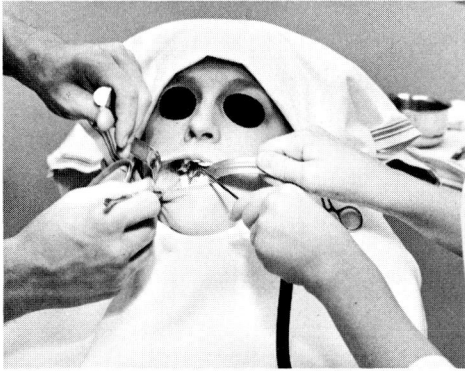

FIG. 8-50. *The assistant uses his right hand to hold the retractor and his left hand to aspirate.*

out interfering with the vision of the surgeon. Because the operator may occasionally see an immediate need for the suction which is not visible to the assistant, the assistant should be prepared to give up the aspirator to the surgeon quickly upon his indication and be ready to accept it from him in the same manner.

The assistant should be aware of the normal sound of the aspirator and able to detect when it is partially plugged or obstructed. Immediate freeing of the ob-

struction is necessary, which may necessitate the changing of the suction tip. These actions must be done quickly and efficiently. The effective use of the aspirator greatly increases the surgeon's efficiency and saves considerable time that otherwise might be utilized by the patient's attempting to use the cuspidor. Following surgery, good irrigation of the suction tip and its tubing prevents blood clotting and general clogging of this instrument.

Tooth Extraction Forceps

Although many kinds of extraction forceps are available, all are designed according to certain basic principles. In general, maxillary forceps are designed so that the beaks are in line with or parallel to the long axis of the handles, and mandibular forceps have the beaks at right angles to the handle. During extractions, every effort is made to keep the beaks of the forceps in line with the long axis of the tooth in order to minimize root fracture. The forceps may be designed to correspond to the anatomy

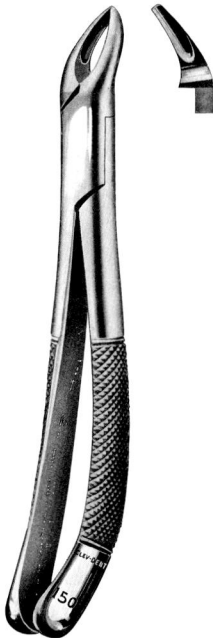

FIG. 8-51. *No. 150 forceps. (Clev-Dent, Div. of Cavitron Corp.)*

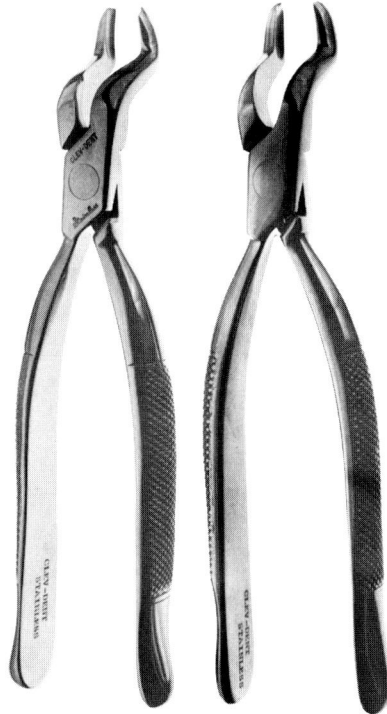

FIG. 8-52. *No. 53R and 53L forceps. (Clev-Dent, Div. of Cavitron Corp.)*

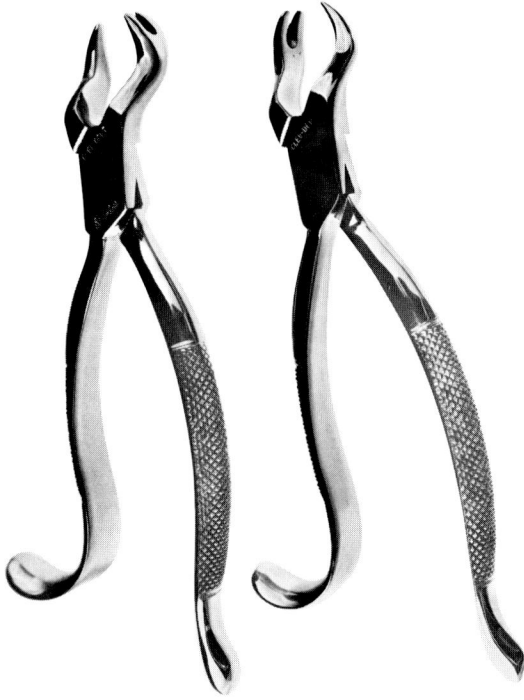

FIG. 8-53. *No. 88R and 88L forceps. (Clev-Dent, Div. of Cavitron Corp.)*

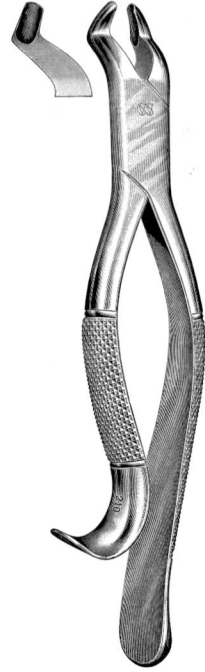

FIG. 8-54. *No. 210 forceps. (S.S. White Div., Penn-walt Corp.)*

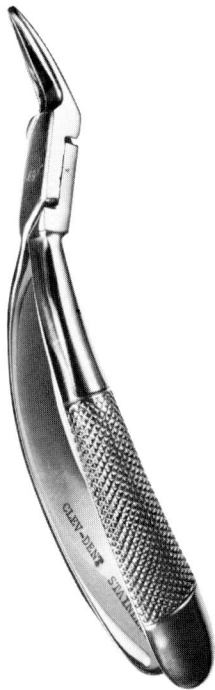

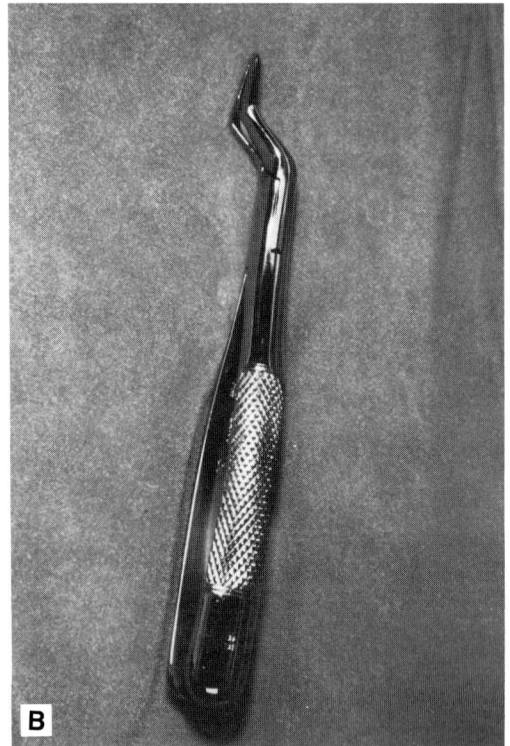

FIG. 8-55. *(A) No. 69 forceps. (Clev-Dent, Div. of Cavitron Corp.) (B) Bayonet root tip forceps. (Hu-Friedy)*

of particular teeth, or they may have a universal design.

The following are some examples of extraction forceps:

Clev-Dent (Stainless Steel) No. 150 (Fig. 8-51)—for maxillary incisors, cuspids, and bicuspids.

Clev-Dent (Stainless Steel) No. 53R and 53L (Fig. 8-52)—anatomic forceps for maxillary molars.

Clev-Dent (Stainless Steel) No. 88R and 88L (Fig. 8-53)—nonanatomic forceps used when alveolar application is necessary in the presence of severely carious crowns or when the forceps beaks fit the bifurcation of the roots.

S. S. White (Tarno) No. 210 (Fig. 8-54)—for maxillary third molars.

Clev-Dent (Stainless Steel) No. 69 (Fig. 8-55)—universal root spicule forceps for grasping a tooth when the crown has fractured leaving a small portion of the root available. Figure 8-55B demonstrates a similar forceps.

S. S. White (Tarno) No. 151 (Fig. 8-56)—for mandibular incisors, cuspids, and bicuspids.

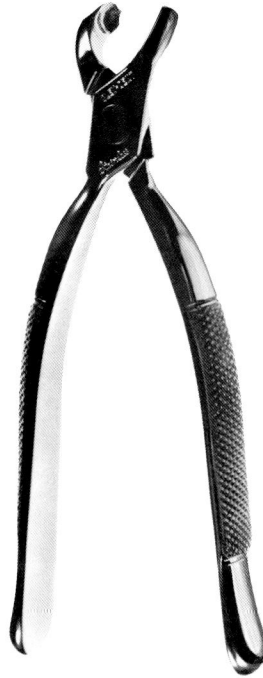

FIG. 8-57. *No. 17 forceps. (Clev-Dent, Div. of Cavitron Corp.)*

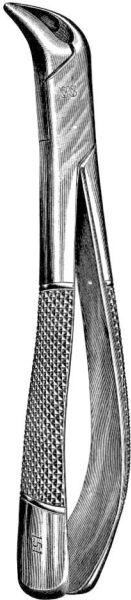

FIG. 8-56. *No. 151 American style forceps. (S.S. White Div., Pennwalt Corp.)*

Clev-Dent (Stainless Steel) No. 17 (Fig. 8-57)—anatomic forceps for mandibular molars.

Clev-Dent (Stainless Steel) No. 23 (Fig. 8-58A)—nonanatomic forceps for broken mandibular molars. Often referred to as cowhorn forceps. The Ash series of forceps is especially good for individual situations as in crowded dentition, but must be handled with considerable experience or fracture of the crown may occur (Fig. 8-58B).

S. S. White (Tarno) No. 101 (Fig. 8-59)—Universal forceps applicable for most deciduous extractions.

When using the extracting forceps, the operator will find the removal of the tooth less difficult if some luxation by means of an elevator has preceded the extraction movement. The forceps is applied to the tooth by means of the "application grasp" (Fig. 8-60). Apply the forceps beak to the most difficult surface first, which is usually the lingual; the ball of the hand forces the beak well on to the surface of the tooth beneath the gingiva. The buccal or labial

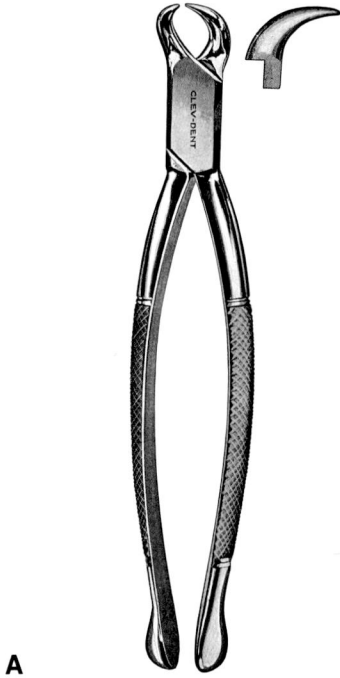

A

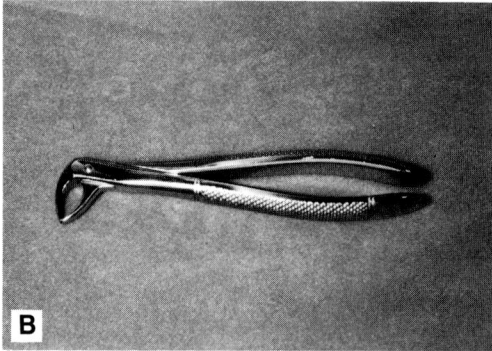

B

FIG. 8-58. *(A) No. 23 forceps. (Clev-Dent, Div. of Cavitron Corp.) (B) Ash forceps. (Walter Lorenz Surgical Instruments, Inc.)*

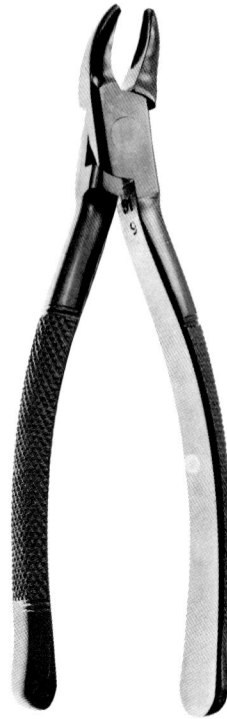

FIG. 8-59. *No. 101 forceps. (S.S. White Div., Pennwalt Corp.)*

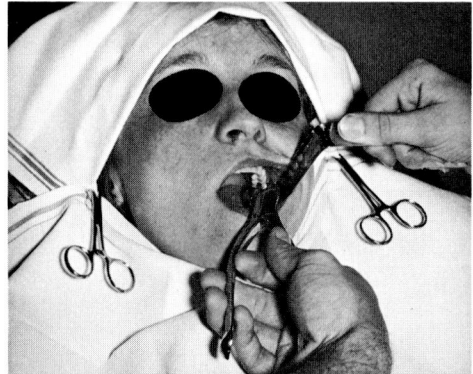

FIG. 8-60. *Application grasp. Note lingual beak seated firmly in the ball of hand.*

beak is then allowed to come into contact with the crown of the tooth, and the fingers encircle the handle to permit a firm grasp referred to as the "extraction grasp" (Fig. 8-61). A crushing force should be avoided, but firm and continuous pressure should be applied as the movements of the tooth extraction are developed.

Basic Forces Exerted During the Extraction of Teeth

A. Maxillary teeth
   1. Central incisors: Labial pressure with mesial rotation
   2. Lateral incisors: Labial pressure with mesial rotation
   3. Cuspids: Labial pressure with mesial

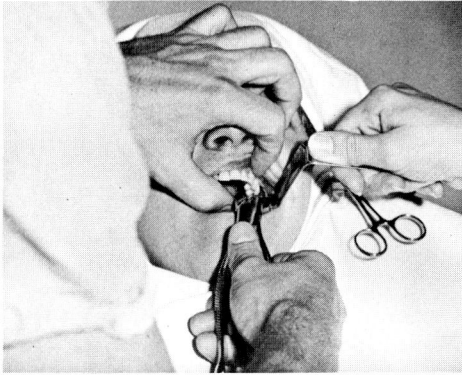

FIG. 8-61. *Extraction grasp. Note position of left hand.*

rotation and downward traction
4. First bicuspids: Slight buccal pressure, lingual pressure, slight rotation, and downward traction
5. Second bicuspids: Slight buccal pressure, lingual pressure, and downward traction
6. First molars: Buccal pressure, lingual pressure, remove to the buccal, with downward traction
7. Second molars: Buccal pressure, lingual pressure, remove to the buccal, with downward traction
8. Third molars: Buccal pressure, remove to the buccal

B. Mandibular Teeth
1. Central incisors: Labial pressure, lingual pressure, slight mesial and distal rotation, and upward movement
2. Lateral incisors: Labial pressure, lingual pressure, slight mesial and distal rotation, remove to the labial, with upward movement
3. Cuspids: Labial lingual movement with slight rotation and upward movement
4. First bicuspids: Buccal pressure with slight mesial distal rotation and upward movement
5. Second bicuspids: Buccal pressure, with slight mesial distal rotation, and upward movement
6. First molars: Buccal pressure, lingual pressure, remove to the buccal with upward movement
7. Second molars: Buccal pressure, lin-

gual pressure, remove to the buccal, with upward movement
8. Third molars: Buccal pressure, remove to the buccal or lingual

In all instances, traction is the final movement.

The patient should be seated comfortably with the head and cervical spine in line with the back. The chair should be tipped back one to two notches from the center. In general, the chair should be low for extractions of mandibular teeth and somewhat higher for maxillary teeth. The operator's elbow should be level with the surgical site. When the forceps has been appropriately applied, his left hand should grasp the alveolar process. Either the right front or right rear position can be used when appropriate (Figs. 8-62 and 8-63).

Before the first movement of the tooth is

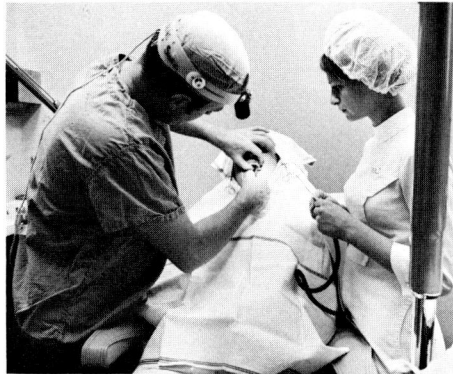

FIG. 8-62. *Right front position for extraction.*

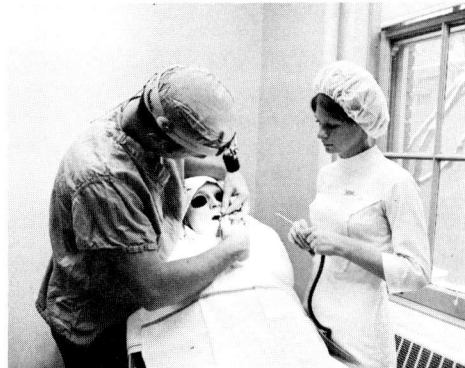

FIG. 8-63. *Right rear position for extraction.*

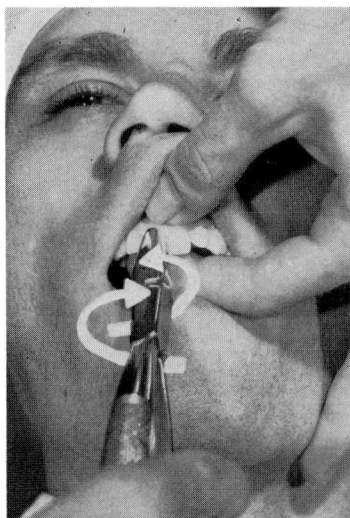

FIG. 8-64. *Extraction of upper anterior tooth (rotation emphasized). (From: Clark, Practical Oral Surgery, Lea & Febiger, 1965)*

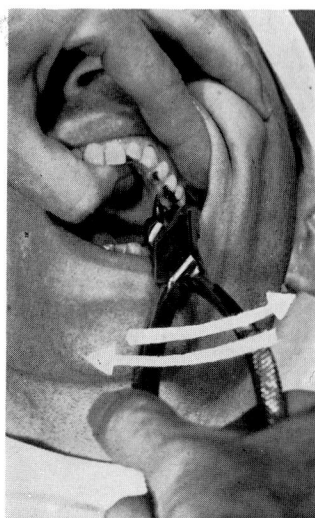

FIG. 8-66. *Extraction of upper molar (buccolingual movement emphasized). (From: Clark, Practical Oral Surgery, Lea & Febiger, 1965)*

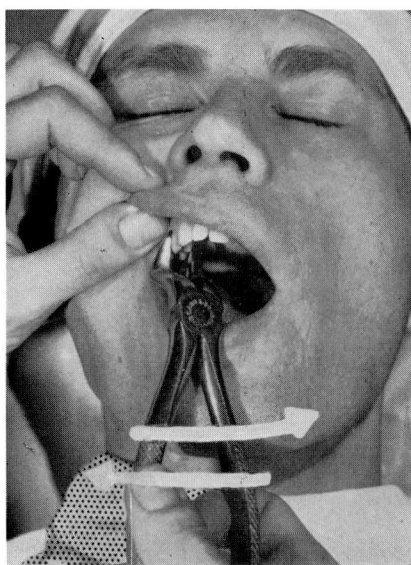

FIG. 8-65. *Extraction of upper bicuspid (buccolingual movement emphasized). (From: Clark, Practical Oral Surgery, Lea & Febiger, 1965)*

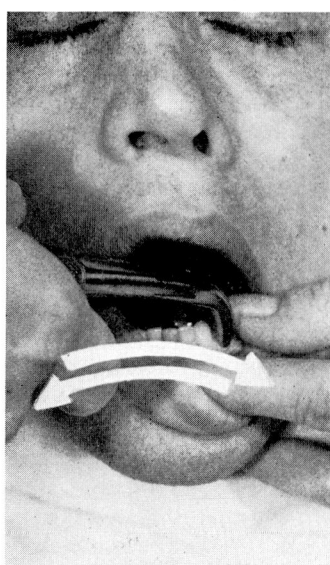

FIG. 8-67. *Extraction of lower bicuspid (rotation emphasized). (From: Clark, Practical Oral Surgery, Lea & Febiger, 1965)*

initiated, take a second look to be sure the forceps is on the right tooth to be extracted. The extraction movements are then instituted, depending on the anatomy of the tooth to be extracted. This, coupled with slight traction as luxation increases, should provide a smooth integrated extrac-tion procedure (Figs. 8-64 through 8-68).

Occasionally, a difficult molar extraction may be accomplished best by the use of no. 23 forceps (cowhorn) (Fig. 8-58A). The beaks of this forceps are round leading to a point, and the two points are inserted into the bifurcation of the tooth just beneath

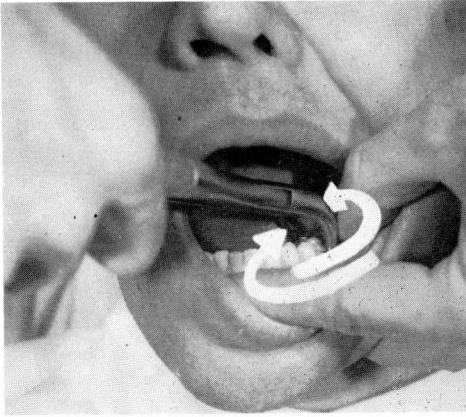

FIG. 8-68. *Extraction of lower molar with cowhorn forceps (handles rotated to give buccolingual movement of tooth). (From: Clark, Practical Oral Surgery, Lea & Febiger, 1965)*

the alveolar crest by gently squeezing the handles together. The instrument is then moved up and down, like a pump handle, which further seats the beaks into the bifurcation, lifting the tooth from its socket. The tooth is then inspected carefully to be sure it is intact, and the curette is used to explore the socket gently. Once the surgeon is satisfied of a clean wound, his thumb and forefinger compress firmly the socket walls expanded during the extraction procedure. Suturing of an uncomplicated extraction site is unnecessary. The procedure is complete when a small moistened gauze is placed over the extraction site and the patient is requested to hold it in position for 20 minutes. Appropriate postoperative instructions are then given.

CHAPTER 9

Multiple Extractions and Immediate Denture Surgery

Daniel E. Waite

For things we have to learn before we can do them, we learn by doing them. ARISTOTLE

Multiple Extractions

Regardless of the surgical procedure, the surgeon should have a definite routine for his evaluation and examination before initiating treatment. The patient's record and radiographic studies should be reviewed carefully at an appointment prior to the time of treatment. The patient's history should be coordinated with specific questions concerning any recent changes in his health status. Once the above have been satisfied, the patient should be seated comfortably in the chair. This usually means tipping back the chair 45 to 60° to give the patient the security of being seated well back into it (Fig. 9-1). When extracting teeth from the mandible, it is best to have the occlusal plane approximately parallel with the floor. For the extractions of the maxilla, the maxillary occlusal plane is best at a 45° angle with the floor. In any event, the patient should be comfortable, as should the operator.

The operator then systematically evaluates the work to be accomplished, deciding what anesthesia to use and meticulously examining the tooth or teeth to be extracted clinically and roentgenologically. Decisions must be made regarding soft tissue flap design and the potential need for bone removal. A general selection of instruments, including a choice of elevators and forceps, may also be considered. It is well to form a mental picture as to how one expects the case to proceed in terms of patient cooperation and of difficulties anticipated.

Operative Guidelines

To achieve uniform success in the technical side of oral surgery, it is important to develop good working habits. A habit is a custom or aptitude acquired by repetition and marked by facility of performance. Good working habits ensure good patient care.

As the prospective dentist contemplates a lifetime of operative work, he would do well to ponder the consequences of failing to operate systematically. Every act of the surgeon should advance the operation closer to its conclusion. An aimless, hit-and-miss approach to a surgical task becomes laborious, time consuming, and uncertain of result.

Some professionals feel it is undignified to standardize the method of caring for patients. Certainly, the total care of the patient cannot be carried through according to an ironclad plan because individual

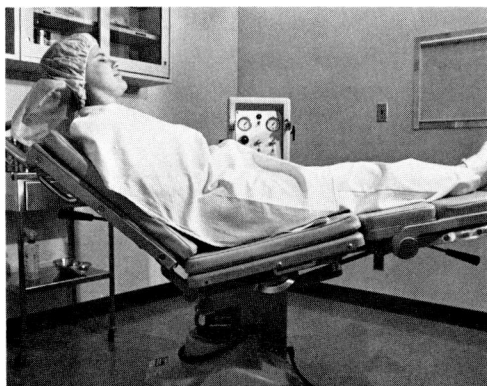

FIG. 9-1. *The chair should be tipped approximately 45 to 60° to allow for patient comfort.*

differences in cases are always present. However, areas of treatment lend themselves well to standard disciplines, and the thoughtful operator is prepared to apply these separate, individual skills to the surgical problem in proper sequence. Serious mishaps are rather uncommon in oral surgery and usually are avoidable. Wasted time, fatigue of the patient and operator, and substandard working conditions are far too common.

Increased efficiency takes effort, thought, and planning, but it is a goal that is worth working toward. As efficiency improves, a reduction in accidents, operating time, and trauma anticipated along with a proportionate increase in the pleasure of operating and in the surgical result.

In order to achieve more efficiency in operating, the following possible measures require consideration:

Assistance. Up to a certain point, competent assistance is necessary. This limit is seldom reached in practice because of the cost of salaries, the continual training of assistants, and unavoidable turnover.

Painstaking Preparation and Planning of Operation. A complete diagnosis—history, examination, radiographs, medical opinion, and the like—is mandatory. When indicated, a review of textbooks or periodical literature to determine the best procedure may be done.

Avoid Unnecessary Motions. This takes discipline, a methodical temperament, and means working in steps.

Working by Direct Vision. This is

achieved by adequate opening of the wound, maintaining a bloodless field, and having brilliant illumination on the field all the time.

H.B. Clark, Jr. has compiled all of these measures into a basic set of operating conditions known as "The Seven Minimum Essentials." Although originally adopted for tooth removal operations, they have come to be regarded as a checklist or set of standards for all oral surgical work, whether performed under local or general anesthesia, and whether conducted in the dental clinic or the hospital operating room.

THE SEVEN MINIMUM ESSENTIALS

R 1. *Radiograph*: a clear, recent radiograph of the tooth and some of the surrounding structures

A 2. *Anesthetic*: a suitable anesthetic agent for the task at hand

F 3. *Forceps and elevators*: appropriate for the teeth to be removed

F 4. *Flap tray*: a tray of instruments for performing flap operations, sterile and ready

L 5. *Light*: brilliant illumination on the site of operation 100 percent of the time. This is best achieved with the headlight (Fig. 9-2)

E 6. *Efficient assistance* throughout the entire operation, on every operation

S 7. *Suction aspiration*

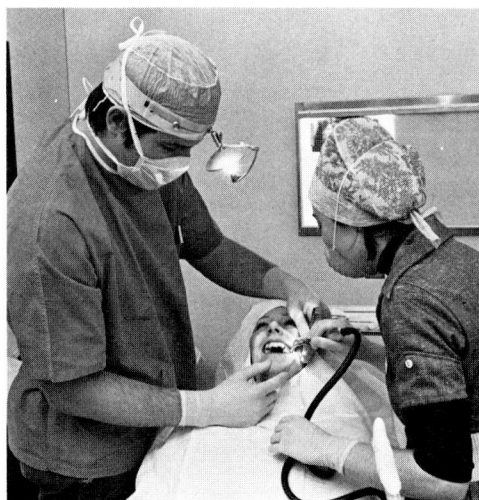

FIG. 9-2. *The headlight provides excellent illumination to the oral cavity.*

For ease in memorization, the initial letters have been arranged to form a key word: RAFFLES.

Radiograph. No tooth extraction operation should be attempted without a clear recent radiograph of the tooth and some of the surrounding area. Time taken to secure a good radiograph is not wasted; on the contrary, it is a good investment in safety and efficiency. The dentist must firmly believe in the principle of working from a good radiograph if he is to convince his patients that it is essential. Some patients are astonished at the thought of "wasting" an x-ray picture on a tooth that is about to be sacrificed. The dentist should refuse to operate if an understanding cannot be reached on this point.

Operating with the constant advantage of good preoperative radiographs affords many benefits. They give a good view of the shape, size, and curvature of the root; the density of bone; the presence of pathologic processes such as cysts, tumors, or fractures that may not have been suspected; and they verify the clinical diagnosis of the condition of the tooth itself in matters of depth of caries, location of pockets, and so forth. Be certain that the object of the surgery appears near the center of the film; do not be forced to read accurately the periphery of any radiograph (Fig. 9-3).

Anesthesia. The anesthetic agent used for an operation must be suitable for the case at hand. The dentist must make this decision; the patient's whim or demands must not be the deciding factor. It is a good

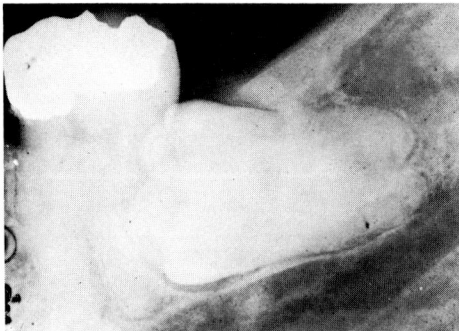

FIG. 9-3. *A good x-ray study of proper density and with the surgical object in the center of the film. One should not be forced to read the periphery of a film.*

plan to ask the patient if he has a preference for any particular agent, and if the choice is suitable, use it. On the other hand, if the patient and the operator disagree, the difference must be resolved. The following are indications for general anesthesia:

1. Children who are too young to adequately understand or who are extremely apprehensive.
2. Brief procedures, in the presence of acute infection, such as incision and drainage or the extraction of a single tooth.
3. Patients who are sensitive or allergic to some component of the local anesthetic solution.
4. Prolonged operations on patients whose physical or mental condition would be inadequate to give the surgeon ideal working conditions—these patients should be cared for by general anesthesia in the hospital operating room.

Forceps and Elevators. It is self-evident that, in the surgical removal of teeth, forceps and elevators must be available and ready for use. The choice of extraction instruments poses few problems when one has mastered the proper method of using each and knows those features of instrument design that afford greatest efficiency. Whenever possible, elevation of a tooth should be attempted, to make the extraction easier and less subject to root fracture.

Flap Tray. This is a standard rectangular surgical tray upon which are the instruments for reflecting a mucoperiosteal flap and performing the usual dentoalveolar surgery involved with the extraction of difficult teeth, recovering roots, alveoloplasty, and other procedures. Because the flap tray may not be needed for every extraction, it is not a part of the regular instrument setup. However, it should be in readiness at all times and added to the basic tray setup when needed (see Fig. 7-14).

Light. Brilliant illumination on the field of operation at all times is imperative. There are many rational arguments for the use of the headlight as the only instrument that can meet these criteria. It eliminates the possibility of shadows caused by the operator's head, and it permits variation of the direction of the beam when the patient's position changes or when a small cavity such as a tooth socket must be illuminated (Fig. 9-1).

To utilize the headlight adequately, the dentist should consider his individual practice and habit. From the standpoint of specialties such as oral surgery, otolarnygology, and ophthalmology, the headlight is a great help and should be used. However, in the general practice of dentistry, it is not customary to use the headlight routinely. Much oral surgery, therefore, will be done under the "regular" light. Good overhead lights are necessary for most general dental procedures and are generally a part of a good dental office.

Efficient Assistant. Attempting to do surgery alone is difficult and invites accidents, frustrations, and wasted energy. It is mandatory to use an assistant who is well-trained in the specific functions and hand motions that are required. The assistant is to:

1. Use the suction aspirator constantly to remove blood, saliva, and debris from the floor of the mouth, the dorsum of the tongue, the right and left retromolar areas, and the wound itself. If this duty is faithfully performed, the patient should never have to expectorate, and the operation proceeds more efficiently and with cleanliness. If the aspirator tip becomes plugged, one must instantly clear the obstruction with the stylet or reaming wire.
2. Use the water syringe (in conjunction with the aspirator) to cool the bur or clear debris or blood from the operative site. This should be done without a specific request from the operator.
3. Provide adequate retraction.
4. Reassure the patient in a pleasant, affirmative manner.

When scrubbed for an operation, the assistant must remain at chairside until completion of the procedure. An additional nonsterile attendant is highly desirable to answer the telephone, receive and discharge patients, make appointments, and procure items that might be needed during the operation. This person is referred to as a circulator.

Suction Aspirator. This is perhaps the greatest contribution to oral surgical technique in recent times. It provides an entirely new concept in operating. Formerly, many arm and hand motions of the operator or assistant were devoted to sponging with gauze or cotton. Use of the aspirator maintains a bloodless field effectively throughout the entire operation.

These "Seven Minimal Essentials" must be used for every oral surgical procedure. In the various operations described in subsequent chapters, it may always be assumed that these facilities are present and functioning. They are equally essential in the dental clinic, office, or hospital operating room.

Instruments

Nurses and dental assistants should know the exact instruments needed for a given operation and the order they should be placed on the tray. The habit of placing an instrument on the tray in the place from which it was picked up should be established. This will ensure a clean and orderly tray during an operation.

The instruments that should be on every tray when single extraction is indicated and a flap procedure not contemplated are shown in Figure 9-4. The instruments that should be included on the tray whenever two or more extractions and a flap procedure are indicated are shown in Figure 7-14.

Alveoloplasty

When difficulty with the extraction is anticipated, or two or more teeth are to be removed, an alveoloplasty may be necessary, including the reflection of the flap (Figs. 9-5 and 9-6). The terms alveolectomy and alveolotomy are often used synonymously with alveoloplasty, the more preferred term. The author defines alveolectomy as the appropriate reduction of the alveolus primarily for the reception of a prosthesis. An important consideration during the alveolectomy procedure is the conservative reduction of bone rather than the radical removal of it. Alveolotomy is defined as removal of specific portions of the alveolar bone to gain access, for example, to retained roots, residual areas of infections, or cysts.

One should mentally review the nerve and blood supply of the incision in order to provide the flap with the maximal blood supply. The incision should be kept on the

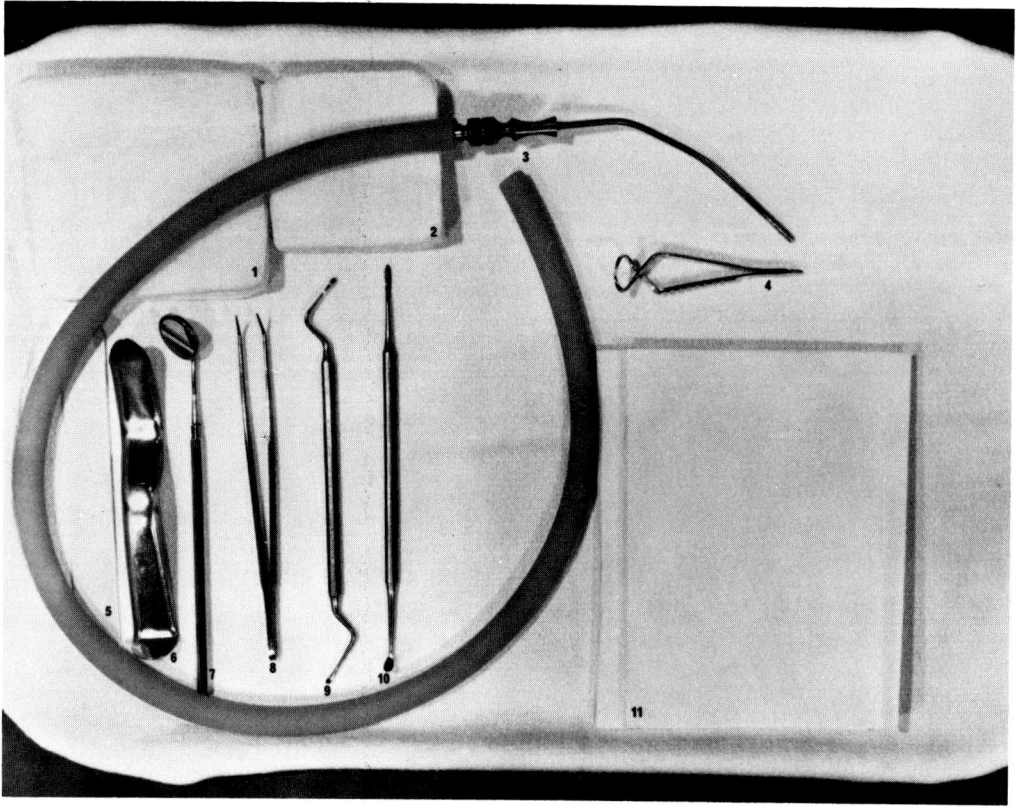

FIG. 9-4. *A basic tray should include 4" × 4" sponges (1); 3" × 3" sponges (2); suction (3); towel clip (4); tongue blade (5); retractor (6); mouth mirror (7); cotton pliers (8); double-ended curette (9); no. 1 Woodson elevator (10); pads to adjust light (11); and forceps and elevators according to the case.*

crest of the ridge whenever possible, and angle cuts are rarely necessary. The flap should always have a wider base than its three margins, and it should be wider than the anticipated bone defect. Once the surgical site has been exposed adequately, the alveolectomy should be done. If an alveoloplasty is indicated to remove thick cortical bone to ease the removal of the teeth, the excessive bone is reduced prior to the extraction by either chisel, rotating bur, or rongeur techniques (Fig. 9-7). If, however, the alveoloplasty must be done to remove gross undercuts or sharpness to the alveolar ridge in order to enhance the reception of the prosthesis, it should be completed following the extraction of the teeth. Under good visualization, bone is reduced in a controlled manner. If rongeurs are used, one blade is placed high on the crest of the ridge with the other blade beneath the undercut; a shaving or planing tech-

nique is used, bringing the one blade to the other (Fig. 9-8). Smoothing is done with bone rasps or files, the area carefully debrided by irrigation, and the flap returned. The entire area is then manually palpated so that no sharpness or loose fragments of bone remain.

When reviewing the tooth or teeth to be extracted, one should pay attention to the degree of caries, severe abrasion, or longstanding attrition that may be evident. In such instances, the root structure and bony relationships may make the extraction more difficult. If large fillings are present, it is wise to counsel the patient that one may hear a crumbling or grating noise which is slippage of the forceps. Should a large filling be adjacent to the tooth to be removed, fracture of it may be unavoidable (Fig. 9-9). In such anticipated instances, the patient should be advised of the possibility of a fracture of these restorations. It

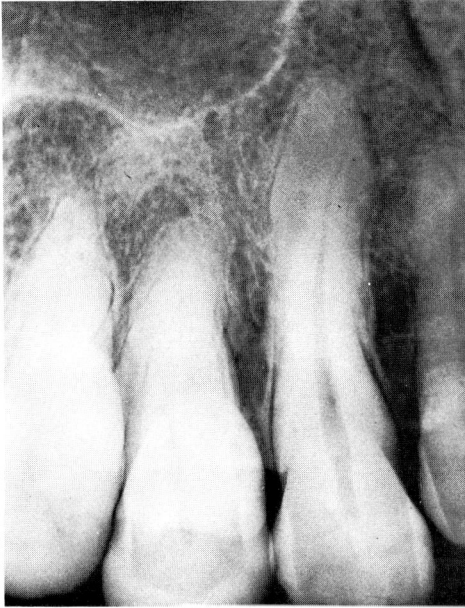

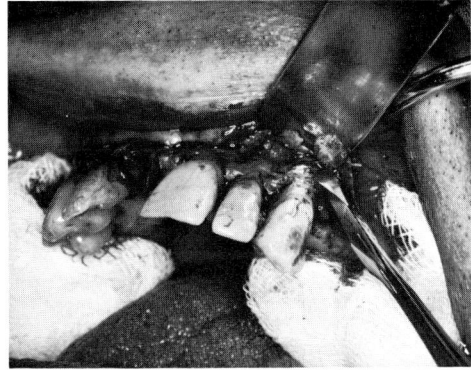

FIG. 9-7. *Envelope flap has been reflected. A bony prominence is evident over the cuspid, and is being reduced by chisel technique.*

FIG. 9-5. *Because of the bulbous curvature of the root of the cuspid, a difficult extraction is expected; therefore, a flap should be anticipated as well as possible root recovery and alveoloplasty.*

is important to review the size of the tooth and its roots, particularly if they have been distorted on the radiograph. The formation and number of roots, the possibility of root fracture, and the type of bone in regard to its density are matters for consideration that would create fewer surgical problems it they are reviewed in advance. The relationship of the tooth to the maxil-

lary sinus or the mandibular canal, and the presence of root canal fillings and large maxillary tuberosities may require a considerable change in the surgical approach (Fig. 9-10).

The examination should also include the supporting hard and soft tissues; low frenum attachments or complete loss of alveolar bone with deep gingival pockets would be significant (Fig. 9-11). The thickness of the labial or buccal cortical plates provides information as to the need for bone reduction. Bone density may also be judged by the age and size of the patient. Teeth are often less brittle in younger patients than in older ones; the bone permits

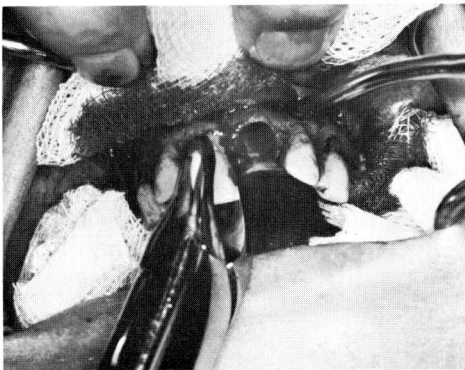

FIG. 9-6. *More than one tooth is being removed, and in order to smooth the alveolar margins and compress the expanded sockets, an alveoloplasty procedure should be anticipated.*

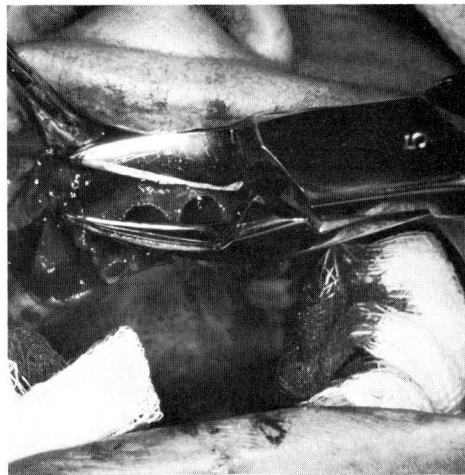

FIG. 9-8. *Bone reduction using no. 5 rongeur: the superior blade is locked on alveolar bone and the inferior blade is brought to it in a planing manner.*

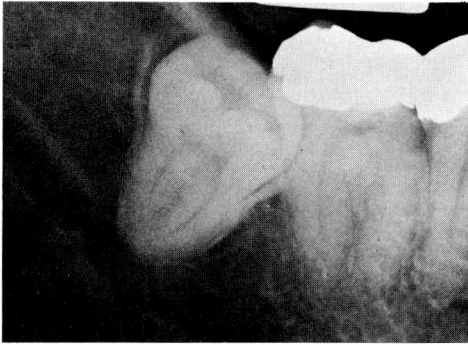

FIG. 9-9. *There is a large filling in the second molar; the third molar is to be extracted.*

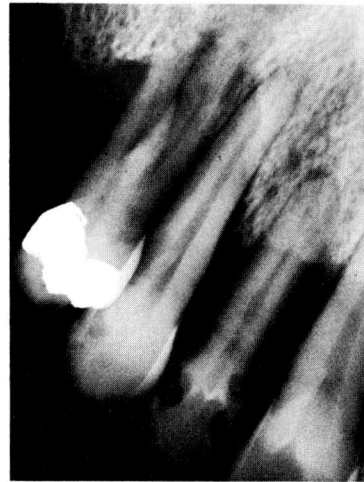

easier expansion of the sockets, and less root fracture occurs.

A technique for the reduction of buccal and labial alveolar undercuts removes the V-shaped area of bone between the buccal and lingual cortical plates. Once this intermedullary bone has been excised, firm pressure is used to collapse the labial and buccal plate toward the lingual plate. This

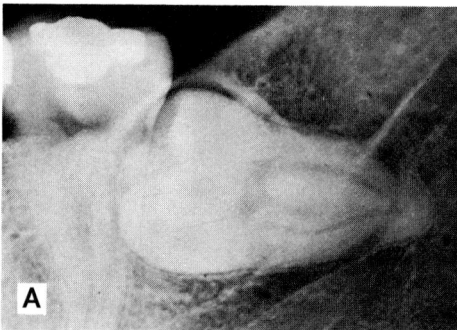

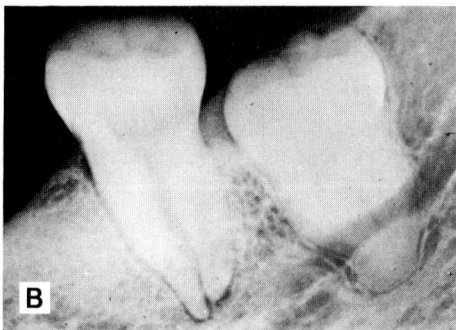

FIG. 9-10. *(A and B) Teeth impinging on the inferior alveolar canal make surgical delivery more difficult and increase the postoperative sequelae.*

FIG. 9-11. *Deep periodontal pocket formation changes the bony fulcrum, often making the extraction more susceptible to root fracture.*

creates a greenstick fracture high in the buccal or labial sulcus; sutures are used to hold the overlying lingual and buccal tissues together (Fig. 9-12). No mucoperiosteal flap is reflected in this procedure. Although the technique does accomplish the reduction of the undercuts and some bony irregularities while avoiding the reflection of the mucoperiosteal flap, it has some essential disadvantages:

1. A fracture is created in the alveolar bone, which we try to avoid as a basic principle.
2. Vital medullary bone, which contributes so much to the healing process, is sacrificed.
3. A sharp, knife-like edge on the ridge may result where the edges of the two cortical bone plates come together.
4. Because both of these plates consist of cortical bone, they are subject to resorption.

While this procedure may be less time consuming and causes less hemorrhage than the other methods, it is not routinely recommended for acceptable alveoloplasty.

The order of the extraction of teeth may be altered and dictated by individual cases, but basic guidelines can be stated. The surgery should be done in opposing quadrants when possible, maintaining the ante-

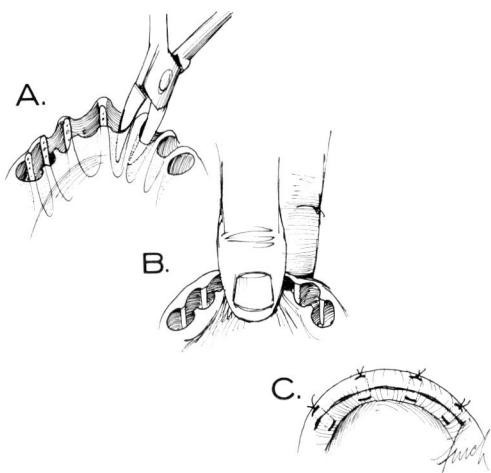

FIG. 9-12. *Intermedullary alveolectomy. (A) Excision of interseptal bone. (B) Compression of cortical plates. (C) Mattress sutures in place.*

rior teeth until the last surgical appointment. Extraction should begin with the most posterior tooth to be extracted, working toward the anterior. Complete each quadrant, including the alveoloplasty and suturing, before proceeding to another arch.

Immediate Denture Surgery

Prosthodontics and oral surgery become closely related in the management of immediate denture patients. The complexities inherent in the construction of the prosthetic appliance make it mandatory that every possible avenue be pursued to present the individual patient with a prosthesis that is both aesthetic and functional. Therein lies one of the major advantages of the immediate denture insertion technique. With this procedure, the anterior teeth are still present in the arch and serve as a guide to the correct and natural positioning of the artificial teeth. The surrounding oral structures are also maintained close to their normal position and vertical dimension. Less postoperative discomfort occurs because the prosthesis acts as a protecting splint. In addition, there is no period of edentulous adjustment—an important consideration for all patients, especially those who by necessity are constantly before the public.

Some disadvantages of immediate denture surgery are:

1. Earlier relining of the denture are necessary, and possibly a new prosthesis.
2. An increased number of office visits are necessary during the first few months.
3. Cost is increased with this type of management.

Prosthodontic Consideration

The most desirable plan is to remove the posterior teeth at an earlier appointment. Care should be taken to assure adequate surgical reduction of the tuberosity area in both vertical and lateral directions so that sufficient space exists for the base plate material and the posterior teeth. If possible, occlusal contacts should be maintained, thus preserving interarch distance during the healing period.

Obviously, appropriate methods of obtaining good impressions, casts, and complete jaw relation records are indicated. As has already been mentioned, the preservation of the exact relation of the teeth in the arch is of great value and advantage in the immediate denture service. Some of this relation may be lost unless the plaster teeth are removed one at a time and replaced by porcelain or plastic teeth. After outlining the gingival margin of the cast with a sharp pencil, remove the maxillary central incisor by cutting away the stone down to the outlined area (Fig. 9-13). Carefully envision the proposed extraction site and trim the stone socket accordingly. Arrange the prosthetic tooth as desired for esthetics and function. This is accomplished by observing the tooth from the incisal as well as from the labial. The adjacent teeth serve as an accurate guide for vertical position, mesiodistal inclination, and rotational position (Fig. 9-14). The stone teeth are removed and replaced one at a time until the anterior teeth are arranged. Once the teeth are set to the clinician's satisfaction, observe the cast for rough areas and any undercuts that may interfere with the path of insertion of the denture. The canine eminence and tuberosity regions can be especially troublesome. Remember, it is better to undertrim than to overtrim the cast.

Prior to the surgical appointment, the occlusion is corrected as much as possible before the processed dentures are removed from their casts. The labial flange

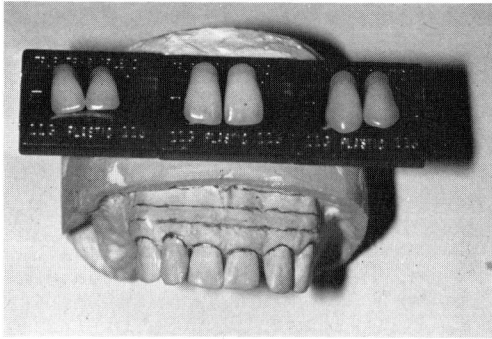

A

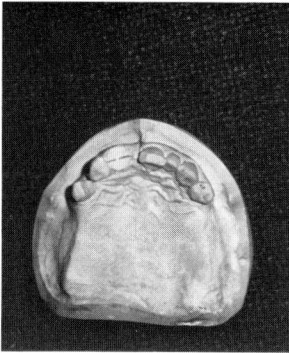

B

FIG. 9-13. *(A) Working cast for a guide in immediate denture surgery. Lines on the cast mark the vestibular depth and divide the labial flange into three equal widths. (B) One tooth at a time is removed from the stone cast. Trim undercuts and sharp areas only and carefully envision the proposed surgery.*

of the denture must be well-rounded, shortened, and thinned. The inner surface of the denture should also be recessed in the region where the socket prominences protrude. A surgical splint is constructed with clear acrylic, using as a model the stone casts from which the anterior teeth

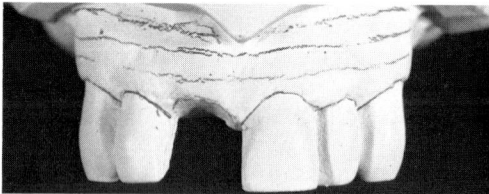

FIG. 9-14. *The prosthetic teeth are viewed from the incisal as they are placed, one at a time, on the stone cast.*

have been cut away and bony trimming simulated by scraping the casts (Fig. 9-14). The splint should be a full palatal splint to record accuracy during the surgical reduction and trimming of bone. The operation then consists of fitting the alveolar process and tissues to the previously constructed splint.

Surgical Procedure

Local anesthesia is injected in both the lingual and labial tissues. This not only supplies adequate anesthesia for patient comfort, but also aids in hemostasis. Premedicating drugs may be used to the great advantage of the surgeon in calming an anxious patient.

If a flap has to be raised during the operation, it should be done initially and conservatively. This permits better vision and access, especially for bone contouring and smoothing, and generally expedites the procedure (Fig. 9-15). Excessive reflection of the surgical flap can result in a potential loss of vestibular height and unnecessary swelling accompanied by hematoma under the tissue at the denture periphery. This would obviously be detrimental to the stability and retention of the prosthesis. The object is to prepare the mouth so that the denture can rest firmly upon normal tissue.

The teeth are then removed by the usual careful techniques, trying to prevent the fracture of the labial plate of bone. Chisels or burs may be used to remove a portion of the labial cortical bone especially in the canine region to help avoid bone fracture and the subsequent loss of this bone. The transparent surgical template is then placed in the mouth after all the teeth have been removed, but before surgical trimming of the bone or soft tissue. The template must be seated perfectly or it will not reveal the proper areas to be trimmed. When the template has been seated securely against the palate and posterior maxillary ridge, the areas at the surgical site that are blanched from the pressure indicate the need for additional reduction (Fig. 9-16). The template is removed and soft tissue or bone is trimmed, as indicated, to relieve areas of excessive pressure. Insufficient or excessive trimming causes the denture to be positioned incorrectly. This

FIG. 9-15. *Minimal envelope flap reflection for controlled reduction of bone if necessary prior to tooth removal.*

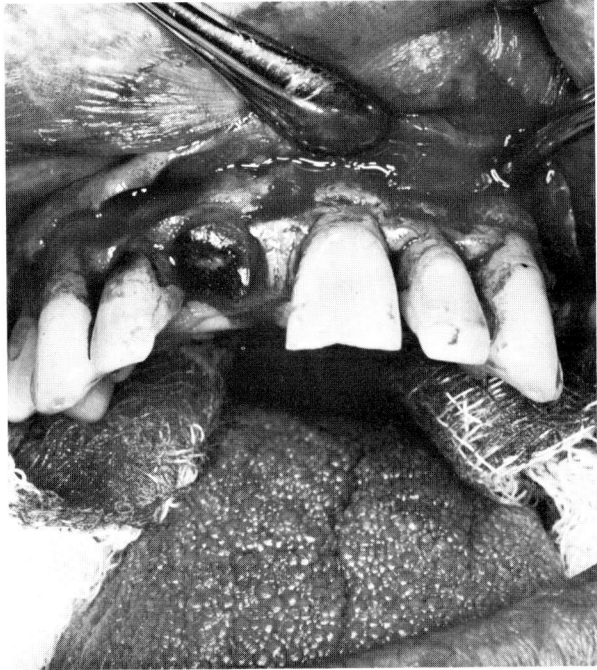

FIG. 9-16. *The surgical template is repeatedly tried in place. Blanched areas indicate where additional reduction may be necessary.*

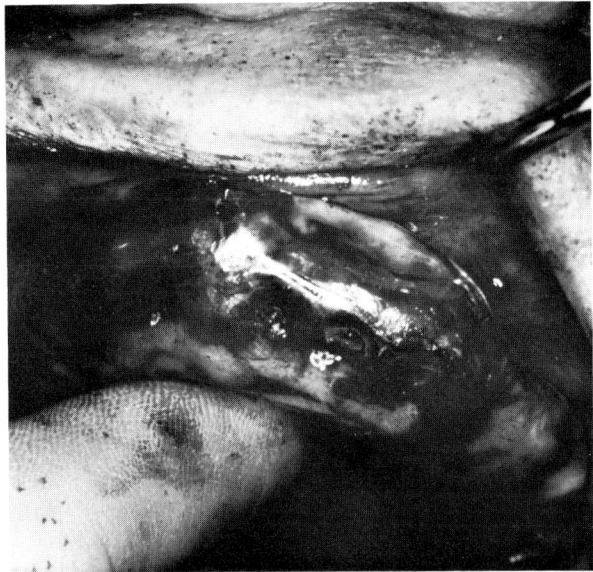

results in improper occlusion and unnecessary pain and discomfort for the patient.

Following the alveoloplasty, the tissue may also have to be reduced in circumference with a pair of soft tissue scissors. The reduction of this excess tissue is easily accomplished by removing a small wedge at the extremity of the incision (Fig. 9-17). The interdental papillae are then trimmed and sutures placed over the interseptal bone. If not adequately reduced and sutured firmly, the tissue is likely to become flabby, predisposing the tissue to subsequent denture injury. The operator must realize, however, that an overzealous attempt at reapproximation of the mucoperiosteal flaps may result in shortening of the vestibule.

FIG. 9-17. *By reducing the bony circumference of the arch, there may be an excess of labial tissue. This can best be reduced by taking a small vertical triangular wedge of tissue from the extremity of the incision.*

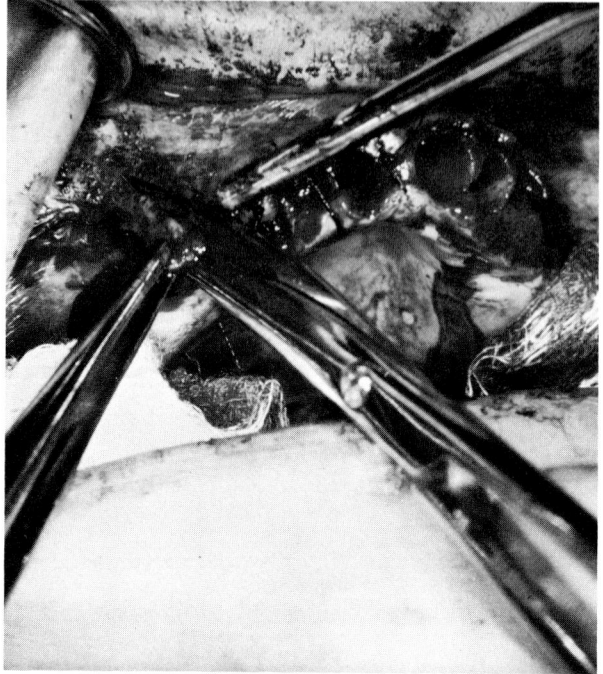

FIG. 9-18. *Immediate denture, 24 hours postoperative.*

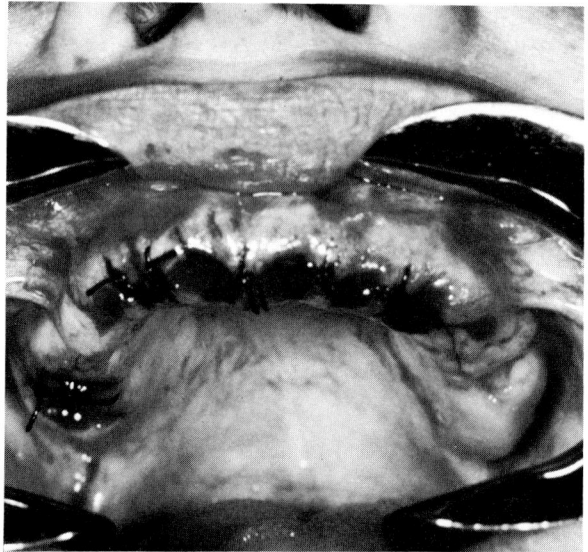

Sutures may be interrupted or continuous, and 3-0 or 4-0 silk is excellent for this purpose. The denture should have been previously placed in an acceptable sterilizing solution, after which it is rinsed in sterile saline solution and placed in the mouth. The occlusion is checked and, if satisfactory, the patient is instructed to keep the prosthesis in position for 24 hours, at which time the dentist performing the surgery will remove it for the first time (Fig. 9-18).

Premature removal may result in swelling that makes reinsertion of the denture impossible or at least extremely painful. It should be emphasized that the trauma of

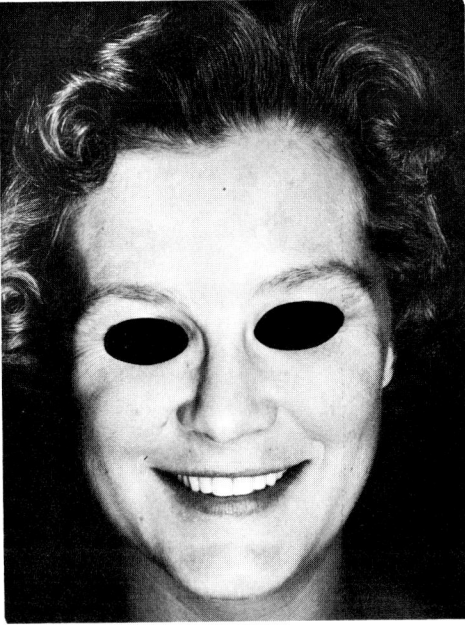

FIG. 9-19. *Five days postsurgery: edema subsided, prosthesis in place, and patient happy.*

surgery is not alleviated by the removal of the denture, and that adequate medication is necessary.

To minimize swelling, the patient should apply ice packs to the face off and on during the first 24 hours subsequent to surgery. Chewing is discouraged during the first 24 hours, and a liquid diet is prescribed. One should remember that the occlusion has not been finally adjusted, and thus mastication is inefficient, painful, and may dislodge the denture. Stability of the denture improves when the occlusion is perfected. If the loss of sleep is contemplated due to nervousness, stress, or discomfort, a sedative should be prescribed.

The prosthesis should be removed 24 to 48 hours subsequent to insertion and the mouth examined for border impingement and excessive pressure areas at the surgical site; the necessary adjustments are made. Sutures are removed in approximately 5 days after surgery. Following adequate postoperative management, the usual follow-up care for prosthesis management and adjustment is indicated (Fig. 9-19).

CHAPTER 10

Impacted Teeth

Hak Joo Kwon

Let each man exercise the art he knows. ARISTOPHANES

This chapter is intended to expand the reader's understanding and knowledge of impacted teeth that present surgical difficulty for removal. It emphasizes the surgical removal of impacted teeth and includes the definition of impacted tooth, prevalence, etiology, indications, and contraindications for surgical removal. Classification, diagnosis, and treatment of impacted third molars and canines, and other postoperative care are presented.

Definition of Impaction

Impaction and *uneruption* need to be defined when discussing impacted teeth. Every impacted tooth is also unerupted. A tooth that has not assumed its normal position relative to the age of the patient is an example of an unerupted tooth. The impacted tooth is one where eruption has been interfered with by other teeth, overlying bone, or fibrous tissue (Fig. 10-1).

Prevalence

Dachi and Howell[1] examined 3874 routine, full-mouth radiographs of patients over 20 years of age and found almost 17 percent of them with at least one impacted tooth. The teeth most often impacted were maxillary third molars (22%), mandibular third molars (18%), and maxillary canines (0.9%). Archer[2] added to the list the fourth through eighth most frequently impacted teeth: mandibular premolar, mandibular canine, maxillary premolar, maxillary central incisors, and maxillary lateral incisors. Impacted teeth are such a prevalent abnormality that all dental practitioners should be familiar with their diagnosis, surgical management, and complications.

Etiology

Durbeck[3] suggested the etiology of impacted teeth should be discussed under three separate theories.

Orthodontic theory. Inasmuch as the normal growth of the jaw and the movement of teeth are in a forward direction, anything that interferes with such development causes impaction. Forward movement is usually retarded by dense bone that can be produced by many pathologic conditions including acute infection, fever, severe trauma, malocclusion, and local inflammation of the periodontal membrane. Constant mouth breathing usually contributes to contracted arches, thus leaving insufficient room for the teeth erupting last. Occasionally, an early loss of deciduous teeth may cause malposition of permanent teeth that results in impactions.

Phylogenic theory. Nature tries to eliminate that which is not used, and the changing nutritional habits of our civilization have practically eliminated humans' need for large, powerful jaws. Thus, over centuries the maxilla and mandible have decreased in size leaving insufficient room for third molars. Congenitally missing third molars in some individuals supports the view that the third molar is a vestigial

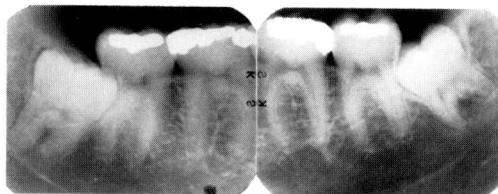

FIG. 10-1. *Impacted mandibular third molars.*

organ without current purpose or function.

Mendelian theory. Heredity is the most common etiologic factor in impaction. The transmission of small jaws from one parent and large teeth from the other would likely result in insufficient space for the teeth and instances of impaction.

Indications for Removal of Impacted Teeth

The retention of impacted teeth poses significant risks, and because neither the time nor the probability of sequelae can be predicted, all impacted teeth should be considered for removal. Removal is certainly indicated when the impacted tooth causes any of the following problems.

Lack of space. A disparity between the size or number of teeth and the size of the jaw is probably the most common indication for removal of impacted teeth. According to Lytle,[4] fewer than 5 percent of young adults with all 32 teeth have sufficient space for the full eruption of third molars. Quite often the mesial cusp of the lower third molar is exposed to the oral cavity but the distal part is still under the bone of the ascending ramus (Fig. 10-2). The gingiva covering the distal part often develops pericoronitis. Even when the distal part of the crown is erupted, high gingival attachment and the position of the third molar may produce chronic inflammation and infection because oral hygiene is difficult to maintain.

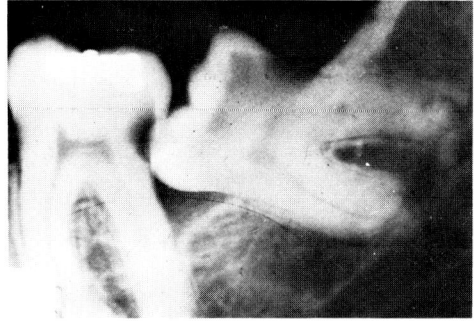

FIG. 10-3. *Mesioangular impaction demonstrates caries within the impacted tooth and the second molar.*

Damage to adjacent teeth. The position of an impacted tooth may result in food entrapment, contributing to caries development in the adjacent tooth (Fig. 10-3). Chronic infections or cyst formations from the impacted tooth may also eliminate bony support to an adjacent tooth. Early removal of the impacted tooth improves the prognosis for adjacent teeth because bony defects created by the surgery fill more rapidly and completely in young adults than in older individuals.

Odontogenic tumors or cysts. About 10 percent of impacted teeth form cysts (Fig. 10-4), according to Dachi and Howell.[1] As a general rule, impacted teeth associated with a cyst will be removed when the cyst is removed. However, in some situations (i.e., an eruption cyst) it is possible to excise the cyst and permit the tooth to erupt normally.

Recurrent infections. The most common indication for removal of impacted third molars is infection (pericoronitis) (Fig. 10-5). Even though pericoronitis can be treated with antibiotics, it usually recurs. The destruction from pericoronitis may extend to the second molar through the development of a periodontal pocket on its distal aspect. The patient is further threatened because the infection may spread to the fascial spaces.

Preparation for irradiation of the jaw and transplants. Partially or fully impacted teeth falling within the treatment zone should be removed prior to radiation treatment. Extraction prevents osteoradionecrosis associated with radiation expo-

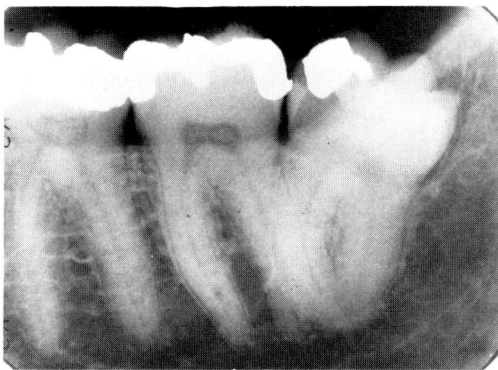

FIG. 10-2. *Partially erupted lower third molar. Note bone on distal part of the crown.*

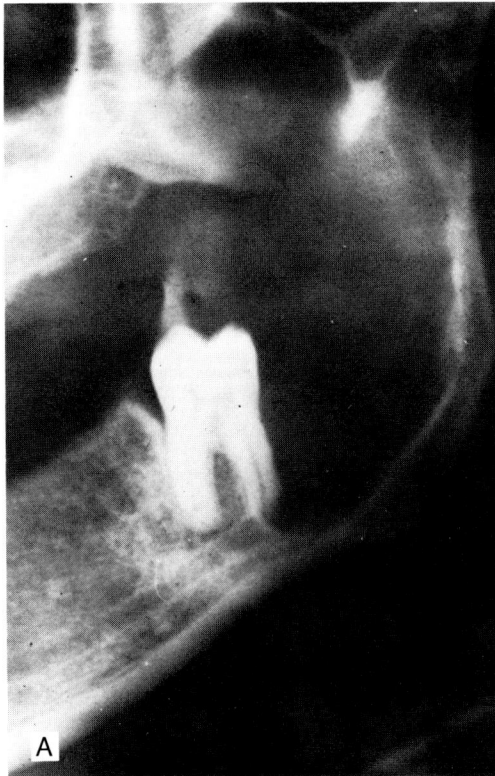

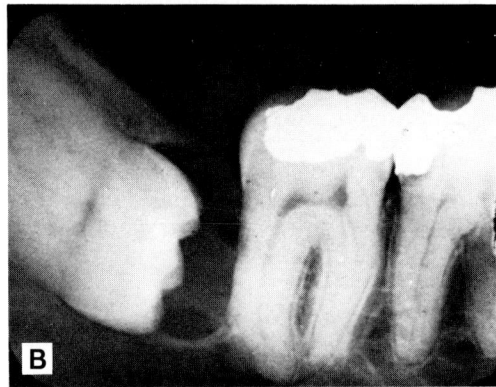

FIG. 10-4. *(A and B) Dentigerous cysts from impacted third molar.*

The density of bone surrounding the tooth increases and the ability of the body to heal decreases with age. During and after middle age medical problems develop that may compromise the patient's ability to withstand anesthesia and surgery.

Contraindications for Removal of Impacted Teeth

Leaving impacted teeth in place is discouraged except under particular circumstances, as follows:

Damage to adjacent structures. A clear risk of damage to the neurovascular bundle, maxillary sinus, or an adjacent functional tooth does not justify the removal of an asymptomatic or nonpathologic impacted tooth. These complications, however, are difficult to predict. Of the surgical procedures to remove impacted third molars, 5 percent involve some degree of nerve damage, but 0.5 percent are prolonged or permanent.[5] Postoperative anesthesia or paresthesia of the lip, cheek, teeth, gingiva, or tongue should be considered potential complications, and should be discussed with the patient before surgery.

Compromised physical status. The most significant contraindication to impaction removal is probably compromised health status. Patients having had a myocardial infarction or cerebrovascular accident within the past six months should delay extraction, if elective. Antibiotics and pain relieving medication can be used to temporarily resolve problems associated with an infected impacted tooth.

Advanced age. Elderly patients should not be subjected to impaction surgery if the tooth is asymptomatic, there is no sign that

sure. The patient who is going to have transplants (kidney, bone marrow, heart, etc.) should have impacted teeth evaluated prior to surgery, and a decision made as to removal or retention.

Lack of function. Unless there are contraindications to surgery, a nonfunctioning impacted tooth should be removed. Delay is not likely to avoid the extraction but rather to increase its difficulty and risks.

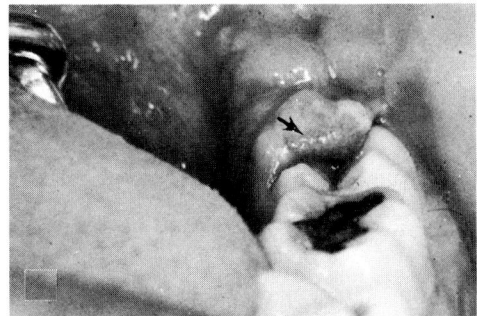

FIG. 10-5. *Pericoronitis.*

a cyst is forming, and the denture base does not ride on the impaction site. These patients should be observed periodically with radiographs to verify any change or worsening position.

Juvenile full mouth extraction. Young patients having all teeth extracted because of rampant caries should retain unerupted third molars. The molars preserve the retromolar pad and the maxillary tuberosity, both of which give support to the prosthesis. Later, if the molars begin to erupt and interfere with the prosthesis, they may be extracted.

Teeth to be moved orthodontically. An impacted canine often can be moved orthodontically into the functional position. When this appears promising, the tooth should be left in place until the potential for orthodontic treatment has been evaluated.

A risk-benefit evaluation should be made prior to recommending treatment for each impacted tooth. Patient age is a significant factor decreasing risks for younger people and increasing them for older individuals. However, the benefit of removing the tooth—especially an asymptomatic one—must be weighed against the risks. Even in the terminally ill and very aged, symptomatic impactions should be removed if the patient can be expected to tolerate the procedure and be made more comfortable. Therefore, most impacted teeth should be removed to correct existing pathologic conditions or to prevent future problems; however, some impacted teeth are left intact because the cure would be worse than the disease.

Impacted Third Molars

Third molars are by far the most commonly impacted teeth. There are no sex differences in the incidence of impacted third molars. While maxillary impactions are more common than mandibular, the impacted mandibular third molar has more problems. Thirty-seven percent of mandibular and 15 percent of maxillary impacted third molars have some type of radiolucency around the crown.[1]

Preoperative Consultation

The preoperative consultation is important in helping the patient develop confidence in the dentist and staff. To gain this confidence, the dentist must communicate well with the patient and prepare him for surgery by describing the surgical procedure, dietary preparation and premedication, choice of anesthetics, possible and probable complications and sequelae, and the postoperative care to be carried out by the patient. The fee for the procedure should be estimated for the patient. This information must be understood before the patient can join the dentist in agreements on whether to perform the surgery at all; whether to do it in the office, an ambulatory surgicenter, or as a hospital inpatient; and which type of anesthesia to use. A patient's thorough understanding of the treatment prior to surgery is as important as the understanding of postoperative instructions. Patients scheduled for general anesthesia or other sedation should be instructed to take nothing by mouth for 6 to 8 hours prior to surgery. Also, the patient must plan to bring someone to the surgical appointment who can take him home and provide postoperative supervision.

The consultation concludes with the patient's signing an informed consent document that may protect the dentist against some litigation.

Separating the surgical visit from the preoperative consultation requires an extra trip to the office by the patient and uses the surgeon's time, but it offers several advantages: the surgical appointment will be more efficient because time will not be taken for extensive explanations; the surgeon can examine the x-rays more thoroughly; the surgery visit may be scheduled more conveniently for the patient; and the patient is likely to be better prepared emotionally for the procedure.

Evaluation of the patient. Knowledge of the patient's medical and dental history is essential before any surgical procedure. Obtaining a good history may help the dentist alter the treatment plan to suit any special needs or conditions of the patient. Even though the patient's written medical history is available, the dentist should spend time interviewing to evaluate the patient's emotional status and to observe his attitude toward the surgical procedure. The patient's age, sex, race, and physical status may affect the difficulty of the surgery even for a tooth in the same position.

Evaluation of anesthesia options. Patient request must not be the only factor in selecting anesthesia. However, if the patient has a preference, and the choice is suitable, the preference may be followed. Local anesthesia with intravenous sedation is a good selection. The oral route for administering the sedation is also used, and it

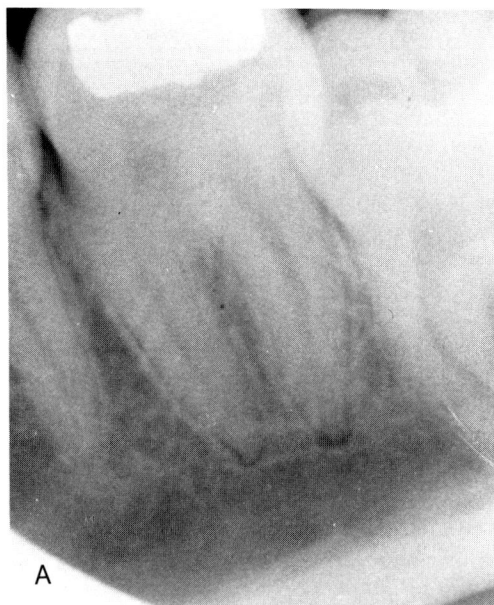

A

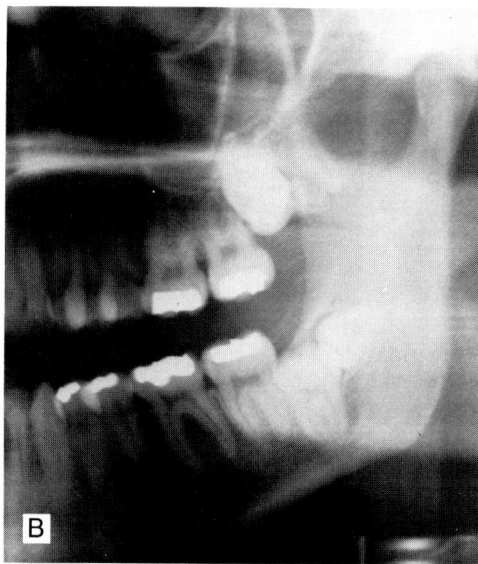

B

FIG. 10-6. *(A) This patient was referred for extraction of all four third molars with full mouth periapical x-rays. This x-ray was for lower left third molar. (B) Ordered panorex. Note impacted fourth molar that did not appear on periapical x-ray.*

may be appropriate to use a general anesthetic. Whatever selection is made, the patient should be fully informed and the risk outlined. The type of anesthesia should be selected on the basis of patient medical problems, emotional status, and difficulty of the procedure.

Evaluation of the tooth to be extracted and surrounding structures. Acute pericoronitis should be diagnosed and treated before surgery. If pericoronitis is present around the lower third molar and the upper third molar is traumatizing the tissue, the upper third molar may be removed first to eliminate further trauma to the pericoronal tissue. The mandibular molar is removed when the infection and pain have subsided, either from treatment with warm salt water rinses, or antibiotic therapy.

Panoramic radiographs are helpful in evaluating the tooth and its relationship to the inferior alveolar canal, maxillary sinus, and any cysts or bone pathology. If the x-ray does not provide adequate information, it should be retaken, or a more appropriate type of x-ray requested. On periapical x-rays, the target tooth should be centered in the film (Fig. 10-6).

Crown and roots are studied on the x-ray. The crown is examined in relation to the enamel cap, pulp, occlusal surface, and the buccal deflection. Caries is an important consideration, as it often complicates removal and alters the treatment plan. The roots vary in size and shape and may extend in any direction (Fig. 10-7).

Surrounding bone density must be evaluated to determine the surgical approach to its removal. The amount of bone to be removed is estimated by evaluating the crown and roots in relation to the bone and the direction of removal.

Mandibular canal position must be known to avoid injury to the nerve and vessels (Fig. 10-8). Richards[6] described the tube shift technique for evaluating the relationship of the impacted tooth and mandibular canal.

Adjacent teeth also should be inspected for caries, large restorations on crowns or periodontal disease.

Classification of Impaction

The dentist should adhere to a classification procedure to determine the types of

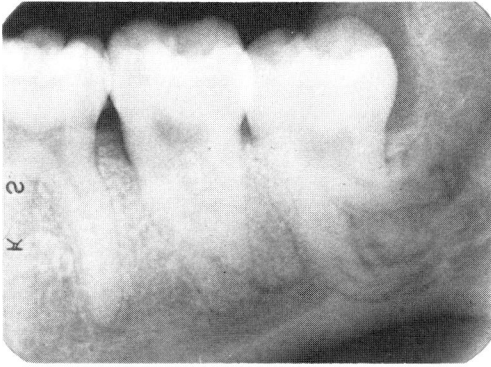

FIG. 10-7. *Note root shape, size, and directions on lower third molar—an extreme case.*

impaction he wishes to handle personally and those to be referred. Careful classification of the impaction may predict the difficulty of the case and helps the surgeon to plan the procedure.

The classification also helps the assistant set up the instruments and schedule the appointment. Consistent use of classifications therefore contributes to success in performing a procedure and overall harmony in the clinic or office. *Pell and Gregory's classification*[7] gives a good classification of mandibular third molar impaction on the basis of the relationship of the second molar to the ascending ramus of the mandible, the relative depth of the third molar in the bone, and the position of the molar in relation to the long axis of the second molar (Fig. 10-9). Radiographic examina-

tion is necessary to determine the anatomic position for classification.

Relation of the tooth to the ramus of the mandible:

Class I. Sufficient space exists between the ascending ramus and distal of the second molar for the accommodation of the entire mesiodistal diameter of the crown of the third molar.

Class II. The space between the ascending ramus and the distal of the second molar is less than the mesiodistal diameter of the crown of the third molar.

Class III. All or most of the third molar is within the ramus.

Relative depth of the third molar in bone:

Position A. The highest portion of the impacted tooth is on a level with or above the occlusal surfaces of the second molar.

Position B. The highest portion of the impacted tooth is on a level with or above the cervical line of the second molar.

Position C. The highest portion of the tooth is on a level with or below the cervical line of the second molar.

Winter's classification[8] considers the position of the tooth in relation to the long axis of the second molar (Fig. 10-10).

Mesioangular
Distoangular
Vertical
Horizontal
Buccoangular
Linguoangular
Inverted

Surgical Technique for Impacted Mandibular Third Molar

At the surgical appointment, the surgeon briefly reviews the medical history to find anything that has changed since the preoperative consultation and confirms the patient's understanding of the treatment plan. Risks and complications should be reviewed with the patient, and the discussion noted in the chart. The impaction tray (Fig. 10-11) should be opened and the patient prepared and draped. The drapes are sterile towels that cover the hair and chest. A mouth grossly deficient in hygiene may require scaling, prophylaxis, or hydrogen peroxide rinses prior to surgery.

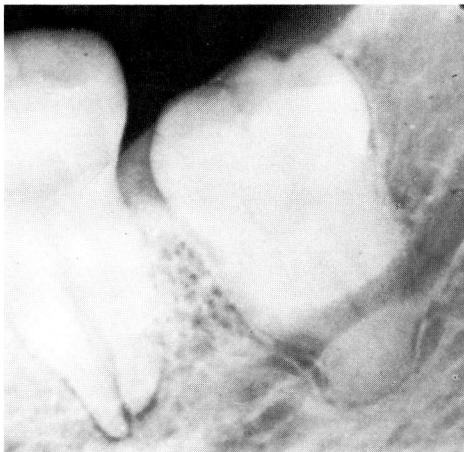

FIG. 10-8. *Note proximity of canal to both second and third molars.*

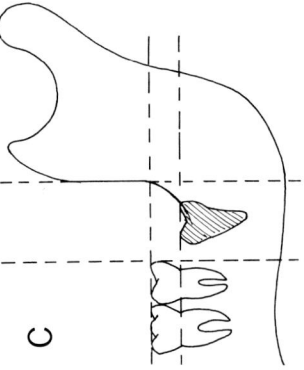
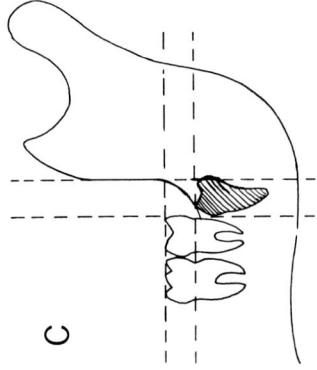
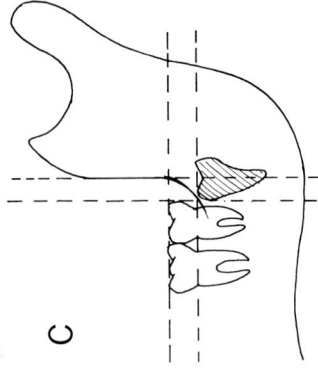

A   B   C

Class I

Space between the distal of the second molar and the ascending ramus is greater than the mesiodistal diameter of the third molar.

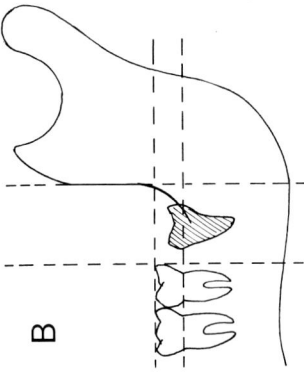
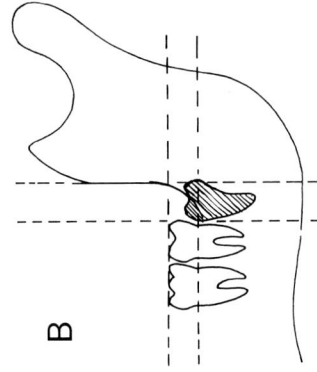
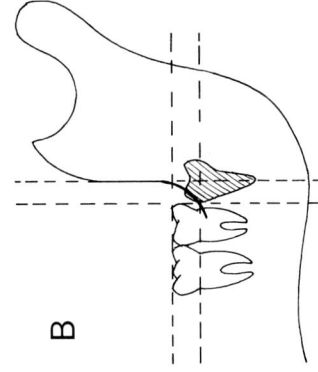

A   B   C

Class II

Space between the distal of the second molar and the ascending ramus is less than the mesiodistal diameter of the third molar.

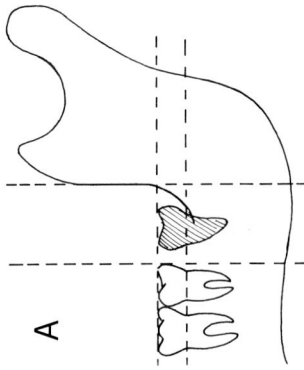
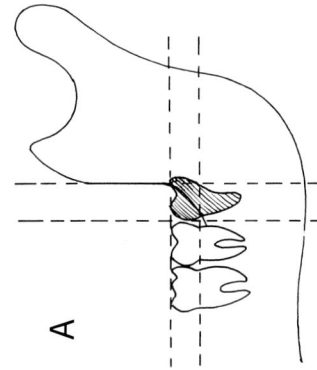
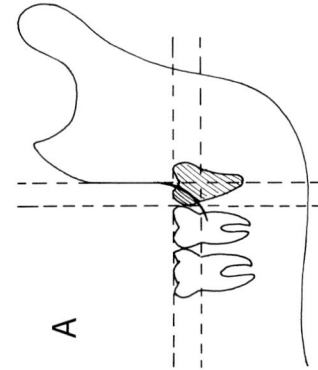

A   B   C

Class III

All or most of the third molar is within the ramus.

FIG. 10-9. *Classification of third molar impactions.*

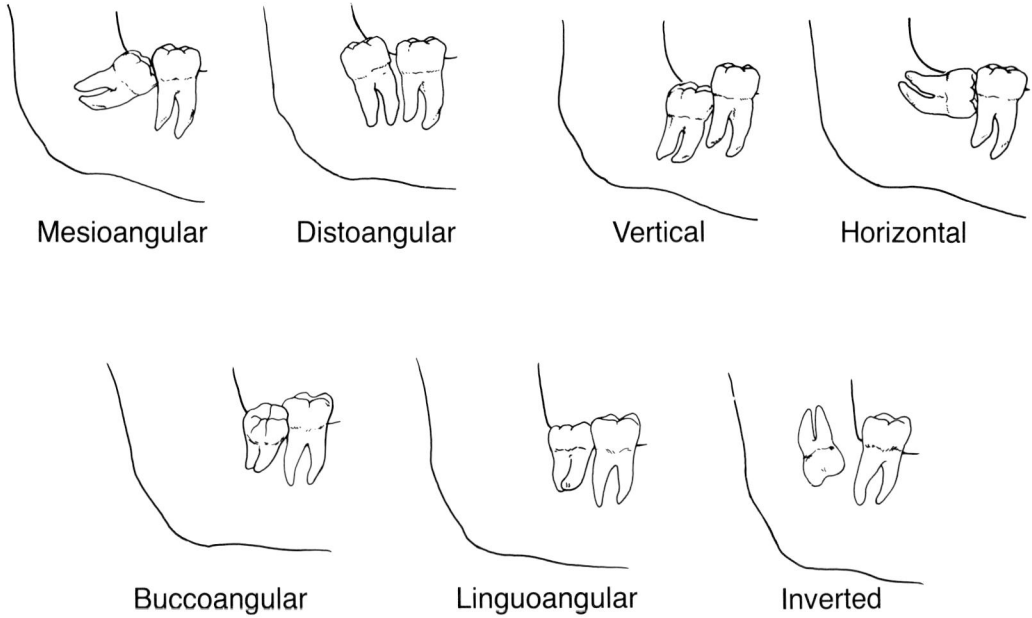

Mesioangular	Distoangular	Vertical	Horizontal

Buccoangular	Linguoangular	Inverted

FIG. 10-10. *Winter's classification of impacted third molar.*

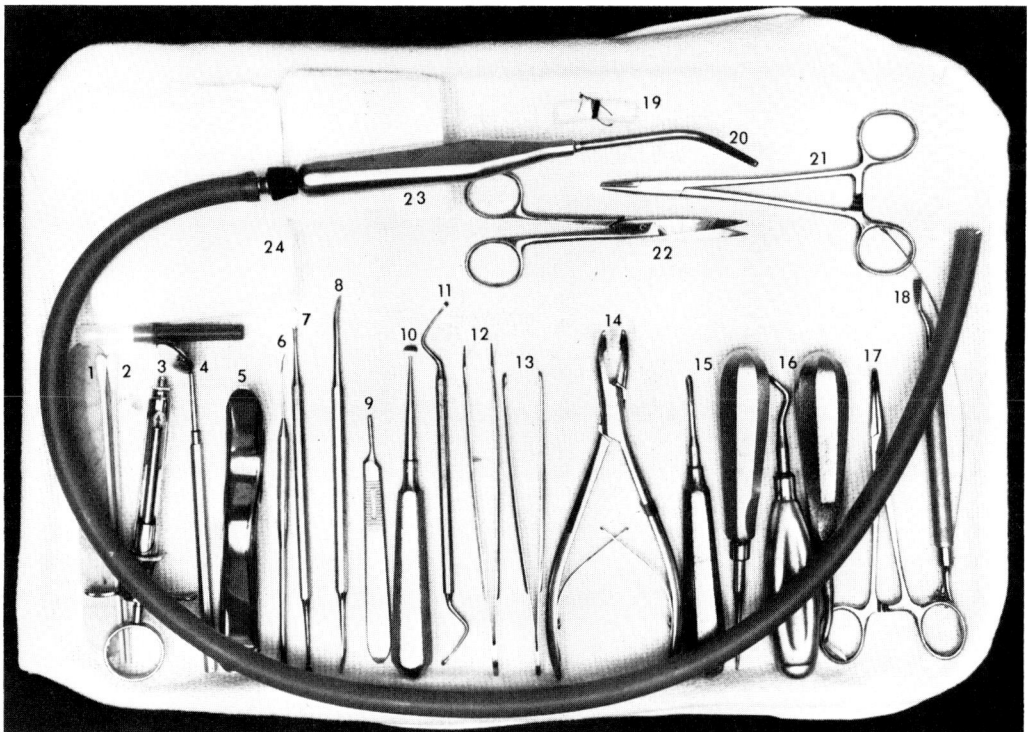

FIG.10-11. *Impaction tray. 1. Tongue blade 2. Applicators 3. Anesthetic needle and syringe 4. Mirror 5. Minnesota retractor 6. Probe 7. Woodson #1 elevator 8. Periosteal #9 9. Bard Parker handle 10. Molt #4 elevator 11. Double-ended curette 12. Cotton pliers 13. Russian forceps 14. Round-nosed rongeurs 15. 301 and 46 elevators 16. 190 and 191 elevators 17. Kelly hemostat 18. Bone file 19. 3.0 silk suture 20. Suction 21. Needle holder 22. Suture scissors 23. 3x3 gauze 24. 4x4 gauze. (not pictured: light handles and drape)*

Anesthesia is administered and the effectiveness established.

Incision and flap design. The flap is designed to provide adequate access and visibility to the surgical field. The base should be wide enough to ensure a good blood supply. A common error in impaction removal is making the flap too small. Tissue does not heal end to end, but in all directions. Therefore, a 1-inch flap takes just as long to heal as a 2-inch flap. For this reason, conservation in flap size does not benefit the patient and may detract from the surgical techniques. Two flap designs may be considered: envelope and vertical.

The envelope flap incision begins lingual to the external oblique ridge and extends approximately 1.5 to 2.0 cm to the distolingual aspect of the mandibular second molar. It continues buccally around the neck of the second molar to the interproximal space between the first and second molars (Fig. 10-12). The incision can be extended farther during surgery to provide more access if necessary.

The vertical flap is identical to the envelope but has an additional vertical incision which extends downward approximately 2 cm toward the mucobuccal fold (Fig. 10-13).

Individual preference determines which flap design is used. The author finds the vertical incision to be necessary only in instances of extremely deep impaction.

For most impaction surgery, the incision is made using the No. 15 Bard Parker blade. The incision must extend to bone, and the entire length is completed in one stroke. The reverse bevel technique should

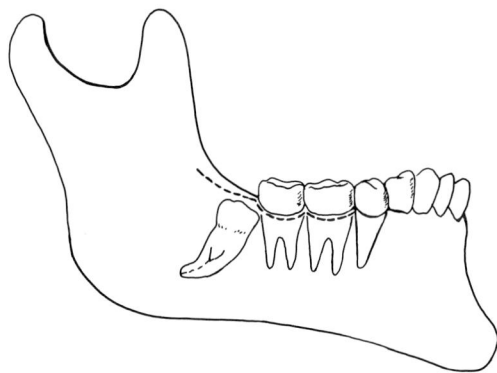

FIG. 10-13. *Vertical flap.*

be used round the neck of the second molar or beyond as needed.

The molt No. 4 periosteal elevator is a good instrument for reflecting the flap. The push stroke for further reflection is applied as soon as it becomes effective, and the total flap is reflected. Care must be taken to strip the periosteum with the mucosa. The flap is held back by a Minnesota retractor, which should be placed lightly against the bone so it does not bear constantly against the flap.

Bone removal and tooth delivery. One should have a mental picture of where the embedded tooth lies within overlying bone. The bone is carefully trephined with the surgical drill under irrigation. The area should be as large as necessary without endangering the second molar. The bur holes are connected and the bed of bone lifted off. Working space and displacement space must then be created. Working space is used for placement of the elevator or the bur for work directly on the tooth. Displacement space is needed if the tooth is to be split or to be moved prior to delivery.

The tooth may be split using a chisel or sectioned using the bur. Either technique works well, but if the patient is conscious, the bur and elevator technique is preferred (Fig. 10-14). Particular sectioning methods should be considered according to the type of impaction (Fig. 10-15).

Lingual split-bone technique. The lingual rather than buccal approach requires bone removal distolingually with final delivery of the tooth to the lingual. Although this technique, developed by Sir William Kelsey Frey and published by Ward,[9] is

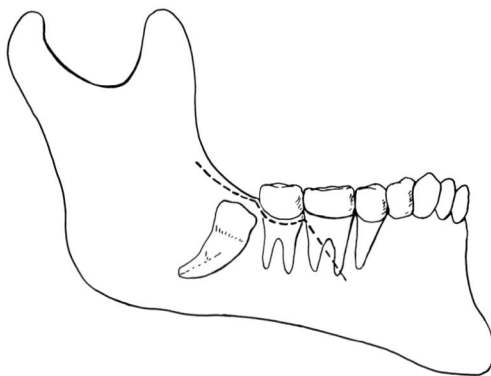

FIG. 10-12. *Envelope flap.*

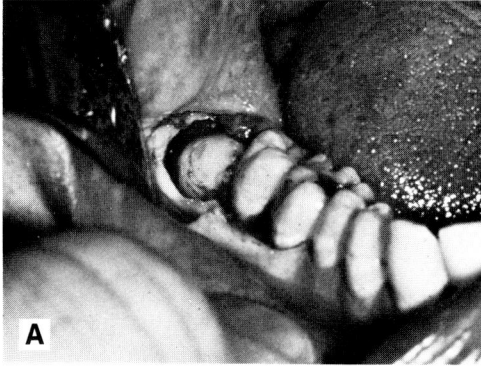

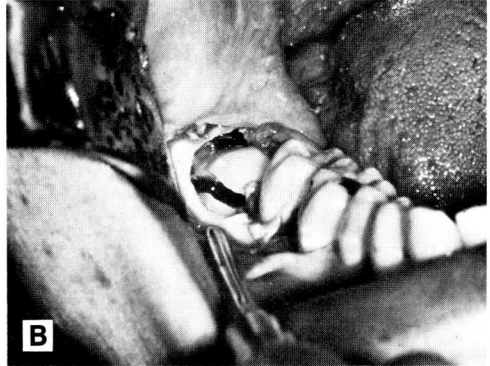

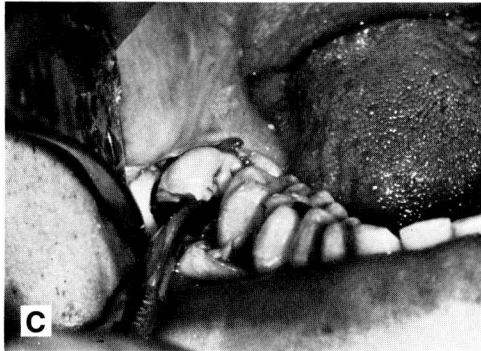

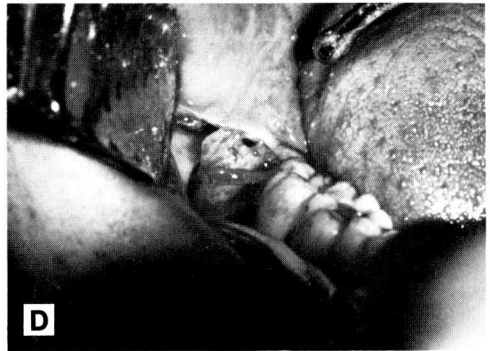

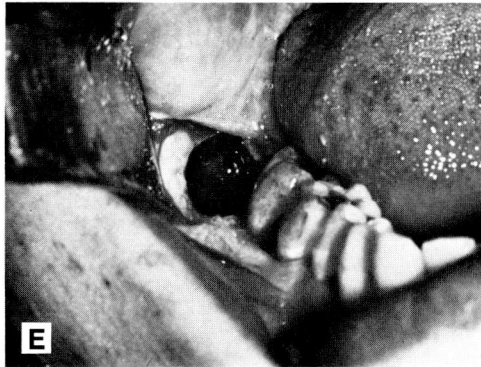

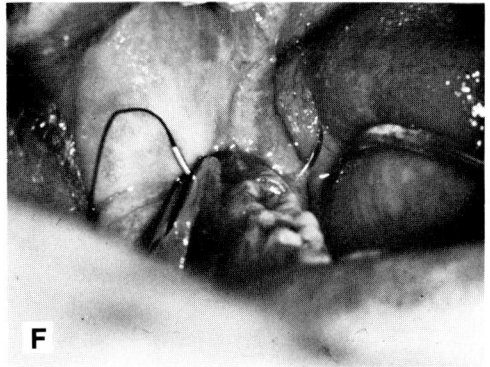

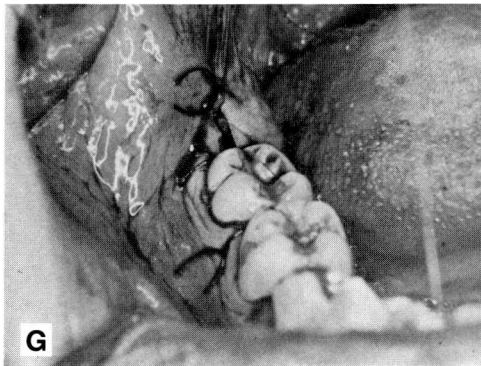

FIG. 10-14. *Envelope has been reflected and overlying bone removed with rotary instruments. (B) Impacted tooth is sectioned with bur in line with long axis of tooth. (C) Elevator is in place and superior portion of tooth is moved forward and out. (D) Inferior portion of tooth is elevated into the superior space and removed. (E) Socket is cleansed and free of debris, ready for closure. (F) Flap is returned and sutured with black silk suture. Suture distal to second molar is placed first. (G) Three sutures adequately position the mucoperiosteal flap.*

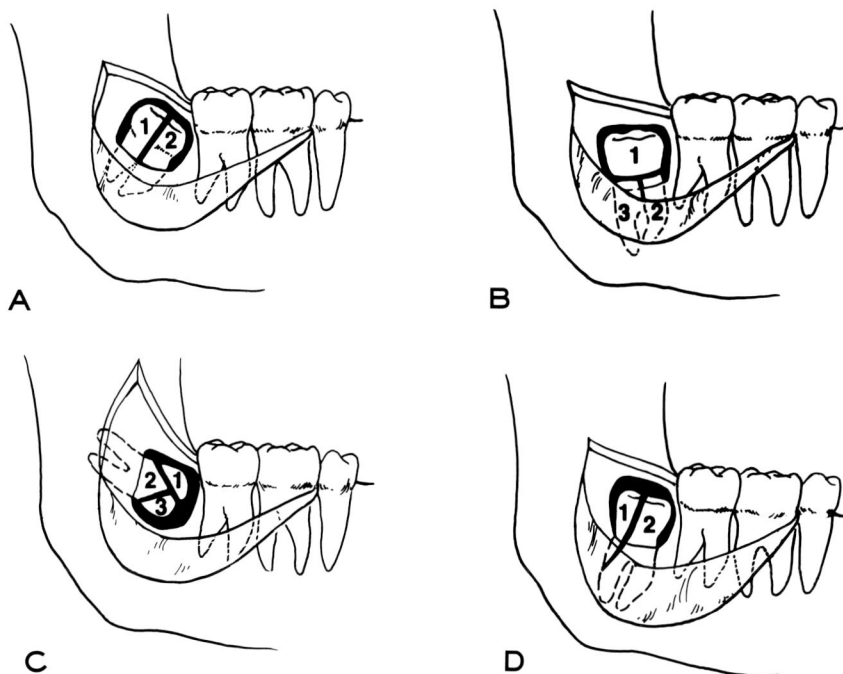

FIG. 10-15. *Sectioning methods of impacted mandibular third molar. (A) Mesioangular impaction. (B) Distoangular impaction. (C) Horizontal impaction. (D) Vertical impaction.*

reported to be a shorter surgical procedure with fewer postoperative complications, it is not recommended for the novice or infrequent operator.[10] Manipulation of lingual soft tissue, the proximity of the lingual nerve, and the severity of postoperative infection occurring in this area are challenges of this procedure. Lingual soft tissue edema, lateral pharyngeal space abscess formation, and trismus frequently accompany surgery involving these tissues.

Completion of extraction. When the tooth has been removed, it must be examined for root fracture. Using a curette and hemostat, remove the follicle. Interseptal areas and other bone margins may need to be smoothed with a bone file. Irrigation is used to remove bone dust and chips. When final inspection assures that no active, severe bleeding is occurring, the flap is returned and sutured with 000 black silk suture material. If the patient is unable to return for suture removal, absorbable suture material may be used. Before applying the pressure pack, the flap is pressed into its original position.

When the surgery is complete, postoperative x-rays will be needed if inspection in a bloodless, well-washed field does not resolve concerns about remaining tooth or root fragments. The surgical notes should reflect any problems or special conditions found during the procedure or on the x-rays afterward. The patient should be informed of any complications that developed during surgery. The fact that this information has been given is then noted in the chart.

Postoperative instructions. The patient should be prepared to perform appropriate postoperative self-care to minimize complications. Information should be given in lay language. Patients who had been under general anesthesia or sedation should be given instructions in the company of another responsible person who can review the information later when the patient is more coherent. All instructions should be given in written form and reviewed orally (Fig. 10-16).

Pain. Most patients are apprehensive about postextraction pain; however, appropriate analgesics are effective in pain control. The patient may start taking the

POSTOPERATIVE INSTRUCTIONS

Postoperative care is important after oral surgery and recovery may be delayed if this is neglected. Some swelling, stiffness and discomfort is to be expected. If this is excessive, please call or return for care.

THE DAY OF OPERATION

Bleeding
a. Keep gauze pack in place 30 minutes with constant, firm pressure.
b. Keep head elevated and rest quietly.
c. Do not suck or spit excessively. If bleeding persists, repeat the above.
d. Some oozing and discoloration of saliva is normal.

Swelling
Apply ice pack to region of surgery at 20-minute intervals for the first 6–8 hours.

Pain
Take prescribed tablets and rest.

Diet
Liquids, soft, or regular (as desired). Do not skip meals.

The Second Day
Brush teeth. Use hot water rinse (½ tsp. salt in glass of hot water [coffee temp.]) 3–5 times per day. Continue tablets for pain if necessary.

A

M_____
has an appointment with

Day	Date	Time
Mon.		
Tues.		
Wed.		
Thurs.		
Fri.		

The above time is reserved for you. If you are unable to keep your appointment, please notify the Clinic 24 hours in advance.

If care is necessary after clinic hours, please call:

000-0000

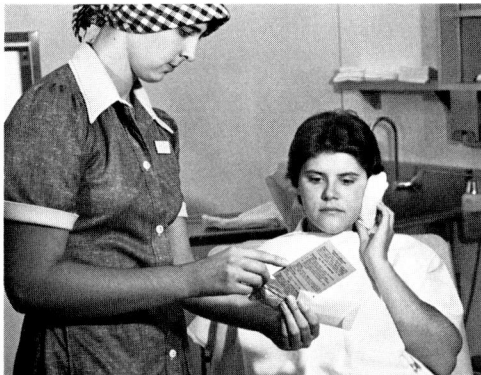

B

FIG. 10-16. *(A) Outline of instructions for postoperative care and postoperative appointment card. (B) Instructions for postoperative care should be explained when they are given to the patient.*

prescribed analgesic before the local anesthetic wears off to prevent the pain from becoming severe. However, if severe pain develops 2 to 3 days after extraction, the patient should be seen to evaluate the possible localized osteitis. (See Chapter 11, Complications of Exodontia, for a discussion of dry socket.)

Bleeding. A limited amount of postoperative bleeding is normal and usually stops within few hours. All patients must be evaluated for bleeding prior to dismissal from the office. Dampened sponges are placed directly over the socket rather than over the teeth, and the patient is instructed to maintain pressure for at least 30 minutes. The most common cause of continued bleeding is probably the failure of the patient to position the gauze pack properly.

Swelling. Most extractions of impacted teeth will produce some swelling. The swelling after difficult impaction removal or all four extraction of third molars will increase for 2 to 3 days postoperatively.

The usefulness of heat and cold to control swelling post-trauma and postsurgery is controversial. Recent research confirms that heat and cold applied intraorally and extraorally produce significant changes in blood flow to facial tissues. The traditional recommendations are therefore supported.[11] When four third molars have been removed, ice packs can be applied on alternating sides at 20-minute intervals for the first 6 to 8 hours.

During the second 24-hour period, warm salt water rinses may be started to remove food debris from the surgical site, and to reduce edema. A usual mixture is ½ teaspoon of salt in one cup of warm water.

Some surgeons believe that steroids used systemically or locally modify the inflammatory reaction, reducing postoperative swelling and pain. Pederson[12] injected 4 mg dexamethasone into the masseter muscle just before starting the third molar extraction and found about a 50 percent reduction in postoperative swelling and trismus.

Diet. Following surgery, the patient should not chew food until the anesthetic is fully worn off. During the first 24 hours, a liquid or soft diet is encouraged. Thereafter, patients should eat whatever is comfortable to them. Postoperative diet should provide an adequate caloric intake.

Emergency telephone number. Patients invariably appreciate the dentist's phone call after surgery inquiring into their well-being. Whether or not this is done, all patients should be encouraged to call the office if unusual signs or symptoms occur. The emergency phone number should be included with the postoperative written instructions in case the patient wants to contact the dentist.

Follow-up visit. Before the patient is dismissed after surgery, a follow-up appointment should be made for 5 to 7 days later for suture removal. While suture removal is not difficult, good lighting, small sharp scissors, and gentle handling of the tissue contribute to patient comfort and confidence in the surgeon. The suture is cut on one side very close to the mucosa so that contaminated suture does not pass through inside the tissue. The suture is then pulled through from the other side.

Surgical Technique for Impacted Maxillary Third Molar

Maxillary third molars are removed with less surgical difficulty than mandibular third molars because the bone of the maxilla is less dense, permitting the use of elevator technique to lift the tooth. Furthermore, maxillary third molars are less likely to require surgical sectioning than is the case with mandibular third molar impactions.

Incision and flap design. Access to the buccal surface of the posterior maxillary alveolar process is very difficult. To improve accessibility in case of removing upper right maxillary third molar, the patient's head should be turned away from the dentist, the mouth partially opened, and the lower jaw deviated toward the dentist. This positions the coronoid process of the mandible laterally and provides a better operative field.

The incision should be made buccal to the crest of the ridge, rather than along the crest into the hamular notch. An envelope flap is usually adequate, but a vertical arm may be added to the flap for increased exposure of a high impaction (Fig. 10-17).

Bone removal and tooth delivery. Frequently, a portion of the crown of the impacted tooth is visible or a bulge in the bone surface overlying the crown identifies the tooth. The bone on the buccal surface of the crown is usually so thin it can be removed using the molt No. 4 curette. If the buccal bone is thick or unyielding, a surgical bur may be used to remove it. Maxillary third molars very rarely need sectioning for removal.

Elevators are usually effective for removing the uncovered maxillary third molar. The straight 301 or 46 elevator, Potts elevator, or 190 and 191 may be used. The choice of elevator depends on the anatomic location of the tooth, its morphology, the condition of the bone, and the operator's preference.

Surgical Technique for Impacted Maxillary Canines

After the third molars, the maxillary canines are most frequently impacted (Fig. 10-18). Maxillary canine impactions occur in both sexes, but are more common in females. Palatal impaction is three times more frequent than buccal, and unilateral is more common than bilateral impaction of the canines.[1]

Removal is only one option for managing impacted canines. Surgical exposure is sometimes performed in preparation for orthodontics; surgical repositioning is sometimes possible; and in some instances, the impacted canine may be removed.

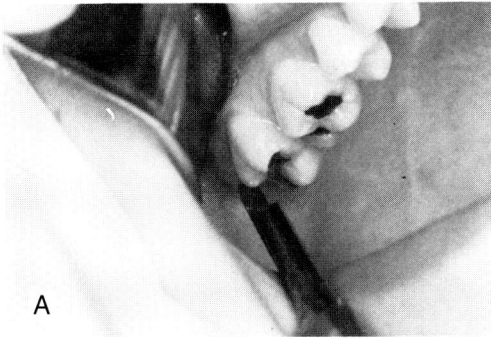

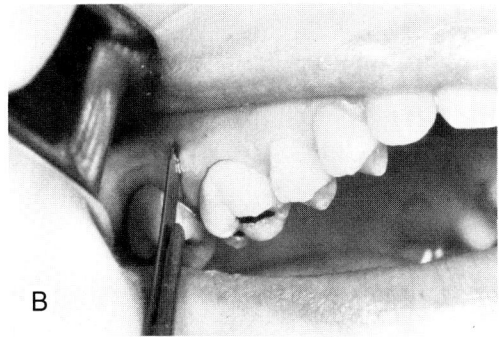

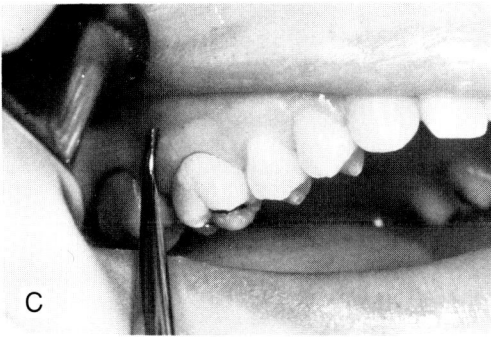

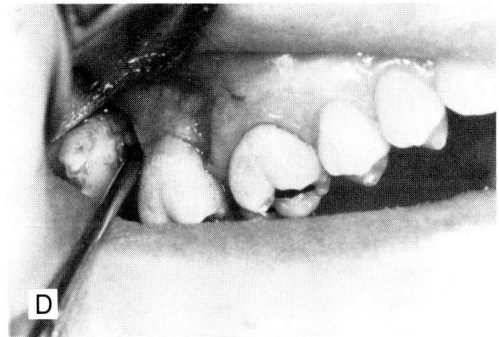

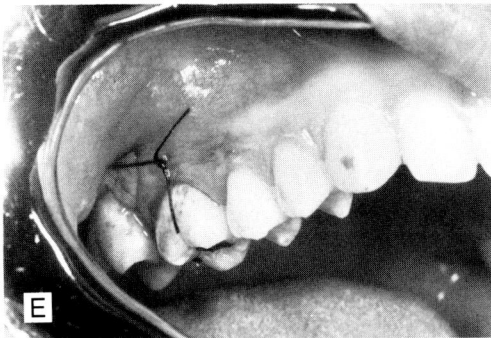

FIG. 10-17. *Maxillary impacted third molar removal. (A) Incision on posterior of second molar. (B) Vertical releasing incision. (C) Flap reflect using molt #4 elevator. (D) Elevating a tooth using Potts elevator. (E) Final sutures on vertical incision area. One more suture needed on posterior incision area.*

Localization of impacted canine. When removal is the chosen option, the exact position of the target impacted canine must be known preoperatively. Inspection often reveals whether the tooth is located on the labial or palatal. Bulges of the mucosa and alveolar bone or displacement of adjacent teeth help define the position of at least the crown of the tooth. Radiographic examination is needed as usual to confirm the clinical impression. Localization of impacted maxillary canines is aided by using the shift technique (radiographic). Remember, if the impacted tooth moves in the same direction as the cone on the machine, it is on the lingual. If the tooth shifts in the opposite direction, it is on the labial or buccal side.

Impacted maxillary canines are most frequently found in the following positions:

1. In the palate with the crown located to the lingual side of the upper lateral incisor and the root extending posteriorly in the palate parallel to the bicuspid roots.
2. With the crown to the lingual side of the maxillary central incisor and the root extending posteriorly in the palate parallel to the bicuspid roots or between the bicuspid roots and extending through to the buccal surface.
3. With the crown of the impacted tooth on the palatal area and the body of the root on the buccal side.
4. With the crown of the impacted tooth on the buccal side and the root extending to the lingual side of the bicuspid roots and the root extending to the lingual side of the bicuspid roots.

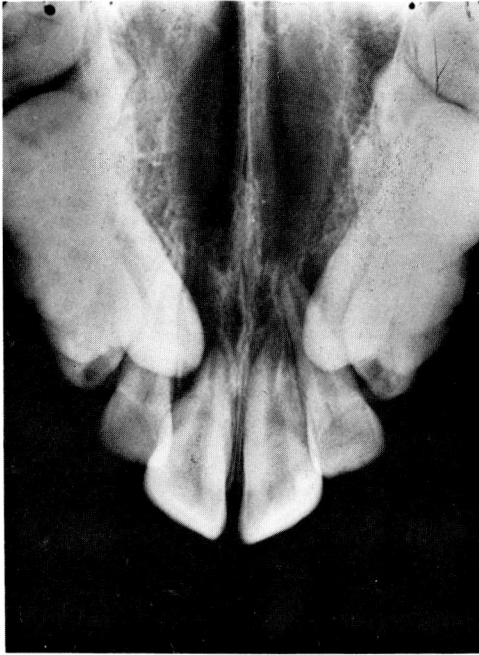

FIG. 10-18. *Occlusal x-ray film of bilateral maxillary impacted canines.*

5. Entire tooth on the buccal.
6. Bilaterally impacted either on palate or on buccal side.

Flap design and tooth delivery. The flap design depends on the location of the impacted canines. If the entire canine is on the palatal or the labial surface of the dental arch, the mucoperiosteal flap is created on the same side, usually originating from the necks of the adjacent teeth. Since the great majority are palatally positioned, this is the usual surgical approach. The heavy palatal tissue is reflected and the bone relieved over the crown of the impaction. The crown can then be sectioned near its cervical line and removed, and the roots

drawn into the space left by the crown (Fig. 10-19). The flap is returned and sutured.

References

1. Dachi, S.F., and Howell, F.V.: A survey of 3,874 routine full mouth radiographs: II. A study of impacted teeth. Oral Surg., *14:*1165, 1961.
2. Archer, W.M.: Oral Surgery. 4th Ed. Philadelphia, W.B. Saunders Co., 1966.
3. Durbeck, W.: Impacted mandibular third molars—etiology of impaction. *In* The Impacted Lower Third Molar. Brooklyn, Dental Items of Interest Publishing Co., Inc. and London, Henry Kimpton, 1945, pp. 4–8.
4. Lytle, J.J.: Indications and contraindications for removal of the impacted tooth. Dent. Clin. North Am., *23*(3):334, 1979.
5. Guralnick, W.G., and Laskin, D.M.: Consensus Development Conference: Removal of Third Molars. Bethesda, MD, Nat. Inst. of Health, November 28–30, 1979.
6. Richards, H.H.: Roentgenographic localization of mandibular canal. J. Oral Surg., *10:*325, 1952.
7. Pell, G.J., and Gregory, B.T.: Impacted mandibular third molars: classification and modified techniques for removal. Dent. Digest, *39:*330, 1933.
8. Winter, G.B.: Impacted Mandibular Third Molar. St. Louis, American Medical Book Co., 1926.
9. Ward, T.G.: The split bone technique for removal of lower 3rd molar. Br. Dent. J., *101:*297, 1956.
10. Rud, J.: The split-bone technique for removal of impacted mandibular third molars. J. Oral Surg., *28:*416, 1970.
11. Kwon, H.J., Rhee, J.G., Song, C.W., and Waite, D.E.: Temperature effects on "blood flow" in facial tissues. J. Oral Maxillofac. Surg., *44:*790, 1986.
12. Pederson, A.: Decadronphosphate in the relief of complaints after third molar surgery. Int. J. Oral Surg., *14:*235, 1985.

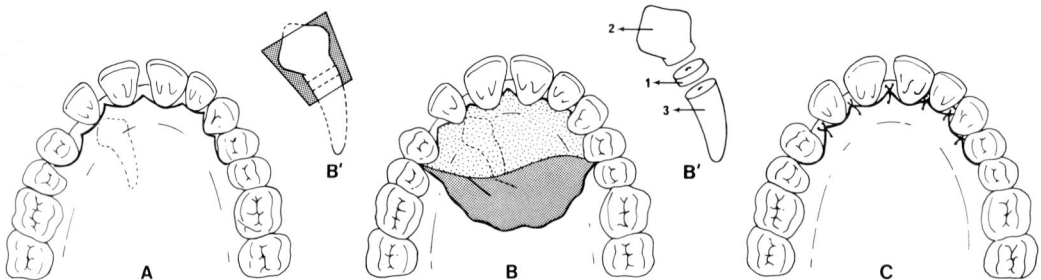

FIG. 10-19. *Sectioning method for removing impacted canines. (A) Flap outline. (B) Flap reflected. (C) Flap returned and sutured.*

CHAPTER 11 # Complications of Exodontia

ROGER A. MEYER

Haste in every business brings failure. HERODOTUS

A complication may be defined as any event during or after an operation that, if unrecognized or untreated, may adversely affect the patient. The removal of teeth, especially those that are malposed, multirooted, or impacted, can be a technically demanding and difficult procedure even in the most skilled hands. Complications occurring during tooth removal should not be unexpected nor considered prima facie evidence of the operator's failure to exercise proper judgment and surgical technique. Rather, the operator should observe surgical principles at all times to prevent or minimize complications. He should have a plan, the necessary instruments, and assistance to manage the more common problems associated with dentoalveolar surgery.

Evaluation and Planning

Careful patient evaluation can prevent or minimize many complications. Potential problems can be anticipated and the surgical approach modified to enhance the likelihood of a favorable outcome.

Assessment of potential difficulty begins with a review of the patient's medical history and a thorough clinical examination. The patient's level of emotional maturity and ability to cooperate are observed. The condition of the tooth or teeth to be removed (extent of caries, soundness of the crown, mobility, position in the arch), status of surrounding soft tissues (inflammation, recession, bleeding), and amount of alveolar bone are given specific attention.

Correlation of radiographic appearance with clinical findings is the cornerstone of diagnosis in exodontia. The first consideration in evaluating an x-ray is the diagnostic quality of the film. The tooth to be removed and its periapical region must be totally visible (Fig. 11-1). The film should not be over- or underexposed so that soft tissue details are "burned out" or normal bone is inadequately penetrated. Proper angulation prevents foreshortening of roots and superimposition of tooth crowns. Correct mounting and labeling of x-rays helps to prevent operating on the wrong side of the mouth or on the wrong patient. A definite routine should be followed in evaluating each x-ray. The tooth, alveolar bone, and associated structures (e.g., maxillary sinus, inferior alveolar canal) are scanned carefully for variations from the normal.

On the basis of the surgical diagnosis, a definite plan of operation should be developed for removal of the tooth, with an alternate plan available if necessary. For example, what initially appears to be a routine forceps removal of a tooth may require the raising of a mucoperiosteal flap, removal of alveolar bone, and sectioning of the tooth after the tooth fails to yield to elevator and forceps.

The patient should be fully informed about the diagnosis, the need for and type of surgical procedure, and the potential risks or complications involved. Many patients' legal actions following surgical complications are based on misunderstanding or lack of prior knowledge of the possibility of a given complication, rather than on the complication itself (in other words, lack of

145

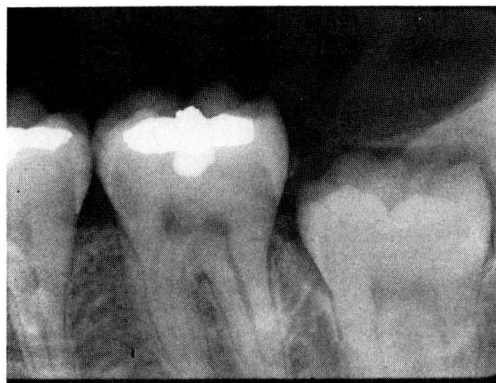

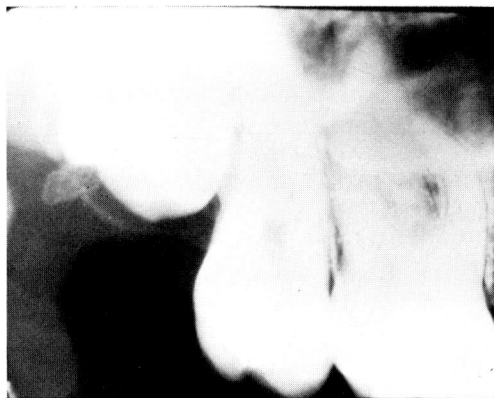

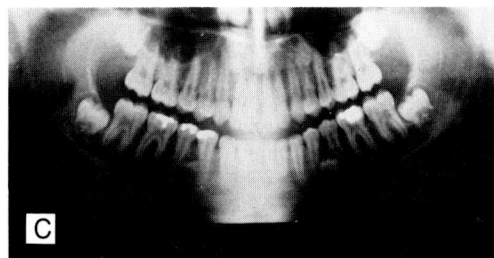

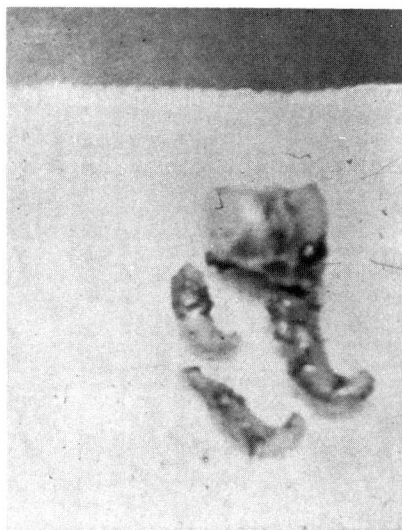

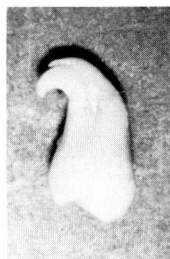

FIG. 11-1. *(A and B) Inadequate periapical views fail to show curvature of impacted third molar roots. (C) Panoramic radiograph provides adequate information on which to judge the difficulty of removal of impacted teeth. Note also multiple supernumerary teeth.*

informed consent rather than surgical negligence).

Clark[1] has advocated the "seven minimum essentials" for the removal of teeth and other oral surgical operations (see Chapter 9). No operator should begin an exodontia procedure without having satisfied Clark's requirements.

Proper draping of the patient protects face, eyes, hair, and clothing (Fig. 11-2). Adherence to principles of asepsis by using mask and gloves greatly diminishes the risk of passing contaminated material or communicable diseases (common cold, hepatitis, AIDS, venereal disease, tuberculosis, etc.) between patient and doctor or assistants.[2,3]

Placement of a bite block between the teeth or edentulous jaws on the side opposite the area to be operated on stabilizes the mandible against sudden or reflex closure (Fig. 11-3). The bite block prevents accidental needle breakage during local anesthetic injection, soft tissue lacerations from scalpels or burs, and blunt trauma from elevators or retractors that might be caused by sudden closure of the mandible. Proper manual support of the mandible with the bite block in place stabilizes and minimizes trauma to the temporomandibular joints during forceps extraction of a tooth.

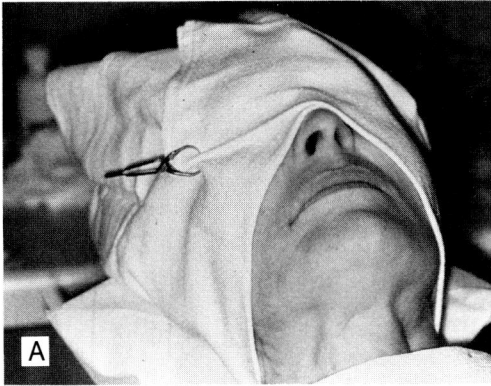

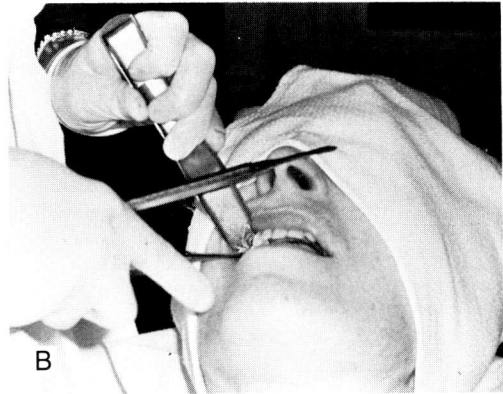

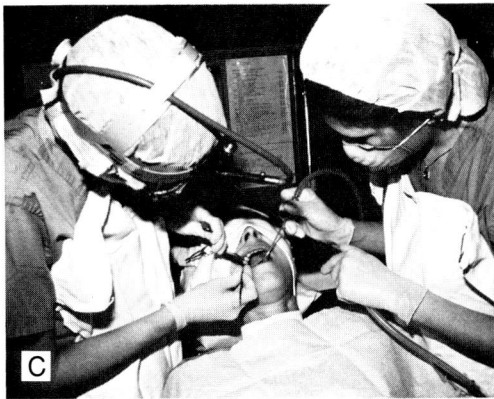

Fig.11-2. *(A and B) Towel drape covers patient's face and hair and protects the eyes from debris of surgical procedure or misguided instruments. (C) Surgeon and assistant follow principles of asepsis by wearing mask, cap, and gloves. Note headlight used for maximal illumination.*

The operator faced with a complication during an exodontia procedure should remain calm and handle it expeditiously. This will occur only as the result of his training, experience, and personal and professional maturity. If the operator perceives that a problem is occurring, the procedure should be stopped immediately. He assesses the situation by clinical observation, and obtains necessary radiographs. A plan of treatment is decided upon. The patient is informed that a situation has arisen requiring a modified or additional surgical approach (e.g., raising of a mucoperiosteal flap and removal of bone for root recovery). There is no mention of a "mistake" or implied negligence by the operator. The patient is reassured as to the intended outcome of the procedure, and the operation is resumed.

Flap Design

The raising of a mucoperiosteal flap (see Chapter 9) is an important adjunct to exo-

dontia procedures, either as part of the original surgical plan or as necessitated for access to recover a fractured root or section a tooth to aid in its removal. Proper flap design avoids injury to important structures (Fig. 11-4). Injury to the lingual nerve is avoided by carrying the incision for exposure of the unerupted mandibular third molar posterolaterally from the second molar. Vertical incision for release of a buccal mucoperiosteal flap in the mandibular premolar area places the mental nerve in jeopardy if carried too far inferiorly.

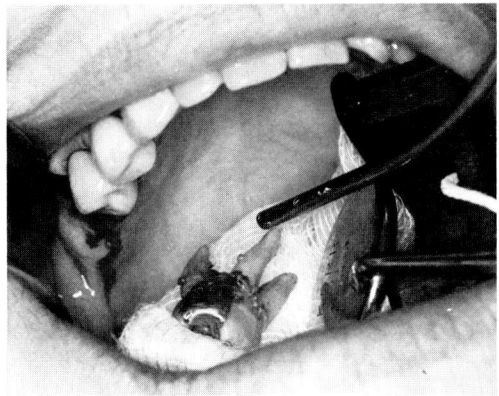

Fig. 11-3. *Bite block in place assists in stabilization of the jaws. Gauze pack has prevented displaced tooth from entering the pharynx.*

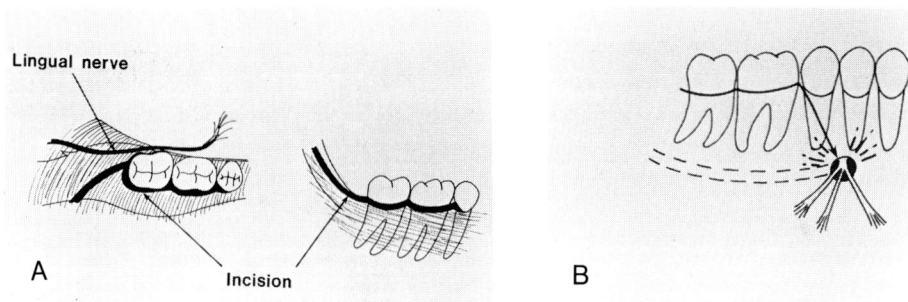

FIG. 11-4. (A) Incision for mucoperiosteal flap in mandibular third molar region is directed postero-laterally behind second molar to avoid injury to lingual nerve. (B) To avoid injury to mental nerve, vertical incision in mandibular premolar area should not be overextended inferiorly.

Tooth Division

Controlled surgical removal of teeth by selective removal of alveolar bone and sectioning the crowns and dividing the roots is often easier and safer than forceps removal. This is particularly true for mandibular and maxillary first molars, where excessive forces generated by uncontrolled application of elevators or forceps might cause loss of large amounts of alveolar bone, tuberosity fracture, or mandibular fracture. It is actually faster, safer, and more conservative to section teeth and remove alveolar bone in a planned fashion in such instances. Surgical tooth removal is indicated for erupted multirooted teeth in the following situations: (1) divergent and curved roots, (2) fractured crown during attempted forceps removal, (3) grossly carious crown without solid tooth structure for forceps application, and (4) tooth not luxated by either forceps or elevators. Surgical removal of teeth generally requires the additional access provided by a mucoperiosteal flap, either the "envelope" or "hockey stick" type. Enough alveolar bone,

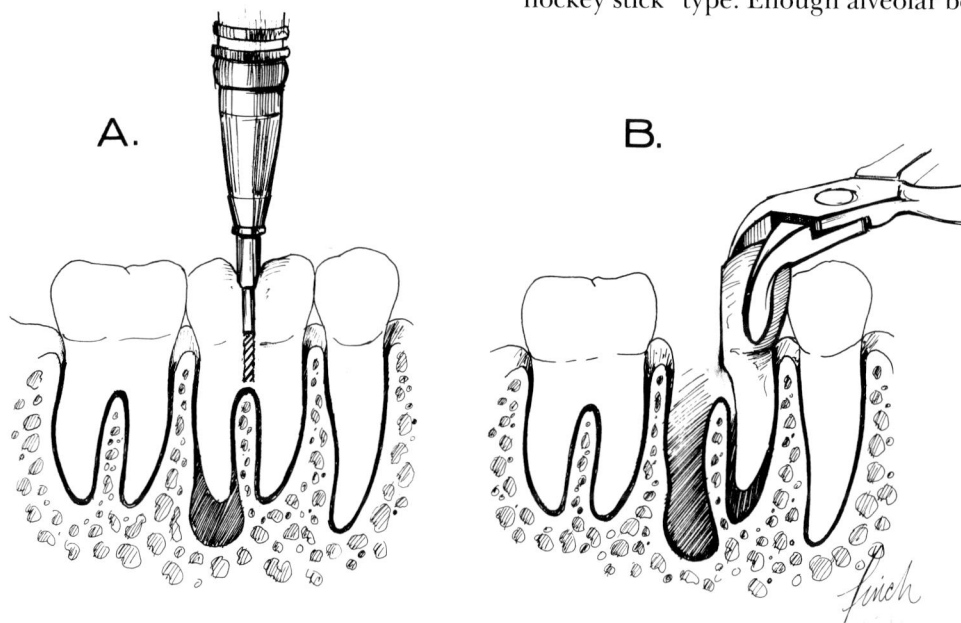

FIG. 11-5. (A) One method of sectioning mandibular molar. (B) After sectioning, removal of the two segments is similar to upper premolar removal.

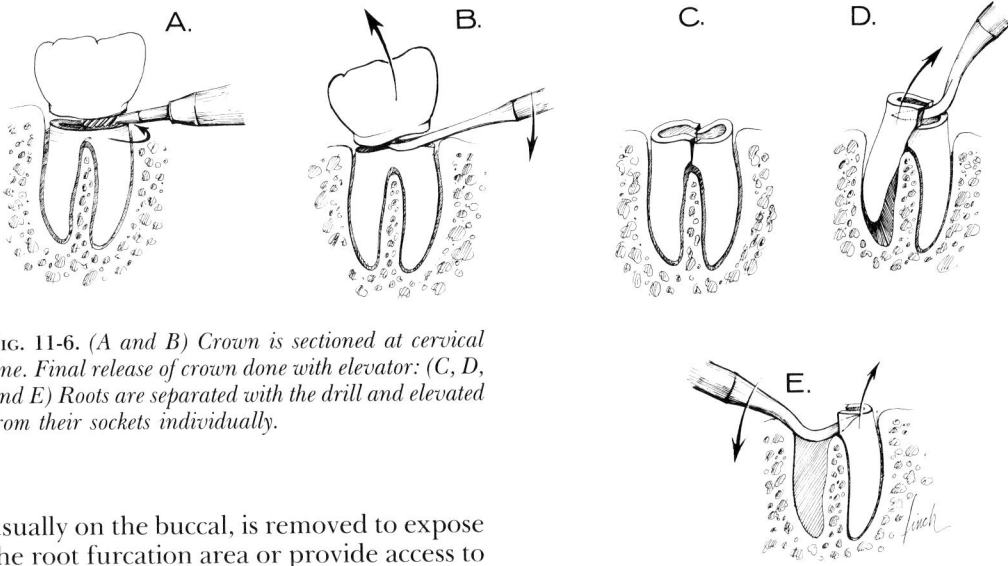

FIG. 11-6. *(A and B) Crown is sectioned at cervical line. Final release of crown done with elevator: (C, D, and E) Roots are separated with the drill and elevated from their sockets individually.*

usually on the buccal, is removed to expose the root furcation area or provide access to place a purchase point for an elevator with the high-speed drill.

The approach to sectioning multirooted teeth varies only slightly, depending on the tooth. For lower molar teeth, the crowns may be sectioned buccolingually and the tooth extracted in two segments. (Fig. 11-5). Other division techniques include: (1) sectioning the crown at the gingival crest and the remaining root structure buccolingually, and recovering the roots separately (Fig. 11-6), or (2) sectioning one root through the bifurcation, removing the crown and the attached root, and recovering the other root separately (Fig. 11-7).

Maxillary molar removal necessitating tooth division can be done by sectioning the crown at the junction of the mesiobuccal and distobuccal roots, removing the crown and the palatal root intact, and recovering the two buccal roots separately (Fig. 11-8). If this method is unsuccessful, the entire crown may be sectioned free and the roots all recovered separately (Fig. 11-9). Remember, however, that the maxillary antrum often dips low into the trifurcation

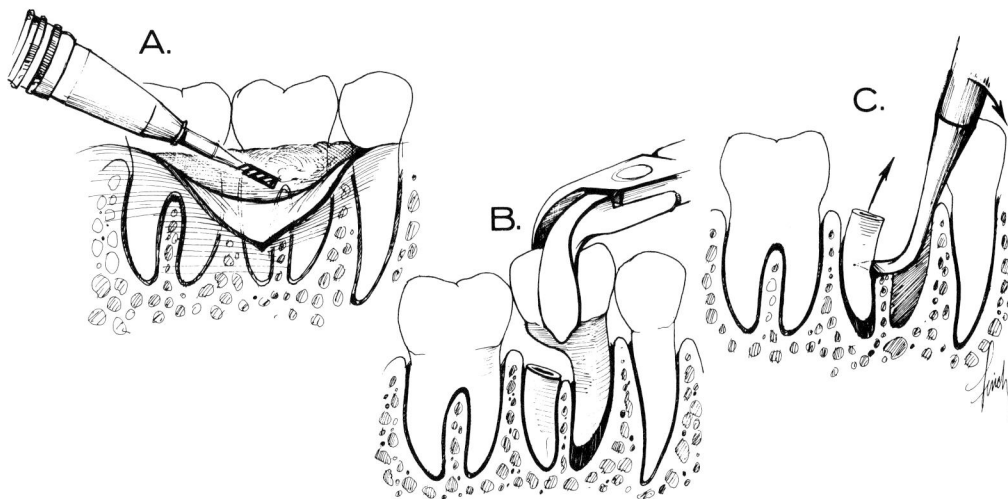

FIG. 11-7. *(A) One root is sectioned at bifurcation. (B) Crown and one root removed. (C) Remaining root luxated with elevator.*

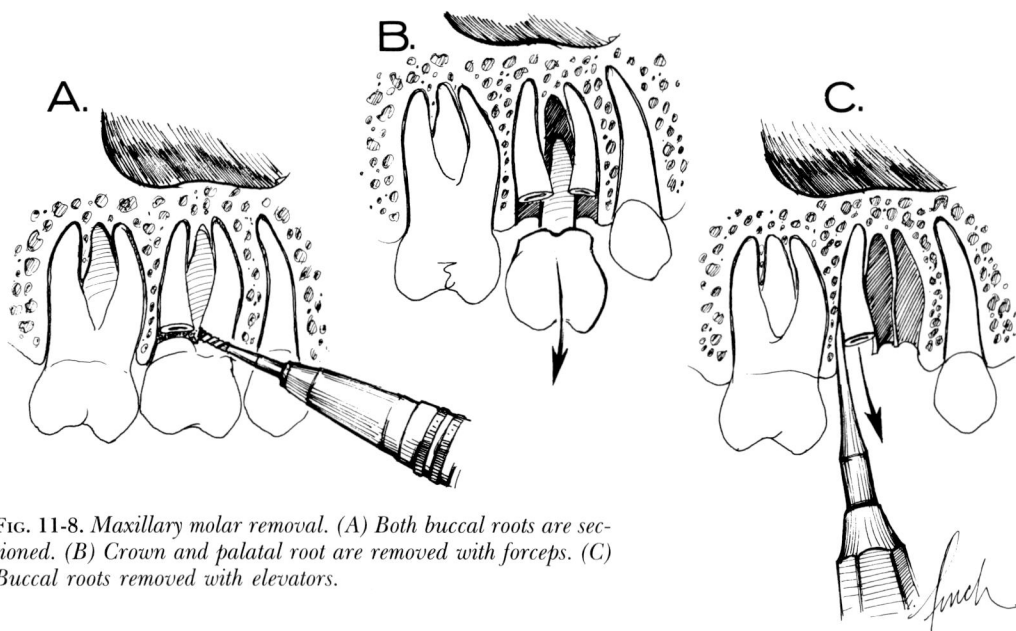

FIG. 11-8. *Maxillary molar removal. (A) Both buccal roots are sectioned. (B) Crown and palatal root are removed with forceps. (C) Buccal roots removed with elevators.*

of the palatal and buccal roots and makes the buccal approach to the palatal root hazardous.

Root Recovery

Broken roots occurring during tooth removal should not necessarily be considered as evidence of careless or faulty surgical technique. A number of factors may make root fracture unavoidable, including: (1) ankylosis of tooth root to bone, (2) hypercementosis, (3) periodontal disease, (4) dense or sclerotic bone, (5) lack of alignment of forceps beaks with long axis of tooth, and (6) long, spiny, curved roots.

As a basic principle, some form of elevation should be applied to the tooth to be extracted. Whenever subluxation of the tooth, no matter how slight, occurs prior to application of forceps, root fracture is less likely and simple extraction with forceps is more easily accomplished. Moreover, if a

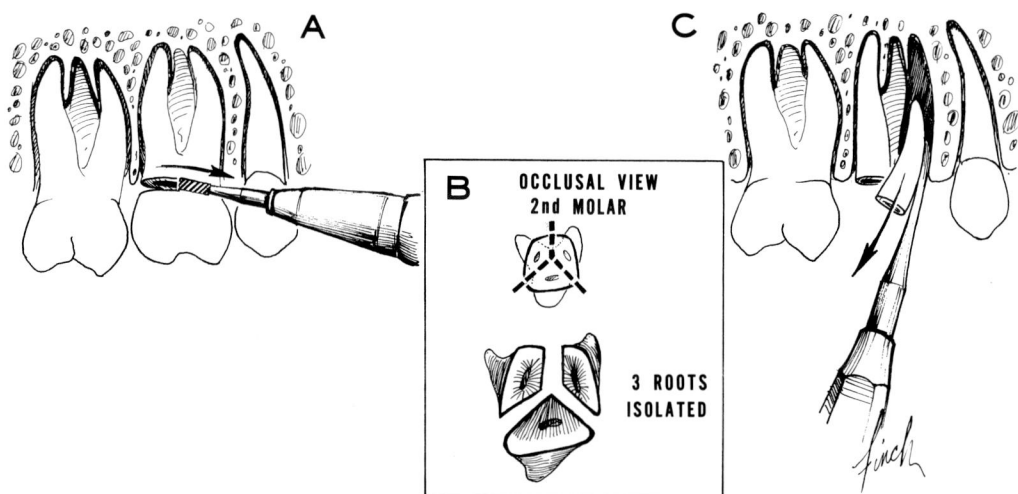

FIG. 11-9. *Alternate method of maxillary molar removal. (A) Entire crown sectioned at cervical line. (B) Roots separated with drill after crown removed. (C) Each of the three roots is removed individually.*

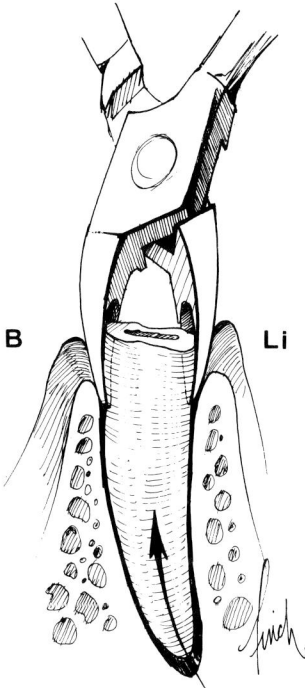

FIG. 11-10. *Root forceps are seated well below cervical line of tooth for good application of extraction maneuver.*

root should fracture, its recovery from the alveolus is facilitated if it has already been mobilized.

When root fracture occurs, the efficient surgeon should have a treatment plan. As the particular problem presents itself, one should immediately move to the step in the root recovery outline that is appropriate to the problem. The use of forceps with a special design should be considered first. A variety of root forceps are available. A standard root forceps is the no. 69. A long narrow beak for application below the cervical line may be all that is needed (Fig. 11-10). If this is unsuccessful, the second procedure entails utilizing the elevator as a displacement instrument. The no. 301 straight-blade elevator works well (Fig. 11-11). The instrument should be carefully inserted between the root and socket, tipping the root, then manipulating the elevator to displace the root, walking it down the socket wall. If a purchase point is indicated or a curved elevator more appropriate, the Hu-Friedy 190 and 191 elevators are excellent.

The third procedure for root recovery is to use the handpiece with a small round bur as a retraction instrument (Fig. 11-12). The size of the bur can be determined by the size of the root to be recovered. Thrust the rotary bur into the center of the root fragment, penetrating down the pulpal canal and binding the bur in the tooth fragment at a slight angle to further increase the lock. Then stop the motor and withdraw the bur with attached root.

The fourth procedure is the window technique (Fig. 11-13). On occasion, the decision to utilize this procedure may be made immediately, bypassing the others. A mucoperiosteal flap will be necessary. Once the flap has been reflected, a window is made with the bur or chisel near the apex of the root to be recovered. An instrument appropriate to the size of the window is then inserted and used to drive the root out of the socket. A primary goal of the window technique is to conserve alveolar bone.

The final procedure is taken only when the others have failed or are not indicated. Raise a full mucoperiosteal flap and remove bone for access to the root (Fig. 11-14). A vertical releasing incision should always be made at least one tooth away from the root to be recovered to assure the return of the flap margin over solid bone.

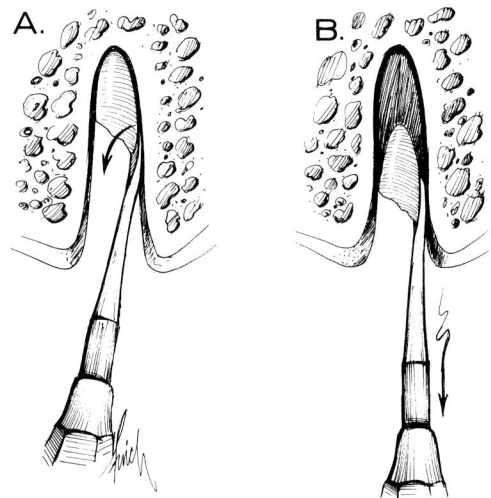

FIG. 11-11. *Proper use of root elevator. (A) Tip of elevator inserted between root and alveolus. Apically directed force on elevator is avoided. (B) Root is dislodged with occlusally directed traction.*

Avoid apically-directed pressure on the root or tooth from elevators or forceps to prevent the tooth or root from being driven from the socket into surrounding anatomic areas, such as maxillary sinus (antrum), infratemporal fossa, inferior alveolar canal, or sublingual or submandibular spaces.

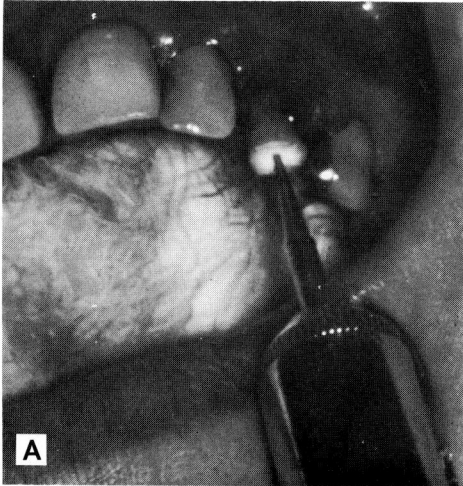

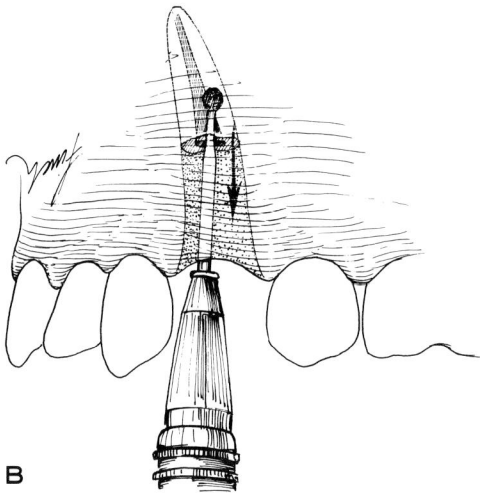

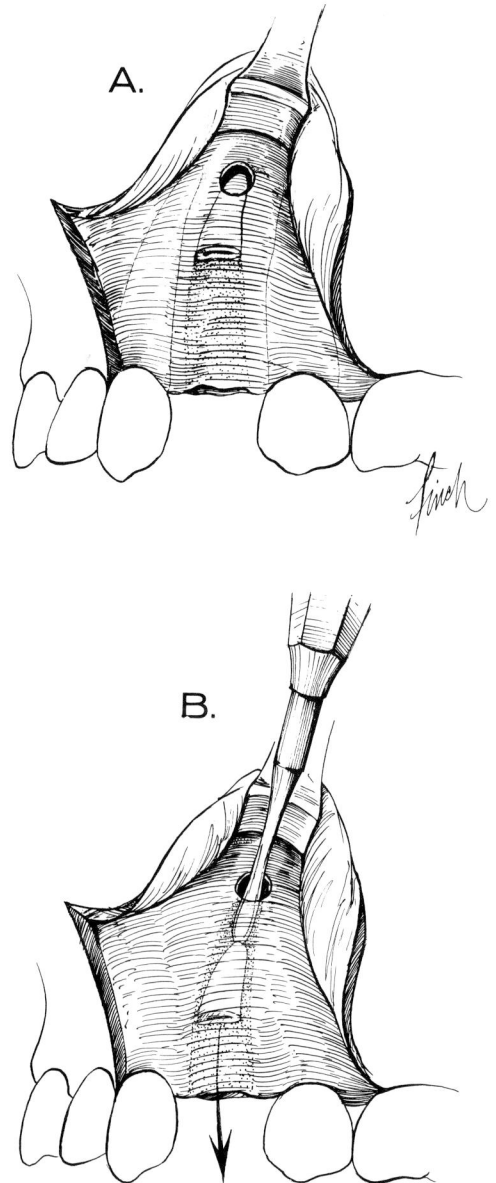

FIG. 11-12. (A) Use of dental drill as root removal instrument. (B) Bur is driven into pulp canal and then into root cementum, drill is stopped, then bur is withdrawn bringing root with it.

In review, the procedures for root recovery are: (1) root forceps, (2) appropriate elevator, (3) bur technique, (4) window technique, (5) flap and removal of bone.

Adequate vision is probably the most important adjunct to recovery of fractured roots. Strong, fine-tipped suction handled by a capable assistant, a good light source (especially from a headlight), and access provided by the well-designed mucoperiosteal flap and judicious removal of alveolar bone are important in providing the operator with the best view of the root.

FIG. 11-13. Window technique for root recovery preserves alveolar bone. (A) Small window created with bur over root apex. (B) Root driven out of socket with elevator.

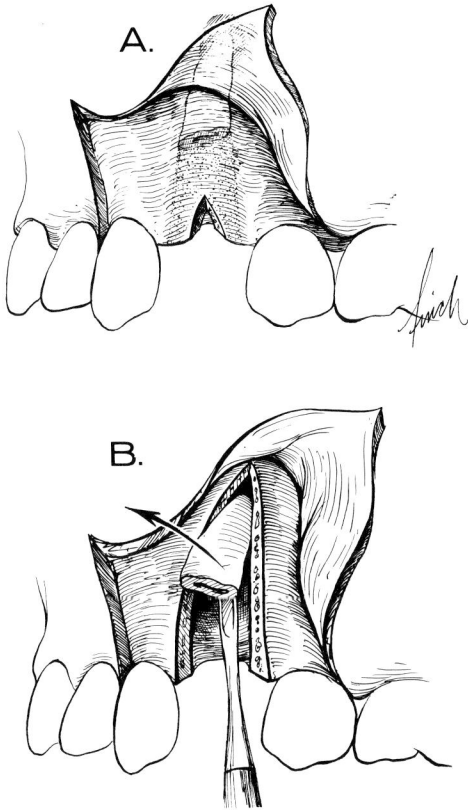

FIG. 11-14. *Direct removal of root. (A) Mucoperiosteal flap raised. (B) After removal of alveolar bone, root is easily luxated with an elevator.*

If a root or entire tooth becomes displaced and is no longer visible, the operator should first obtain a radiograph to verify its position. For example, it may be impossible to tell on clinical examination alone whether a maxillary molar root rests in the infratemporal fossa or the maxillary sinus (Fig. 11-15). Further, the antrum

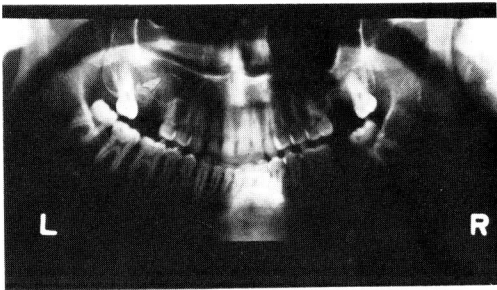

may be compartmentalized by bony septae making exact location of the displaced fragment critical to its removal.

If a root fragment or tooth is forced into the maxillary sinus, do not enlarge the socket opening into the antrum to facilitate attempted recovery. This only increases the size of the oroantral opening, which will have to be surgically closed. An initial attempt, however, should be made with a fine suction tip through the socket to recover the root that may lie just above the socket on the antral floor. If this fails, the antrum should be approached through the standard Caldwell-Luc operation (see Chapter 16). The root can then be recovered under direct vision with antral curettes, irrigation, or suction (Fig. 11-16). The socket and buccal openings into the

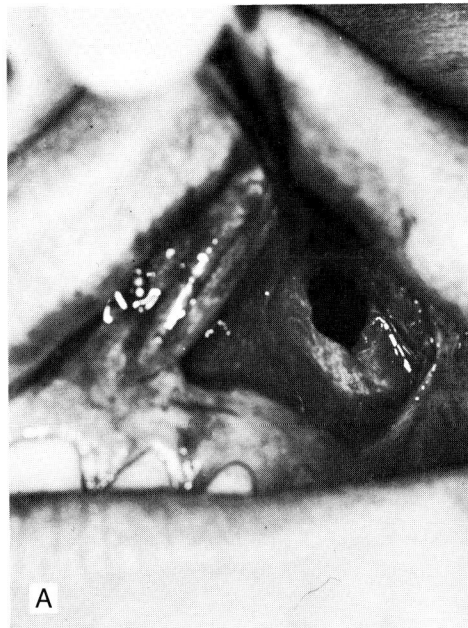

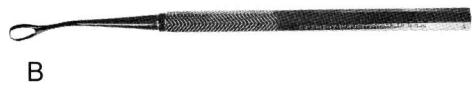

FIG. 11-15. *Displaced root in left maxillary sinus.*

FIG. 11-16. *(A) Access to the maxillary sinus is via an incision placed in mucosa over apices of premolar teeth. (B) The antral curette is often helpful in retrieving a displaced root.*

sinus are closed primarily by advancing and suturing the mucoperiosteum. The patient is provided with antibiotic cover because of oral contamination of the sinus and nasal decongestants to assure normal drainage from the antrum into the nasal cavity.

Root tips forced into the inferior alveolar canal are difficult to recover (Fig. 11-17). Complications during their removal include hemorrhage and inferior alveolar nerve injury, discussed later in this chapter. Special microneurosurgical instruments and magnification with either loupes or the operating microscope are required to avoid these complications. The procedure may be lengthy and require general anesthesia to render the patient perfectly still. Such operations are best done by the specialist.

Because of the thin lingual bone in the molar region of the mandible, root tips may be displaced medially into the sublingual or submandibular space (Fig. 11-18). Attempts at removal only displace the root further into the soft tissues unless control is exercised. Place a finger extraorally against the skin over the submandibular space, and exact superiorly directed pressure to create a counterforce during exploration which will elevate the root against the lingual surface of the mandible. An extensive lingual mucoperiosteal flap is raised to adequately visualize the root tip, which is grasped with an alligator or other fine forcep and removed. Uncontrolled displacement of the root inferiorly into the neck may cause a serious fascial space infection and require more extensive surgical procedures to remove it.

Fractures

Injudicious application of force by elevators or forceps, rather than breaking the tooth or roots, may result in fracture of the maxillary tuberosity, alveolar segment, or mandible. These fractures may occur in spite of the best surgical technique, especially with the long-rooted molar located in a tuberosity with low-lying maxillary antrum or in the atrophic mandible.

When the maxillary tuberosity has been fractured during exodontia, the bone should be preserved if possible. If the fractured tuberosity remains attached to periosteum, its blood supply is intact and it should be repositioned. It is stabilized by suturing the overlying mucosa and, if a tooth or teeth are present in it, by a fracture arch bar or acrylic splint. The fractured tuberosity thus treated should heal normally, prevent oroantral communication and preserve ridge form for construction of a dental prosthesis. If, however, the fractured segment of tuberosity has been completely detached from periosteum, it has lost its blood supply and will become necrotic (Fig. 11-19). If it is left in place, it will most likely cause an infection and se-

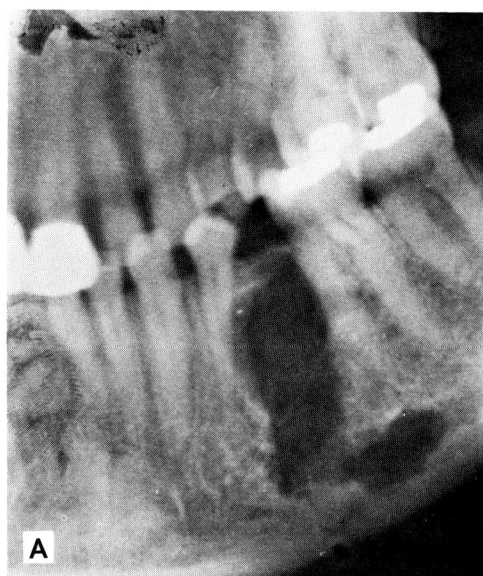

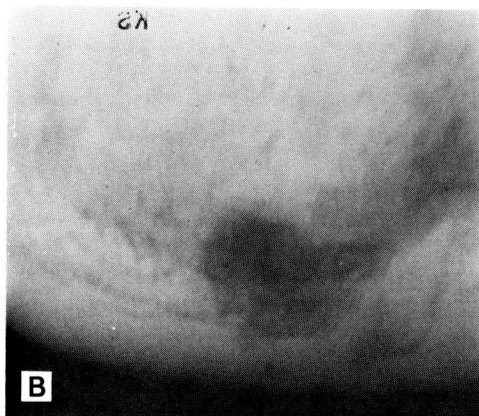

FIG. 11-17. *Root tip dislodged into the inferior alveolar canal.*

with an arch bar, acrylic splint, or bonded orthodontic brackets and arch wire. Antibiotic cover should be instituted immediately to protect tuberosity or alveolar bone exposed to saliva-borne bacteria.

A complete fracture of the mandible is a more serious condition that may occur during tooth extractions, especially long-rooted molars, where a radicular or dentigerous cyst has replaced a large area of bone or when the mandible is atrophic. Diagnosis and management of fractures is discussed thoroughly in Chapter 19. As in fractures of the tuberosity or alveolar bone, antibiotic therapy should be initiated immediately as prophylaxis against contamination of the bone by saliva-borne bacteria (principally streptococci) before prompt referral to a specialist for definitive treatment.

Hemorrhage

Persistent or uncontrolled bleeding, a sequel not uncommon to exodontia procedures, may occur in either the early (first few hours) or late (up to 10 days) postoperative period. Careful identification and control of sources of bleeding during surgery and proper instructions to patients concerning the use of gauze pressure packs reduce the possibilities of postoperative hemorrhage.

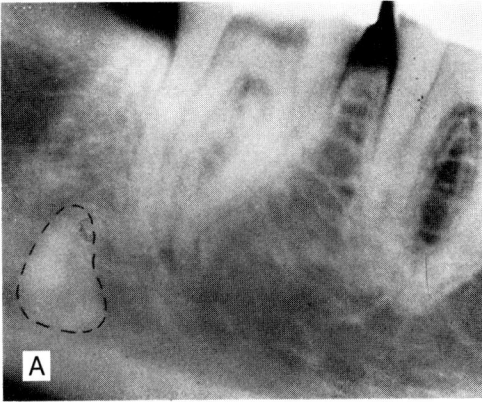

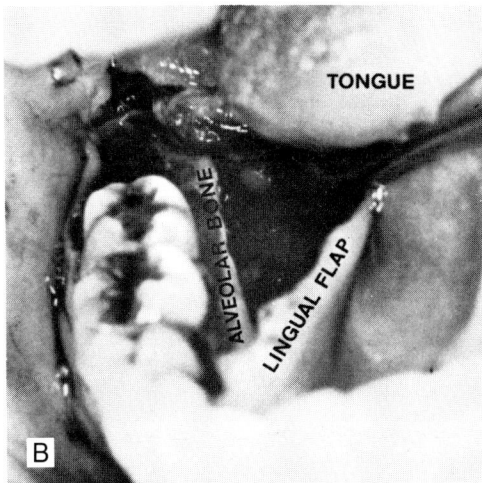

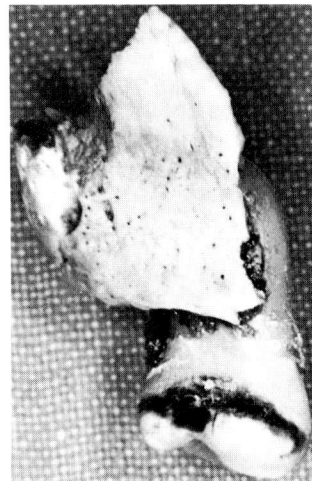

FIG. 11-18. *(A) Mandibular third molar root tip forced through lingual alveolar plate into submandibular space. (B) Lingual mucoperiosteal flap is raised to provide access to displaced root.*

questrate. Therefore, the detached bone should be removed, a mucoperiosteal flap reflected bucally and/or palatally, the sharp alveolar bony margins smoothed with rongeurs and bone file and a watertight closure of the mucosa performed to prevent orantral communication.

Fracture of an alveolar segment containing teeth other than the one being extracted may occur in the maxillary canine or mandibular incisor region. This incident is identified by the sudden mobility of the adjacent teeth, and immediate treatment is required to preserve the loosened alveolar bone and teeth. The teeth are stabilized manually in normal position and fixated

FIG. 11-19. *Tuberosity luxated during extraction of maxillary third molar. This segment has become completely devitalized and should not be replanted.*

Bleeding following any surgical procedure is due to systemic or local causes. Systemic causes can often be suspected on the basis of a careful history. Most patients with deficiencies in clotting factors or platelets have a history of previous prolonged hemorrhage requiring active treatment following procedures such as tooth extractions, tonsillectomy, or relatively minor lacerations. Easy bruising without significant trauma or bleeding into joints can be signs of coagulation deficiencies. Hereditary conditions such as hemophilia or Von Willebrand's disease are suspected from the family history. Anticoagulant medications (e.g., Coumadin) interfere with normal clotting and cause clinically significant bleeding following dentoalveolar surgery, if not discontinued sufficiently in advance of operation. Certain disease states are known to be associated with the presence of a circulating anticoagulant (e.g., systemic lupus erythematosus).

Local causes of hemorrhage originate in either soft tissue or bone. Soft tissue bleeding is either arterial, venous, or capillary. Arterial bleeding is bright red and spurting in nature. Arteries in the soft tissues at risk during exodontia procedures include the greater palatine artery and the buccal artery which lies lateral to the retromolar pad area. Surprisingly, the nasopalatine artery bleeds very little when it is transected, as it usually is during exposure of a palatally impacted canine tooth. Venous blood, dark red in color, flows steadily and heavily if the vein is large. Slow minimal ooze, and bright red color characterize capillary bleeding. Troublesome bone bleeding originates either from nutrient canals in the alveolar region, central vessels, such as the inferior alveolar artery, or from central vascular lesions (hemangioma, arteriovenous malformation).

The patient who reports on continued bleeding after surgery should be questioned carefully. If bleeding has just begun and the patient is cooperative, application of firm pressure over the bleeding site by biting down firmly on a gauze sponge or a tea bag (tannic acid aids in coagulation of blood) for one hour at home may secure good hemostasis (Fig. 11-20). Persistent bleeding should be evaluated and treated by the dentist.

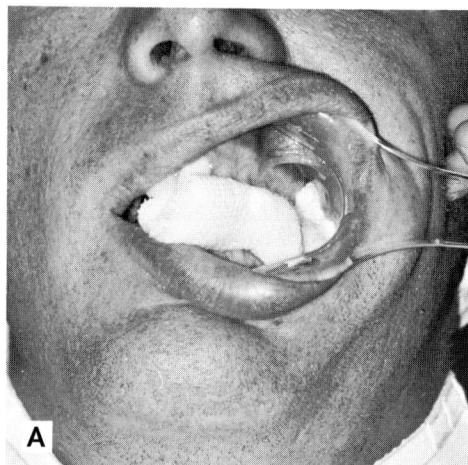

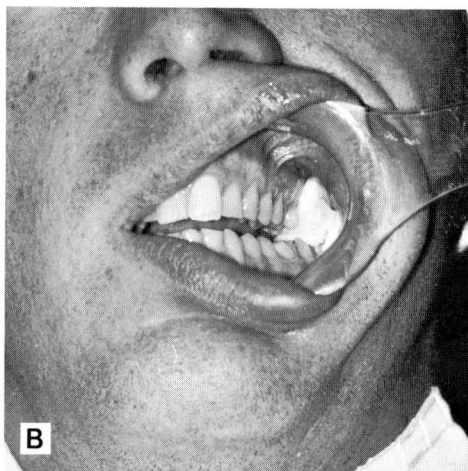

Fig. 11-20. *Gauze pack placed after extraction of third molars. (A) Gauze placed too far anteriorly to exert pressure over extraction sockets. (B) Pack is placed directly over extraction sockets to produce maximal effect on hemostasis.*

Try to quantify the amount of blood lost and its character (blood clots are more significant than blood-tinged saliva). The patient's general condition related to the amount of blood loss can be determined by his answers to questions about dizziness, weakness, nausea, and thirst, all of which might indicate significant reduction in circulating blood volume (see Chapter 5 for a discussion of shock). On examination, the patient who has lost more than 10 to 15 percent of circulating blood volume exhibits pallor, diaphoresis, and anxiety. Blood

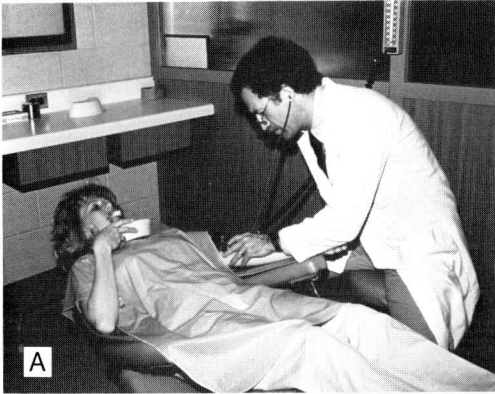

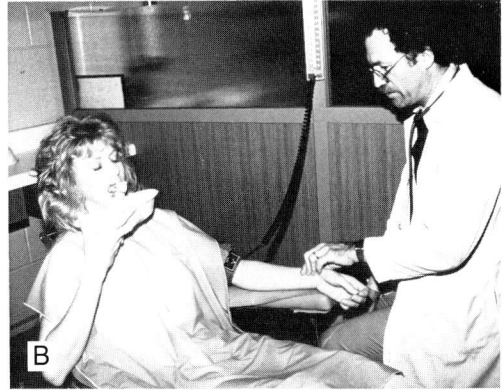

FIG. 11-21. *Checking vital signs in a bleeding patient. If significant decrease in circulating blood volume has occurred, the pulse rate increases and the blood pressure may drop when the patient is changed abruptly from the (A) supine to the (B) upright position.*

pressure decreases and pulse rate increases and has weaker amplitude when a patient who has sustained significant blood loss is changed from the supine to the upright position (Fig. 11-21). Of the two, pulse rate reflects blood volume deficiency earlier than blood pressure.

Management of bleeding requires proper equipment. An emergency tray set up with the necessary instruments and supplies should always be readily available in the clinic, office, or hospital emergency room (Fig. 11-22). Requirements include good suction, adequate light, local anesthetic with a vasoconstrictor, instruments such as retractors, hemostats, scissors, needle holders, and supplies such as Gelfoam or Surgicel, powdered thrombin, gauze sponges, bone wax, and sutures. An assistant is invaluable to retrieve needed supplies or extra instruments and to retract and suction.

Everything should be done to reassure the patient and any accompanying relatives or friends. The dramatic appearance of blood is frightening to most of the lay public. Proceed in an orderly, deliberate, and calm manner. Local anesthesia of the general area from which the bleeding originates is applied first to render further manipulations painless. Often the vasoconstrictor itself slows or even stops the bleeding. Clear the patient's mouth of blood and clots. Remove any sutures to facilitate retraction of mucoperiosteal flaps raised during the original surgery. Conduct a thorough search of the soft tissue and bone to identify the source of bleeding. If the bleeding seems to be capillary in nature, place a gauze pack over the area held by firm biting pressure for 15 minutes. This is often all that is necessary to control or stop capillary oozing. Larger vessels, arteries, or veins require direct clamping with a hemostat and tying off with a suture, placement of a stick-tie or, if small in diameter, coagulation with the electrocautery.

Bleeding from the inferior alveolar canal presents a special problem because access is limited and blood tends to gush vigorously from the extraction socket. Use strong suction to clear the socket of blood as completely as possible. Avoid blind clamping with a hemostat to prevent injury

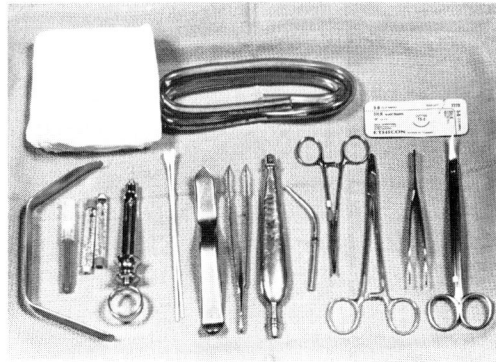

FIG. 11-22. *Standard tray set-up for the control of hemorrhage. Gelfoam, Surgicel, powdered thrombin, or bone wax are added, if needed.*

to the inferior alveolar nerve. Working rapidly, pack the depth of the socket firmly with Gelfoam or Surgicel, cover with a firmly placed gauze pack and apply firm pressure. This should control the bleeding and allow a clot to form at the interface of the vessel and the Gelfoam or Surgicel. Brisk bleeding from nutrient canals within the alveolar bone is controlled easily by crushing the bone over the canal or packing it with bone wax.

Once bleeding is controlled, attention can be paid to the patient's overall status. If symptoms and/or signs of hypovolemia resulting from blood loss exist, an intravenous line should be established for fluid administration. In some cases hospitalization and blood transfusion may be necessary for adequate stabilization of the patient. Patients in whom good hemostasis cannot be achieved, despite seemingly adequate measures, must be screened for the possible presence of a coagulation defect. Prothrombin time, partial thromboplastin time, and bleeding time are basic tests for defects in the intrinsic, extrinsic, and platelet mechanisms of coagulation. An abnormal bleeding time is followed by a platelet count to determine whether a quantitative or qualitative platelet deficiency exists. Further sophisticated coagulation tests should be ordered under a hematologist's supervision. All patients who have lost considerable amounts of blood should have a baseline complete blood count taken at the time of the bleeding episode. Although the magnitude of blood loss is not reflected in the initial blood count, a subsequent test in 2 to 3 days will show a drop in hemoglobin and hematocrit that indicates how much bleeding has occurred. Consideration for replacement iron therapy can be given to patients whose blood counts are found to be below acceptable levels and are symptomatic (weakness, fatiguability, tachycardia).

Nerve Injuries

Injuries to peripheral branches of the trigeminal nerve—particularly the inferior alveolar, lingual, and mental—occur during the removal of teeth despite the best surgical judgment and technique. Such injuries are not necessarily evidence of negligence or carelessness.[4] The resulting

numbness, tingling, or burning of the affected area can be quite disturbing to the patient. A report from the National Institute of Dental Research indicates that some type of nerve injury occurs during impacted third molar removal in 5 percent of cases and that the sensory loss is prolonged or permanent in 0.1 percent.[5] Presently, the most frequent cause of litigation against dentists is a nerve injury.

Prevention of nerve injuries is based upon knowledge of the anatomy of the nerves located in the area of surgery. The inferior alveolar nerve usually crosses from medial to beneath the lateral cortex of the mandible at or near the third molar region. The relationship of the inferior alveolar canal to the third molar roots can be determined from an x-ray.[6] When the canal and roots appear on x-ray to be in close relationship, the condition may be either one of superimposition without real proximity, or the root may be grooved, notched, or actually perforated by the canal (Fig. 11-23). When the canal is in contact (groove or notch) with the root, the root appears less radiopaque where it is crossed by the canal. The canal narrows where it perforates the root. Recognition of such relationship of root to inferior alveolar canal alerts the astute clinician to the increased risk of inferior alveolar nerve injury.

The mental nerve branches from the inferior alveolar nerve, exits the mandible laterally by way of the mental foramen located inferior to the premolar root apices, and divides into three separate branches. Incisions in the mucobuccal fold or retraction of a mucoperiosteal flap must be done with consideration for the location of the mental nerve.

The lingual nerve leaves the mandibular nerve in the pterygomandibular space and takes one of three courses as described by Mozsary.[7] The nerve may pass inferior to the submandibular salivary duct and medially into the tongue, inferior to the submandibular gland and medially into the tongue, or come to lie against the periosteum of the medial surface of the mandible in the second and third molar region before it swings medio-anteriorly into the tongue. The lingual nerve is in jeopardy in this last-mentioned position during removal of third molars. Carrying mucosal

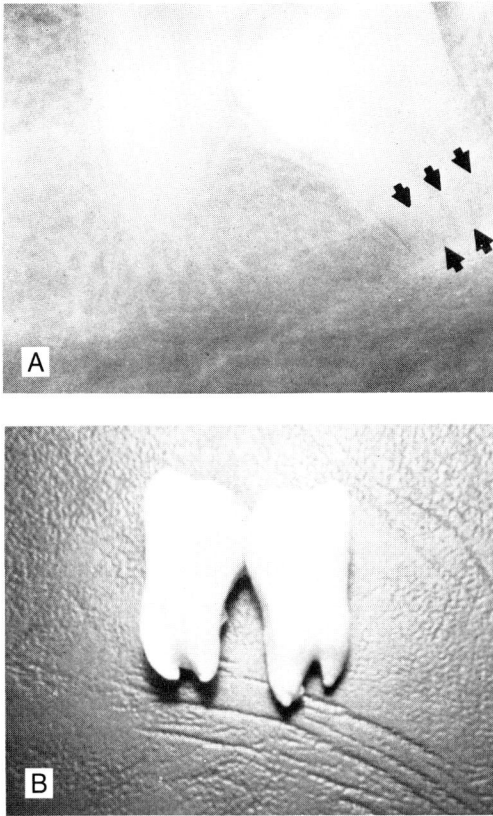

FIG. 11-23. *(A) Notching of third molar roots by inferior alveolar canal is suspected on x-ray and (B) confirmed after the teeth have been removed.*

incisions buccally in the retromolar area and protecting the lingual soft tissues during use of osteotomes or the high-speed drill minimizes surgical risk to the lingual nerve.

Seddon's classification helps the clinician evaluate nerve injuries, assess prognosis for recovery, and determine when and if surgical intervention is indicated.[8] *Neurapraxia* is a temporary conduction failure without anatomic disruption of the nerve. Complete recovery can be expected within four weeks, and surgical repair is not required. *Axonotmesis* is a more serious injury in which a prolonged conduction failure is due to disruption of some of the axons within the nerve. However, the endoneurial sheaths remain intact to guide the pathway of regenerating axons. Return of nerve function may not begin before 4 weeks, but some return should be clinically apparent by 8 weeks after injury. Recovery from axonotmesis may be partial or complete, but some degree of deficit commonly persists, particularly unpleasant sensations (paresthesias) such as spontaneous burning or tingling, or hyperpathia (painful response to the application of ordinary stimuli). *Neurotmesis* is a complete loss of nerve function due to crushing, stretching, or severing of the entire nerve. Sensory loss is profound and generally permanent without surgical intervention.

Evaluation of nerve injuries requires a careful history and a thorough physical examination to document the sensory deficit. The date of the injury is important in timing surgical repair.[9] Following nerve severance the distal axons undergo Wallerian degeneration and the axonal (endoneurial) tubules are cleared of necrotic debris in preparation for new axonal growth from proximal axons. This process is completed by about 6 weeks post-injury, and up to this time nerve repair will be most effective. Endoneurial tubules that are not recannulated eventually begin to atrophy and are replaced by scar tissue, making recannulation impossible. The exact time beyond which repair of nerve severance is not possible has not been determined clinically, and it is probably highly variable. However, clinical experience has shown atrophy of all distal nerve tissue to have occurred by 1 year post-injury. Nerves which are compressed (axonotmesis) rather than severed have a much longer time (perhaps years) during which surgical intervention can produce improvement because all axons and/or endoneurial tubules will probably not have undergone degeneration.[10]

The progress of symptoms that has occurred since injury is important. Levant has shown that neurapraxia following inferior alveolar nerve injury exhibits a predictable pattern of recovery that includes in succession anesthesia, tingling and crawling sensations, hyperpathia, hypoesthesia, hyperpathia and return to normal by 4 weeks.[11] If the patient remains totally numb after 4 weeks, the injury is either axonotmesis or neurotmesis. If no sensation returns after 8 weeks, the injury may be neurotmesis and no recovery without surgery can be expected.

Although there are many anecdotal accounts of recovery of sensation 1 to 2 years after nerve injury, it is doubtful whether such patients had objective findings of a neurologic examination to document the degree of sensory deficit actually present. The physical examination is, therefore, critical to the proper assessment of nerve injuries. Sensory response to sharp and dull stimuli, two-point discrimination, electric pulp-testing, and percussion of affected teeth are used to map out an area of sensory deficit which should be recorded in the patient's chart (Fig. 11-24). An x-ray of the area of injury may show bone or root fragments displaced into the inferior alveolar canal. At a subsequent examination findings should be compared to determine whether or not the area of sensory deficit is diminishing in size or in intensity.

Treatment of nerve injuries is based upon their classification as determined by the documented sensory deficit and progress since injury. Neurapraxia requires no surgical intervention. Axonotmesis may benefit from surgical intervention, if abnormal sensations have not resolved after a

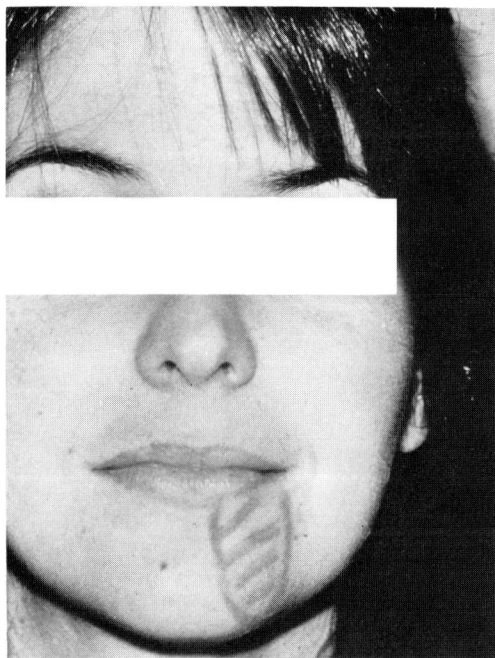

FIG. 11-24. *Area of sensory deficit following injury to the inferior alveolar nerve.*

reasonable period of time (probably several months). Neurotmesis requires surgical repair, if there is to be any hope for return of sensation. Timing is critical to success. Any nerve known to have been severed must be repaired as soon as possible, preferably within 24 hours of injury. Instances in which complete nerve disruption is suspected but not directly observed can be followed for 6 weeks. If complete sensory loss persists, exploration and repair should be carried out between the sixth and eighth weeks, when the distal endoneurial tubules will have maximal receptivity for regenerating proximal axons.[9]

Because the lingual and inferior nerves are only 2 to 3 mm in diameter and branches of the mental nerve each about 1 mm in diameter, nerve operations require magnification with the operating microscope or loupes. A high degree of manual skill, developed by practice on laboratory animals and assisted by special instruments, is essential. Microneurosurgical operations are carried out under general anesthesia in the hospital operating room as the patient must remain absolutely motionless during the lengthy surgical procedures (often several hours). The inferior alveolar nerve is approached by a submandibular skin incision and decortication of the lateral surface of the mandible, while the lingual and mental nerves are exposed intraorally. The basic principles of microneurosurgical repair include good hemostasis, good visualization, proper alignment of the nerve ends to be repaired, and suture without tension.

Depending upon what is found at operation, one or more of the following may be done: excision of neuroma, decompression by removal of impinging scar tissue, bone or tooth fragments, primary nerve repair by suturing or nerve grafting (Fig. 11-25). Nerve severances are repaired by fine sutures (8-0 or 10-0) of nonreactive material such as silk or nylon. Repair of the outer connective tissue layer (epineurium) or individual fascicles (perineurium) within the nerve is done. In mixed (motor and sensory) nerves, intrafascicular repair has given better results, but in purely sensory nerves such as the lingual or inferior alveolar that advantage has not been established. If a segment of nerve is missing,

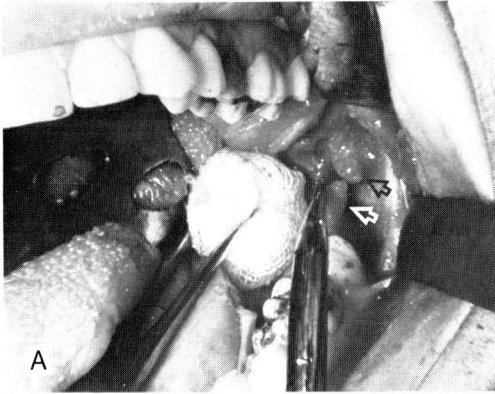

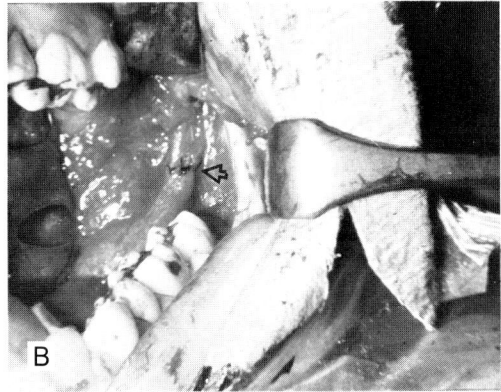

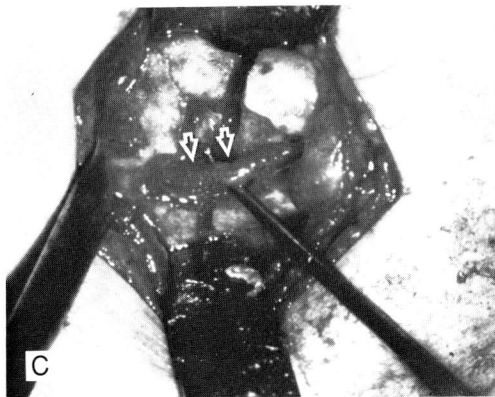

FIG. 11-25. *Nerve injuries. (A) Severed proximal and distal ends of lingual nerve identified. (B) Lingual nerve after primary repair (neurorrhaphy) with nylon sutures. (C) Inferior alveolar nerve compressed in malunited mandibular fracture has been dissected free of impinging bone and scar tissue. Osteotomy has been done to reposition fracture segments.*

necrotic, or replaced by scar tissue, the two ends of the nerve may not be able to be brought together without tension across the suture line. In such cases, the gap is replaced with an autogeneous nerve graft. The greater auricular nerve in the neck or the sural nerve in the posterior calf are suitable donor nerves.

Currently, microneurosurgery for repair of peripheral branches of the trigeminal nerve is specialized surgery available at only a few medical centers in the United States. Clinical results indicate that the repair of neurotmesis is most successful if surgery is performed within the first 2 months after injury, while axonotmesis due to compression may be repaired successfully several months or even years later.[10]

Alveolar Osteitis

Delayed healing of the extraction socket is a painful condition known as alveolar osteitis, postextraction alveolitis, or "dry socket." Alveolar osteitis results from a disintegration of the blood clot exposing the bony walls of the extraction socket to saliva and other contaminants which institutes a painful localized inflammatory process (Fig. 11-26).

Symptoms begin on the third to sixth postoperative day and include throbbing jaw pain (often with radiation to the ear), fetid odor to the breath, and a bad taste in the mouth. Examination reveals a liquefied blood clot or exposed alveolar bone. Alveolar osteitis can occur in any extraction site, but it is most common in the mandibular third molar socket. Incidence overall is approximately 5 percent. However, patients at unusually high risk include those with pericoronal infection within 10 weeks prior to extraction[12] and patients taking an estrogen-containing medication (e.g., birth control pills). Use of epinephrine-containing local anesthetics does not play a causative role in the development of alveolar osteitis.[13]

Birn demonstrated the importance of the fibrinolytic system in the breakdown of extraction socket blood clots and the development of alveolar osteitis.[14] Estrogen, for example, is known to have a fibrinolytic effect.[15] Inhibiting lysis of the fibin clot has a prophylactic effect on alveolar osteitis. A

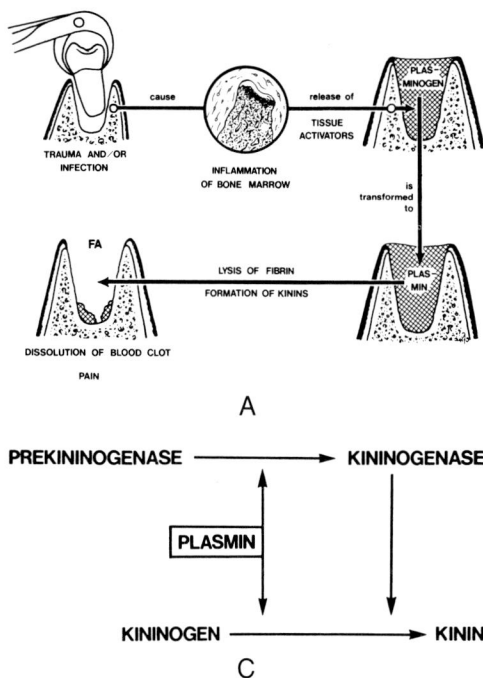

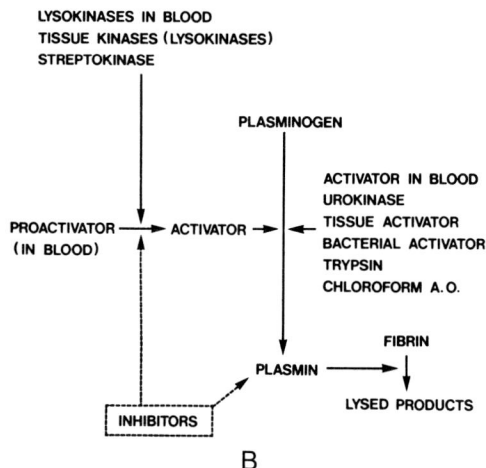

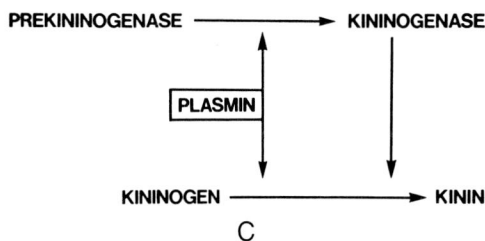

FIG. 11-26. *Alveolar osteitis. (A) Etiology and pathogenesis. (B) Components of the fibrinolytic system and their relationships. (C) Main components of the kinin-forming system. Plasmin is the activator. (From: Birn, H.: Etiology and pathogenesis of fibrinolytic alveolitis ["dry sock socket"]. Int. J. Oral Surg. 2:211, 1973.)*

propylic ester of p-hydroxybenzoic acid[16] and polylactic acid[17] applied topically both have been used successfully in clinical studies to prevent alveolar osteitis.

Other methods of reducing the incidence of alveolar osteitis include preoperative rinsing with an antiseptic mouthwash (Chloraseptic), vigorous irrigation of the socket with sterile saline at the conclusion of surgery[18] and placement of antibiotics such as tetracycline[19] topically into the socket. Prophylactic systemic antibiotic cover has a beneficial effect only on patients with a recent pericoronitis.

Once alveolar osteitis is established, 10 to 14 days are required for exposed bone to become covered with new granulation tissue. During this period, if untreated, the pain that accompanies the condition is often more severe than that of the original surgical procedure. Treatment must be prompt and vigorous to allay the patient's discomfort, and it is directed at the socket itself. In some cases, local anesthesia is administered so that the patient can tolerate treatment. The socket is isolated, irrigated with sterile warm saline, and cleared of debris with gentle suctioning. Curetting of the socket is painful and of no benefit. A dressing is applied loosely to the socket to produce local analgesia and prevent further contamination with food and saliva (Fig. 11-27). Iodoform gauze saturated with a eugenol-containing solution is a simple and effective analgesic dressing. With a properly applied dressing, relief of symptoms usually occurs in 15 to 20 minutes and lasts for 48 to 72 hours. Little or no narcotic analgesia medication is necessary. The patient is seen every 2 or 3 days for dressing changes until the socket walls are covered with granulation tissue at which time painful symptoms should have ceased. After discontinuance of the dressings, a defect in the socket area will require irrigation with a syringe after meals by the patient until it has filled in with new tissue, usually about 3 weeks.

Although multiple bacteria have been isolated from dry sockets, the condition is only a surface inflammation, not a true infection. Therefore, antibiotics are generally of little value in the treatment of an established alveolar osteitis.

Aspiration

The loss of foreign material (e.g. blood, tooth, filling material, or bone) into the pharynx can become an acute emergency if the airway is obstructed mechanically by

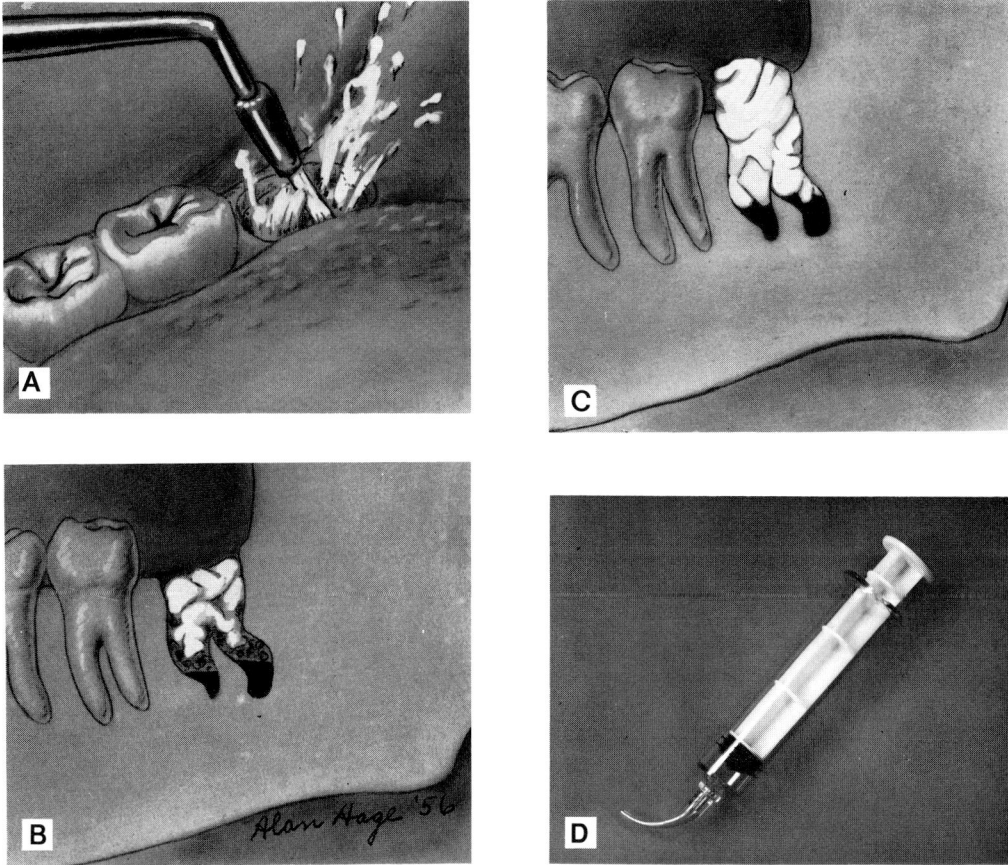

FIG. 11-27. *Treatment of alveolar osteitis. (A) Irrigation of the socket. (B and C) Placement of analgesic dressing to occlude (B) but not overfill (C) socket. (D) Disposable plastic syringe used to irrigate socket defect after discontinuance of dressings. (A and B from Waite, D.E.: Dry Socket. Practical Dental Monographs, Year Book Publishers, Inc., 1957.)*

the material or reflexly by acute laryngospasm. This complication is best prevented by placing a gauze pack between the tongue and hard palate to catch any displaced material, application of strong suction by a diligent assistant, and a good light source to enhance visualization.

Once foreign material reaches the base of the tongue or soft palate, the awake patient reflexly swallows passing the material into the pharynx. The initial sign is usually gagging or brief coughing. If the material passes into the esophagus, no further signs or symptoms may occur other than the vague sense of a "lump in the throat." Foreign material entering the respiratory tract by way of the larynx in the patient not obtunded by general anesthesia or sedatives initiates violent coughing, laryngospasm,

and respiratory stridor. Sustained laryngospasm or mechanical obstruction of the larynx or trachea rapidly leads to hypoxia. The patient is placed in Trendelenberg position, and attempts are made to clear the pharynx manually or by large-bore suction (Fig. 11-28).

To prevent cardiac arrest, cricothyrotomy must be done immediately if the airway is not established. If the material is small enough to pass through the vocal cords and enter one of the mainstem bronchi (usually the right), the airway will not be totally obstructed, but audible wheezing respirations will occur. Once the airway is secured, the operator must arrange for location of the foreign material by chest x-rays and for its removal by bronchoscopy or open thoracotomy (Fig. 11-29).

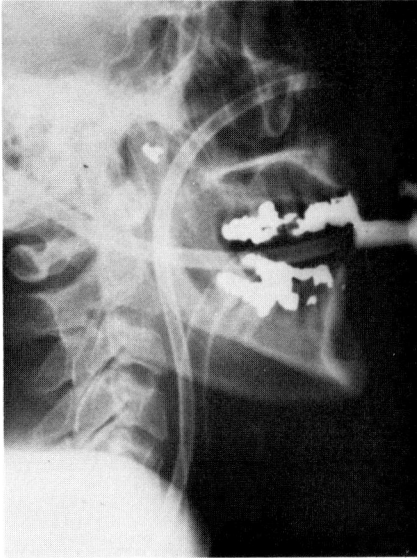

FIG. 11-28. *A gold inlay, dislodged during a surgical procedure, is displaced into the nasopharynx.*

Foreign material that passes into the gastrointestinal tract causes little acute distress. Most patients pass the swallowed object in the stool within a few days (Fig. 11-30). However, the operator must arrange for chest and abdominal x-rays to locate the object and document its passage. Occasionally, endoscopy or open operation is necessary to remove an object that be-

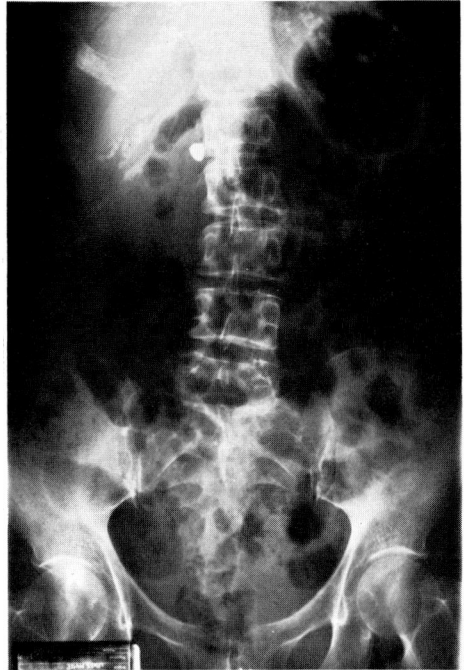

FIG. 11-30. *A cast gold crown was inadvertently swallowed by this patient. Its presence in the bowel and subsequent passage are documented by serial abdominal radiographs.*

comes lodged in or perforates the gastrointestinal wall.

Other Complications

Additional mishaps that can occur during the removal of teeth include injuries to adjacent teeth, soft tissue injuries, injection hematoma, and broken anesthetic needles. Although not as potentially serious as those complications discussed above, knowledge of their possibility will alert the operator to methods of prevention and recognition.

Injuries to adjacent teeth include broken restorations, fractured crowns, and luxation. An amalgam or cast gold restoration may have a proximal overhang that abuts against the tooth to be removed in a way that inevitably damages the restoration. Cusps of adjacent teeth may have been improperly undermined and weakened by poorly designed restorations. Occasionally, an adjacent tooth is dislodged or completely luxated out of the socket, or the wrong tooth may be removed. If the tooth is not completely developed, it should be

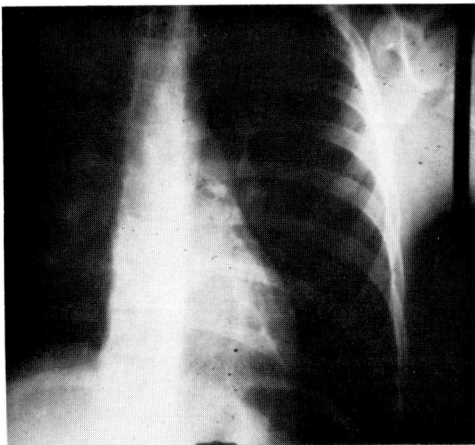

FIG. 11-29. *A tooth, displaced into the pharynx during extraction, was aspirated into the lung. The chest x-ray documents the presence of the tooth in the left mainstem bronchus.*

immediately repositioned and splinted. The wide open root apex gives maximum potential for revascularization of the pulp, which is essential for survival and retention of the replanted tooth.[20] The luxated fully developed tooth has a less certain prognosis, but replantation should be attempted.

Soft tissue injuries during tooth removal are produced by the dental drill, scalpel, or elevators. The tongue or lip not properly protected by retractors can be severely lacerated or burned by the rapidly rotating dental bur during bone removal or tooth sectioning (Fig. 11-31). Reflex jaw closure by the patient when a bite block is not in place can displace the scalpel into the soft tissues of the tongue, cheek, lip, or palate. If a periosteal, tooth, or root elevator is not properly applied with a finger stop, slippage of the instrument may cause it to be driven deeply into the soft tissues. Such injuries should be thoroughly irrigated with sterile saline, carefully inspected to ascertain whether significant structures (e.g., salivary gland duct) have been injured, and closed with sutures to prevent secondary contamination and infection, if they penetrate beneath the mucosa.

Soft tissue injuries may occur postoperatively in children who have been given local anesthesia. The anesthetized lip, cheek, or tongue becomes the object for pernicious morcellization by the unwary child. Placement of a gauze pack between the teeth for an hour, using lidocaine or mepivacaine without vasoconstrictor whenever possible, and specific advice to the parent about watching for this incident usually prevent its occurrence.

Laceration of a blood vessel during local anesthetic injection is a rare but unsettling experience for the patient and the operator. During the posterior superior alveolar nerve injection injury to the pterygoid plexus of veins or a branch of the maxillary artery causes a sudden, often painful release of blood with swelling and sometimes blanching of the cheek. Pressure over the area and application of an ice bag controls the swelling and eases any associated pain. If a large hematoma forms, any contemplated surgical procedure in the area should be postponed (Fig. 11-32). Immediate incision into this area might release the pressure formed by the hematoma and

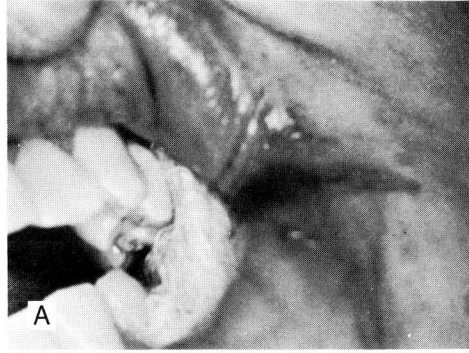

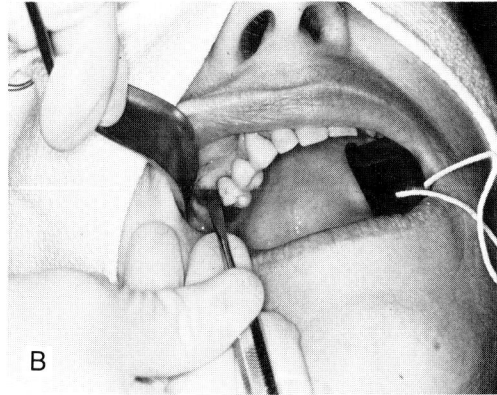

FIG. 11-31. *(A) Lip burn at oral commissure caused by contact with rotating dental bur. (B) Use of the bite block and finger stop when holding instruments prevents many inadvertent soft tissue injuries.*

allow troublesome and difficult-to-control hemorrhage to occur. In 2 weeks the area will have organized and healed, and planned surgery can be performed.

Injury to vessels in the pterygomandibular space seldom occurs during local anesthetic injection and may not even be recognized at that time. Postoperative trismus may be the only sign of such incident. Physical therapy, including application of heat and jaw opening exercises, may be required to resolve trismus persisting for more than 1 week after hematoma from either posterior superior alveolar or inferior alveolar injection.

Since the introduction of disposable local anesthetic needles, the breaking of a needle during injection has been rare. Occasionally, however, an inherent physical weakness in the needle or its connection to the hub, or reflex closure of a patient dur-

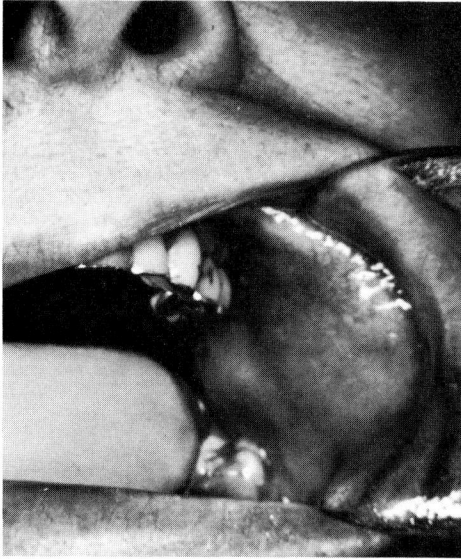

FIG. 11-32. *Hematoma from injury to the pterygoid plexus during posterior superior alveolar local anesthetic injection.*

ing injection without a bite block in place causes needle breakage. Recovery of a broken needle from the soft tissues is a challenging and frustrating surgical experience. The first step in management is accurate localization of the needle by radiographs. The decision regarding removal should be made in consultation with an oral and maxillofacial surgeon. In some cases removal is delayed to allow fibrous tissue reaction to immobilize the needle and facilitate its removal. If the needle is not near vital structure and poses no symptomatic problem for the patient, it may be left in place as long as it continues to do no harm.[21]

Accidents or complications occur during exodontia despite the most careful planning and meticulous surgical technique. The prudent operator will be cognizant of potential risks associated with exodontia procedures, take all reasonable steps to prevent injury to the patient, and act promptly and properly whenever a complication arises. Regular drills of all office personnel assist in developing and maintaining an orderly approach, no matter

how serious the situation. Each person in the office should have an assigned task to perform during an emergency or complication. A list of telephone numbers for ambulance and emergency room and for those specialists who might be needed should be at hand.

References

1. Clark, H. B., Jr.: The seven minimum essentials for tooth removal operations. J. Wisc. State Dent. Soc., 25:155, 1949.
2. Ahtone, J., and Goodman, R.A.: Hepatitis B and dental personnel: transmission to patients and prevention issues. JADA, 106:219, 1983.
3. Cooley, R. L., and Lubow, R. M.: AIDS: An occupational hazard? JADA, 107:28, 1983.
4. Kipp, D. P., Goldstein, B. H., and Weiss, W. W., Jr.: Dysesthesia after mandibular third molar surgery: a retrospective study and analysis of 1,377 surgical procedures. JADA, 100:185, 1980.
5. Guralnick, W. C., and Laskin, D. M.: Consensus development conference: removal of third molars. Bethesda, MD, National Inst. of Health, 1979.
6. Hooley, J. R., and Whitacre, R. J.: A Self-Instructional Guide to Oral Surgery in General Dentistry. 2nd Ed. VI. Assessment of and Surgery for Impacted Mandibular Third Molars. Seattle, Stoma Press, 1980.
7. Mozsary, P. G., and Middleton, R. A.: Microsurgical reconstruction of the lingual nerve. J. Oral Maxillofac. Surg., 42:415, 1984.
8. Seddon, H. J.: Nerve lesions complicating certain closed bone injuries. JAMA, 135:691, 1947.
9. Merrill, R. G.: Prevention, treatment and prognosis for nerve injury related to the difficult impaction. Dent. Clin. North Amer., 23:471, 1979.
10. Meyer, R. A.: Clinical experience with surgical repair of nerve injuries (Abstract Session). (Paper presented to Amer. Assn. Oral and Maxillofac. Surg., Washington, DC, October 4, 1985.)
11. Levant, B. A.: Mental anesthesia and its prognosis. Brit. J. Oral Surg., 4:206, 1967.
12. Kay, L. W.: Investigations into the nature of pericoronitis. Brit. J. Oral Surg., 4:52, 1966–1967.
13. Meyer, R. A.: Is local anesthesia responsible for alveolar osteitis? Medicine et Hygiene, 1073:1745, 1973.
14. Birn, H.: Etiology and pathogenesis of fibrinolytic alveolitis ("dry socket"). Int. J. Oral Surg., 2:211, 1973.

15. Coope, J., et al.: Effects of "natural estrogen" replacement therapy on menopausal symptoms and blood clotting. Brit. J. Med., *4*:139, 1975.

16. Ritzau, M., and Swangisilpa, K.: The prophylactic use of propylic ester of p-hydroxybenzoic acid on alveolitis sicca dolorosa. A preliminary report. Oral Surg., *43*:32, 1977.

17. Brekke, J. H., et al.: Influence of polylactic acid mesh on the incidence of localized osteitis. Oral Surg., *56*:240, 1983.

18. Butler, D. P., and Sweet, J.B.: Effect of lavage on the incidence of localized osteitis in mandibular third molar extraction sites. Oral Surg., *44*:14, 1977.

19. Hall, H. D., et al.: Prevention of dry socket with local application of tetracycline. J. Oral Surg., *29*:35, 1971.

20. Andreasen, J. O., and Hjortung-Hansen, E.: Replantation of teeth. Radiographic and clinical study of 110 human teeth replanted after accidental loss. Acta Odontol. Scand., *24*:263, 1966.

21. Orr, D. L.: The broken needle: report of case. JADA, *107*:603, 1983.

CHAPTER 12 # Biopsy Technique

DONALD G. CHILES

If the only tool you have is a hammer, you tend to see every problem as a nail.   ABRAHAM MASLOW

"Biopsy is the removal and examination, usually microscopic, of tissue from the living body, performed to establish precise diagnosis."[1] Unfortunately, many patients consider biopsy a test for cancer. They should be reassured that although cancer is the most serious condition detected, most biopsies reveal benign lesions. Many practitioners use terms such as "tissue examination of laboratory study" instead of biopsy when suggesting the necessity for the procedure.

Marcello Malpighi (1628-1694) formulated basic microscopic technique and is considered to be the founder of microscopic anatomy of animal and vegetable tissues. Rudolph Virchow (1821-1902) is considered by some to be the father of microscopic pathology.[2] However, Georianni Margagni (1682-1771) published a book of *The Sites and Causes of Diseases,* which laid the foundation of pathologic anatomy. Margagni's discoveries in this area are too many to enumerate. His extensive work and discoveries have earned him the title of "founder of modern pathology."[3]

The primary indication for biopsy is to confirm a clinical impression of a lesion. Biopsy may be recommended when a lesion does not respond to conservative therapy. It may also be indicated for determination of the more definitive treatment of the lesion. A general rule is, "When in doubt, biopsy!" An ulceration that bleeds easily and doesn't heal (within 10 to 14 days); a lump or thickening; a reddish or whitish patch that persists—all are warning signs for potential oral cancer. Difficulty in chewing, swallowing, or moving the tongue or jaws are often late changes.

In 1985, an estimated 29,000 new cases of oral cancer occurred in the United States. The incidence is more than twice as high in males than females and most frequent in men over age 40. Lips, tongue, mouth, and throat can be affected by oral cancer.[4]

Early detection is of the utmost importance in the success of treatment and survival of oral cancer patients. The dentist is in an ideal position to aid in the diagnosis of this disease through the regular examinations and recall visits of patients.

A thorough history and examination should always precede the determination for biopsy. Inspection of adjacent tissues, both clinically and radiographically, may indicate more involvement of the lesion than initially suspected. One should carefully palpate the lesion to determine whether it is fixed or freely movable, tender or nontender, superficial or extending to surrounding tissues. Any lymphadenopathy (size and location) should also be noted. Findings of the evaluation help to establish a good working differential diagnosis. This, in turn, should influence the decision as to what type of biopsy is indicated.

The type of biopsy to be performed depends on the location, size, and clinical impression of the lesion. Basic types of biopsy include excisional, incisional, cyto-

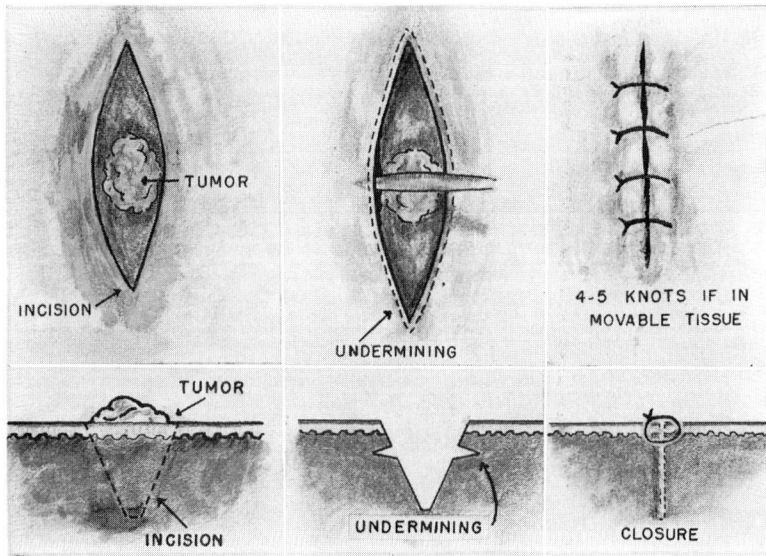

FIG. 12-1. *Technique for excisional biopsy. (From: Clark,* Practical Oral Surgery, *Lea & Febiger, 1965)*

logic smear, and exploratory. Although most oral biopsies are performed under local anesthesia, the patient's medical condition and the size, location, and character of the lesion may require a hospital admission for general anesthesia.[5]

Excisional Biopsy

The preferred technique for most lesions is excisional biopsy. Removal of the entire lesion with adequate margins accomplishes the goal of biopsy as well as treatment (Figs. 12-1 through 12-4).

Technique

1. Obtain anesthesia. Avoid distortion of the tissue with local anesthetic infiltration.

2. Isolate the lesion and immobilize tissues. A traction suture (Fig. 12-3), hook, or forceps may be used for immobilization. Avoid crushing the specimen.
3. Make an elliptical incision around the lesion. The margins should be at least 5 mm from the lesion in width and depth.
4. Place the excised specimen in a 10 percent formalin solution immediately.
5. The biopsy site may be sutured or allowed to heal by secondary intention, depending somewhat on the size of the incision.

Incisional Biopsy

Incisional biopsy is partial removal of a lesion and used when the lesion is large

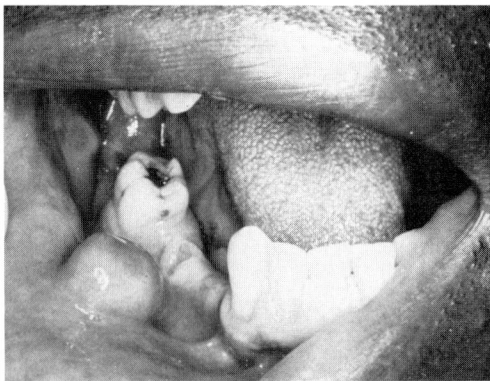

FIG. 12-2. *Lesion for excisional biopsy.*

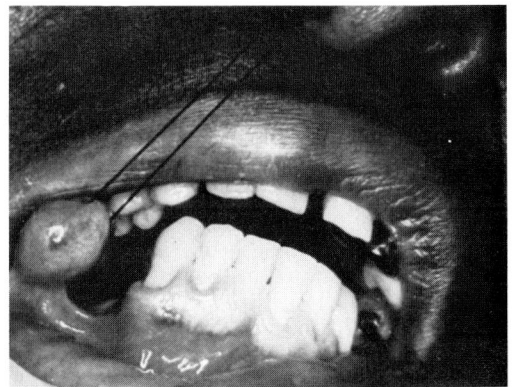

FIG. 12-3. *Traction suture for immobilization of lesion.*

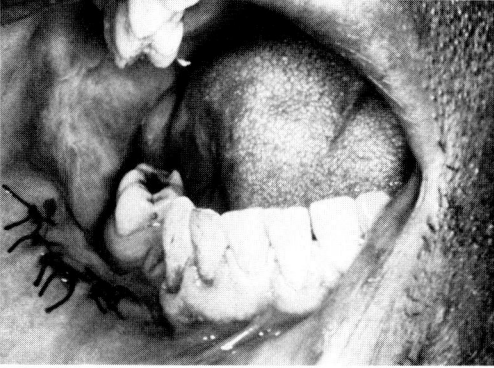

FIG. 12-4. *Biopsy site sutured after excisional biopsy.*

and total removal would be a major procedure (Figs. 12-5, 12-6, and 12-7). After establishment of the diagnosis, either further surgery or conservative management of the lesion is indicated. The incisional biopsy is essentially the same as an excisional biopsy except that the elliptical incision merely includes a portion of the lesion with adjacent normal tissue (Fig. 12-5).

Other techniques that result in partial removal of the lesion are needle or aspirational and punch biopsy (Fig. 12-8). Both techniques may be used for lesions in locations where conventional instrumentation is impossible. Tissue from the needle biopsy may be an aspirant of fluid or a core of the lesion. Special forceps are used in the punch biopsy and may crush the speci-

men (Fig. 12-9). The results of the histopathologic study are often uncertain and not dependable for a definitive diagnosis when the tissue has been crushed or mishandled.

Exfoliative Cytology

Exfoliative cytology may be indicated if the patient refuses an excisional or incisional biopsy procedure. It is not a substitute for biopsy! The technique is atraumatic and painless. A positive cytology report should be confirmed by biopsy prior to any definitive treatment.

Technique
1. A sample of superficial cells is scraped from the area in question and smeared evenly on a glass slide.
2. The slide is immediately fixed either by immersing it in 95 percent ethyl alcohol and ether or by spraying it with commercial fixative or with a hair spray (Aqua-Net, in its present formulation, has been useful).[6]
3. The slide is then delivered to the laboratory for evaluation.

Specimen Handling

As previously stated, the tissue submitted for histopathology must be handled carefully to avoid distortion interfering with adequate evaluation. Crushing of the specimen during biopsy, dehydration secondary to delay in fixation, or improper

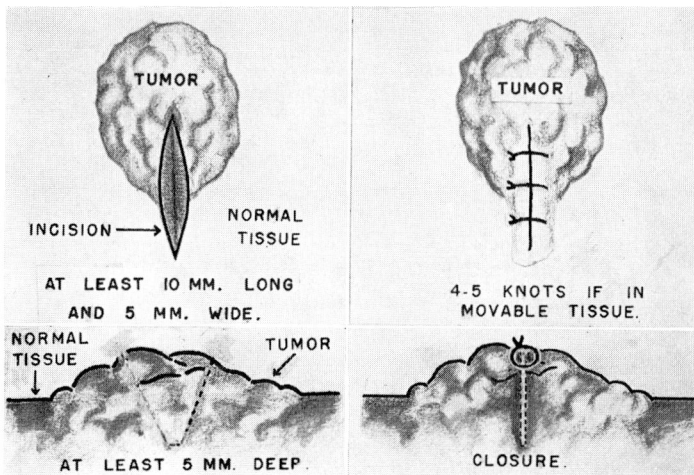

FIG. 12-5. *Technique for incisional biopsy. (From: Clark,* Practical Oral Surgery, *Lea & Febiger, 1965)*

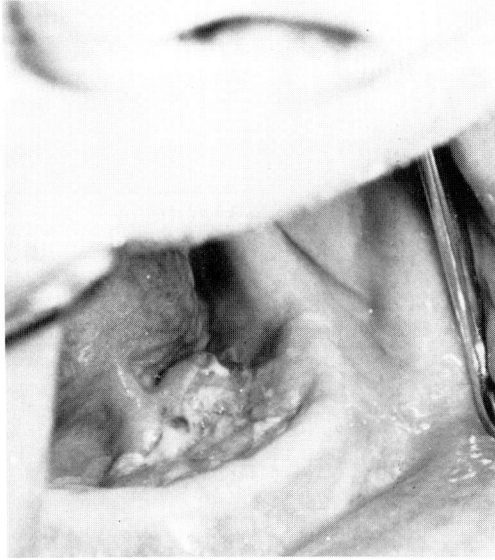

Fig. 12-6. *Highly suspicious lesion for incisional biopsy.*

fixation (inadequate volume or type of fixative) may make the biopsy useless.

The most common fixative utilized is 10 percent formalin (4 percent formaldehyde).

Approximately 20 times the volume of formalin relative to the size of the specimen should be used. If formalin is not available immediately, an isotonic solution of saline or local anesthetic may be used and the specimen refrigerated until the proper solution is available.

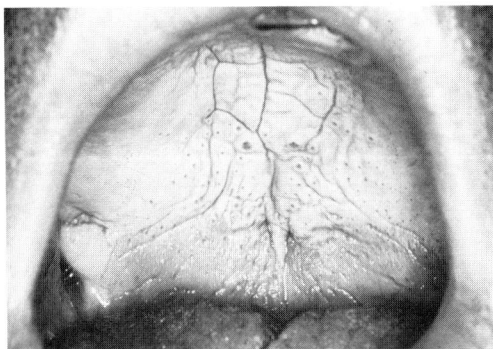

Fig. 12-7. *Indication for incisional biopsy (lesion involves entire palate).*

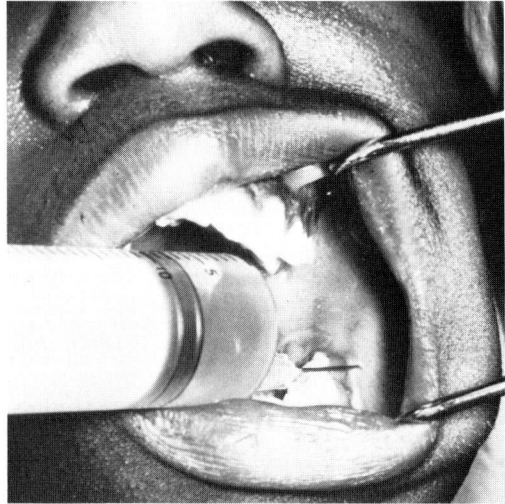

Fig. 12-8. *Aspirational biopsy.*

Fixation Technique

1. Carefully blot the specimen of any excess blood.
2. Orient the specimen by identifying appropriate margins. A suture is helpful to label a specific area of the specimen.
3. Immediately place the specimen into the appropriate fixative.

Biopsy Request Form

The biopsy request form should identify the submitting doctor, patient, and pertinent facts about the lesion. A history of growth rate, duration, or previous treatment is helpful. The location, size, regional lymph node involvement, or superficial vs. invasive character of the lesion with the clinical impression are also beneficial to the pathologist.

The specimen container should be marked clearly with the patient's and doctor's names and date to avoid confusion in the laboratory. Diagnosis of tissue of questionable source is of no benefit to the doctor or patient.

Biopsy of bone lesions may require surgical flaps or may be obtained through the socket of a recently extracted tooth (Fig. 12-10). The basic principles previously stated in this chapter apply to bone biopsies. A major difference is the laboratory time to process the specimen. Bone must be decalcified prior to cutting the tissue in preparation for microscopic examination.

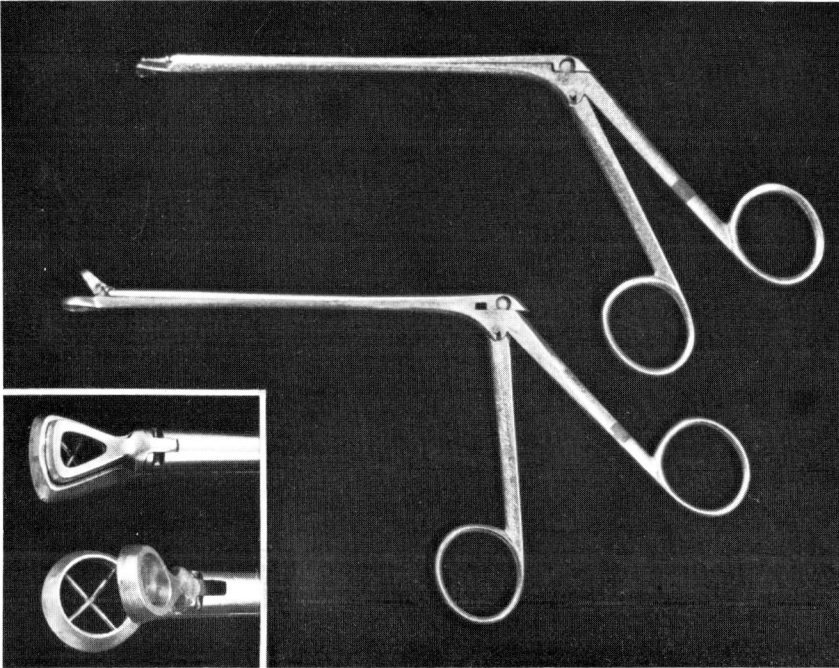

Fig. 12-9. *Punch biopsy forceps.*

This results in a longer period of time to learn of the pathologic diagnosis.

The decision to perform a biopsy or refer for treatment depends on the primary practitioner who discovers the lesion in question. In general, if the lesion is obviously malignant or highly suspect, the patient should be referred to the practitioner who will do the definitive treatment. Otherwise, the biopsy may be performed by the primary practitioner who is comfortable and adequately trained in the procedure.

When the decision to refer the patient to a specialist is made, the referring practitioner should reassure the patient regarding the need for referral. A letter explaining the reason for referral, x-rays, lab studies or any other available information about the patient should be sent to the specialist. It is customary for the specialist to send a letter or copy of the pathology report to the referring practitioner for follow-up and information for the patient's records. It is important that the patient is followed to be certain that the appropriate treatment has been accomplished.

The beginning of this chapter noted that the most common lesions detected by biopsy were benign. However, because of the seriousness of the malignancies, proper classification and staging of oral cancer is useful in the treatment of the disease. The TNM staging system is used to classify the

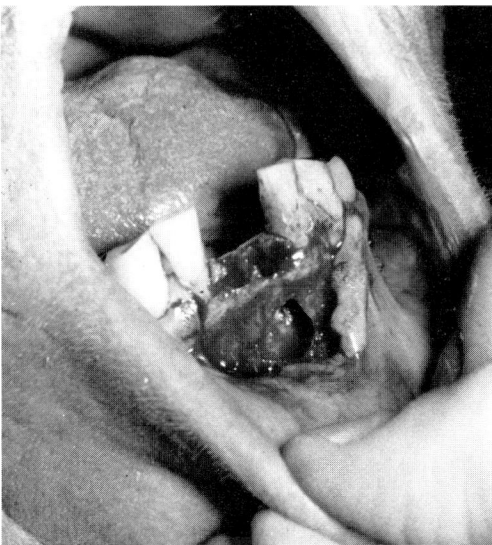

Fig. 12-10. *Bone biopsy.*

three significant events in the natural history of a cancer: tumor growth (T), spread to primary nodes (N), and metastasis (M). This system indicates the degree of extension of the tumor.

An oral primary tumor is designated T_1 if it is 2 cm or less in size, and T_2 if more than 2 cm but not more than 4 cm. T_3 refers to a lesion that exceeds 4 cm, and T_4 describes a massive tumor more than 4 cm in diameter with deep invasion involving the antrum, pterygoid muscles, base of tongue, or skin of the neck.

Neck node status (N) depends on the presence or absence of lymph node enlargement, whether the enlargement is solitary or multiple, and the estimated size of the largest node in either the homolateral or contralateral side of the neck. By adding (M_o) or (M_1) to indicate the presence or absence of distant metastasis, the TNM status of a disease is defined by one of four stages[7] (Fig. 12-11).

Of all oral diseases, oral cancer is the most serious threat to life. Because both the survival of patients and the quality of life following treatment vary significantly with the stage of the disease at time of treatment, it is essential that cancer detection occur at an early stage of the disease.

The various types of cancer treatment involve surgery, radiation, chemotherapy, or combinations of these modalities.

Complications of Cancer Treatment

It has been estimated that 35 percent of the adults and 90 percent of the children with malignant conditions develop oral complications related either to the disease or to therapy. Ulceration, mucositis, and xerostomia were the most frequent complications. Bacterial and fungal infections were also noted.[8]

FIG. 12-12. *(A and B) Radiation dermatitis and skin necrosis.*

Stage I	$T_1N_0M_0$
Stage II	$T_2N_0M_0$
Stage III	$T_3N_0M_0$ or
	$T_1N_1M_0$ or
	$T_2N_1M_0$ or
	$T_3N_1M_0$
Stage IV	T_4N_0 or N_1M_0
	Any T N_2 or N_3M_0
	Any T; any N M_1

FIG. 12-11. *Stage grouping of oral cancer.*

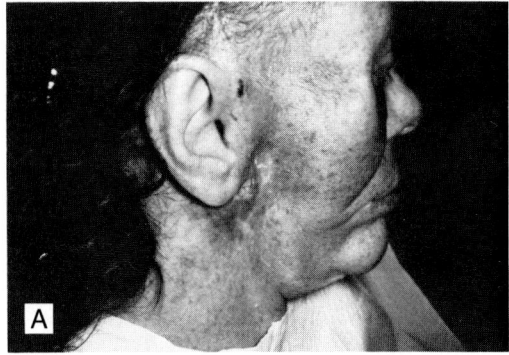

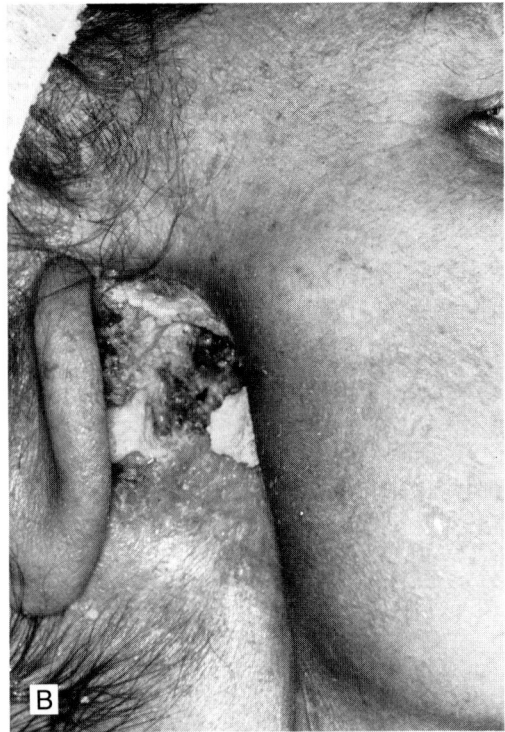

Ionizing radiation therapy in doses high enough to produce cancericidal effects to the tumor cause unavoidable effects on the adjacent normal tissue. Radiation treatment of the head and neck may cause dermatitis and delayed skin and subcutaneous tissue damage (Fig. 12-12). Trismus of the muscles of mastication may occur. Damage to salivary glands (major and minor) may result in decreased and altered saliva. The patient may be more susceptible to oral in-

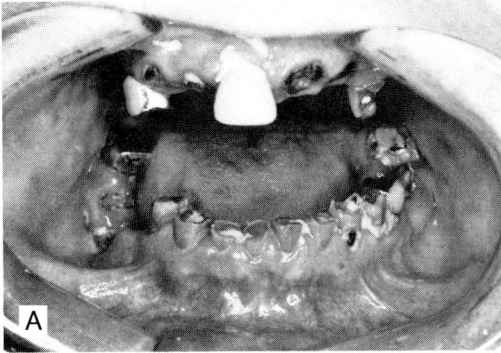

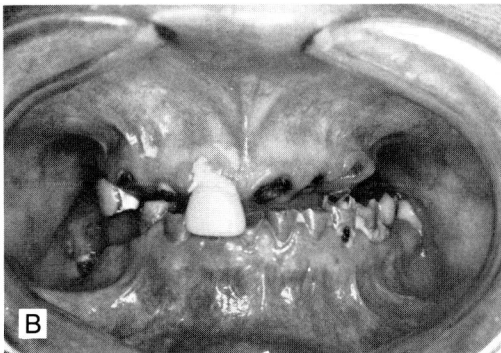

Fig. 12-13. *(A and B) Radiation caries.*

prosthodontist, and surgeon is frequently needed to accomplish a satisfactory result.

The dentist should be constantly alert when evaluating and examining patients regarding oral pathology. Recognition of premalignant or early malignant lesions may ultimately save a life! Biopsy is one of many tools available for good patient care.

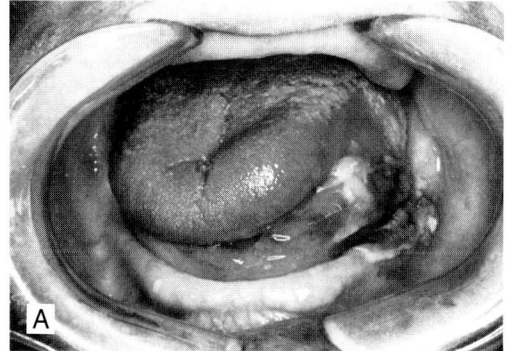

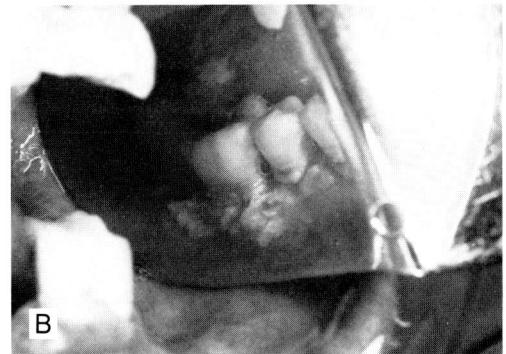

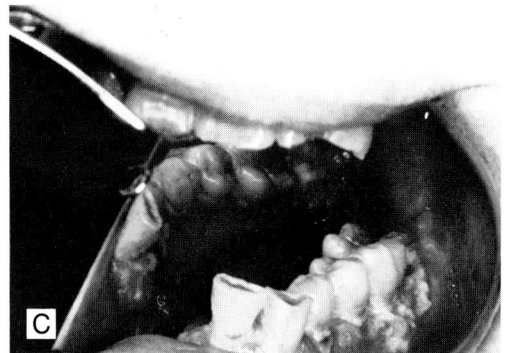

Fig. 12-14. *(A, B, and C) Oral infection secondary to chemotherapy.*

fections, especially those due to Candida albicans. The decreased and chemically changed saliva probably contributes to the increased caries activity seen in postirradiated patients (Fig. 12-13). Cervical caries is typically noted. In some cases, the salivary function may recover in 6 to 12 months.

Chemotherapy is used to treat the cases of disseminated micrometastasis. Stomatitis and hemorrhagic complications are most often seen as side effects of chemotherapy. Bacteria, fungi, and viruses are involved in the oral infections noted in the immunosuppressed and granulocytopenic patient (Figs. 12-14 and 12-15). Chemocaries is also seen and resembles the cervical caries of radiation therapy.

Surgical resection of tumors of the jaws and oral cavity often results in large defects accompanied by disfigurement and dysfunction (Fig. 12-16). This often necessitates extensive rehabilitative efforts to restore appearance and function. The combined management of the dentist,

FIG. 12-15. *(A and B) Infection secondary to a combination of chemotherapy and radiation therapy.*

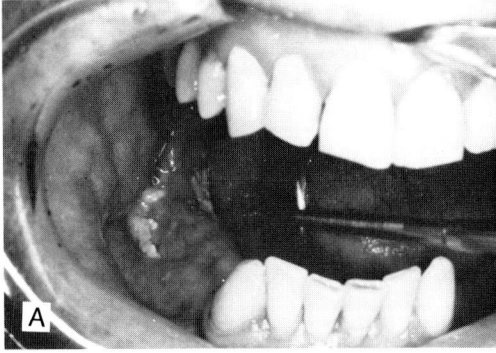

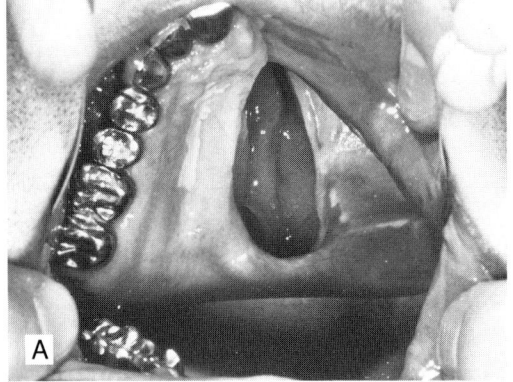

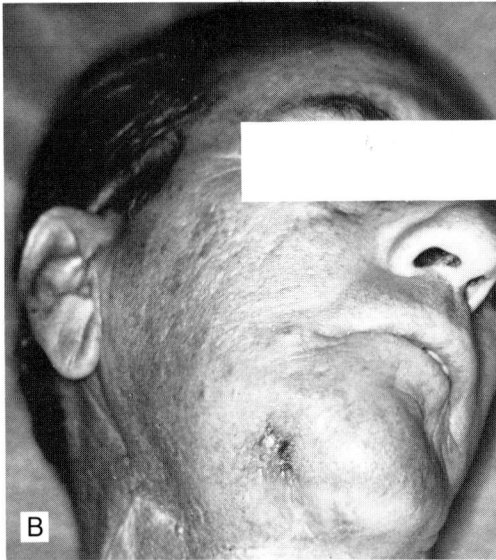

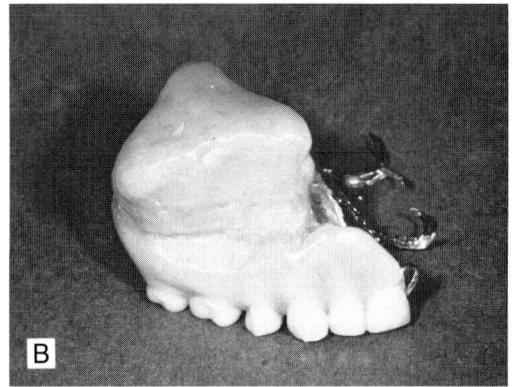

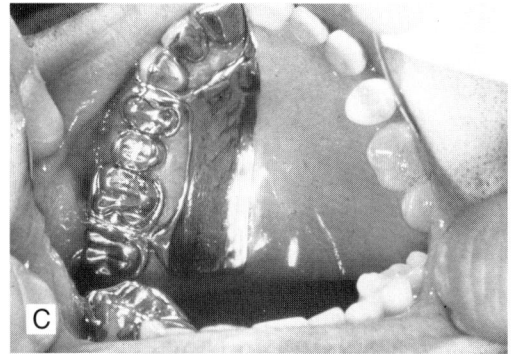

FIG. 12-16. *(A) Defect from ablative tumor surgery. (B) Maxillary prosthesis for surgical defect. (C) Maxillary prosthesis in place.*

References

1. Dorland, W.A.: Dorland's Illustrated Medical Dictionary. 26th Ed. Philadelphia, W.B. Saunders Co., 1981.
2. Steiner, R.B., and Thompson, R.D.: Oral Surgery and Anesthesia. Philadelphia, W.B. Saunders Co., 1977.
3. Margotta, A.: The Story of Medicine. New York, Golden Press, 1968.
4. 1985 Cancer Facts and Figures. New York, American Cancer Society, 1985.
5. Thomas, K.H.: Oral Surgery. St. Louis, C.V. Mosby Co., 1963.
6. Rickles, N.H.: Oral exfoliative cytology: an adjunct to biopsy. *In* Oral Cancer. New York, American Cancer Society, 1972–73.
7. Steckler, R.M., and Spiro, R.H.: Cancer of the oral cavity. *In* Copeland, E.M.: Surgical Oncology. New York, John Wiley & Sons, 1983.
8. Fischman, S.L.: Oral health status in the United States: oral cancer and soft tissue lesions. J. Dent. Educ., *49:*379, 1985.

CHAPTER 13

Cysts of the Oral Cavity

DONALD R. MEHLISCH

There is only one good, knowledge, and one evil, ignorance.
                                        SOCRATES

A cyst is a pathologic space or sac usually containing fluid. Some have been found to be void; others contain soft tissue. Most lesions are uniform and consistent in their histologic features and are characterized by an epithelial lining of the lumen. Cysts of the oral regions may arise in any of the soft or hard tissues in the area of the mouth but are most frequently observed within the maxilla or mandible and quite commonly have several origins (Fig. 13-1). Some arise in association with the tooth or its primordium, the tooth germ. Others arise from the reduced enamel epithelium of a tooth crown, the epithelial rests of Malassez, or the remnants of the dental lamina. Still others arise from the extension of an inflammatory response in the pulpal tissues into the apical region and stimulate the residuals of Hertwig's sheath to proliferate. Another group may be due to embryonic inclusions and injury.

The clinician should have a working knowledge of basic principles of classification of benign cystic lesions in the oral cavity. Classifications originally were based upon clinical and roentgenographic features, but new findings and ideas regarding origin and growth have led to modifications. The following classification serves as a guide to our discussion.

Intraosseous Cysts
  I. Odontogenic
    A. Periodontal
      1. Inflammatory
        a. Apical periodontal (radicular)
        b. Residual
      2. Developmental
        a. Lateral periodontal
    B. Follicular (dentigerous)
    C. Primordial
    D. Odontogenic Keratocyst
      1. Parakeratinized variant
      2. Orthokeratinized variant
    E. Calcifying Odontogenic (Gorlin cyst)
  II. Nonodontogenic
    A. Developmental
      1. Fissural
        a. Median mandibular
        b. Median palatal
        c. Globulomaxillary
      2. Incisive canal (Nasopalatine duct)
  III. Nonepithelial Bone Cysts ("Cyst-like" Conditions)
    A. Traumatic bone (Solitary bone cyst)
    B. Aneurysmal bone
    C. Stafne's bone cavity (Mandibular salivary gland depression)
Soft Tissue Cysts
  I. Salivary Gland
  II. Gingival
  III. Dermoid
  IV. Lymphoepithelial
    A. Cervical (Branchial cleft)
    B. Intraoral
  V. Thyroglossal duct
  VI. Nasolabial

Periodontal Cysts

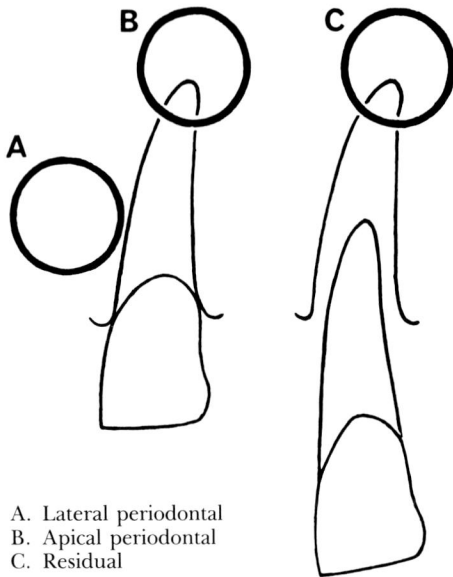

A. Lateral periodontal
B. Apical periodontal
C. Residual

Developmental and Soft Tissue Cysts

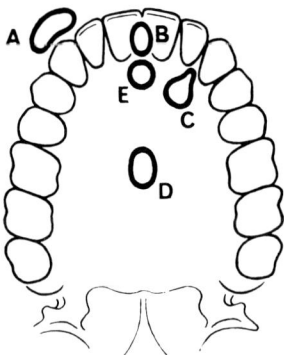

A. Nasolabial   C. Globulomaxillary
B. Median alveolar   D. Median palatal
  (Median mandibular)
      E. Nasopalatine

Intraosseus Cysts—Odontogenic

Periodontal

INFLAMMATORY

Inflammatory cysts originate developmentally or as a result of inflammation. Developmental cysts are those that form

DENTIGEROUS and PRIMORDIAL CYSTS

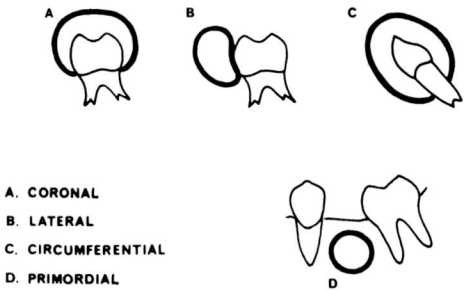

A. CORONAL
B. LATERAL
C. CIRCUMFERENTIAL
D. PRIMORDIAL

BONE CYSTS

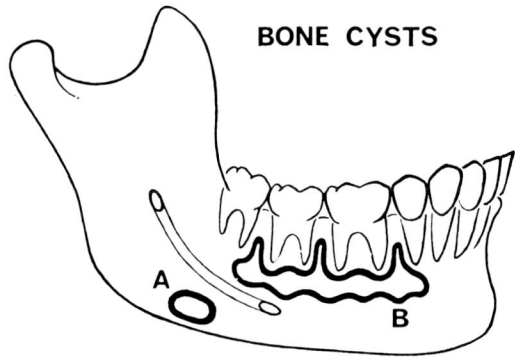

A. Stafne's Idiopathic Cavity

B. Solitary Bone Cyst

FIG. 13-1. *Schematic drawings showing locations of cysts. (Killey, H.C., and Kay, L.W., courtesy of Int. Surg.)*

during the process of odontogenesis and vary according to the particular stage at which the cystic change occurred. Inflammatory cysts result from infection extending from the pulp into surrounding periapical tissues.

Apical Periodontal (Radicular)
Incidence. Of all cystic lesions in the jaws this is the most common and, therefore, the most common of all cysts of odontogenic origin. Males tend to be affected more than females, presumably because the latter are more conscious of appearance and seek attention sooner. This cyst is found more frequently in the maxilla than in the mandible (Fig. 13-2).
Etiology. Extension of inflammation into periapical tissues from the root canal forms a localized mass of chronic inflammatory granulation tissue, the apical granuloma. If

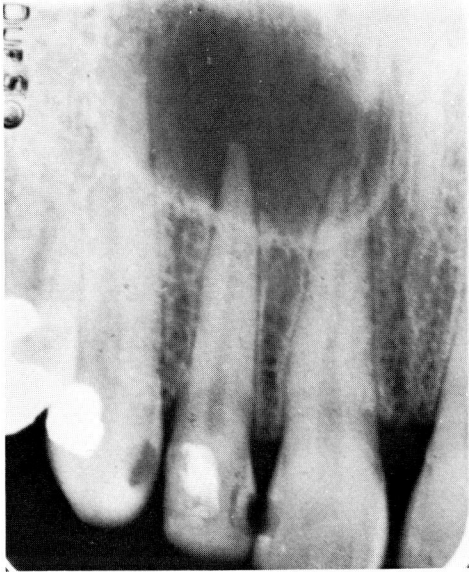

Fig. 13-2. *Apical radicular cyst: lateral incisor does not respond to pulp testing. (Courtesy of Dr. D.E. Waite)*

the central cells degenerate due to inadequate blood supply, an epithelium-lined lumen results, the radicular cyst.

Features. Although often a painful condition initially as a result of inflammation, the cyst itself is frequently symptomless. The tooth in association with the cyst is nonvital. Generally, it does not grow to large dimensions and little if any expansion to the jaw occurs. Radiographically, an area of translucency, which is often well circumscribed, exists at the root apex. The walls are of varying thickness, the lining of which may be smooth or roughened. Contents consist of fluid or a rather thick cheese-like material. The cyst is lined by squamous epithelium with many processes penetrating into the underlying connective tissue. Chronic inflammatory infiltration of the cyst wall is usually well marked.

Treatment and Prognosis. The most commonly applied procedure is enucleation. Nonvital teeth that are associated should be treated by root canal and apicoectomy procedures or, if retention is not desirable, extracted. External sinus tracts must be excised. Marsupialization is indicated when there is a possibility of traumatic penetration of the maxillary sinus and the nose or involvement to some other structure such

as the inferior alveolar nerve. Complete removal of the epithelial lining and elimination of the cause will be followed by bone deposition and resolution of the defect.

Residual

When an apical cyst is overlooked after extraction of the causative tooth or root, it has the potential to enlarge and is called a residual cyst (Fig. 13-3).

Incidence. It is less common than the radicular cyst, as it most often is a missed radicular. Most patients are middle-aged or elderly and there is an equal sex predilection. The incidence is greater in the maxilla than in the mandible.

Etiology. The following causes have been given as probable ones:

1. It develops upon either a deciduous tooth or a retained root that later exfoliates or is extracted without knowledge of the underlying pathologic process
2. If a tooth associated with a dentigerous cyst is removed but the cyst is unrecognized, the residual cyst will persist and increase in size
3. Incomplete removal of a periapical cyst or granuloma

Features. It is typically present in an edentulous area. The majority are asymptomatic and found on routine radiographic examination. Pathologic fracture or encroachment on associated structures may be the presenting symptoms. Histologically, it is like the underlying process that was initially present.

Treatment and Prognosis. The technique for

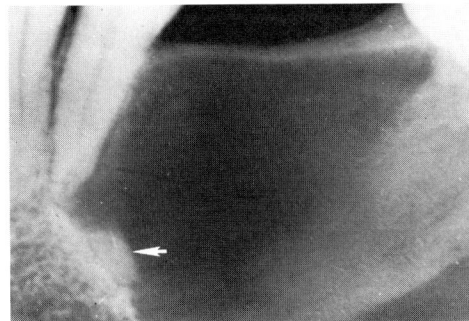

Fig. 13-3. *Residual cyst originating from a root of a tooth previously extracted. (Courtesy of Dr. D.E. Waite)*

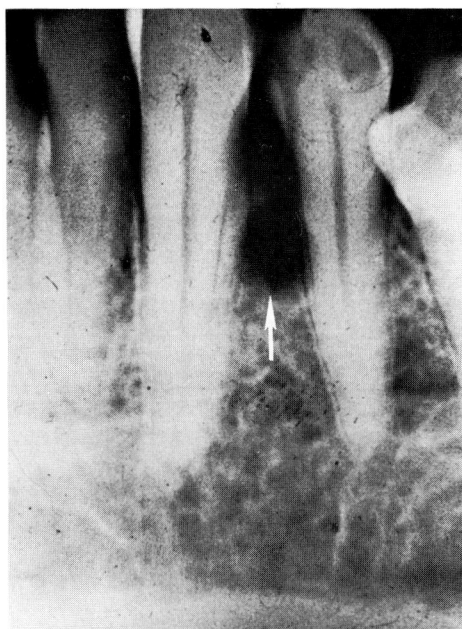

FIG. 13-4. *Lateral periodontal cyst. (Courtesy of Dr. D.E. Waite)*

removal is the same as that employed for an apical cyst, but it is important to preserve the contour of the edentulous ridge.

DEVELOPMENTAL

Lateral Periodontal

These lateral inflammatory cysts must be distinguished from a minority of cysts which are developmental in character (Fig. 13-4).

Incidence. This is a rare but recognized entity. It is chiefly found in adults but it occurs so rarely that no significant conclusions can be drawn regarding specific age or sex. It occurs more often in the mandible than in the maxilla. Although found occasionally in the incisor region, it is most often related to the cuspid, bicuspid, or molar teeth.

Etiology. It appears to arise directly in the lateral periodontal membrane of an erupted tooth. Epithelial debris of Malassez in the periodontal membrane is suspected, but the stimulus for epithelial proliferation is undetermined.

Features. The majority of cases have no clinical signs or symptoms and, therefore, are discovered during routine roentgenographic examination. The associated teeth are vital. It may have a serous caseous content. This cyst usually has a well-formed stratified squamous epithelial lining, often keratinized. This is supported by a connective tissue wall that has a heavy inflammatory cell infiltration.

Treatment and Prognosis. Enucleation with preservation of the adjoining teeth is the procedure of choice. Diagnosis should be established due to similarity in appearance in an early stage between this cyst and other more serious lesions such as the ameloblastoma.

Follicular (Dentigerous)

The occurrence of cystic change arising from the enamel organ after amelogenesis has been completed leads to the formation of a dentigerous cyst. Three positional variations of cyst to tooth are of much academic interest but little clinical signifi-

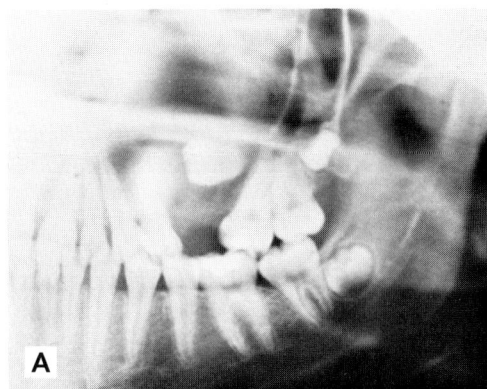

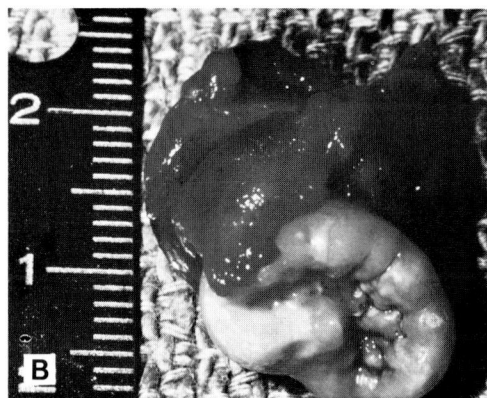

FIG. 13-5. *(A) Radiograph of dentigerous cyst of maxilla. (B) Gross specimen of cyst with tooth.*

cance. These include the *central or coronal type,* which is most common. The *lateral type* is ascribed to activity in the lateral portion of the enamel organ. In the *circumferential dentigerous cyst,* the whole enamel organ around the neck of the tooth becomes cystic (Fig. 13-5).

Incidence. The dentigerous cyst is a far more common type of odontogenic cyst than the primordial but less common than the apical types. Incidence appears to be equal in the two sexes, and the commonest age periods for diagnosis are childhood and adolescence, although sometimes they are found in adults. It occurs in the mandible more frequently than in the maxilla. Late erupting teeth are those frequently concerned in formation of a dentigerous cyst, and in descending order of importance are the lower third molar, upper cuspid, upper third molar, and lower bicuspid teeth.

Etiology. The cause is unknown, although two theories have been suggested which include perifollicular inflammation and retrograde changes in the stellate reticulum of the enamel organ. The cyst forms as a result of fluid collecting within the cell layers of the reduced enamel epithelium or between the crown and the enamel epithelium. Since the expanding cyst space is enveloped by a follicle, the term *follicular cyst* is sometimes substituted for its commoner counterpart.

Features. Progressive enlargement of the jaw occurs, although it is generally painless. Some degree of deformity may result as the lesion is capable of much enlargement with concomitant destruction of the bone. Facial asymmetry may eventually induce the patient to request treatment. Pain may be a symptom if infection is superimposed. Those who wear dentures may have a sudden or gradual alteration in denture fit as the first intimation of the pathologic condition. Roentgenographic examination shows a well-defined translucency associated with the crown of an impacted or unerupted tooth. This is generally unilocular, but a multilocular effect can be present when the cyst is of irregular shape.

The cyst contents consist of clear yellowish fluid, in which cholesterol crystals may be present, or purulent material if infection has occurred. Mural thickenings may prove on microscopic investigation to be ameloblastic changes.

The cyst wall is composed of fibrous connective tissue in which the inflammatory infiltrate is usually minimal. The lining is stratified squamous epithelium, generally in a uniform thin layer, a few cells in depth. This cyst lining is seen to be continuous with the reduced enamel epithelium covering the crown. Occasionally, the epithelium is cornified.

Treatment and Prognosis. Treatment, to some degree, is dictated by the size of the lesion and whether or not it is desirable to save the involved tooth. If the tooth is to be maintained, a Partsch-type procedure should be performed. Therefore, marsupialization as a method of treatment is strongly advocated in the child when the tooth and/or adjacent teeth are being prevented from assuming their normal positions in the arch. Alternatively, a dentigerous cyst should be carefully enucleated along with the tooth of origin. It is widely held that ameloblastomas frequently arise in dentigerous cysts. Recurrence is a possibility if some epithelium remains.

Primordial

Cystic change that occurs in the enamel organ before the formation of calcified structures have developed results in the primordial cyst. Thus, this cyst is found in place of a tooth instead of associated with one (Fig. 13-6).

Incidence. This is the least common type of odontogenic cyst and perhaps accounts for 10 percent of all epithelium-lined cysts of the jaws. The age of identification has ranged from the very young to the very old, but it is found predominantly in the adolescent and young adult group with males and females affected equally. It is found most frequently in the mandibular third molar region but may arise elsewhere in the jaws.

Etiology. The stellate reticulum disintegrates to leave a cystic space bounded by the inner and outer enamel epithelium, which becomes a stratified squamous epithelial lining. It may, therefore, take the place of a missing tooth or develop from the primordial cells of a supernumerary tooth.

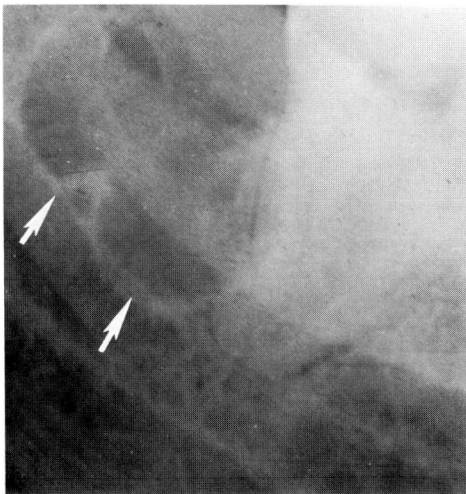

FIG. 13-6. *Primordial cyst; no history of previous third molar removal. (Courtesy of Dr. D.E. Waite)*

Features. It is often asymptomatic until it reaches considerable size or becomes secondarily infected. Expansion of the jaw and displacement of neighboring teeth may occur. Generally, the cyst does not reach as large or as expansile a size as does the dentigerous cyst, although it maintains the potential of displacing adjacent teeth by pressure.

A diagnostic feature of the primordial cyst observed at operation is the extreme thinness of the capsule when compared with other odontogenic cysts. The wall may be thickened by chronic infection.

It differs little in histologic appearance from the dentigerous cyst. Basal layers of the epithelium generally show a regular appearance without rete pegs or proliferation into the subjacent connective tissue. A thin layer of keratin is often present.

Treatment and Prognosis. Surgical removal by enucleation with thorough curettage of the bone and primary closure will render excellent long-term results and a recurrence rate that is negligible. Tendency to regrowth will follow marsupialization.

Odontogenic Keratocyst

PARAKERATINIZED AND
ORTHOKERATINIZED VARIANTS

Keratinization of the epithelial lining sometimes occurs in cysts of the jaws. For some time it was thought that this keratinization was not characteristic of any one particular type of odontogenic cyst, but rather it could be found in dental cysts, either radicular, residual, dentigerous, and, indeed, in nonodontogenic inclusion cysts as well. It has now been well documented and proved that certain characteristic histologic features warrant consideration as a particular entity believed to be primordial in origin. This cyst is the odontogenic keratocyst.

Incidence. It comprises between 5 and 10 percent of odontogenic cysts of the jaws. A relatively higher incidence in the second, third, and fourth decades of life is noted but it can occur in any age group. Slightly more males than females have been diagnosed. It has a strong predilection for the mandible and the most common site is the third molar region. In both the maxilla and mandible, the majority of cysts occur posterior to the first bicuspids.

Etiology. Primordial cysts of the jaws are derived directly from the undifferentiated dental lamina. Thus, primordial cysts may develop from Serres' pearls, which are retained portions of the dental lamina, or from any suppressed tooth anlage, either from normal dentition or from a supernumerary tooth. Because almost all primordial cysts are keratinized, it has been assumed that keratocysts are actually primordial cysts.

Features. In approximately 50 percent of cases expansion of surrounding bone occurs, not infrequently of both medial and lateral borders. Roentgenographic evidence of resorption of the roots of related teeth has also been shown. Recurrent inflammatory episodes in the region of a recently extracted tooth may be part of the clinical picture and help establish the diagnosis. Less common features include numbness of the lower lip on the related side. Other abnormalities may be associated and give consideration for the diagnosis of multiple basal cell nevi syndrome.

The cyst wall and lining are usually smooth and somewhat thinned. Occasional small projections of granulation tissue may be present. Not infrequently, bony septa divide the lining into loculations, and in multilocular lesions separate cyst cavities may be present. Cortical bone may be quite thin or perforated by the cyst.

Usually, the epithelium consists of five or ten rows of cells with an accentuated basal layer and occasionally vacuolated cells in the spinal cell layers. Rete pegs are rarely seen. Frank atypia (dysplasia) may characterize a basal cell hyperplasia, and increased mitotic activity may be seen. A number of cysts may have keratinization of the epithelium lining the cyst cavity. The odontogenic keratocyst may have the keratin formed by the epithelial lining present in two variants. It may be parakeratin in which there is persistence of the nuclei or an orthokeratin in which the nuclei are absent. Clinically, the parakeratinized variant appears to have a much higher incidence of recurrence.

Treatment and Prognosis. It is of surgical interest that keratocysts seem to have a pronounced tendency to recur. Recurrences may be over 50 percent in some cases and may be repeated. Recurrences may be due to daughter-cyst formation of the cyst wall or to the proliferation of the cyst epithelium into connective tissue that has been left behind after enucleation of the delicate cyst membrane. Treatment is by complete enucleation of the cyst and to be even more careful in removal of the cyst lining in keratocysts than in unkeratinized cysts. Aspiration of the cyst contents may prove to be an important aid in the diagnosis of the odontogenic keratocyst. The fluid removed shows a markedly reduced content of soluble protein when compared with serum from the patient. Therefore, electrophoresis of the cyst contents appears to be a valuable preoperative method of distinguishing the odontogenic keratocyst from other odontogenic cysts.

Calcifying Odontogenic (Gorlin Cyst)

The calcifying odontogenic cyst is an uncommon epithelial lesion characterized by unusual keratin production and dystrophic calcification. It bears a marked similarity to the cutaneous calcifying epithelioma of Malherbe. It may also be confused with a variety of cutaneous, odontogenic, and other tumors. Although the term calcifying odontogenic cyst may not be entirely accurate on a histomorphologic basis, the apparent limited growth potential and strictly benign behavior of the lesion make this designation reasonable on a clinical basis.

Incidence. This relatively rare new odontogenic lesion has been described as a separate and distinct oral lesion for about 20 years. Patients of any age may be affected, but a significant number of lesions have been reported in children and adolescents. There appears to be no sex predilection. Calcifying odontogenic cysts have been described in either jaw and no particular region shows a dominance.

Etiology. although histogenesis has not been definitely established, there appears to be strong evidence suggesting an odontogenic origin. The occasional association of an unerupted tooth or odontoma, the ameloblastic basal-cell layer with areas resembling stellate reticulum, epithelial rests resembling remnants of dental lamina, and almost exclusive occurrence in the gingiva or alveolar processes of the maxilla or mandible support an odontogenic origin.

Features. A peripheral or intraosseous lesion causing nonspecific signs and symptoms is the usual feature, although resorption of adjacent teeth may occasionally be seen. Roentgenographic findings, while not distinctive, are the means to detecting most of these tumors. The appearance is a monoloculated radiolucency with variably defined borders that may or may not have perforated cortical bone. Small radiopacities can appear within the lesion, suggesting the possibilities of ossifying fibroma, odontogenic adenomatoid tumor (adenoameloblastoma), ameloblastic odontoma, and calcifying epithelial odontogenic tumor, among others.

A marked resemblance exists among cases, and all have a cystic cavity lined by a stratified epithelium. The basal layer of cells is distinct and takes up more stain than that of the ordinary cyst. These cells are cuboidal to columnar, resembling enamel epithelium, and have big "ghost" epithelial cells scattered among them which appear to be aberrant keratinization. The presence of melanin in this lesion is not unique.

Treatment and Prognosis. Calcifying odontogenic cysts seem to have a limited growth

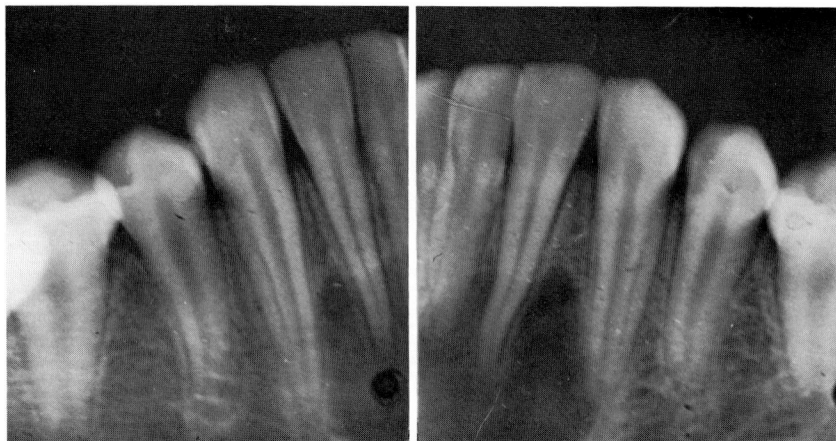

FIG. 13-7. *Median mandibular cyst; all teeth are vital. (Courtesy of Dr. D.E. Waite)*

potential, and surgical enucleation has been the preferred therapy. Some tendency toward recurrence has been noted, and close follow-up care is indicated. More extensive surgery including resection may be necessary in recurring cases.

Intraosseous Cysts—Nonodontogenic

Developmental

FISSURAL

Cysts classified as fissural are believed to arise from remnants of the epithelium that covered the developing facial processes during the embryonic period of life. Various factors have been postulated suggesting the origin. These include epithelial entrapments in the lines of closure of the processes, which perhaps give rise to cleft palate and cleft lip as well.

Median Mandibular

Incidence. This cyst is rare and only a few examples have been recorded. It is certainly less common than the other fissural cysts. There is no distinctive distribution between the sexes. It is found symmetrically in the midline of the mandible (Fig. 13-7).

Etiology. It arises from epithelial inclusions in the area of the symphysis, or from the enamel organ of supernumerary tooth germs. The epithelium proliferates and then becomes cystic. Inflammation and trauma may be considered as factors in the development of this lesion, as well as in all other fissural cysts.

Features. This cyst remains relatively small (1 to 3 cm) and is therefore usually discovered on roentgenographic examination. A detectable swelling may occur in the labial sulcus. Although it appears to involve the apices of adjoining teeth, which may be in close relationship with the inclusion cyst, the lamina dura remains intact and the teeth are vital. It has a well-defined but variable shape, being ovoid, circular, or irregular. The cyst lining consists of stratified squamous epithelium. The wall consists of fibrous connective tissue that usually reveals little or no evidence of an inflammatory response.

Treatment and Prognosis. Treatment is careful enucleation without involvement of the apices of the incisors. Teeth that have had some divergence of the roots from the cyst may gradually improve their positions.

Median Palatal

Incidence. This cyst is rare and occurs mainly in adults of either sex in the midline of the maxillary alveolus or the hard palate, between the lateral palatal processes. Generally it is present between the incisive fossa and the posterior border of the hard palate.

Etiology. It arises from the epithelial rests in the suture line, and is probably the result of inflammation or trauma. It has been suggested that this cyst is probably a nasopalatine cyst which has extended backward into the palate.

Features. There is no clinical evidence unless it becomes extremely large and causes expansion of surrounding bone with palpable swelling. It is well-defined, ovoid in outline, and essentially appears the same as the median alveolar cyst. The cyst is lined by stratified squamous or ciliated columnar epithelium. There may be some chronic inflammatory infiltration in the subepithelial connective tissue.

Treatment and Prognosis. Treatment and prognosis are the same as for median alveolar cysts.

Globulomaxillary

The term globulomaxillary cyst is really no longer appropriate, since the globular process is now referred to as the premaxillary process in embryologic terminology. However, the term lateral fissural cyst, which has been proposed as an alternative designation, has not gained general acceptance (Fig. 13-8).

Incidence. It is uncommon, appearing in adults of either sex. The cyst forms at the junction of the globular portion of the medial nasal process with the maxillary process (between lateral incisor and cuspid teeth).

Etiology. The conventional view is that the cyst develops from residual epithelium in the areas of contact of the globular process of the frontonasal bone with the adjacent maxillary processes of palatine bones. These can be visualized as two upright triangular plates that angulate posteriorly to join each other immediately behind the upper central incisor teeth.

Features. It is possible to make a presumptive diagnosis of the globulomaxillary cyst if the lateral and cuspid teeth are tilted together coronally, and each tooth gives a normal response to pulp testing. Roentgenographically, it appears as a pear-shaped radiolucent lesion with a prominent cortical margin and with the lamina dura of adjoining teeth preserved.

When the cyst is small, it is spherical in shape. With elongation, it ultimately resembles an inverted pear with the inferior, narrow V-shaped end extending into the interdental bone, and it may even reach the alveolar crest.

The epithelial lining of the cyst is more often from the nasal mucosa than from the oral covering; hence, it is pseudostratified columnar ciliated epithelium, or some modification thereof. The wall is usually thick with scattered lymphocytes and plasma cells concentrated along the lining.

Treatment and Prognosis. Enucleation, whenever possible, is the treatment of choice. However, if the lesion is extremely large, it may be prudent to perform a preliminary marsupialization to allow decompression and some bone regeneration. This should be followed by enucleation and primary closure to accelerate the healing process and reduce the risk of a residual defect.

FIG. 13-8. *Globulomaxillary cyst. (A) Occlusal view. (B) Periapical view. (Courtesy of Dr. D.E. Waite)*

INCISIVE CANAL (NASOPALATINE DUCT)

Nasopalatine

The generic term nasopalatine cyst refers to both the cyst of the incisive canal and that designated the cyst of the palatine papilla. Distinction between these two is based on whether the lesion is intraosseous or located solely within the soft tissues in the region of the papilla. The nasopalatine duct connects the oral and nasal cavities in

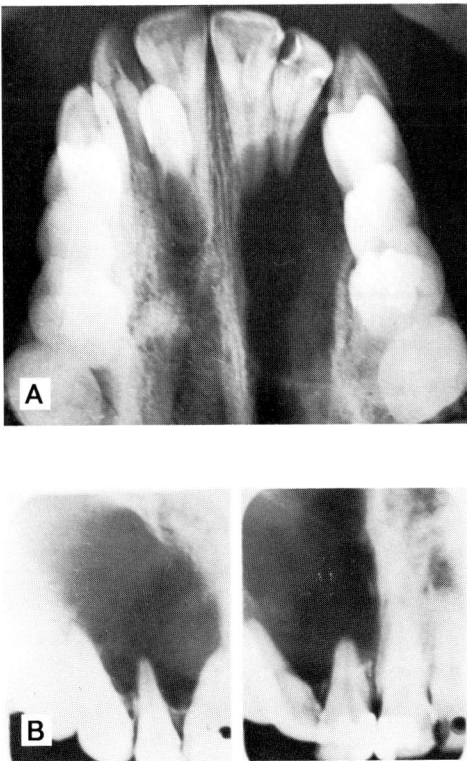

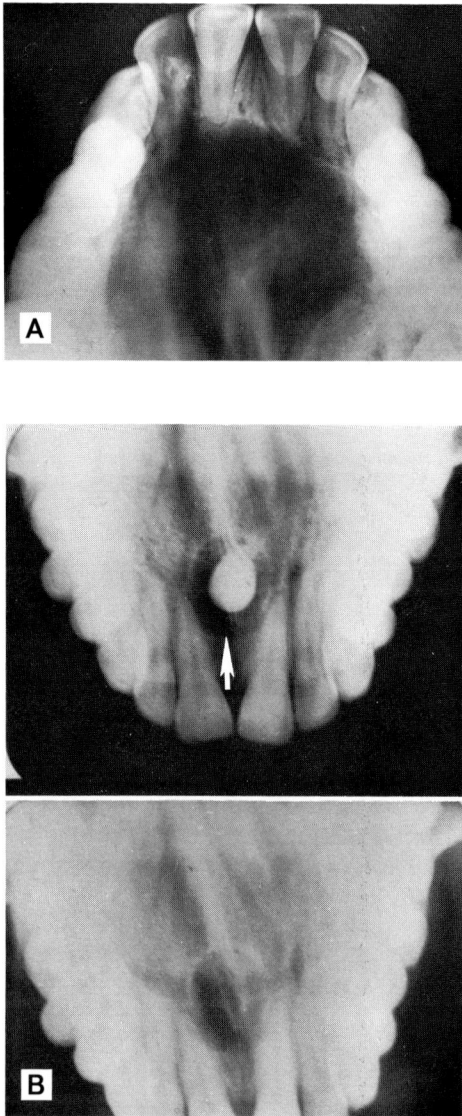

FIG. 13-9. *Nasopalatine cyst.* (A) Occlusal view. (B) Lipiodol indicates the internal cyst size and the thickness of the nasopalatine cyst wall. (Courtesy of Dr. D.E. Waite)

many mammals, and in the embryonic stage of the human. Cyst formation may occur from the epithelial remnants of the ducts that normally persist in the adult. Those cysts forming either within the palatine papilla or in the incisive canal will be considered together (Fig. 13-9).

Incidence. Asymptomatic cysts of this type have been found in 1 percent of persons on roentgenographic survey. One out of every 66 cadaver specimens examined in

another study had identifiable incisive canal cysts. This is the most common type of maxillary developmental or fissural cyst. It is predominantly found in adulthood with no apparent sex distribution. The cyst may arise at any point along the canal, but most originate in the lower portion of the maxilla between the apices of the central incisors.

Etiology. In the embryo, two wide tracts, the nasopalatine ducts, extend between the nasal and oral cavities. They do not normally persist as such into adult life, although some portion of these pathways may frequently remain. Cysts arise from the epithelial debris of these vestigial nasopalatine ducts.

Features. The majority remain asymptomatic and even those that demonstrate insidious symptoms follow no consistent pattern. The most frequent complaint is a lump in the midline of the palate anteriorly, and on palpation the cyst is usually fluctuant. Infection may be responsible for a pronounced swelling of the palatal soft tissues which occurs secondarily. There may be pain, which is either well localized or neuralgic in character, radiating to the side of the nose or the eyes. Adjacent teeth should be normal in color and nonsensitive to percussion, but a periapical condition should be ruled out with the aid of vitality testing.

A well-defined cyst outline is situated apparently between or above the roots of the maxillary central incisor teeth and may be bilateral, giving the characteristic heart shape. However, it can be round or ovoid.

The presence of mucous glands in the walls of the cyst is highly indicative of their origin within the incisive canal. The cysts are usually lined with a modified-type or respiratory epithelium, although cysts of the papillae may be partly lined by squamous epithelium. Unexpected diversions from this descending pattern in epithelial type may be due to metaplastic transformation. Cartilage may also be identified in the wall of the cyst and incorporated as part of the specimen.

Treatment and Prognosis. When there is irrefutable clinical evidence of an incisive canal cyst with or without abnormal roentgenographic enlargement of the fossa, surgical removal should be instituted, which is

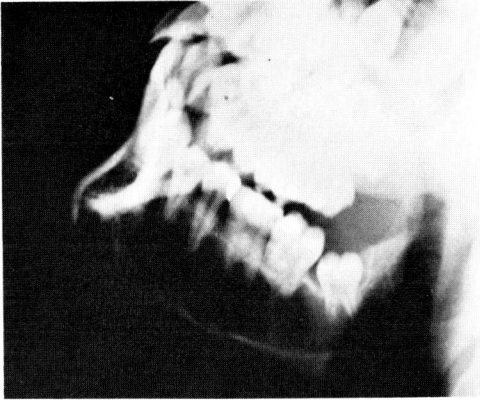

FIG. 13-10. *Radiograph of solitary bone cyst.*

usually adequate. Several cases of adenocystic carcinoma have been reported developing in the glands in the cyst wall and should be considered in the differential diagnosis.

"Cyst-Like" Conditions

Nonepithelial Bone Cysts

TRAUMATIC BONE CYST (SOLITARY BONE CYST)

The solitary bone cyst occurs most often elsewhere in the body, principally the upper part of the diaphysis of the humerus and other long bones. It is an unusual lesion that appears with disturbing frequency and has been termed hemorrhagic bone cyst, extravasation cyst, and progressive bone cavity. The term "cyst" in relation to this lesion is controversial and probably a misnomer (Fig. 13-10).

Incidence. It is relatively common during the first two decades of life. The relative infrequence of this lesion in later decades of life has given speculation that the cavities tend to undergo a natural cure. Lesions occur particularly in children and adolescents between 10 and 20 years of age. Males are affected more often than females, probably because of an increased exposure to traumatic injuries. The majority are located in the subapical region of the posterior portion of the mandible between the cuspid and the third molar. It is this area in which the marrow cavity of the jaw is situated in young persons. Occasion-

ally, a lesion may develop in the incisor region.

Etiology. The cause and mode of formation of solitary bone cysts are still unknown, but a number of theories have been given. These include (1) trauma and hemorrhage with failure of organization, (2) spontaneous atrophy of the tissue in a central benign giant-cell lesion, (3) abnormal calcium metabolism, (4) chronic low-grade infection, and (5) necrosis of fatty marrow secondary to ischemia. Little positive evidence supports these theories, and perhaps the best explanation is that, relative to cysts in all locations, it represents the results of an aberration in the development and growth of the local osseous tissue.

Features. The condition is usually symptomless and frequently discovered accidentally on routine roentgenography. There is often a history of trauma to the jaw though it is not always recent. Expansion of the bone is not common but may occur. Teeth that may be associated with the cyst retain their vitality and are not loosened despite extensions of the cyst into the surrounding bony spaces.

Surgical exploration reveals a space in the bone that contains a little clear or perhaps blood-stained fluid, shreds of necrotic blood clot, a thin connective tissue membrane lining, or nothing. Accordingly, the material available for pathologic examination comprises simply a mass of bone fragments, blood clot, and small scraps of soft tissue.

Treatment and Prognosis. Surgical exploration of the area is required for diagnosis and usually constitutes treatment. Any cyst lining should be enucleated and the area curetted. Curettage should stimulate hemorrhage which results in rapid obliteration of the defect and eventually healing by new bone formation.

ANEURYSMAL BONE CYST

The aneurysmal bone cyst was first described and characterized as such by Jaffe and Lichtenstein in 1942. It occurs most often in long bones and the vertebral column. It may occur in other bones but is rare in the jaws. Previously, it has been described under such terms as hemorrhagic osteomyelitis, ossifying hematoma, osteitis fibrosa cystica, and aneurysmal giant-cell tumor.

Incidence. It is rare and reports of lesions in the jaws are limited but cases have been described. The abnormality occurs mainly in children, adolescents, or young adults with an overwhelming majority in those under 20 years of age. There is no marked sex predominance. The mandible is generally affected, but the lesion may also occur in the maxilla.

Etiology. Factors that may cause an aneurysmal bone cyst are still unknown. Even though a history of trauma is often obtained, it is not certain that it can be directly related to the development of this lesion. A possible relationship with the giant-cell lesion has been postulated. Another widely accepted theory is that the condition is caused by some variation in the hemodynamics or vascular supply of the area. This lesion has no relationship to the solitary bone cyst, and it occurs in bone that has previously been apparently normal.

Features. Pain is not a feature with lesions in the mandible or maxilla, as is frequently the case in other bones that are involved. A firm enlargement of the jaw may be tender. Characteristically, this benign solitary lesion causes local expansion, but the growth is not infiltrative and a thin layer of overlying subperiosteal new bone is preserved in most cases. The soap-bubble appearance seen roentgenographically in long bones is not evident in the jaw lesions. Instead, a radiolucent expansile lesion which may destroy the cortical plate is seen.

The lesion is soft, fusiform or round in shape, tender, of firm or springy consistency, and contains numerous blood-filled spaces. Resultant bleeding is a persistent ooze that may be difficult to control, rather than a sudden spurting or vigorous free hemorrhage.

The area involved by the lesion is honeycombed and consists of numerous blood-filled spaces lined by a single layer of compressed flattened cells and giant cells. The intervening septa and stroma consist of young fibroblasts, giant cells, blood vessels, and foci of hemosiderin. In general, it is similar to that of the peripheral and central giant-cell reparative granulomas.

Treatment and Prognosis. The lesion is amenable to treatment by curettage or surgical enucleation and this is the method of choice in a surgically accessible lesion. Recurrence may follow inadequate removal and require additional therapy.

STAFNE'S IDIOPATHIC BONE CAVITY (MANDIBULAR SALIVARY GLAND DEPRESSION)

Stafne's idiopathic bone cavities can be mistaken for cysts in the mandible. Although not actually cysts of the jaw, they have been included because of their clinical and roentgenologic similarity to the cystic lesions that have been discussed. This similarity frequently presents a problem in differential diagnosis (Fig. 13-11).

Incidence. It is relatively uncommon, with the largest series of cases reported by the author for whom the lesion is named. Few defects have been observed in children and no sex distinction has been suggested. It is consistently situated beneath the mandibular canal and adjacent to the lower border of the jaw between the bicuspid region and the angle.

Etiology. The cause is unknown but several plausible theories have been suggested. Stafne believed that such cavities might arise during development of the jaws by failure of the normal deposition of bone in an area formerly occupied by cartilage or by failure of subperiosteal apposition at the lower border. Other theories suggest that the cavities might be constricted remains of solitary bone cysts, an eosinophilic granuloma, or embryonic defects.

Features. This is a symptomless lesion dis-

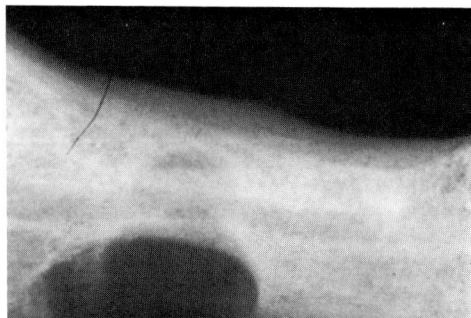

Fig. 13-11. *Stafne's latent bone cyst, below the inferior alveolar canal. (Courtesy of Dr. D.E. Waite)*

covered during routine roentgenography in which it appears as a round or oval radiolucent defect. The area of rarefaction is well demarcated by a dense radiopaque line. Sometimes the lesion extends from cancellous tissue into cortical bone and may perforate the inferior margin of the body of the mandible. Cavities may vary between 1 and 3 cm in diameter. Generally, there are constancy of position, uniform appearance, failure to change with time, and an occasional bilateral occurrence. All these factors strongly favor a developmental origin.

Because these are idiopathic bone cavities, no diagnostic tissue can be mentioned. These cavities may, in fact, be empty. Contrary, they may contain normal salivary gland tissue, lymph node tissue, or abnormal glandular tissue. Published reports have stated that the outer plate was thin and that perforations had occurred along the inner cortical plate.

Treatment and Prognosis. In view of the fact that the lesions are symptomless and nonprogressive, surgical exploration is hard to justify. Apart from the diagnostic problem the lesions present, these idiopathic cavities are of no particular concern. They are nonpathogenic and require essentially no treatment, although regular follow-up roentgenographs should be taken. This defect in the mandible may constitute a point of weakness and pathologic fracture may occur.

Soft Tissue Cysts

Salivary Gland

Salivary glands of the oral regions may give rise to small cysts in connection with the complex ductal system and may be found anywhere in the oral submucosa. Any disruption of the flow of salivary secretions may result in retention of fluid, which will produce the lesion.

Incidence. The salivary gland cyst is common in connection with the minor salivary glands, but has no predilection for age or sex. Common sites are the lips, cheeks, undersurface of the tip of the tongue, and the floor of the mouth (ranula). With the exception of the anterior half of the hard palate, which is devoid of salivary glands, it can occur anywhere in the oral cavity.

Etiology. Origin is probably dual in nature. First, cyst formation may result from trauma to the ducts of mucous glands with escape of secretions into the surrounding connective tissue. Second, retention of the secretion results in dilatation of the duct system, and an epithelium-lined cyst.

Features. It appears as a small, circumscribed, usually elevated, translucent, bluish lesion on the mucosa. Spontaneous rupture often occurs, with the liberation of a viscous fluid. In the course of a few weeks or perhaps longer, additional fluid may accumulate and the lesion reappears. This cycle of rupture, collapse of the cyst, and refilling may continue for months.

Early lesions may not have a definite cystic cavity. A fully developed one consists of a cystic cavity filled with a lightly basophilic homogeneous material. The cyst-like space is lined by a thin layer of flattened cells that may resemble an epithelial lining, but which are in fact compressed connective tissue cells. In some cases only granulation tissue is present and no lining is seen.

Treatment and Prognosis. Salivary gland cysts are treated by surgical excision, together with the associated salivary tissue. If the cyst is due to a defect in the duct and close to the mucosal surface, a Partsch procedure may be indicated. Recurrence following excision is occasionally seen but becomes less likely if the associated salivary gland acini are also removed.

Gingival

Gingival cysts may not be deserving of a specific category and should not be confused with eruption cysts. The only specific criterion for the lesion is its location in the gingival tissues.

Incidence. It is relatively rare and of infrequent occurrence. It is found in infants and adults, with the largest incidence in the sixth decade. There is no sex predilection. It appears particularly in the cuspid and bicuspid areas of the mandible but occasionally in the anterior part of the jaw. Mandibular gingival tissues are involved twice as frequently as are the maxillary gingival tissues.

Etiology. Causation is obscure but the possible mechanisms by which the cyst may form are (1) traumatic implantation of epithelium, (2) surface epithelium that proliferates in a down-growing manner and undergoes cystic changes, or (3) dental lamina remnants, enamel organ or epithelial islands from the surface epithelium.

Features. It is a slowly growing and circumscribed swelling of the gingivae, which is usually radiolucent. Occasionally, large lesions occur and pressure may cause erosion of the adjacent cortical plate of bone. The lesion is lined by stratified squamous epithelium, the periepithelial collagen being free of inflammatory cells.

Treatment and Prognosis. Surgical excision is almost always curative.

Dermoid
(Dermoid Inclusion Cyst)

The dermoid cyst is similar to the epidermal or epidermoid cyst, but with the addition of skin appendages such as hair, sebaceous glands, or teeth. It is, therefore, a form of cystic teratoma. In the oral regions the term *dermoid inclusion cyst* is used to indicate a lesion derived from ectoderm only. Because of the differences in histogenesis and clinical significance, distinction between the dermoid cyst and dermoid inclusion cyst needs to be made (Fig. 13-12).

Incidence. The dermoid cyst is uncommon. The majority occur in young adulthood and show no sex predilection. The floor of the mouth and submandibular and sublingual regions are the most common sites.

Etiology. The dermoid cyst is thought to arise from epithelial rests persisting in the midline after fusion of the mandible and hyoid branchial arches. The dermoid inclusion cyst is derived from ectoderm only and capable of producing epidermoid tissue. The dermoid cyst, on the other hand, is derived from primordial germ cells and is comprised of a combination of ectodermal, mesodermal, and endodermal elements. In approximately 5 percent of cases, one of the tissue elements in the dermoid cyst becomes malignant. The importance of the distinction between these two cysts, therefore, is significant.

Features. The typical lesion produces a bulge in the floor of the mouth if it is above the geniohyoid muscle and may become large enough to elevate the tongue, causing difficulty with mastication and speech. Cysts inferior to the geniohyoid muscle and above the mylohyoid muscle produce a submental swelling. This cyst may also arise below the mylohyoid muscle. Typically, a "dough-like" feel is present on palpation of the lesion. The cysts vary in size but generally approach several centimeters in diameter.

Microscopically, dermoid inclusion cysts are lined by keratinizing stratified squamous epithelium and contain keratin scales and sebaceous material. Sebaceous glands, sweat glands, and hair follicles may be found in the cyst wall, and occasionally other structures are present.

Treatment and Prognosis. Complete excision is curative treatment for such lesions.

Lymphoepithelial

CERVICAL (BRANCHIAL CLEFT)

Branchial arch remnants may give rise to a lesion in the lateral aspect of the neck in the form of a fistula or cyst.

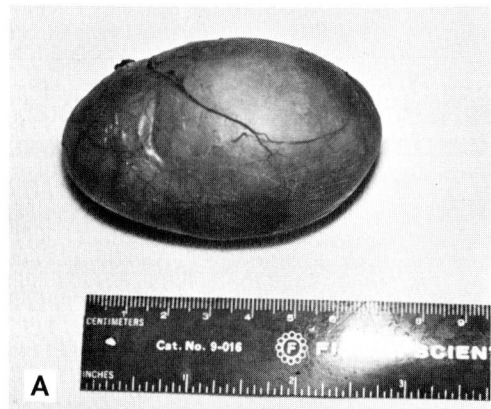

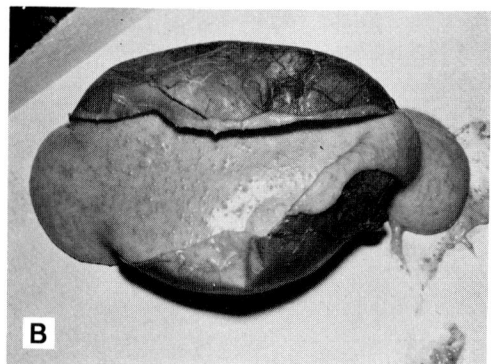

FIG. 13-12. *(A) Gross specimen of dermoid inclusion cyst. (B) Gross specimen of dermoid inclusion cyst cut.*

Incidence. This is not a common lesion overall; however, 10 to 15 percent are seen at the angle of the mandible. Patients are most frequently young adults between 20 and 40 years of age. It does occur in children, but usually after sexual maturity. There is no known sex preference. It usually occurs on the lateral side of the neck, but some are seen at the angle of the mandible. Rarely, a branchial cyst may occur in the floor of the mouth.

Etiology. This cyst may arise from ectodermal or endodermal remnants associated with the branchial arches, usually between the second and third. It has also been shown to obtain histogenesis from residual cervical sinus epithelium or epithelial inclusions within lymph nodes in the region.

Features. It presents as a soft fluctuant mass that historically appears in the lateral aspects of the neck anterior to the sternocleidomastoid muscle or may involve the parotid region. It may slowly increase in size and may also develop a fistulous tract. The tract will drain externally in most cases; however, in rare instances it will drain intraorally.

Microscopic sections of superficial lesions reveal cysts that are usually lined by stratified squamous epithelium and contain a watery fluid. Lymphoid tissue may surround the cyst and show all the characteristics of a lymph node. Lesions located in the deeper structures of the neck are lined by pseudostratified columnar epithelium, and beneath the epithelium there is a dense infiltrate of lymphocytic cells which frequently contain well-developed germinal centers. In a deeper lesion the lumen may contain a great deal of mucus instead of the watery fluid.

Treatment and Prognosis. If these lesions are aspirated or drained, they will recur because the cyst itself has not been removed and will persist. The lesion is best treated by complete surgical removal.

INTRAORAL

The intraoral component of the lymphoepithelial cyst is an uncommon lesion.

Incidence. The floor of the mouth or ventral surface of the tongue have been the predominant locations for this tumor. Other areas involved include the soft palate and mandibular vestibule.

Etiology. Glandular epithelium is included in oral lymphoid accumulations during embryogenesis and has undergone cystic degeneration.

Features. It may occur at any age and both sexes appear to be affected equally, although the number of cases reported is small. Microscopically, a well-circumscribed mass of lymphoid is seen with a stratified squamous epithelium lined cystic cavity within.

Treatment and Prognosis. Conservative local surgical excision is the treatment of choice. There is rarely a recurrence.

Thyroglossal Duct

The thyroglossal duct cyst is an uncommon developmental cyst that can occur anywhere along the course of the embryonic thyroglossal duct, which extends from the foramen cecum of the tongue into the deep fascia near the thyroid isthmus.

Incidence. It is relatively rare and there are no significant data on age or sex predilection. As stated, it can occur anywhere along the course of the thyroglossal duct, the commonest area of involvement, however, being close to the hyoid bone in the midline. It may also be found beneath the foramen cecum in the musculature of the tongue.

Etiology. The thyroid gland rudiment appears during the fourth embryonic week between the derivatives of the first and second branchial arches that, in part, form the tongue. A hollow stalk, the thyroglossal duct, extends from the foramen cecum in the base of the tongue down through the neck to the thyroid gland. By about the tenth week this duct breaks up and disappears, but cysts may form from residues of this duct.

Features. It appears as a soft fluctuant mass unattached to the surrounding tissues unless fistulous tracts develop, which occurs in approximately 25 percent of cases. Dysphagia may be the initial symptom, but usually the cyst is painless and varies from 1 to 5 cm in diameter.

Cysts occurring above the level of the hyoid bone are lined by stratified squamous epithelium and those below this level by ciliated respiratory-type or columnar epithelium. However, the histologic pattern is variable and a single cyst may show different types of epithelium from one area to another.

Treatment and Prognosis. Complete surgical removal of the cyst with its tract is essential to prevent recurrence. Because of the relationship to the hyoid bone, this bone may need to be divided during surgery.

Nasolabial

The nasolabial cyst is strictly a soft tissue lesion and does not occur within bone. Its inclusion in certain classifications with fissural cysts of the jaws has been a convenient and accepted practice. Alternative designations of naso-extra-alveolar cyst, nasal vestibule cyst, nasal wing cyst, and mucoid cyst of the nose have been used (Fig. 13-13).

Incidence. The condition is uncommon with less than 200 cases reported in the literature. It is found in the young and the elderly, but most are in persons in the third, fourth, and fifth decades. An overwhelming majority of cases reported have occurred in females, almost 80 percent. Cysts of this type develop at the junction of the globular, the lateral nasal, and the maxillary processes. There is no predilection for one side of the midline or the other. In fact, 12 percent of cases will be bilateral, and in these the female again is affected most frequently.

Etiology. These lesions are thought to arise from epithelium of the embryonal clefts of the face at the point where the maxillary, the median nasal, and the lateral nasal processes fuse. The frequency of bilateral cysts seems too high to be accounted for by possible external etiologic factors, and

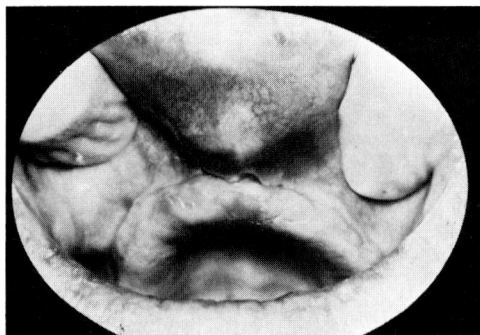

FIG. 13-13. *Inflammatory (nasolabial) cyst.*

helps substantiate the theories advancing developmental disturbances as the cause of nasolabial cysts.

Features. This lesion produces a visible external swelling of the lip, can displace the ala cartilage, may distort the shape of the nose, and may obliterate the nasolabial fold. Swelling is mentioned as the chief complaint in 60 percent of cases and upward extension into the nasal vestibule may cause eventual obstruction of the airway, interfering with breathing. Protrusion downward between the lip and alveolus may allow palpation of the lower border of the cyst in the labial vestibule. Since the cyst occurs in soft tissue only, it is not visible roentgenographically unless it has caused some resorption of the maxilla by pressure, as occasionally occurs.

The cyst usually lies just beneath the epithelium of a thin layer of condensed connective tissue that contains only a few vessels and fibroblasts. The connective tissue capsule is lined by stratified squamous or columnar epithelium and the cyst contains straw-colored mucinous fluid.

Treatment and Prognosis. Treatment of the nasolabial cyst is surgical removal from an intraoral approach. The operation can be complicated by perforation of the nasal mucosa and great care needs to be taken when separating the cyst lining from the surrounding mucosa. This will be more difficult if the cyst has previously drained into the nose, and sometimes the sac is firmly attached to the margin of the ala.

General Principles of Treatment of Cysts of the Oral Cavity

Obvious reasons exist for treatment of benign cysts of the oral cavity. Foremost, cysts increase in size and have a tendency to become infected. Their location in the jaw also constitutes an area of weakness which may cause a pathologic fracture. Further, it is not possible to be certain of the benign nature of a cystic lesion until it has been explored surgically and examined histologically.

The treatment of benign cysts of the oral cavity is predominantly surgical, and there are two basic types of operative procedures: (1) enucleation and (2) marsupialization.

Enucleation

Enucleation allows for the opening to the cyst cavity to be covered by a mucoperiosteal flap and the space filled with blood clot which will eventually organize and form normal bone. Undoubtedly this is the most satisfactory method of treatment of a cyst. In many instances a window in the bone already exists from expansion of the cyst. However, if the bone covering the cyst remains intact, a window will be necessary and can be made through the cortical plate using either mallet and chisel or bone burs. Rongeurs are helpful in enlargement of the opening and are less likely to puncture or tear the cyst wall, which should remain intact. The margins of the cyst are easier to define if the membrane is not ruptured, and enucleation is simplified because the lining can be separated more readily from the bony cavity if the fluid content remains compressed. Curettes and small periosteal elevators can be used to thoroughly strip the cyst from its bony walls. After the cyst lining has been removed, the bony defect should be thoroughly inspected and the surface dried. The empty cyst cavity should then be gently irrigated with warm saline solution and the flap sutured back into position.

In some extensive lesions a biopsy may be indicated. At the time of opening, overlapping or excessive tissue is trimmed away from the buccal mucoperiosteal flap. The remainder of the flap is then turned into the cavity to cover part of the bare area of bone and packed with iodoform gauze dressing. This procedure collapses the body of the cyst but permits filling of the cystic space by compression from the formation of new bone external to the cyst. When sufficient bone has formed, the entire cyst should be enucleated and primary closure effected.

Marsupialization (Partsch Operation)

Marsupialization of cysts consists of surgically producing a window by removing a generous section of the overlying mucoperiosteum, bone, and adjacent cyst wall to decrease intracystic tension. The border of the incised mucosa is then sutured to the border of the cyst wall that has been cut completely around its circumference. After this procedure, the cystic cavity should slowly decrease in size. Ideally the window should be as large as possible, because if the diameter of the opening is small, continuity of the cyst membrane may be reestablished and the cyst will refill and expand again.

In general, marsupialization, or the Partsch operation, of cysts within the jaws should be avoided. The marsupialization method is indicated when a cyst is too large to enucleate with safety, to avoid devitalizing involved teeth, or if it is anticipated that unerupted teeth in a dentigerous cyst will erupt into position. In the case of fissural cysts, marsupialization is an unsatisfactory procedure because obliteration of the cavity does not occur. Another disadvantage to consider is that only a small portion of the cyst membrane can be submitted for biopsy examination, in contrast with the complete specimen that is obtained by extirpation.

Vitality of Teeth

Regardless of the method of treatment employed, it is essential to perform routine preoperative and postoperative vitality tests on all teeth related to the cyst.

Aspiration

Aspiration of a suspected cyst can be a valuable diagnostic aid, especially when doubt still exists about the nature of the lesion after careful clinical and roentgenographic examination. This investigation is helpful in distinguishing between a maxillary cyst and the maxillary sinus. If it is impossible to withdraw the plunger of the syringe during attempted aspiration, a solid lesion should be considered. The presence of blood under considerable pressure in a suspected cystic formation is probably indicative of the existence of an aneurysmal bone cyst, whereas in a central cavernous hemangioma the pressure of the blood is considerably less marked.

In the case of a solitary bone cyst, either a minute quantity of serous or sanguineous liquid is aspirated or the cavity is found to be devoid of fluid.

Infected cysts usually contain pus as well as normal cyst fluid. After longstanding infection the cyst is likely to contain a thick, semisolid mass of pus together with cholesterol crystals which cannot be aspirated.

Complications

Fracture. Although relatively rare, a pathologic or spontaneous fracture can occur as a result of cyst formation. The presence of a cystic lesion in the mandible weakens the bone, and a fracture may occur from comparatively minor trauma. Occasionally, an undiagnosed cyst may become so large that a fracture may occur during normal mastication. When the traumatic fracture of a cystic area does occur, management may become a problem. The cyst must be completely removed and the fracture parts reduced and immobilized. A small cyst of the mandible usually leaves sufficient bone on either side of the fracture line to ensure an area of contact sufficient for healing. However, when the cyst is extremely large, as it usually is in pathologic fractures, so much bone may have been destroyed that little remains in apposition across the fracture line after the fragments are reduced, and therefore satisfactory resolution is less likely to occur at the fracture site. Replacement of the missing portion of bone by a bone graft may be necessary.

Infection. Two-stage treatment of this problem may be necessary. First, control the infection, and second, render definitive surgery to eradicate the cyst. The infection will probably require establishment of drainage and use of antibiotics. Chronically infected cysts may be removed without initial drainage since localization of the infection exists. Antibiotic coverage is indicated. Postoperative infections should be controlled locally by irrigations, iodoform packing of the bone cavity, and use of systemic antibiotics. Bone cavities that remain open must be irrigated frequently to prevent accumulation of food and debris until healing by secondary intention is complete.

Selected Reading

Bhaskar, S.N., and Laskin, D.M.: Gingival cysts. Oral Surg., *8*:803, 1955.

Browne, R.M.: The odontogenic keratocyst. Br. Dent. J., *128*:225, 1970.

Buchner, A., and Hansen, L.S.: The histomorphologic spectrum of the gingival cyst in the adult. Oral Surg., *48*:532, 1979.

Dahlin, D.C.: Bone Tumors, 2nd ed. Springfield, Charles C Thomas, 1967.

Fantasia, J.E.: Lateral periodontal cyst. Oral. Surg., *48*:237, 1979.

Finn, P., Hjorting-Hansen, E., Gorlin, R.J., and Vickers, R.A.: Calcifying odontogenic cyst: Range, variations and neoplastic potential. Acta Odontol. Scand., *39*:227, 1981.

Gorlin, R.J.: Potentialities of oral epithelium manifest by mandibular dentigerous cysts. Oral Surg., *10*:271, 1957.

Hayward, J.R.: Dentigerous cysts. Am. J. Orthod., *32*:140, 1946.

Jaffe, H.L.: Giant-cell reparative granuloma, traumatic bone cysts, and fibrous (fibro-osseous) dysplasia of the jawbones. Oral Surg., *6*:159, 1953.

Killey, H.C., and Kay, L.W.: An analysis of 471 benign cystic lesions of the jaws. Int. Surg., *46*:540, 1966.

Payne, T.P.: An analysis of the clinical and histopathologic parameters of the odontogenic keratocyst. Oral Surg., *53*:538, 1972.

Shafer, W.G., Hine, M.K., and Levy, B.M.: A Textbook of Oral Pathology, 4th ed. Philadelphia, W.B. Saunders Co., 1983.

Toller, P.: Origin and growth of cysts of the jaws. Ann. R. Coll. Surg., *40*:306, 1967.

Vap, D.R., Dahlin, D.C., and Turlington, E.G.: Pindborg tumor: the so-called calcifying epithelial odontogenic tumor. Cancer, *25*:628, 1970.

Weathers, D.R., and Waldron, C.A.: Unusual multilocular cysts of the jaws (botryoid odontogenic cysts). Oral Surg., *36*:235, 1973.

Wysocki, G.P.: The differential diagnosis of globulomaxillary radiolucencies. Oral Surg., *51*:281, 1981.

CHAPTER 14

Tumors of the Oral Cavity

DONALD R. MEHLISCH

There are some remedies worse than the disease.

PUBLILIUS SYRUS

This account of lesions of the oral tissues is directed especially to the student of dentistry and the general dental practitioner. For the most part, it is concerned with benign tumors involving tissues that are observed frequently in the course of care rendered to every patient seen in the dental office. Although the list of potential lesions that could be amassed is extensive, lesions discussed are considered essential from the standpoint of frequency, severity, potential for initial recognition, and differential diagnosis. Some tumors that occur in this location are similar to neoplasms found elsewhere, whereas others are peculiar to the head and neck area.

Naturally, the full assessment of each patient's malady depends on the integration of various sources of available information. These include clinical, roentgenographic, historical, and laboratory parameters that require consideration in arriving at a diagnosis. To provide a full description of all aspects that need to be taken into account in arriving at a diagnosis is beyond the scope of this chapter but the information is available in a number of excellent texts, for those who require a more comprehensive description.

Neoplasms of Epithelial Origin

Squamous Cell Papilloma

The squamous cell papilloma is a common tumor occurring at all ages and found anywhere in the oral cavity. Common sites are the mucosae of the cheeks, lips, palate, tongue, and gingivae. It may be attached to the underlying tissues by either a narrow or a broad pedicle and projects well above the adjacent mucosa in a cauliflower-like pattern. Irritation, infection, and viral and metabolic disturbances have been mentioned as causes. Microscopically, papillary projections of stratified squamous epithelium cover a thin core of connective tissue. Treatment consists of excision and should include the pedicle and base. Recurrence is rare and these lesions do not undergo malignant change.

Malignant counterpart: squamous cell carcinoma

Papillomatosis (Pseudoepitheliomatous Hyperplasia, Inflammatory Papillary Hyperplasia)

Under the influence of a variety of conditions such as chronic inflammation, irritation, chronic ulcers, fungal or viral infections, bony sequestra, poor oral hygiene, and poor-fitting dentures, several discrete tumors may arise and be scattered over the mucosae. The palate is the most commonly affected area but the lips, tongue, alveolar ridges, and occasionally, the cheeks are involved. Clinically, numerous papillary projections consist microscopically of a core of connective tissue covered by acanthotic squamous epithelium. On rare occasions, inflammatory papillary hyperplasia may undergo malignant change. These lesions, which appear to occur in males more frequently than in females during the

195

fourth to fifth decades, should be treated first by removal of the cause and then with surgical excision.

Malignant counterpart: squamous cell carcinoma

Pigmented Cellular Nevus (Pigmented Mole)

A tumor-like malformation that occurs on the skin and mucous membrane, the nevus may be congenital or developmental. *Intradermal, junctional, compound, juvenile,* and *blue* are the different types of recognized nevi. Pigmented moles are congenital, occurring generally after puberty. Histologically, nevus cells are large distinct cells situated within the connective tissue and separated from the overlying epithelium by a well-defined band, except in the junctional type. The fact that this zone is not present in the junctional nevus has serious implications—a tendency for this nevus to develop into a malignant lesion. For moles that require removal because of cosmetic or irritational considerations, surgical excision is indicated. Junctional nevi require close follow-up care, because 10 percent of all malignant melanomas are believed to arise this way.

Malignant counterpart: malignant melanoma

Leukoplakia

The definition of leukoplakia, white plaque, unfortunately has been used loosely with various interpretations by clinicians and pathologists alike. The diagnosis of leukoplakia should be reserved for a microscopic examination demonstrating dyskeratosis and premalignancy. This lesion, like oral cancer, occurs more frequently in males than in females, and generally in patients over the age of 40. Causative factors are various forms of tissue irritations, chief of which is smoking. Primary sites are the lower lip, tongue, cheeks, and floor of the mouth (Fig. 14-1). Microscopic findings are those of varying degrees of hyperkeratosis, parakeratosis, acanthosis, and dyskeratosis, the latter being the important factor. Other white lesions that may appear similar include frictional keratosis, lichen planus, familial white dysplasia, moniliasis, and stomatitis nicotina. Treatment is directed at elimina-

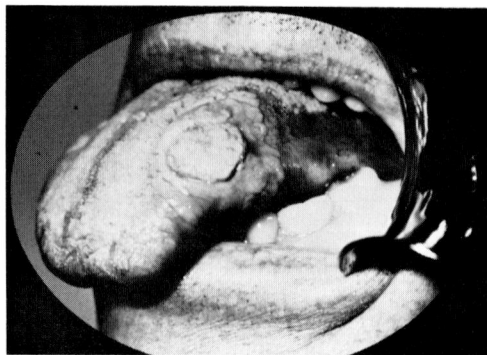

FIG. 14-1. *Leukoplakia of the tongue.*

tion of recognizable irritating factors and *total* excision.

Malignant counterpart: squamous cell carcinoma

Squamous Cell Carcinoma (Epidermoid Carcinoma)

The most common malignant neoplasm of the oral cavity, constituting 5 percent of all malignant tumors in the body, the squamous cell carcinoma accounts for 90 percent of oral malignant neoplasms. Tobacco, alcohol, syphilis, dental and oral infections, exposure to sunlight, ionizing radiation, occupational factors, as well as intraoral lesions such as leukoplakia, herpes simplex, lichen planus, median rhomboid glossitis, and Plummer-Vinson syndrome have been implicated as etiologic factors. Carcinoma of the oral cavity demonstrates a striking sex predilection, occurring much more frequently in men than in women with the peak age between 50 and 70 years. Location of the neoplasms has a strong influence on the clinical appearance, histology, and prognosis (Figs. 14-2 and 14-3). Papillary, ulcerative, nodular, or wart-like growths may be seen, and the microscopic findings can vary between a well-differentiated to highly invasive malignancy. Tumors of the lip have generally the more favorable prognosis, for these metastasize to the regional lymph nodes much less frequently than those in other locations. Surgery, x-ray radiation, and chemotherapy have been used alone or in combination. Depending upon the location of the cancer, radiation can be hazardous because of the damaging effects of the

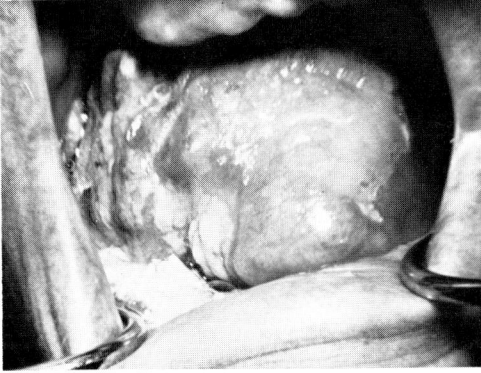

FIG. 14-2. *Cancer of the tongue and floor of the mouth.*

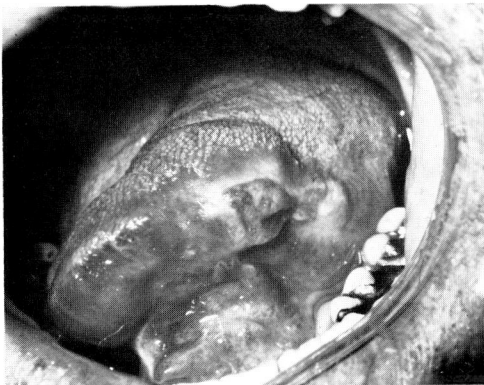

FIG. 14-4. *Basal cell carcinoma of the face.*

x-rays on the bone and potential osteora-dionecrosis.

Basal Cell Carcinoma

Basal cell carcinoma occurs in the skin of the face and possibly in the oral mucosae (Figs. 14-4 and 14-5). Exposure to the ul-traviolet rays in sunlight has been recog-nized for many years to be carcinogenic. It is probably the most common type of can-cer that occurs in men, especially those exposed to the weather. This tumor fre-quently begins as a small papule that ul-cerates, heals, and ulcerates again, giving foundation to the name "rodent ulcer" which it has been termed. Basal cell carci-noma exhibits essentially no tendency for metastasis, and good results can be antici-pated from surgical excision or from x-ray radiation. Multiple nevoid basal cell carci-nomas, keratocysts of the jaws, vertebral

and rib anomalies, most commonly bifid rib, make up the *basal-cell syndrome*, which was first reported in 1951. Lesions associ-ated with this syndrome have malignant potentiality. The multiple nevoid basal cell carcinoma cannot be differentiated from the ordinary basal cell carcinoma.

Neoplasms of Connective Tissue Origin

Lesions of fibrous and connective tissue are common in soft tissues of the oral cav-ity. Most of these growths are probably hyperplasias although some may be true neoplasms. These tumors may also appear as central lesions within the jaws, but they are much less common than are their counterparts in the soft tissues.

Fibroma

Fibroma is the most common benign neoplasm of connective tissue that occurs in the oral cavity (Fig. 14-6). It is often related to some form of chronic irritation.

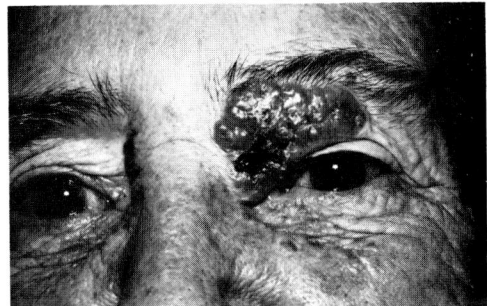

FIG. 14-3. *Cancer of the tongue.*

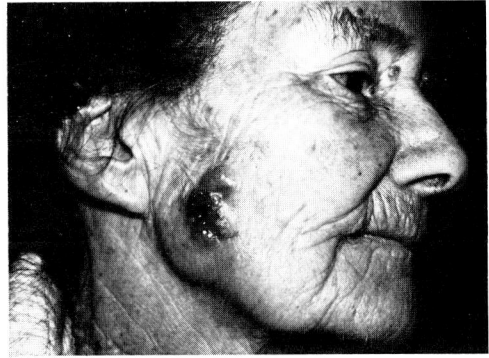

FIG. 14-5. *Basal cell carcinoma of the eyelid.*

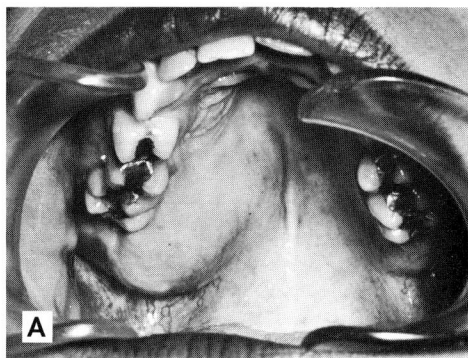

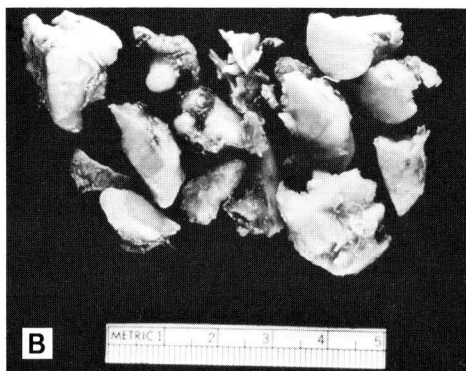

FIG. 14-6. (A) Fibroma of maxilla causing expansion of palate. (B) Gross specimen of fibroma. (Courtesy of Dr. D.E. Waite)

It has been given a variety of designations such as fibrous hyperplasia, fibroepithelial polyp, fibrous epulis, epulis fissuratum, epulis granulomatosa, and others. Fibrous growths occur at any site in the

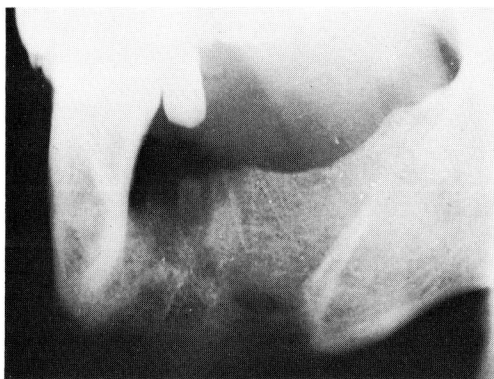

FIG. 14-7. Fibrosarcoma. Note discontinuity of bone at inferior border. (Courtesy of Dr. D.E. Waite)

oral tissues, appearing in all age groups and affecting both sexes equally. The gingivae are affected most often and in this location it is more common in women than in men. The major part of the lesion is composed of connective tissue, which ranges from highly cellular fibroblastic proliferation to masses of collagen. A slow-growing, deep or superficial, sessile or pedunculated lesion, it is not associated with any apparent single etiologic factor. Fibrous growths of the oral tissues are readily dealt with by simple excision but recurrence is not unusual if the entire lesion is not removed, together with any causal factors.

Malignant counterpart: fibrosarcoma (Fig. 14-7).

Peripheral Giant Cell Reparative Granuloma

Peripheral giant cell reparative granuloma is a not uncommon lesion of the oral tissues that has been described under a variety of terms denoting confusion relative to the true nature of the tumor. Although it occurs at any age, the average is between the third and fourth decades. Overall, females are affected several times more frequently than are males. Characteristically of deep red or purple appearance, the cuspid and bicuspid regions are the common site of development. If the lesion is ulcerated, which is not uncommon, it is covered by fibrin. Microscopically, large numbers of giant cells in a stroma of collagen fibers and spindle cells with osteoid tissue, bone, and inflammatory infiltrate are the usual findings. Believed to be granulomatous and reparative in nature instead of neoplastic, the lesion is benign and unencapsulated. It does not recur if completely removed by surgical excision, but complete removal of deep lesions may not be possible. Similar lesions are *pyogenic granuloma* and *pregnancy tumor* (granuloma gravidarum).

Malignant counterpart: fibrosarcoma, osteogenic sarcoma

Myxoma (Fibromyxoma; Lipomyxoma)

The myxoma is a true neoplasm composed of tissue resembling primitive mesenchyme, but few examples have been recorded in the oral soft tissues. Some are

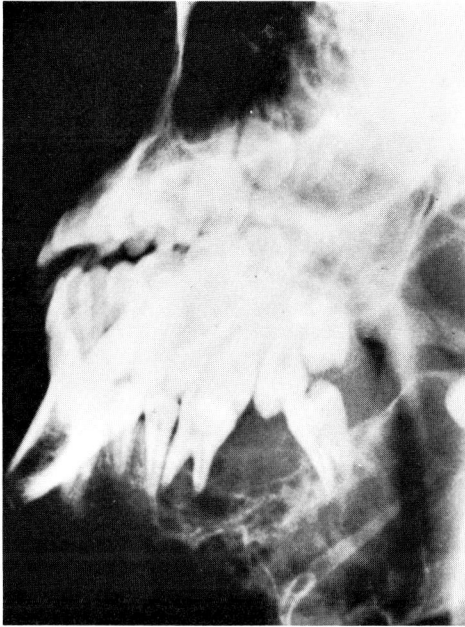

FIG. 14-8. *Myxoma in a 20-year-old woman. (Courtesy of Dr. D.E. Waite)*

sessile or pedunculated lesions having specific origin in the gingivae, lips, palate, or less frequently buccal mucosa (Figs. 14-8 to 14-10). Generally, they are thought to be myxomatous degeneration of a fibrous neoplasm, so it is difficult to discuss the nature of these growths on the basis of the few, incomplete reports available. Treatment is essentially surgical and in some cases wide excision. Myxomas tend to infiltrate the surrounding bone tissue, and therefore, an adequate margin of normal tissue is necessary (Fig. 14-11).

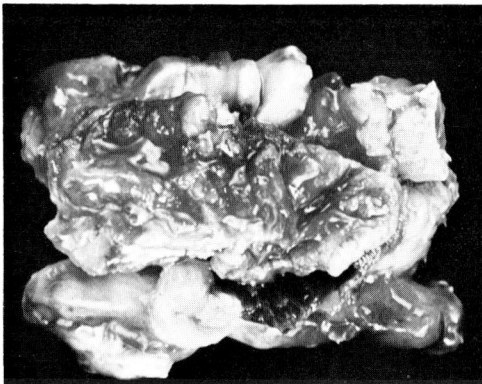

FIG. 14-9. *Gross specimen of fibromyxoma.*

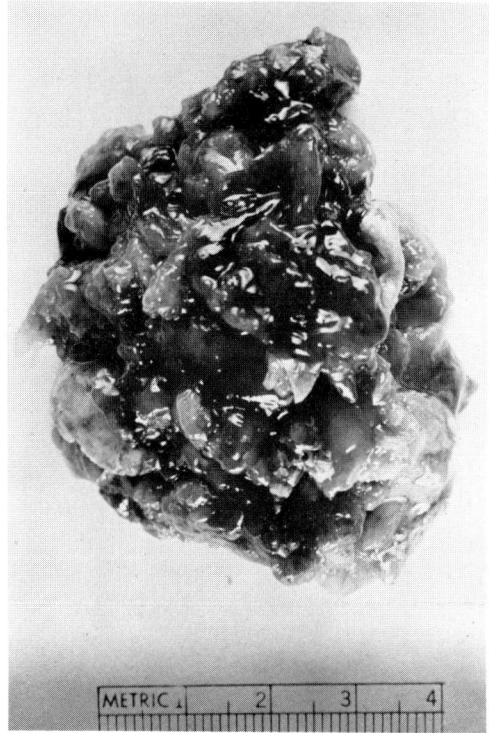

FIG. 14-10. *Gross specimen of myxoma.*

Malignant counterpart: myxosarcoma, fibromyxosarcoma

Lipoma (Fibrolipoma; Myxolipoma)

Tumors of adipose tissue are uncommon in the oral tissues, but occur with considerable frequency in other areas. A benign, slow-growing neoplasm that is usually solitary, the lipoma occurs generally in middle-aged adults. Congenital fatty lesions reported in infants are probably developmental in nature. The tongue is frequently involved as is the buccal mucosa where the lesion appears as a lobulated tumor with thin overlying epithelium allowing the yellow color of fat to be seen. Microscopically, the tumor consists of lobules of mature fat cells, with a varying proportion of connective tissue. The fibrolipoma and myxolipoma have more fibrous or myxomatous tissue than the true lipoma but all are considered essentially the same tumor. Treatment of this pedunculated, encapsulated, elastic-type lesion is surgical excision and recurrences are rare. Slightly

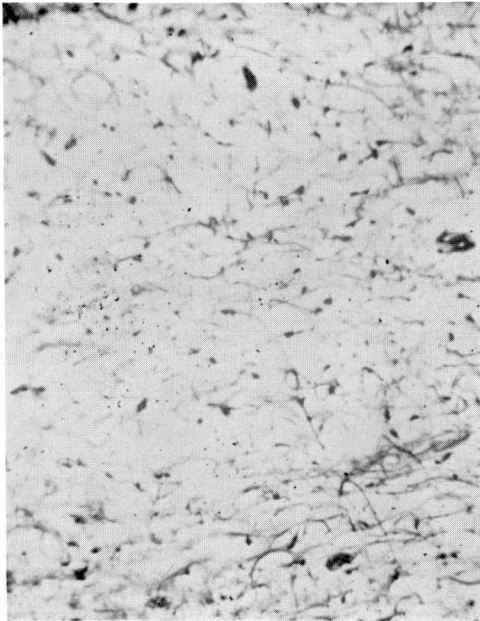

FIG. 14-11. *Histologic section of myxoma.*

wider margins may be necessary for poorly encapsulated lesions.

Malignant counterpart: liposarcoma

Neoplasms of Vascular Tissue

Hemangioma

The hemangioma is characterized by proliferation of blood vessels and occurs more frequently in the head and neck region than in any other part of the body. Of the several types of vascular lesions (capillary, cavernous, sclerosing, cellular), some are relatively aggressive but benign. These lesions are considered by many to be ham-

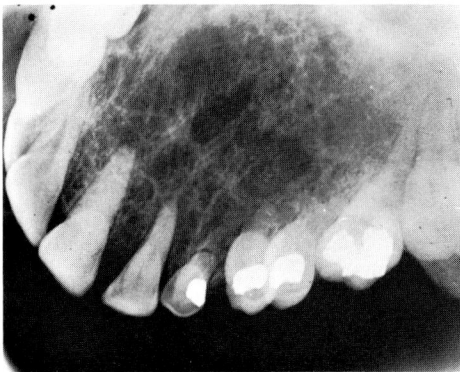

FIG. 14-12. *Hemangioma of maxilla. (Courtesy of Mayo Clinic)*

artomas or developmental malformations rather than true neoplasms. The majority of oral lesions are situated in soft tissues but also found in muscle and bone (Fig. 14-12). The vast majority are present at birth or arise at an early age. A history of recent rapid growth is not uncommon. Pain is usually not part of the clinical findings. These dark reddish blue or purple lesions are smooth and soft, frequently becoming traumatized and suffering ulceration and secondary infection. The central hemangioma located in the mandible or maxilla, although rare, deserves special attention, since patients can die from sudden massive hemorrhage if the lesion or the teeth associated with the lesion are manipulated. The honeycombed radiolucency, with fine fibrillar networks, is distinctive on the roentgenogram. Treatment for this lesion usually includes resection with carotid ligation. Aggressive surgery is also indicated for the *hemangiopericytoma* and possibly the *hemangioendothelioma*. The *sclerosing hemangioma, endothelioma,* and *nevus flammeus (port-wine stain)* are treated like the hemangioma, which is surgical resection, and perhaps sclerosing agents. It is important to know that many congenital hemangiomas have been found to undergo spontaneous regression.

Malignant counterpart: angiosarcoma, hemangiopericytoma, Kaposi's sarcoma

Lymphangioma

Lymphangioma is similar in many respects to the hemangioma, and the two are considered essentially the same. A benign tumor of lymphatic vessels, it is far less common than its counterpart the hemangioma. The lips, cheeks, palate, and most especially the tongue are involved. The majority of lesions are present at birth, but are distributed equally in the sexes, which is different from the hemangioma in which the female develops the lesion more often than the male. Because they are superficial, they are circumscribed, rather diffuse, ill-defined masses consisting of lymph spaces and treated best with surgical excision. They will not respond to sclerosing solutions.

Malignant counterpart: malignant lymphoma (follicular lymphoma, reticulum-cell sarcoma, lymphosarcoma, Hodgkin's disease)

Tumors of Nerve Tissue

Neuroma

The neuroma, a tumor-like, irregularly shaped mass of nerve tissue, is not a true neoplasm but rather an exuberant attempt at repair of a damaged nerve trunk. It most commonly results from the accidental or planned sectioning of a nerve and is remarkably rare in the oral tissues, considering the frequency with which teeth are extracted and nerves consequently severed. The lips, tongue, and mental foramen are common sites of involvement. The dominant feature is pain, and reflex neuralgia with distant radiation has been recorded. Because of the pain and progressive nature of the lesion, it is best treated with surgical excision of the nodule.

Malignant counterpart: neurogenic sarcoma

Neurofibroma

Often referred to by a variety of names such as neurogenic fibroma, perineural fibroblastoma, and neurogenic fibroblastoma, the neurofibroma is a benign tumor of nerve tissue origin arising either from the fibrous connective tissue of the nerve sheath or from the sheath of Schwann. A circumscribed mass surrounded by a capsule, it usually occurs on the skin but is also found in the mouth with the tongue the most common site. On oral mucosa, they appear as small sessile, smooth-surfaced growths. Men are affected more than women with most lesions occurring in the first three decades. Multiple neurofibromas of the skin and other tissues in conjunction with café au lait spots and skeletal abnormalities are characterized in *multiple neurofibromatosis (von Recklinghausen's disease)*. Oral lesions in this disease occur in about 10 percent of cases. Microscopic features of these lesions are the same as those of the solitary neurofibroma and nearly always that of a plexiform neuroma. Treatment for the single neurofibroma is excision but the great number in the multiple disease precludes a surgical cure. Malignant degeneration of a sarcomatous nature occurs in approximately 50 percent of patients with von Recklinghausen's disease.

Malignant counterpart: neurofibrosarcoma

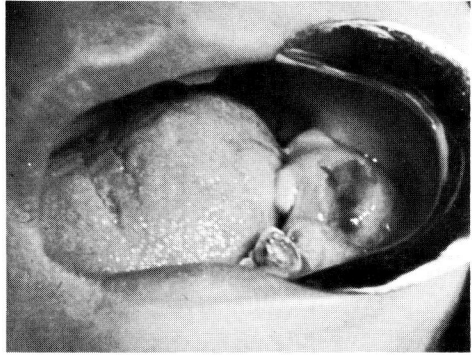

Fig. 14-13. *Neurilemmoma. (Courtesy of Dr. D.E. Waite)*

Neurilemmoma (Schwannoma; Neurinoma)

A tumor that may occur along any of the peripheral cranial or sympathetic nerve routes, the neurilemmoma is derived from the cells of Schwann in the nerve sheath and behaves like a benign neoplastic tumor (Fig. 14-13). Oral tumors give rise to relatively few symptoms, aside from those caused by reason of their size or location. Generally of slow growth and long duration, they are soft on palpation and may be tender. All age groups and both sexes are involved with virtually any area of the head and neck being susceptible, including retropharyngeal, nasopharyngeal, and retrotonsillar. An encapsulated tumor, it consists microscopically of two parts which are interspersed yet discrete. The solid portion is made of cells with elongated or spindle-shaped nuclei and a palisading pattern (Antoni type A), whereas the other areas (Antoni type B) do not exhibit palisading and have a rather unorganized arrangement of cells and fibers with the formation of microcysts. Treatment is surgical excision. The neurilemmoma does not undergo malignant transformation as does the neurofibroma.

Malignant counterpart: malignant Schwannoma

Neoplasms of Muscle Tissue

Leiomyoma

A true neoplasm arising from embryonic nests of smooth muscle cells, the leiomyoma is an extremely rare tumor of the oral cavity, much more rare than in other parts of the alimentary canal. The posterior part of the tongue is the usual site, but it may involve the soft palate. It is a slow-growing circumscribed lesion that is painless, and it grossly resembles the ordinary fibroma. Histologically, it is composed of interlacing bundles of smooth muscle fibers supported by a delicate fibrous connective tissue stroma. Treatment is best accomplished by complete surgical excision.

Malignant counterpart: leiomyosarcoma

Rhabdomyoma

The rhabdomyoma, another rare tumor in the oral cavity, develops from skeletal muscle. It generally occurs in children and infants with the most frequent site being the tongue. Less commonly, it involves the uvula and palate. The microscopic picture is one of varying degrees of pleomorphism of the muscle cells. This slow-growing lesion is poorly encapsulated and owing to its aggressive histologic nature needs to be removed in its entirety with a wide margin of normal tissue.

Malignant counterpart: rhabdomyosarcoma

Myoblastoma (Granular Cell Myoblastoma)

An uncommon tumor of controversial origin, the myoblastoma occurs equally in males and females at all ages. The tongue is the commonest site, but it has been re-ported in the lip, gingivae, soft palate, and uvula. It appears as a slowly growing nodule of the submucosal tissue and is usually small (hardly exceeding 0.5 cm in diameter), well circumscribed, and firm. A growth of similar structure, though not of similar nature, occurs as a congenital lesion in the gums of infants, the *congenital epulis of newborn*. The histogenesis of myoblastoma is still debatable, with several theories, including one of myogenous origin, one of histiocytic origin, and one of neural origin being advocated. Although the nature of the myoblastoma remains obscure, little doubt exists as to its behavior and treatment. The lesion is entirely benign and local excision effects a cure. Pseudo-epitheliomatous hyperplasia may occur in the overlying epithelium in many tumors and may give the lesion the appearance of squamous cell carcinoma which does not develop.

Malignant counterpart: alveolar soft part sarcoma

Neoplasms and Dysplasias of Bone and Cartilage

Osteoma

Osteoma is a benign neoplasm characterized by slow growths of cancellous or compact bone that increase in size by continuous formation in an endosteal or peri-

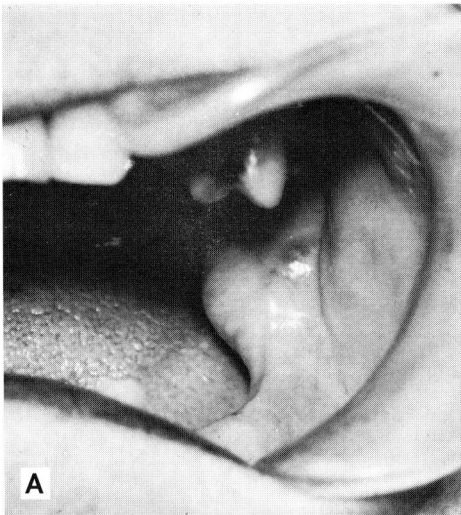

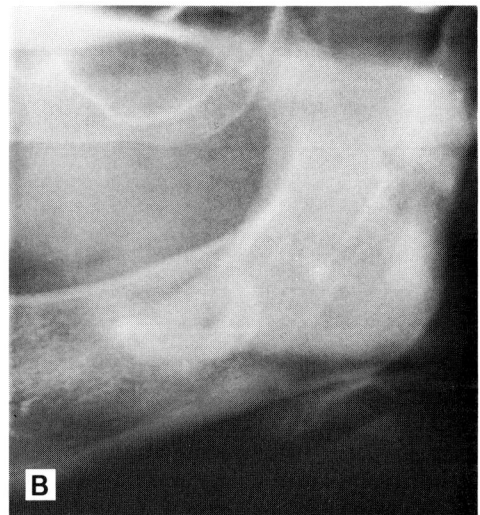

FIG. 14-14. *Osteoma. (A) Osteoma projecting lingually from mandible. (B) Radiograph of osteoma. (Courtesy of Dr. D.E. Waite)*

osteal location. It occurs as a circumscribed hard protuberance growing outward from the bone, or as a dense mass growing centrally within the bone, and is capable of causing facial asymmetry. The mandible is more often involved than is the maxilla (Fig. 14-14). All ages can be affected but it is more common in adults past the fourth decade. Roentgenographically, a dense radiopaque mass protruding from the bone is seen in the peripheral type, whereas a well-circumscribed sclerotic mass appears with the central lesion. Trabeculae of mature lamellar bone with varying amounts of intervening fatty or fibrous marrow are seen microscopically. Surgical removal is indicated if the lesion produces symptoms or interferes with a prosthesis. Skeletal "osteomas" of various bones, but often prominently involving the skull and jaws, are associated with intestinal polyps, fibromatous and other connective tissue lesions, and epidermoid cysts in *Gardner's syndrome*.

Malignant counterpart: osteogenic sarcoma (Fig. 14-15)

Exostoses and Tori

Exostoses and tori, dense bony overgrowths, are non-neoplastic lesions of unknown origin occurring in the mandible and maxilla. The midline of the palate is the most frequent area of involvement, occurring there in about 20 percent of the population, where it is termed *torus palati-*

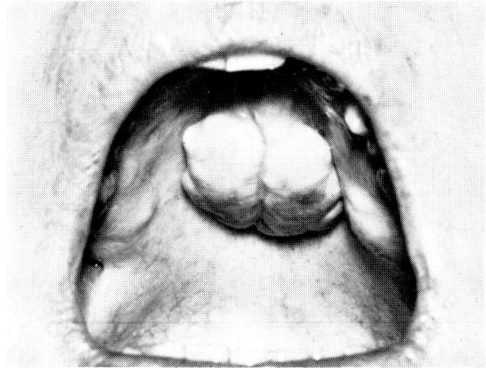

FIG. 14-16. *Torus palatinus.*

nus (Fig. 14-16). Those of the mandible are termed, appropriately enough, *torus mandibularis*, and are seen in only 8 percent of persons, but frequently they are bilateral on the lingual aspects of the jaw. Some studies indicate the palatal lesions are more common in females than in males but no sex incidence holds in the mandible. Formation in both jaws is generally before the age of 30 years, although frequently they are discovered quite late in life. Histologic sections show dense normal bone. Because the general rate of growth is slow, these lesions are not usually treated actively unless interfering with speech, or with fabrication of prosthetic appliance, or overlying mucosa demonstrates chronic irritation or ulceration. Exostoses occur on either side of the maxilla or mandible alveolar processes and deserve the same considerations as tori. Treatment, when indicated, is by excision, generally with a mallet and chisel or surgical bur.

Malignant counterpart: osteogenic sarcoma

Osteogenic Fibroma (Osteofibroma; Central Fibroma)

Osteogenic fibroma, a rare benign tumor in the jaws, is composed of fibroblasts and collagen fibers without formation of bone or osteoid. If bone is being formed, the tumor should be termed ossifying fibroma, although it will be of no significance relative to treatment or behavior. It is reported so infrequently that little is known of the lesion. It causes few symptoms and is found during routine roentgenographic examination. It has

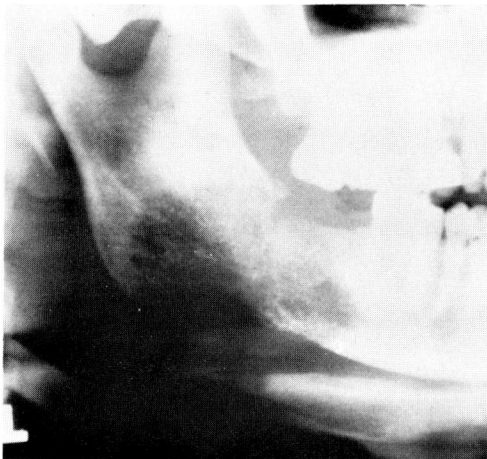

FIG. 14-15. *Radiograph of osteogenic sarcoma of the left mandible.*

well-defined margins and is encapsulated. Histologically, it may be difficult to decide whether the tumor is of odontogenic or osteogenic origin. Treatment is by simple excision.

Malignant counterpart: fibrosarcoma

Osteogenic Myxoma (Fibro-osteogenic Myxoma)

Osteogenic myxoma may occur in any part of the skeleton, but the jaws are the most common site. It is one of several unusual tumors occurring in the jaws and needs to be distinguished from its odontogenic counterpart, the odontogenic myxoma. There is neither a sex nor an age preference, and it may involve either the maxilla or mandible equally. It is thought to arise from vestigial embryonic tissue within the jaw or from degeneration of a central fibroma. It is slow growing but capable of producing considerable facial deformity. A soap-bubble-like area of radiolucency is seen on the roentgenogram. Microscopic examination reveals a myxomatous structure containing few cells and consisting mainly of mucus. The tumor is not encapsulated and infiltrates the marrow, which is important. It is benign and does not metastasize but because of its infiltrative nature requires wide excision for treatment.

Malignant counterpart: myxosarcoma

Fibrous Dysplasia of Bone and Ossifying Fibroma

A group of central lesions of the jaws is included in the general category of fibrous dysplasia in which normal bone is replaced by fibrous tissue from which new calcified tissue subsequently forms by metaplasia (Fig. 14-17). These include the typical lesions of fibrous dysplasia, ossifying fibroma, fibro-osteoma, fibrocementoma, the familial condition of cherubism, and polyostotic fibrous dysplasia, or Albright's syndrome.

"Fibro-osseous dysplasia" is a term that is gaining acceptance for many of the defects of this type that involve the jawbones. Here, these lesions are considered separately, although their histology, roentgenographic features, and treatment make it convenient to group them together (Figs. 14-18 and 14-19).

1. Ossifying fibroma (monostotic fibrous dysplasia) has an equal predilection for males and females, but is more common in children and young adults. Painless and nontender, it appears as a localized hard swelling of either jaw, occurring in the mandible more frequently than in the maxilla. Growth is generally slow with gradually increasing facial deformity.

2. Polyostotic fibrous dysplasia (Albright's syndrome) often occurs in the bones of

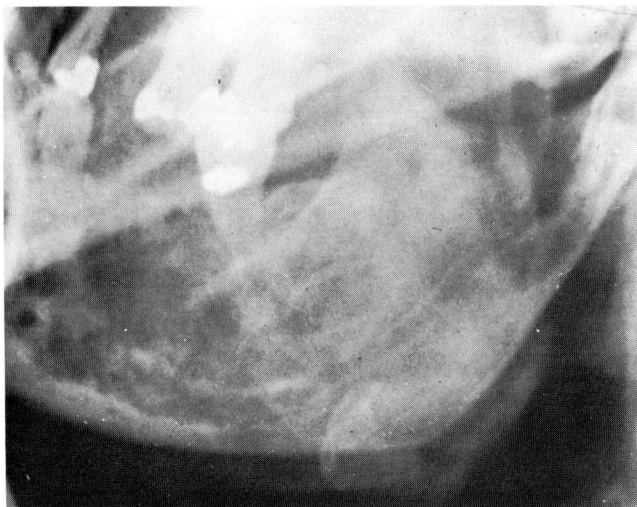

FIG. 14-17. *Fibrous dysplasia of ramus of mandible. (Courtesty of Dr. D.E. Waite)*

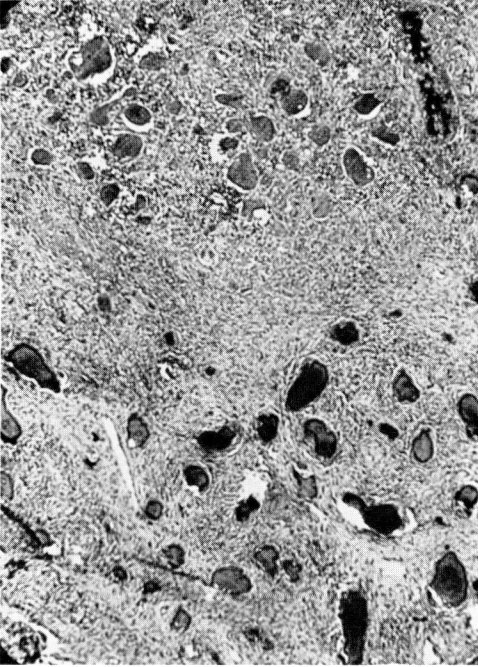

FIG. 14-18. *Histologic section of fibro-osseous lesion.*

one limb, particularly a lower one. The skull bones and jaws are affected when the upper limb is affected most generally. Polyostotic disease affecting more than a few bones is almost always seen first during childhood. The disease is relatively common and, if accompanied by such manifestations as cutaneous pigmentation, endocrine disorders, precocious puberty, and premature skeletal maturation, is termed Albright's syndrome, which is a relatively uncommon disease. The endocrine disturbances

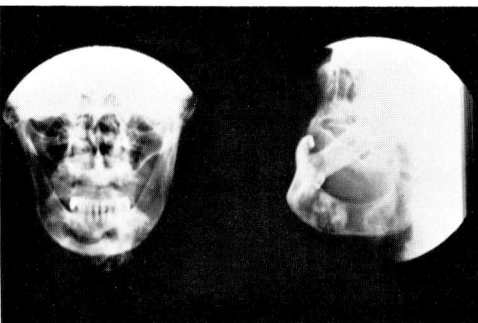

FIG. 14-19. *Radiograph of fibro-osseous lesion of the mandible.*

may alter the time of eruption of the teeth.

3. Familial fibrous dysplasia (cherubism; disseminated juvenile fibrous dysplasia) affects children, who appear to be normal at birth. Males are affected twice as often as females, and swellings are initially seen at about the ages of two and four years. The mandible is almost always affected and often also the maxilla, with bilateral occurrence the rule rather than the exception in both jaws. The deciduous and permanent dentitions show many abnormalities including premature exfoliation, lack of eruption owing to nondevelopment of tooth germs, and irregularly spaced teeth as a result of the expanded bone. Of interest is the fact that the lesions will increase in size quite rapidly to the age of about seven years and then enter a static phase until puberty. Facial deformity is the chief complaint.

Microscopically, the major feature is proliferation of fibroblasts that produce a dense collagenous matrix. Varying amounts of osteoid or bone trabeculae are seen and have no meaning relative to function. Mitotic figures may be seen.

Roentgenologically, the defects of fibrous dysplasia are well-defined zones of rarefaction. Expansion with thinning of the cortex is especially likely and those lesions with a large osseous component will be radiopaque in areas.

Treatment should be conservative since the lesions commonly stop growing at puberty. Primarily, therapy should be directed toward restoring normal configuration to the jawbones. The prognosis in fibrous dysplasia is generally good.

Malignant counterpart: osteogenic sarcoma, fibrogenic sarcoma

Central Giant Cell Tumor of Bone

Few lesions of bone have provoked the controversy that the central giant cell tumor has. It is considered to be a true neoplasm. Giant cell tumors occur almost exclusively between the ages of 20 and 40. The principal symptom is swelling, accompanied in some cases by pain. Slight to moderate swelling of the jaw due to expansion of the cortical plates may occur in the

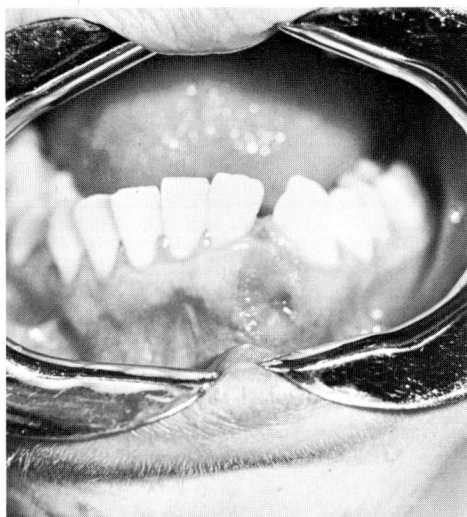

FIG. 14-20. *Giant cell tumor causing separation of teeth. (Courtesy of Dr. D.E. Waite)*

involved area. The tumor forms a maroon or reddish-brown mass that replaces bone, and microscopically consists of numerous giant cells lying in a cellular matrix of spindled-shaped cells and scanty collagen (Figs. 14-20 and 14-21). Roentgenographically, the appearance is not pathognomonic but does present several features suggestive of the diagnosis: the location of the radiolucent area, no periosteal new bone formation over the involved area, "soap-bubble" appearance, thinning of the cortex and expansion of the bone. Removal of the tumor by curettage is the most widely accepted type of therapy. There are recurrences, in rather high percentages, at times, and more radical surgery may be necessary for this, as well as for malignant change which can complicate the course in approximately 10 percent of cases outside the jawbones.

Malignant counterpart: fibrosarcoma, osteogenic sarcoma

Giant Cell Reparative Granuloma

Giant cell reparative granuloma is peculiar to the jawbones. Understandably, it has been confused with the benign giant cell tumor of bone. The giant cell reparative granuloma occurs in adolescents and young adults between the ages of 10 and 25. Found in the female more than in the male, it occurs more frequently in the

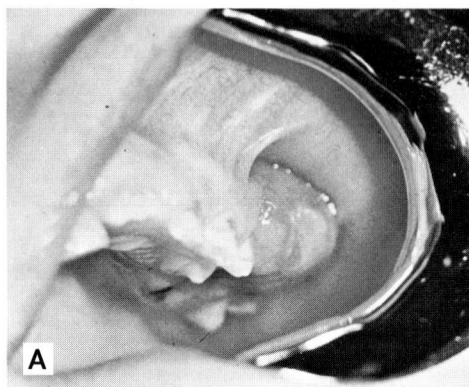

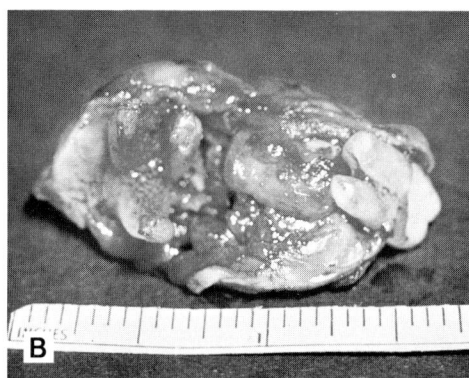

FIG. 14-21. *(A) Giant cell tumor in an 8-year-old boy. (B) Gross specimen of giant cell tumor. (Courtesy of Dr. D.E. Waite)*

mandible than in the maxilla and is confined to the tooth-bearing area of the jaw (Fig. 14-22). Microscopically, the distinguishing features of the giant cell reparative granuloma are the scarcity and irregular distribution of the giant cells, compared to the giant cell tumor. A variable amount of vascularity and microcyst formation may be seen. Similar histologic findings are present in the *"brown tumor" of hyperparathyroidism*. A benign condition, the reparative granuloma can be treated satisfactorily by curettage and only rarely will there be a recurrence.

Malignant counterpart: fibrosarcoma, osteogenic sarcoma

Chondroma

Chondroma is a rare benign tumor of cartilaginous tissue occurring in the jaws. It may occur at any age with cases reported in infants and children. Commonest in the

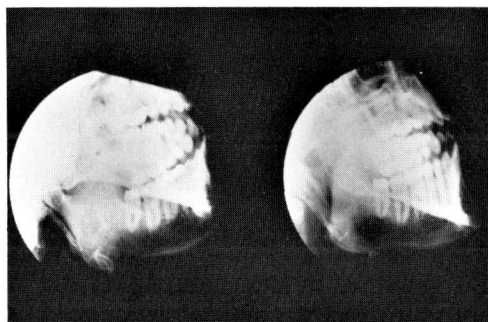

FIG. 14-22. *Radiographs of giant cell reparative granuloma. (Courtesy of Mayo Clinic)*

maxilla, where the anterior alveolar area is the usual site, the maximum incidence is in the fifth and sixth decades. Males are affected more often than females. The presenting symptom is usually the presence of a mass, as there is no pain in the initial stages. Roentgenographically, there is an area of irregular bone destruction, and resorption of roots can occur. Cartilaginous tumors vary considerably in histologic appearance from area to area. Hyaline cartilage, bone formation, myxomatous changes, and cystic degeneration may all be seen. Surrounded by a fibrous capsule, the tumor may break through indicating aggressive growth and, therefore, should be excised with a safe margin. In a number of cases chondromas have been reported to gradually transform into malignant lesions.

Malignant counterpart: chondrosarcoma (Fig. 14-23)

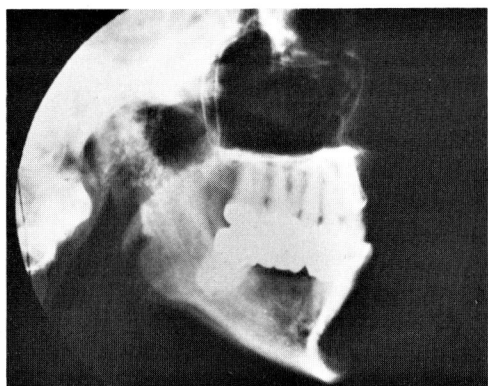

FIG. 14-23. *Radiograph of chondrosarcoma of the neck of the mandible. (Courtesy of Mayo Clinic)*

General Principles Related to Tumors of the Oral Cavity

The study of tumors of the oral cavity, indeed of the head and neck region, is important to practitioners in several different fields. General surgeons, otolaryngologists, radiologists, plastic surgeons, dentists, oral surgeons, and at times, ophthalmologists and neurosurgeons are included in this group. Tumors are encountered in each of these specialties, either as a matter of diagnosis or during therapy. Surgical procedures may be complicated, demanding a wide range of technical ability. There can be no place for the occasional operator who may fail to provide uniformity of treatment or to seek out that therapeutic modality most likely to succeed in a specific case. Many times, this is best achieved by a group approach. A dental contribution is of great importance. Dentists have an opportunity to recognize early lesions and to play a significant role in carrying out cytologic diagnostic techniques. The removal of decayed and infected teeth before surgery or prior to radiation therapy may also be required. The dentist can also provide responsibility for intraoral splints and prosthetic appliances.

Signs and Symptoms. The nature of the symptoms produced varies according to the location of the lesion. Oral lesions in the asymptomatic stage may, in fact, be first recognized by the patient, especially tumors of the lip, anterior tongue, or floor of the mouth. An irregularity or abnormality of contour may be discovered while brushing the teeth, or bleeding may draw attention to impending trouble. Loosening of one or more teeth may occur if the alveolar ridge is involved. Tongue movement may be influenced and protrusion limited because of infiltration and fixation of the lesion in the floor of the mouth. Lesions arising from the palate, tonsillar fossa, or base of the tongue usually are first manifested by the development of a persistent sore throat. Initially, pain may be intermittent but becomes progressively more intense and prolonged.

Local pain eventually develops as the tumor invades adjacent structures, but is only rarely an early symptom. Pain is frequently referred to the ear from numerous primary sites, including tumors of the floor of the mouth, tongue, alveolar ridge, palate, tonsillar fossa, and hypopharynx.

The clinical characteristics of oral tumors are:

SIGN	BENIGN	MALIGNANT
History	Long	Short
Induration	Absent	Present
Ulceration	Rare	Frequent
Margin	Well-defined	Irregular
Mobility	Freely moveable	Fixed
Papillary outgrowth	Frequent	Infrequent
Regional adenopathy	Absent	Frequent

(From: Sharp, G. S., Bullock, W. K., and Hazlet, J. W.: Oral Cancer and Tumors of the Jaws. McGraw-Hill Book Co., 1965. Used with permission of McGraw-Hill Book Co.)

Examination of the oral cavity. The examination must always be performed in a methodical manner to avoid the possibility of incompleteness. Dentures, both partial and complete, are removed first. Maximum illumination is essential. It should be from either a fixed light or headlight in order to leave the examiner's hands free for manipulation of tongue blades and palpation.

The examination should start with the lips and proceed to the mucous membrane of the cheek back to the anterior pillars. The mandibular gingiva is observed, then the floor of the mouth and tongue, which can be examined together. The tongue should be shifted back and forth to examine first one side and then the other, starting anteriorly and progressing posteriorly to the glossopalatine fold. The maxillary gingiva and hard palate follow, then the soft palate and uvula. Finally, the tonsillar fossa, anterior and posterior pillars, posterior pharyngeal wall, and hypopharynx are examined.

Palpation with a gloved finger must be a routine part of the oral examination. In the floor of the mouth attention to the submaxillary ducts is necessary, and these glands need to be felt and salivary flow determined. The parotid gland is similarly examined. Palpation is especially important for that part of the tongue behind the circumvallate papillae.

Biopsy. A biopsy specimen of an accessible lesion in the oral cavity may be obtained with the use of local anesthesia. Areas of slough or obvious inflammation should be avoided. When the tumor underlies an intact mucosal surface, care should be taken that the specimen is removed at a deep enough level to include any malignant tissue. At times, with small lesions suspected of being cancerous, excisional biopsy may be undertaken, but in this instance, a wide margin of normal tissue must be removed.

Staging and grading are two methods of assessing cancers. The TNM method is useful in describing the anatomic involvement of the lesion. The letter T indicates a primary tumor. N implies regional lymph node involvement, and M indicates distant metastasis. Broder's grading method separates the histopathologic appearance of tumors into four groups.

Grade I: Tumors composed of 25 percent or less abnormal cells.

Grade II: Tumors composed of 25 to 50 percent abnormal cells.

Grade III: Tumors composed of 50 to 75 percent abnormal cells.

Grade IV: Tumors composed of 75 percent or more abnormal cells.

Odontogenic Tumors

Lesions that arise from the odontogenic apparatus or that are associated with it form a complex group. It is necessary to recognize the distinctive histologic features of these lesions and certain others for which they may be mistaken. Some oral tumors develop from dental structures and may simulate neoplasms of osseous derivation. The basis for a clear interpretation of odontogenic tumors demands first a basic understanding of normal odontogenesis.

There is some question whether odontogenic tumors are true neoplasms. Many lesions of the oral tissues that appear clinically as tumors are not neoplasms but are non-neoplastic developmental anomalies or overgrowths of inflammatory or other causation.

In a discussion of odontogenic tumors and tumor-like lesions, the following simple classification is offered.

I. Ectodermal
  A. Ameloblastoma
  B. Calcifying Epithelial Odontogenic Tumor
  C. Adenomatoid Ameloblastoma
  D. Calcifying Odontogenic Cyst
  E. Squamous Odontogenic Tumor
II. Mesodermal
  A. Central Odontogenic Fibroma
  B. Odontogenic Myxoma
  C. Cemental Lesions
    1. Peripheral Cemental Dysplasia
    2. Central Cementifying Fibroma
    3. Benign Cementoblastoma (true cementoma)
    4. Gigantiform Cementoma
III. Mixed (Ectodermal and Mesodermal)
  A. Ameloblastic Fibroma
  B. Ameloblastic Fibro-odontoma
  C. Odontoma

Although dentinomas are included in many classifications, it seems likely that they are but variants of some of the hamartoma-like tumors such as the ameloblastic odontoma.

Ectodermal Tumors

AMELOBLASTOMA

A true neoplasm of enamel organ tissue, the ameloblastoma is the most common of the epithelial odontogenic tumors that does not undergo differentiation or induction of mesodermal derivatives. The term *ameloblastoma* was introduced by Ivy and Churchill in 1930, although first mention of the tumor can be dated back to 1868 and Broca's report. Baden found more than 50 terms associated with this tumor, and greater diversity of opinion has existed concerning all aspects of this neoplasm than perhaps any other found anywhere in the body.

Incidence. This lesion comprises approximately 1 percent of the tumors and cysts seen in the mandible and maxilla and is the most common of the epithelial odontogenic tumors. Sixty-five percent occur in the 20 to 50 year age range, with nearly half in the third and fourth decades of life. Ages can vary from the young to the old. More males than females have generally been reported in the literature, although

studies with a slight predominance of female patients at the time of histologic diagnosis have also been documented. An overwhelming majority occur in the mandible, with well over 75 percent in the body and ramus regions. Maxillary tumors are generally in the posterior regions with possible antrum and/or floor of the nose involvement.

Etiology. Many theories have been advanced about causal factors, most of which have not been shown conclusively to be correct. Trauma, extraction of teeth, ill-fitting dentures or bridges, malocclusion, periodontal disease, loose teeth, rickets, oral infection, unerupted third molars, and supernumerary teeth have all been implicated. Whether these conditions give rise to the tumor or only cause symptoms leading to its detection is debatable. The latter conclusion is probably more correct. They appear to arise from epithelium endowed with the potentiality of odontogenesis.

Features. Swelling is the single most common symptom, occurring in as many as 85 percent of cases. Pain, while not a frequent symptom, has been found in 41 percent of cases in some studies. The ameloblastoma grows slowly, and it is important to realize that patients may be asymptomatic in the early stages of the neoplasm. Panographic roentgenographs have been of great help in the discovery of this tumor in this early asymptomatic state during the routine dental examination. In maxillary tumors, sinus problems or nasal obstruction may be the first symptom. Draining sinuses, unhealed extraction sites usually associated with red granulation tissue within the tooth socket, bleeding, trismus, neural involvement, and other dental problems may be the chief complaint. Roentgenographic aspects typically show a coarsely trabeculated zone of osseous destruction that has the appearance of a multilocular cystic cavity. Bone often appears to be replaced by a number of well-defined radiolucent areas that give the lesion a honeycomb or soap-bubble configuration. Maxillary tumors produce a monocystic cavity in most instances. Thickening of membranes, cloudiness, and destruction of the walls are usual findings when sinus involvement is present. The roentgenographic examination

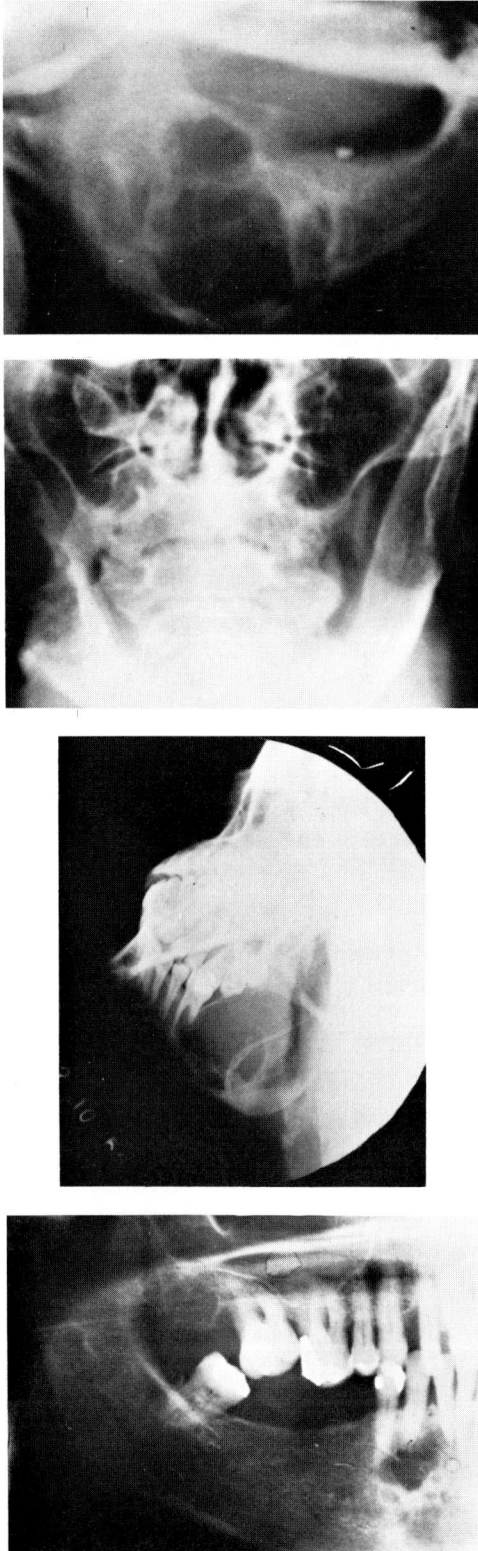

FIG. 14-24. *Radiographs of ameloblastoma.*

and diagnosis, as with any tumor, are nonspecific, and diagnosis cannot be made solely from the roentgenographic evidence (Fig. 14-24).

Although ameloblastomas have been described as solid or cystic, the degree of cyst formation is so variable as to preclude division on this basis. The tumor appears as a grayish-white or grayish-yellow mass replacing bone and containing no calcified tissue. A tumor commonly contains solid areas with microcystic formations together with larger cysts. Partitions between cysts may be bone or, more frequently, soft connective tissue. Clear to straw-colored fluid or a gelatinous material is contained in the cystic spaces. Both the inner and outer cortical plates of the jaw are often thinned and expanded.

Essentially, the ameloblastoma is an epithelial tumor composed of irregularly anastomosing strands, nests, islands, and cords of epithelium separated by variable amounts of connective tissue. All tumors show a follicular, plexiform, or mixed follicular and plexiform pattern (Fig. 14-25). It appears to serve no useful purpose to separate "follicular" from "plexiform" ameloblastomas. Many tumors show at least some foci of squamous differentiation and are commonly called "acanthomatous," and such neoplasms have been mistaken for squamous carcinoma. Granular cells, which usually occur in large masses within the follicle, may replace part or all of the stellate reticulum and sometimes the basal layer of cells as well.

Behavior. The ameloblastoma is a neoplasm that causes expansion more than destruction of bone. However, there is a certain degree of local invasion of the surrounding bone. In the absence of proper treatment, this tumor can grow to a great size, but still remain localized. Recurrences are common, depending on the tumor's size, location, length of duration, and initial forms of treatment. Recurrent tumors demonstrate the same histologic pattern as that of the primary tumor and there is no correlation between histologic pattern and the clinical course. Metastasis is unlikely, and if it does occur it is probably a result of aspiration rather than of lymphatic or hematogenous dissemination.

Treatment and Prognosis. When the results

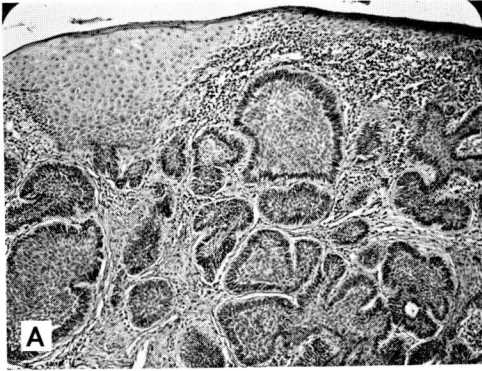

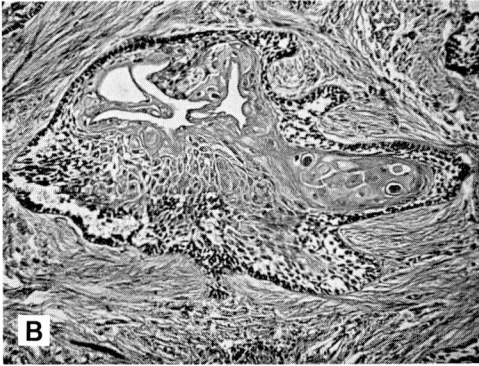

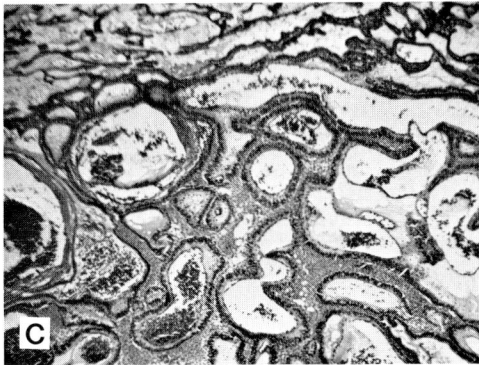

Fig. 14-25. *Histologic sections of ameloblastoma. (A) Follicular pattern. (B) Acanthomatous pattern. (C) Plexiform pattern.*

of treatment of ameloblastomas are assessed, several factors are important. First, long-term follow-up is essential. This neoplasm can continue to grow and extend beyond the margin of what appears to be normal tissue. The relationship between the type of treatment and the rate of recurrence is basic to much of the controversy concerning treatment of this tumor. Exci-

sion, cautery, and curettement are forms of treatment generally considered conservative and are associated with the highest degrees of recurrence. However, when they are used in combination with each other or with other modes of therapy, effectiveness is increased. Curettement is the least desirable form of therapy, whereas resection, whether en bloc or segmental, with an adequate margin of uninvolved tissue, gives the best overall prognosis.

CALCIFYING EPITHELIAL ODONTOGENIC TUMOR

Prior to 1958 when Pindborg described it under its present designation, the calcifying epithelial odontogenic tumor was considered a type of ameloblastoma or odontoma. It has distinctive pathologic features.

Incidence. It is a rare lesion, with relatively few cases being reported in the literature. Men between the ages of 25 and 50 have been affected primarily in the cases thus far reported. The bicuspid-molar region of the mandible has been predominantly involved and may be involved with an unerupted tooth.

Etiology. Its invariable occurrence in relation to an embedded tooth suggests its dental nature, and it has been indicated to develop from the reduced enamel organ of the embedded tooth.

Features. The growth is symptomless, apart from progressive swelling of the jaw, and examination shows a hard tumor that may be diffuse or well defined. The roentgenogram shows an impacted tooth with radiolucency around the crown. This translucent zone has areas of radiopacity which may not be well demarcated from surrounding normal tissues.

The tumor is well circumscribed in most cases, and the apparent cystic spaces seen on the roentgenogram are filled with soft tumor tissue. This is an invasive tumor that destroys surrounding bone, a feature generally noted at operation.

Sheets of polyhedral epithelial cells tend to be closely packed in a connective tissue stroma. Calcification is the most striking feature of the tumor, as its name would suggest. The calcium is deposited in and around epithelial cells which appear to be undergoing degeneration.

Treatment and Prognosis. This neoplasm appears to behave in much the same manner as does the ameloblastoma, recurring if not completely removed. Conservative therapy will most likely result in recurrence, and once the diagnosis of calcifying epithelial odontogenic tumor is made follow-up care is essential, with recurrent lesions receiving aggressive treatment.

ADENOMATOID AMELOBLASTOMA
(ODONTOGENIC ADENOMATOID TUMOR)

First recognized as an entity by Stafne at the Mayo Clinic in 1948, odontogenic adenomatoid tumor has been reported in the literature under varying designations. This neoplasm is a distinctive lesion with characteristic clinical and pathologic features apart from the ameloblastoma.

Incidence. Slightly more than 100 cases have been recorded in the literature denoting the uncommon occurrence of this tumor. Noteworthy is the fact that the adenoameloblastoma occurs in a young age group, over 75 percent of patients being under 20 years of age, and rarely beyond the third decade. Females are affected about twice as often as are males. Generally, adenoameloblastoma is situated in the lateral incisor, cuspid, or bicuspid region of the jaw. Well over half of these tumors are in the maxilla.

Etiology. The actual point of origin of the tumor remains a matter of considerable doubt. Columnar cells, which bear a close resemblance to ameloblasts, and the frequent association of the tumor with unerupted teeth suggests its origin from dental epithelium. Because the adenoameloblastoma is frequently associated with an impacted tooth or originates in a cyst wall, it could theoretically be derived from the enamel organ or its remnants, or from a dentigerous cyst.

Features. It is frequently, but by no means constantly, associated with unerupted teeth and may also occur in a normally erupted dentition. Few symptoms apart from swelling occur and pain is not a usual finding. Expansion of the bone from the gradually increasing swelling may occur, and fluctuation may be evident. Roentgenographically, the lesion reveals a destructive process that is poorly outlined in the jaw. While there is no characteristic roentgenographic finding, the tumor most commonly occurs as a single radiolucent area which varies considerably in size (Fig. 14-26).

Generally the tumors are small, measuring less than 3 cm in diameter. A well-defined fibrous capsule exists, and on cut section small areas of hemorrhage in a grayish-white tissue are demonstrated. Cystic spaces of various sizes containing a yellowish gelatinous material may be present. Teeth may be embedded in the tumor or attached to it.

These tumors are composed of sheets and strands of epithelial cells which whorl and appear active. The characteristic feature of the adenoameloblastoma is columnar cells which appear to be similar to ameloblasts and form tubular spaces. These columnar cells are supported by a scant fibrous connective tissue stroma and have nuclei situated toward the ends of the cell body farthest from the central space. Small foci of calcification are scattered throughout the tumor.

Behavior. The tumor is benign and does not recur after enucleation. It has been noted to show continued growth and can attain a fairly large size before detection.

Treatment and Prognosis. Conservative surgical excision is indicated. Enucleation has also been used successfully in certain instances. Of great importance is the fact that this tumor lacks the propensity for recurrence, as does the ordinary ameloblastoma, and does not demand radical surgery.

CALCIFYING ODONTOGENIC CYST

The calcifying odontogenic cyst (Gorlin cyst) is discussed in Chapter 13.

SQUAMOUS ODONTOGENIC TUMOR
(BENIGN EPITHELIAL ODONTOGENIC TUMOR)

Relatively few cases of this odontogenic tumor have been reported. It was not until 1975 that this lesion was first named and reported.

Incidence. Like the calcifying epithelial odontogenic tumor, it is a rare lesion that occurs in the third decade most frequently. The sex distribution and involvement of maxilla and mandible are equal. However, the maxillary lesions are more anterior than are those located in the mandible.

Etiology. The most agreed-upon cause of this benign odontogenic tumor are the

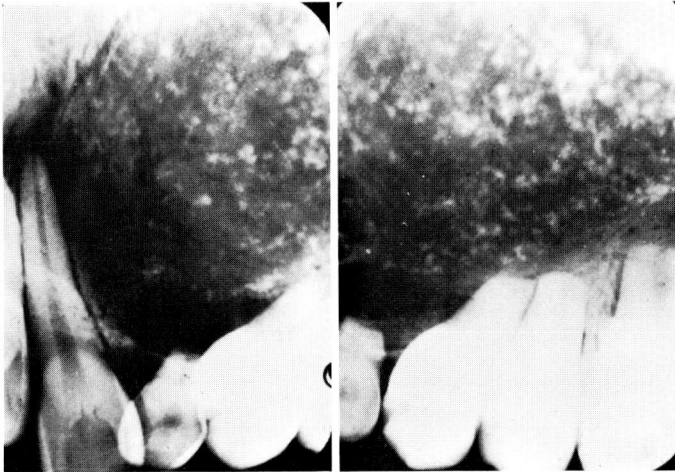

FIG. 14-26. *Odontogenic adenomatoid tumor in 18-year-old patient. (Courtesy of Mayo Clinic)*

rests of Malassez. Proliferations of epithelial tissue have been suggested.

Features. Most likely to be asymptomatic. Pain, tenderness and mobility of the teeth in the involved area can be seen. The roentgenogram will not show any characteristics to suggest a diagnosis.

A very important consideration of this tumor is the histologic similarity to an acanthomatous ameloblastoma or even a low-grade epidermoid carcinoma. Islands of squamous epithelium is the main feature without palisading. Keratinization of individual cells will be seen on occasion, but no epithelial pearls.

Treatment and Prognosis. No recurrence is usually seen after conservative excision. In the few cases reported, maxillary lesions have tended to be more diffuse and may require a little more aggressive excision.

Mesodermal Tumors

CENTRAL ODONTOGENIC FIBROMA

The odontogenic fibroma is similar in many respects to the myxoma and is perhaps only a more cellular form of that lesion. Its great frequency has not been well recognized because it resembles or is identical to the dentigerous cyst on the roentgenograph.

Incidence. The odontogenic fibroma is probably one of the most common odontogenic tumors of the jaws but one that has been reported so infrequently that little is known of the characteristic clinical features. It occurs with equal frequency in both male and female and the majority are diagnosed during the second decade of life. The mandible is affected more frequently than is the maxilla, with the most common site being the third molar and the cuspid regions.

Etiology. The odontogenic fibroma is considered to arise from the mesenchymal dental tissue (periodontal membranes, dental papilla, or dental follicle) on the grounds of its proximity to the teeth and structural appearance. In the protracted period during which odontogenesis takes place, from about the sixth week of intra-uterine life to approximately the twenty-fifth year, one or more of the 52 teeth is being formed and therefore, this embryonic tissue persists in the jaws into adult life.

Features. Because of its origin, the odontogenic fibroma is in close proximity to the tooth, either the root, or in the case of an unerupted tooth, the crown. It grows slowly and painlessly and follows a benign course. A slight enlargement of the area may occur, most often associated with an impacted tooth. Being asymptomatic they may go unnoticed for years, only to be discovered on roentgenographic examination which reveals a radiolucent lesion of varying size associated with the crown of the tooth (Fig. 14-27).

A solid rather than a cystic lesion is usually found on histologic examination. The tumor forms a circumscribed mass that is

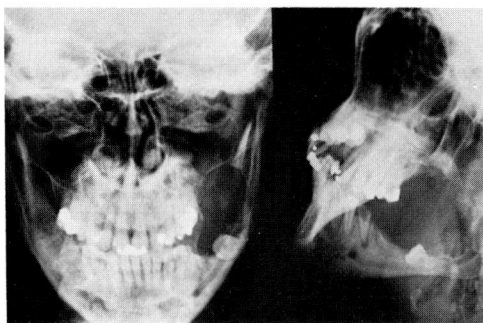

FIG. 14-27. *Radiograph of odontogenic fibroma.*

moderately firm depending on the fibroblastic component. The cut surface of the tumor is pinkish-white.

The histologic pattern of the tumor, particularly the mesenchymal component, belies its clinical behavior and it should not be regarded as malignant. Primitive-appearing fibroblastic connective tissue similar to that of the developing dental pulp is seen. Collagen formation may be marked and distributed throughout the plump fibroblasts. Small clumps of epithelial cells that represent nests of dental epithelium are scattered in the tumor and emphasize the odontogenic origin of the growth (Fig. 14-28).

Treatment and Prognosis. The indicated treatment for this neoplasm is conservative surgical removal or curettage and complete removal will effect a cure. Although it is true that failure to recur may be considered as evidence of adequate surgery, malignant tumors in this area show a marked tendency to recur and metastasize even after unusually extensive surgery.

ODONTOGENIC MYXOMA

Odontogenic myxoma of the jaws constitutes a definite clinical and pathologic entity. Myxomas of bone practically always

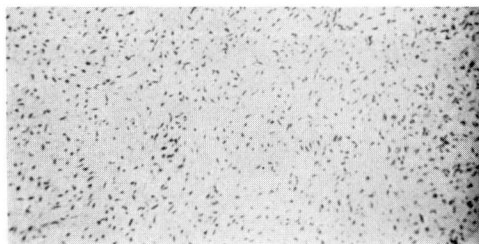

FIG. 14-28. *Histologic section of odontogenic fibroma.*

occur in the jaws, which suggests that they are probably of odontogenic origin.

Incidence. The incidence of myxoma as a neoplasm of bone varies in different studies of bone tumors. The odontogenic myxoma is one of the rare odontogenic neoplasms, and it must be distinguished from the true myxoma. It has been reported to be one sixth as common as the ameloblastoma. Odontogenic myxomas of the jaws occur chiefly in children and young adults with the majority of patients being in the second decade and usually under 35 years of age. The sexes are equally affected. The upper and lower jaws appear to be affected about equally, but there are conflicting studies claiming the mandible or maxilla to be the common site. The molar and bicuspid regions of either jaw are particularly involved.

Etiology. The fact that this tumor is generally associated with unerupted or missing teeth and in young people with abundant odontogenic epithelium supports the theory that in most cases it arises from the mesenchymal portion of the tooth germ.

Features. It is a slowly growing, painless central lesion of the jaw. Expansion of the bone may cause destruction of the cortex as well as facial deformity. Roentgenographically, a radiolucent defect that is often multilocular due to occasional intraosseous septa of bone radiating throughout the tumor is seen. This finding is similar to that produced by other tumors such as the ameloblastoma and giant cell tumor.

The tumor is soft, semitranslucent, and appears as a fusiform swelling in the jaw that may be covered by a layer of thin bone. The cortex is only rarely perforated and the overlying mucosa is normal. The cut surface appears grayish or yellowish-white and has the characteristics of myxomatous tissue. Occasionally, a capsule will be found but it is usually lacking if the growth is infiltrative.

Loosely arranged triangular or spindle shaped cells, many with long fibrillar processes that tend to intermesh, are found in a loose mucoid intercellular material. The intercellular substance may be somewhat granular and basophilic and mitotic figures are few.

Treatment and Prognosis. Current evidence suggests that myxomas of the jaws have a capacity to recur in a manner similar to the ameloblastoma, but do not metastasize. The goal of treatment, therefore, should be directed toward complete local removal. Conservative block resection should be used to minimize the possibility of recurrence. Curettage has seldom been found to be adequate.

CEMENTAL LESIONS (PERIPHERAL CEMENTAL DYSPLASIA, CENTRAL CEMENTIFYING FIBROMA, BENIGN CEMENTOBLASTOMA, GIGANTIFORM CEMENTOMA)

Cementum is a calcified mesenchymal tissue formed in the late stage of odontogenesis and deposited on the roots of teeth continuously throughout life. The morphologic appearances of the proliferated cementum also vary, and terms such as benign cementoblastoma (true cementoma), central cementifying fibroma, gigantiform cementoma, periapical cemental dysplasia (periapical fibrous dysplasia), and others have been used. Unfortunately, there is not yet a generally agreed upon nomenclature. All these will be considered as cementomas even though all are probably not of the same nature.

Incidence. Cementoma is classically described as a lesion of rather common occurrence, and incidence data are difficult to obtain because of the practice of grouping all types together. The commonest type of lesion occurs more often in women (almost ten times that of men) and the majority of patients are over 30 years of age. Over 90 percent occur in the mandible, usually in connection with the anterior teeth. The maxilla is rarely involved.

Etiology. The cause of the cementoma is unknown, although pulpal and periodontal infections, as well as abnormal occlusal forces, have been suggested as contributing factors. However, the lesions are often seen when these factors are not present. The cementifying fibroma (periapical fibrous dysplasia) derives from the specialized bone around the dental roots and thus is not strictly odontogenic.

Features. The condition generally produced no symptoms and is usually detected on roentgenographic examination. Lesions may be single or multiple and do not en-

large sufficiently to expand the jaw. Their evolution continues over a period of many years. Occasionally, they are superficially situated where they are prone to become infected. The roentgenographic appearance depends on the stage of development of the tumor. Early, it will be radiolucent and similar to a dental granuloma or radicular cyst. Later, with the beginning of calcification in the radiolucent area of fibrosis, specks of radiopacity are seen which will appear as circumscribed areas of dense radiopacity with time and maturity of the lesion.

The microscopic features vary with the stages mentioned in the roentgenographic examination. The early stage demonstrates young fibroblasts and a moderate amount of collagen. As the lesion matures more cementum is produced and incorporated into the lesion. Eventually the entire lesion consists of deeply basophilic calcified masses of cementum. Cementum can be distinguished from surrounding bone, which it closely resembles, by the irregularity of incremental growth lines and the paucity of cementocytes. The lacunae tend to be oval rather than round and often extend only in one direction.

Treatment and Prognosis. Caution is urged in the interpretation and treatment of the early radiolucent area which may resemble a granuloma. The cementoma requires only recognition and periodic observation. It is *not* necessary to extract teeth or institute endodontic procedures. Lesions that can be diagnosed as cementifying fibroma may require removal, sometimes aggressive surgery, owing to expansion and involvement of large areas.

Mixed (Ectodermal and Mesodermal)
AMELOBLASTIC FIBROMA

The ameloblastic fibroma contains both odontogenic epithelium and odontogenic mesenchymal tissue elements, the former deriving from the enamel organ and the latter from the dental papilla or the dental follicle.

Incidence. The ameloblastic fibroma is much less common than the ordinary type of ameloblastoma. Although it is a relatively uncommon neoplasm of odontogenic origin, it is the most common of the tumors that contain both ectodermal and mesodermal components. It occurs in younger patients, typically 15 to 25 years of age. Males have been affected slightly more often than females in the reported cases. It arises most commonly in the bicuspid-molar region of the mandible. Overall, it is similar to the ameloblastoma in this respect.

Etiology. The ameloblastic fibroma is a slow-growing tumor often associated with disturbed odontogenesis or embedded teeth. Since no calcified substances are produced, its development from tissues representing the early stages of odontogenesis is indicated. It may well develop from the dental follicle after the onset of calcification of the tooth.

Features. The tumor grows slowly and painlessly, expanding the jaw. It exhibits a somewhat slower clinical growth than the ameloblastoma and does not tend to infiltrate between trabeculae of bone. It enlarges by gradual expansion so that the periphery of the lesion often remains quite smooth. Unerupted teeth may at times be associated with the tumor. No significant difference exists roentgenographically between the appearance of the ameloblastoma and that of the ameloblastic fibroma. It produces a well-circumscribed cyst-like radiolucent zone with well-defined borders. Spreading of the roots of adjacent teeth may be noted occasionally in the roentgenogram (Fig. 14-29).

There may or may not be a definite capsule, but the growth is circumscribed and has a smooth surface. A cut section has the appearance and consistency of a soft fibroma, and grossly the tissue is a soft fibrous mass.

The ameloblastic fibroma is composed of strands and nests of proliferating odontogenic epithelium, which seldom undergoes cystic degeneration. This epithelium tends to take on the physical characteristics, as well as the cellular features, of the dental lamina or enamel organ and resembles to some extent the strands and nests seen in the ameloblastoma. The connective tissue element generally takes the form of a cellular fibroblastic tissue that resembles the dental papilla in the developing tooth, although in some cases, thick collagen bands may be present.

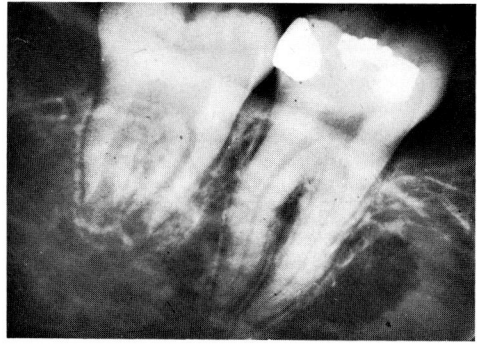

FIG. 14-29. *Ameloblastic fibroma in a 20-year-old patient. (Courtesy of Dr. D.E. Waite)*

Treatment and Prognosis. Its clinical behavior in most cases has been almost entirely benign. Therefore, treatment is somewhat more conservative than that of the ameloblastoma, as it does not appear actively to infiltrate the bone. Removal by curettage is usually adequate since the tendency for recurrence is limited. En bloc resection may be employed if the tumor recurs. The histologic pattern of the recurrent lesion is identical with that of the initial tumor.

AMELOBLASTIC FIBRO-ODONTOMA (ODONTOAMELOBLASTOMA)

The ameloblastic fibro-odontoma occupies a place between the ameloblastic fibroma and compound composite odontomas. In fact, the ameloblastic fibro-odontoma has been regarded as an early stage of the complex or compound composite odontoma. The lesion is quite unusual in that a relatively undifferentiated neoplastic tissue is associated with a highly differentiated tissue, both of which may show recurrence following inadequate removal.

Incidence. The ameloblastic fibro-odontoma is less common than either the ameloblastoma or the composite odontomas. It is considered to be a rare clinical entity. The ameloblastic fibro-odontoma occurs at any age but is particularly prevalent among children under 11 years of age. No sex predilection is known. Any part of either jaw may be affected, but there is a predilection for the bicuspid and molar areas. It appears to occur in the maxilla more than in the mandible.

Etiology. Odontogenic epithelium and odontogenic connective tissue are involved in this tumor, as in the ameloblastic fibroma. The mesenchymal and epithelial elements attain the capabilities for which they were intended and are able to produce calcified portions of a tooth. It should not be inferred that this tumor represents two separate neoplasms growing in unison; rather, there exists a peculiar proliferation of tissue of the odontogenic apparatus in an unrestrained pattern including complete morphodifferentiation, as well as apposition and even calcification.

Features. Most ameloblastic fibro-odontomas are larger than other odontogenic tumors, although this is not always the case. The tumor grows slowly and painlessly to form a hard, nontender mass in the jaw. It is an expanding lesion of bone that can produce facial deformity or asymmetry if left untreated. Since it is a central lesion, considerable destruction of bone may also occur. Roentgenographically, the tumor appears as a translucent area containing irregular radiopaque areas, some of which may be tooth-like in outline. The borders of the translucency are generally smooth, but occasionally indications of bone destruction may be found. Associated teeth may be unerupted or impacted.

The tumor forms a firm, fibrous-appearing mass that contains a variable amount of calcified material, and there may be a fibrous capsule. The dental tissues are produced in a fairly normal pattern.

The histologic pattern is striking, for all stages of development involving dental tissues can be seen. Proliferating odontogenic epithelium is present in nests, strands, or compact masses. Dentin and enamel, which are present in poorly organized states, differentiate it from the ameloblastoma and indicate its basically hamartomatous nature.

Treatment and Prognosis. Nearly all these well-circumscribed tumors are readily cured by conservative surgical means but a margin of normal tissue is indicated, as the tendency for recurrence is marked. Sometimes an en bloc removal or resection is necessary. Sarcomatous change in the connective tissue has been observed only on extremely rare occasions.

ODONTOMA

The term "odontoma" refers to any tumor of odontogenic origin. This tumor is composed of more than one type of tissue and, for this reason, has been called a composite odontoma. Two types of composite odontoma are customarily described—the complex and the compound. The former consists of a mass of irregularly arranged dentin, enamel, cementum, and connective tissue. The latter has large numbers of small though morphologically recognizable teeth. The complex and compound odontomas are discussed together. (Fig. 14-30).

Incidence. The odontoma is a common odontogenic tumor with the capability of its odontogenic epithelium and mesenchyme reaching a degree only slightly below that of normal odontogenesis. Odontomas may be discovered at any age in any location of the dental arch, maxillary or mandibular. The complex odontoma is found most often in older children and in young adults. It is considered to be somewhat more common in females than in males. At least 60 percent of compound odontomas are diagnosed in the second to third decades and more often in females than in males. The complex odontoma has a predilection for the molar portion of the lower jaw, whereas compound odontomas tend to occur in the incisor-cuspid region most commonly.

Etiology. The origin of the odontoma is unknown. Local trauma and infection have

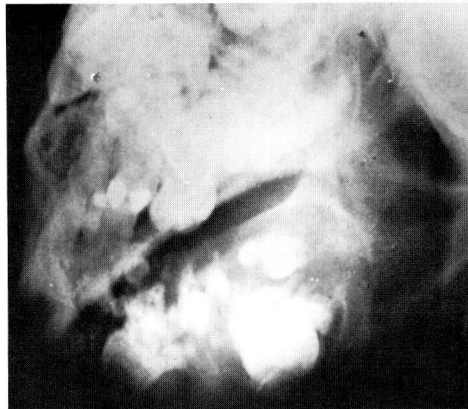

Fig. 14-30. *Compound composite odontoma in 8-year-old patient. (Courtesy of Dr. D.E. Waite)*

been suggested as possible causes. They may also be developmental malformations of dental organs or of tissue with odontogenic potential. However, the odontoma often replaces a missing tooth, suggesting that the dental organ gives rise to the malformation instead of to a normal tooth.

Features. Generally, the lesions are quite small and cause no symptoms although occasionally they may attain quite large dimensions. These tumors grow slowly, often reaching a certain stage and becoming quiescent for many years. The lesion is usually an incidental roentgenographic finding that appears as an area of opacity similar to osteosclerosis. The mass of calcified dental tissues of which it is composed appears as an irregular dense area. The compound odontoma shows numerous small tooth-like structures, but a great variety of appearances can occur.

The complex odontoma is surrounded by a fibrous capsule that is partially separated by fluid. The compound odontoma is also generally enclosed in a fibrous capsule and consists of a number of separate small teeth or denticles embedded in fibrous tissue in which some trabeculae of bone may exist.

The complex odontoma consists of enamel, dentin, and cementum, forming an extensive mass arranged quite irregularly. Much of the enamel is fully calcified. These substances demonstrate a strong tendency to establish an interrelationship with each other similar to that in the normal development of the tooth. In the compound odontoma, enamel, dentin, and cementum are arranged into small separate teeth, most of which are oddly shaped. Each small tooth is an independent structure, and the number of teeth may vary from a few to many. They are bound together with a fibrous tissue capsule, and the entire mass is embedded in bone.

Treatment and Prognosis. Both the complex and compound odontomas are benign in spite of the size they sometimes attain. Surgical removal is indicated, with little expectancy of recurrence.

Selected Reading

Abrams, A.M., and Howell, F.V.: Calcifying epithelial odontogenic tumors: report of four cases. JADA, 74:1231, 1967.

Anderson, H.C., Byunghoon, K., and Minkowitz, S.: Calcifying epithelial odontogenic tumor of Pindborg: an electron microscopic study. Cancer, 24:585, 1969.

Barros, R.E., Dominguez, F.V., and Cabrini, R.L.: Myxoma of the jaws. Oral Surg., 27:225, 1969.

Broders, A.C.: The grading of carcinoma. Minn. Med., 8:726, 1925.

Brannon, R.B.: The odontogenic keratocyst. A clinicopathologic study of 312 cases. Part I: Clinical features. Oral Surg., 42:54, 1976. Part II: Histologic features. Oral Surg., 43:233, 1977.

Browne, R.M., and Gough, N.G.: Malignant change in the epithelium lining odontogenic cysts. Cancer, 29:1199, 1972.

Chaudhry, A.P., Robinovitch, M.R., Mitchell, D.F., and Vickers, R.A.: Chondrogenic tumors of the jaws. Am. J. Surg., 102:403, 1961.

Courtney, R.M., and Kerr, D.A.: The odontogenic adenomatoid tumor. Oral Surg., 39:424, 1975.

Dahl, E.C., Wolfson, S.H., and Haugen, J.C.: Central odontogenic fibroma: review of literature and report of cases. J. Oral Surg., 39:120, 1981.

Franklin, C.D., and Pindborg, J.J.: The calcifying epithelial odontogenic tumor. Oral Surg., 42:753, 1976.

Gardner, D.G.: The central odontogenic fibroma: an attempt at clarification. Oral Surg., 50:425, 1980.

Gardner, D.G.: A pathologist's approach to the treatment of ameloblastoma. Oral Surg., 42:161, 1984.

Goldblatt, L.I., Brannon, R.B., and Ellis, G.L.: Squamous odontogenic tumor. Report of five cases and review of the literature. Oral Surg., 54: 187, 1982.

Gorlin, R.J., Chaudhry, A.P., and Pindborg, J.J.: Odontogenic tumors. Classification, histopathology, and clinical behavior in man and domesticated animals. Cancer, 14:73, 1961.

Larsson, A., Forsberg, O., and Sjogren, S.: Benign cementoblastoma-cementum analogue of benign osteoblastoma? Oral Surg., 36:299, 1978.

Mehlisch, D.R., Dahlin, D.C., and Masson, J.K.: Ameloblastoma: a clinicopathologic report. Oral Surg., 30:9, 1972.

Morgan, G.A., and Morgan, P.R.: Periapical osteofibrosis—differential radiological interpretation. J. Ontario Dent. Assoc., 45:532, 1968.

Pullon, P.A., et al.: Squamous odontogenic tumor. Oral Surg., 40:616, 1975.

Shear, M., and Altini, M.: Malignant odontogenic tumors. J. Dent. Assoc. S. Afr., 37:547, 1982.

Silverman, S., Jr., and Chierici, G.: Radiation therapy of oral carcinoma effects on oral tissues and management of the periodontium. J. Periodontol., *36*:478, 1965.

Slootweg, P.J.: An analysis of the interrelationship of the mixed odontogenic tumors—ameloblastic fibroma, ameloblastic fibro-odontoma, and the odontomas. Oral Surg., *51*:266, 1981.

Slootweg, P.J., and Mullen, H.: Central fibroma of the jaw, odontogenic or desmoplastic. Oral Surg., *56*:61, 1983.

Waite, D.E.: Inflammatory papillary hyperplasia. Oral Surg., *19*:211, 1961.

CHAPTER 15 # Salivary Glands: Anatomy, Development, and Diseases

MARK T. JASPERS

Happy the man who could search out the cause of things.
VIRGIL

Gross Anatomy

PAROTID GLAND

The parotid gland (Fig. 15-1) is the largest of the three paired salivary glands. It is shaped somewhat like an inverted pyramid, with an apex, base, and lateral, anterior, and posterior surfaces. The gland's apex lies between the sternomastoid muscle and the mandibular angle. The base lies near the zygomatic bone and the condylar neck of the mandible.

The anterior surface is grooved by the mandibular ramus and the masseter muscle. The posterior surface is grooved by the mastoid and styloid process and the sternomastoid and digastric muscles. Laterally, the gland may present a detached portion known as the accessory parotid gland. Medially, the gland contacts the internal pterygoid muscle and approximates the lateral pharyngeal wall (Fig. 15-2).

The entire parotid gland is invested with a connective tissue capsule or sheath that is derived from portions of the deep cervical and masseteric fascia.

The facial nerve, emerging from the stylomastoid foramen, enters the gland and courses ventrolaterally, forming the parotid plexus within the gland.

The parotid gland empties into the oral cavity by way of Stensen's duct. This duct emerges from the gland, passes anteriorly, lateral to the masseter muscle, and turns abruptly medially around the masseter's anterior border to pierce the buccal fat pad and the buccinator muscle. It terminates intraorally at the parotid or Stensen's papilla. This opening is located opposite the crown of the maxillary second molar. Stensen's duct has a relatively uniform diameter of approximately 1.5 mm throughout its course.

Each salivary gland is innervated by both parasympathetic and sympathetic fibers. The parotid gland receives its parasympathetic (secretory) fibers from the otic ganglion via the auriculotemporal nerve. Sympathetic innervation to all the salivary glands is probably entirely vasomotor.

The secretion of the adult parotid gland is purely serous. The volume of saliva secreted by the parotid assumes an interme-

220

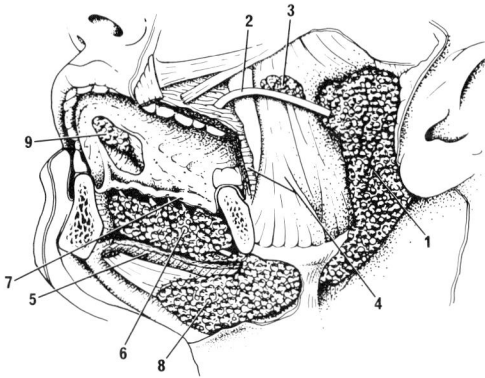

FIG. 15-1. *The major salivary glands and surrounding structures. Parotid gland (1); Stensen's duct (2); accessory lobe of parotid (3); masseter and buccinator muscles (4); mylohyoid muscle (5); sublingual gland (6); plica sublingualis (7); submandibular gland (8); gland of Blandin-Nuhn (9). (Redrawn from H. Ferner (Ed.): Atlas of Topographical and Applied Human Anatomy. Philadelphia, W.B. Saunders Co., 1963)*

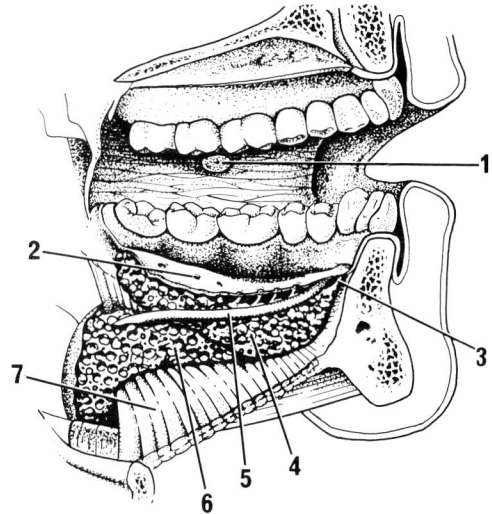

FIG. 15-3. *The submandibular and sublingual salivary glands and surrounding structures. Stensen's papilla (1); plica sublingualis (2); sublingual duct (3); sublingual gland (4); Wharton's duct (5); submandibular gland (6); mylohyoid muscle (7); (Redrawn from H. Ferner (Ed.): Atlas of Topographical and Applied Human Anatomy. Philadelphia, W. B. Saunders Co., 1963)*

diate position in relation to the total volume secreted by all glands. With an increase in stimulation, the relative proportion of the parotid contribution increases.[1]

SUBMANDIBULAR (SUBMAXILLARY) GLAND

The submandibular gland, second largest of the three main salivary glands (Figs.

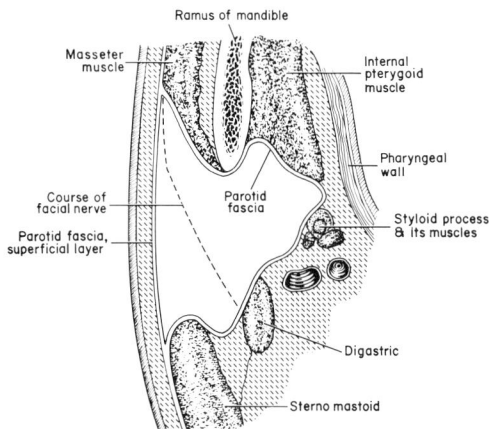

FIG. 15-2. *Transverse section of parotid space and related structures. Note the close relationship between the parotid and the lateral pharyngeal wall. (Redrawn from J. P. Schaeffer (Ed.): Morris' Human Anatomy, 11th ed. New York, McGraw Hill Book Co., 1953)*

15-1 and 15-3), consists of a larger superficial part and a smaller deep process. The two parts are continuous with each other around the posterior border of the mylohyoid muscle. The larger portion lies in the digastric triangle. It is bounded superficially by skin and platysma muscle, laterally by the mandible and medial pterygoid muscle, and inferiorly by the mylohyoid, stylohyoid, and digastric muscles.

The smaller, deep process of the gland is a tongue-like extension that passes around the posterior edge of the mylohyoid muscle. The deep process is bounded by the mylohyoid laterally, the hyoglossus medially, the lingual nerve superiorly, and the hypoglossal nerve inferiorly.

The entire gland is surrounded by a capsule similar to the one that surrounds the parotid. This capsule is derived from portions of the external cervical, digastric, and styloid muscle fascial layers.

The excretory duct of the submandibular gland is Wharton's duct. It arises from the junction of the superficial and deep processes, turns at a right angle superiorly, and courses under the oral mucosa to open at the sublingual caruncle. This sublingual caruncle or papilla is located at the side of the lingual frenulum. Wharton's duct has an average diameter of 1.5 to 3.5 mm; occasionally, however, at the point of turn around the mylohyoid muscle, the ductal lumen may enlarge considerably.

Parasympathetic secretory fibers that supply the gland are derived mainly from the submandibular ganglion.

The submandibular gland secretes a mucous and serous saliva; the serous element predominates. This gland accounts for the largest fraction of the total salivary secretion in the unstimulated state; upon stimulation, this relative proportion decreases.[1]

SUBLINGUAL GLAND

The sublingual gland is the smallest of the major salivary glands. Actually, it is a group of glands forming an elongated mass in the floor of the mouth, lateral and inferior to the tongue (Figs. 15-1 and 15-3).

The superior border of this gland forms a distinct ridge called the plica sublingualis in the floor of the mouth. Inferiorly, the gland rests on the mylohyoid muscle; its lateral surface contacts the mandible and medially it is related to the genioglossus and the submandibular duct.

The connective tissue capsule surrounding the submandibular gland is ill-defined. This gland lies rather independently within the general submandibular space.

The principal excretory duct of the sublingual gland, Bartholin's duct, may fuse with the submandibular duct to share a common opening on the sublingual caruncle. More commonly, however, Bartholin's duct opens independently also on the sublingual caruncle. In addition to Bartholin's duct, from 5 to 30 smaller ducts, the ducts of Rivinus, drain the sublingual gland. These ducts open along the crest of the plica sublingualis at the superior border of the gland.

Parasympathetic innervation to the sublingual gland is similar to the submandibular gland; it is derived from the submandibular ganglion.

The secretion of the sublingual gland is mucous and serous; mucous being the predominant type. The sublingual gland accounts for the smallest fraction of total unstimulated salivary flow.

MINOR SALIVARY GLANDS

Numerous additional and smaller salivary glands (450 to 750)[2] are located within the mucosa throughout the oral cavity. These glands, on an anatomic basis, are classified into the labial, buccal, glossopalative, and palative glands. Some secrete a mucoserous saliva (labial and buccal) while others (glossopalative and palatal) secrete only mucus.

The tongue also contains minor salivary glands. Near the apex on the inferior tongue surface is the gland of Blandin-Nuhn, which secretes mucus and serous saliva (Fig. 15-1). The base of the tongue contains mucous glands. Ebner's glands, located near the valliate papillae, produce a serous secretion.

The minor salivary glands throughout the oral cavity contribute a variable amount of secretion to the total salivary flow. Their total relative contribution has been estimated from 8 to 53 percent of the total salivary volume.

Development And Microscopic Anatomy

Salivary glands begin development through a proliferation of oral epithelium into the underlying connective tissue. This epithelial proliferation develops into an extensively branched system of cords of cells. As development proceeds, lumina form within the cords to form a system of ducts. The smallest, terminal branches of this system differentiate into the secretory portions of the gland.

The secretory portion of a salivary gland, the acini, consists, in general, of a layer of secretory cells lining a narrow lumen. These secretory cells are of two types: mucous and serous. The acini are connected to intercalated ducts which, in turn, connect with striated ducts. The striated ducts, so named because of cellular striations, empty into excretory or interlobular ducts and thence into the oral cavity.

Situated between the basement membrane and the ductal or glandular cells are spindle-shaped cells termed myoepithelial cells. These cells are believed to be contractile; their function is apparently to facilitate salivary flow.

Each major salivary gland is separated into segments called lobes by involutions of the surrounding connective tissue. Lobes are further divided into lobules by connective tissue septa. These septa bind and support the salivary elements which comprise the lobule: acini, their intercalated ducts, myoepithelial cells, and the striated ducts.

Salivary Flow

The secretion of saliva is continuous, even at rest. The quantity secreted is subject to considerable variation and ultimately dependent upon the control exerted by the central nervous system. Secretion is subject to reflex stimulation; stimuli from touch and taste receptors of the oral cavity, or psychic stimuli from other sensory centers or body zones, converge on the salivary nuclei in the medulla oblongata. Efferent pathways from this salivary center are the parasympathetic and sympathetic parts of the autonomic nervous system.

The total quantity of salivary secretion produced per day has been estimated from 500 to 1500 ml.[3] A large variation in flow rate occurs between individuals; it is therefore safe to assume that there will also be a large range for the normal salivary secretion volume.

The salivary flow rate is affected by a number of psychologic, physiologic, and environmental factors. Mental stress, systemic dehydration, and increased room temperature diminish the flow rate, and hyperhydration and cigarette smoking increase it.

The major salivary glands secrete into the oral cavity and contribute to the mixed saliva with its several important functions. Saliva provides lubrication for, enhances the taste of, and begins the digestion of food. It also serves as a cleansing, buffering, and antibacterial agent.

Diagnostic Methods

Clinical Examination

Physical examination of the salivary glands involves a large portion of the cervicofacial region. The examination should assess gland size and consistency, the nature of the salivary flow, and, if necessary, explore the salivary duct and its orifice.

The initial step should consist of a face-to-face observation of the patient. The examiner should note any signs of facial asymmetry, discoloration, visible pulsation, or discharging sinuses. This inspection, especially when judging asymmetry and discoloration, should be conducted from a distance of three to four feet from the patient. Following this initial general examination, the individual glands are examined.

PAROTID GLAND

A parotid gland enlargement usually presents as a diffuse swelling that, when viewed from the front, may overlap the tragus of the ear giving the patient a full-cheeked appearance. This type of diffuse swelling may be quite obvious if it is unilateral, but may be more difficult to detect if it is bilateral (Fig. 15-4).

Palpation of the parotid gland is accomplished using the finger tips with a circular, firm, but delicate pressure. The entire area occupied by the gland should be palpated (Fig. 15-5). The examiner should note any well-defined nodular or diffuse enlargements within the gland substance.

When the parotid gland is examined, it is important to bear in mind the "stylomandibular tunnel" and the parotid tissue it may contain. As will be recalled, a portion of the parotid gland approaches the lateral pharyngeal wall through a "tunnel" formed by the base of the skull, the internal pterygoid muscle, and the styloid process and its muscles. Occasionally, parotid tumors may assume a "dumbbell" configuration, growing in a parapharyngeal direc-

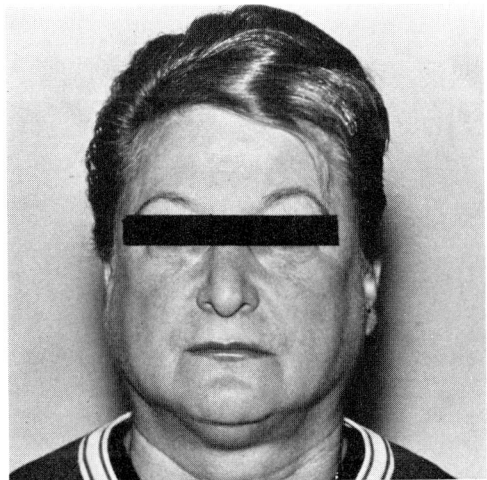

Fig. 15-4. *Bilateral parotid enlargement.*

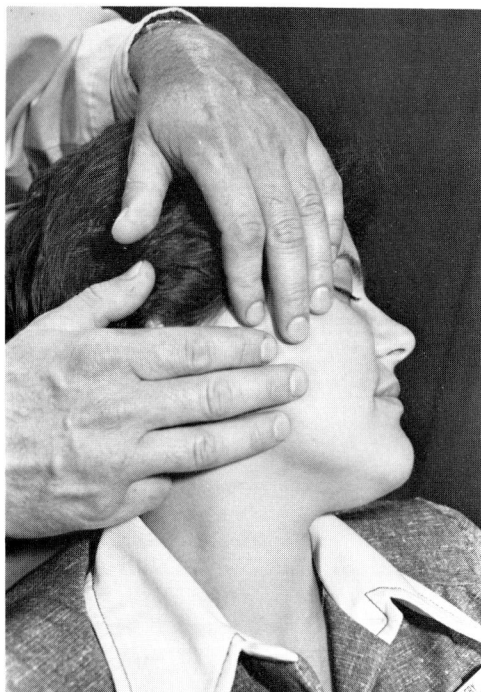

FIG. 15-5. *Palpation of the parotid gland.*

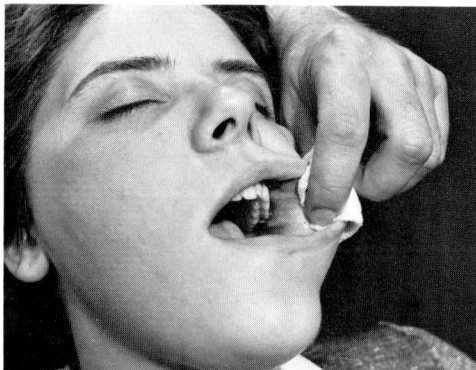

FIG. 15-7. *Salivary duct or lacrimal probes.*

tion to clinically present as a mass in the lateral pharyngeal or the retromandibular fossa area. Considering this, a complete examination of the parotid should include a visual examination for a medial protrusion from the lateral pharyngeal wall or into the retromolar fossa area.

The nature of the parotid flow may be examined by "milking" the gland. The patient's cheek is slightly everted, the duct orifice dried with gauze, and the saliva expressed by a gentle but firm forward-moving pressure initiated immediately anterior to the ear and extending forward (Fig. 15-6). In this manner, saliva may be expressed or "milked" from the gland. A normal gland easily yields watery clear saliva; in diseased states it may contain purulent material, debris, or thick mucous.

Occasionally, it may be necessary to probe the parotid duct to determine the presence of ductal obstruction or strictures. This procedure is best accomplished by everting the patient's cheek, which usually reveals the ductal orifice, and inserting a lacrimal probe (Figs. 15-7 and 15-8). By careful manipulation of this probe, Stensen's duct may be tactilely examined proximally to the point of its right-angle turn through the buccinator muscle.

SUBMANDIBULAR GLAND

An enlargement of the submandibular gland may be diffuse, simply adding fullness to the submandibular region, or nod-

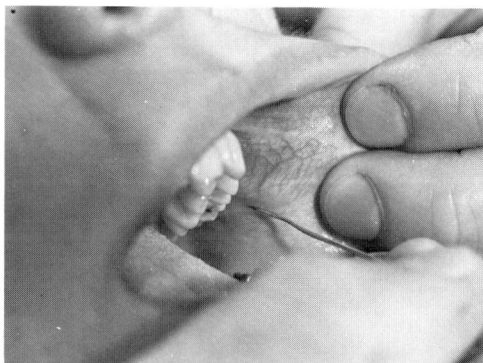

FIG. 15-6. *Eversion of cheek to expose the orifice of Stensen's duct.*

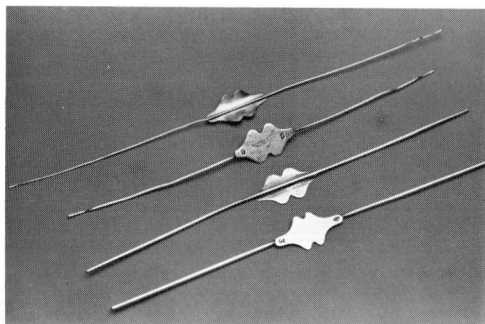

FIG. 15-8. *Insertion of salivary duct probe into Stensen's duct.*

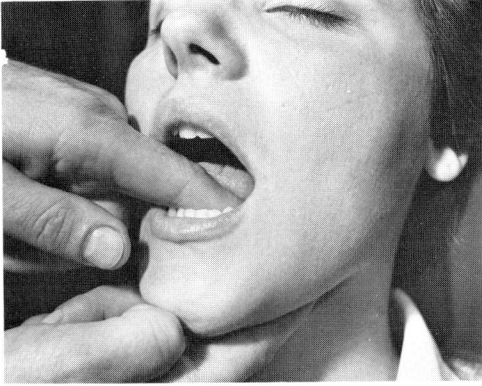

Fig. 15-9. *Bidigital palpation of the submandibular gland.*

ular. As with the parotid, unilateral enlargements are more easily detected due to the resultant asymmetry.

The submandibular gland is best palpated bimanually, using both an intra- and extraoral approach. With the patient's head inclined slightly downward (to flex the neck and relax the tissues in this area), the examining fingers are positioned as illustrated in Figure 15-9. With an upward pressure on the external finger (to raise the contents of the floor of the mouth), the submandibular gland may be palpated between the fingers.

The salivary flow from the submandibular gland should be evaluated. With the patient's tongue elevated as shown (Fig. 15-10), the sublingual papilla may be dried with gauze. Saliva may be "milked" from the gland by a gentle but firm upward

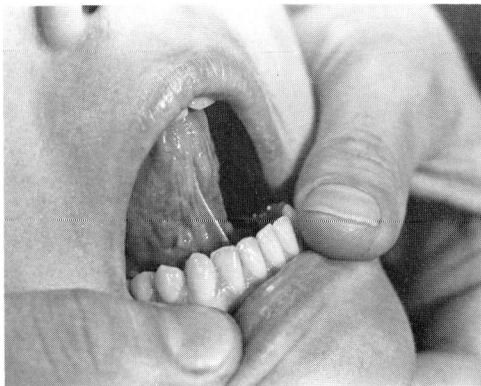

Fig. 15-10. *Elevation of tongue; the sublingual caruncle is thus exposed.*

pressure medial to the mandibular ramus with one or two fingers, beginning at the angle of the mandible and extending forward. Saliva thus expressed should be somewhat viscous and clear.

Wharton's duct not infrequently needs to be probed; to examine the duct proper for obstructions or strictures and to accurately determine its course prior to minor surgical procedures on the floor of the mouth. The orifice of the submandibular duct may be located by expressing saliva as outlined above. Following the location of the orifice, a thin lacrimal probe is carefully inserted and advanced along the duct. Caution should be exercised because of the thinness of the duct walls. This procedure is frequently difficult; several attempts may need to be made.

SUBLINGUAL GLAND

Enlargements of the sublingual gland present as elevations in the floor of the mouth. Again, unilateral enlargements are more easily detected.

The sublingual gland may be palpated bimanually; one finger exerting upward pressure in the submental region and the second placed intraorally as shown (Fig. 15-11). Salivary flow from the sublingual gland is usually examined with the same procedure utilized in the examination of the submandibular flow. With careful drying and observation of the crest of the plica sublingualis, small drops of saliva may usually be seen. Owing to the small size, probing the sublingual gland's ducts is not possible.

MINOR GLANDS

Enlargements of the minor salivary glands usually present as discrete nodules within the substance of the submucosa.

Palpation of the minor glands of the lips, cheeks, and other areas should be done bidigitally whenever possible. With one examining finger intraorally and one extraorally, the cheeks, lips, and parts of the tongue may be examined (Fig. 15-12). The minor glands of the palate may be examined by compressing them against the palate. Examination of salivary flow and the ducts proper of minor salivary glands is usually not attempted in a routine physical examination of the oral regions.

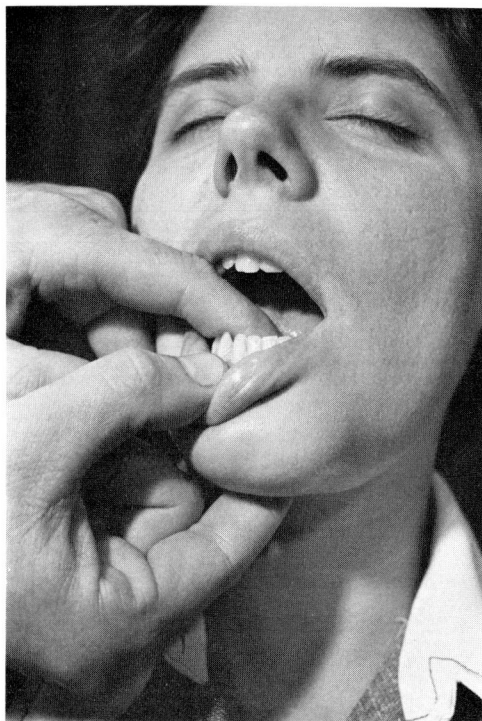

FIG. 15-11. *Bidigital palpation of the sublingual gland.*

Radiologic Examination

Radiologic examination is useful frequently in the diagnosis of calculi within Stensen's or Wharton's ducts.

Radiographic visualization of calculus within the distal portion of Stensen's duct is possible utilizing a periapical film held by the patient against the buccal mucosa along the course of the duct. The patient's

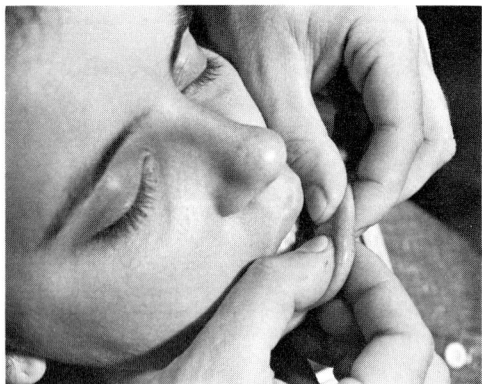

FIG. 15-13. *Calcification in the region of Stensen's duct. This calculus is visualized on a routine periapical film of the second molar area. (Courtesy of Dr. D.E. Waite)*

head is positioned vertically and the central ray directed through the cheek toward the first molar area (Fig. 15-13).

Visualization of calculus within the distal portion of Wharton's duct or the sublingual gland is frequently possible. The patient's mandibular occlusal plane is inclined backward 45 to 50° to the horizontal. An occlusal film is centrally placed as far backward as possible and the central ray directed under and behind the chin so that it strikes the film at a right angle (Figs. 15-14 and 15-15).

Occasionally, it may be necessary to examine radiographically for a calculus within a minor salivary gland. The technique utilized is similar to that utilized for calculi

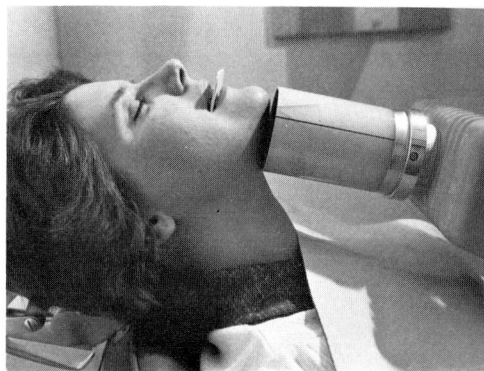

FIG. 15-12. *Bidigital palpation of the minor salivary glands of the lower lip.*

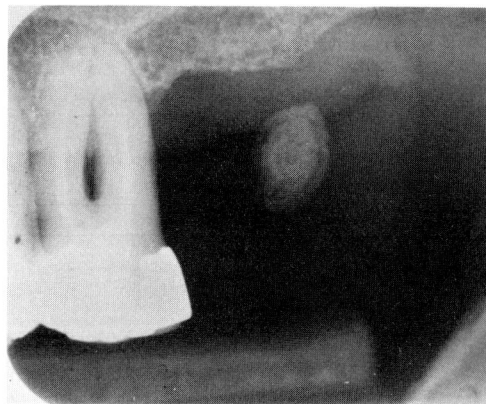

FIG. 15-14. *Radiographic examination of Wharton's duct. The patient's head is inclined approximately 50° from the horizontal. The central ray is directed −20° in the midline.*

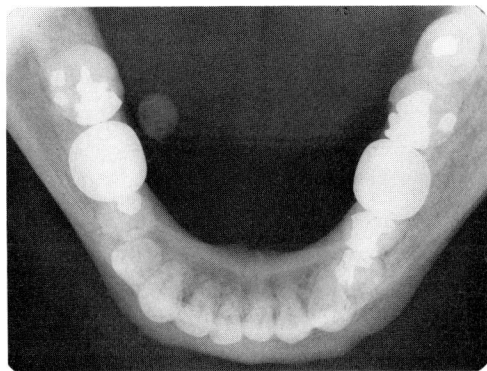

FIG. 15-15. *Calculus within Wharton's duct. The patient experienced no symptoms; the calculus was clinically palpable. (Courtesy of Dr. R. Kuba)*

within Stensen's duct. Obviously, this technique is only adaptable for the lip and cheek regions.

To prevent a "burnout" of a small or poorly calcified intraductal calculus, it is necessary to reduce the radiological exposure time from one third to one half of the normal utilized for dental and osseous tissues.

Intraductal calculus may be exhibited infrequently on a routine panographic radiograph. Figure 15-16 illustrates a large calculus within Wharton's duct.

Sialographic Examination

Sialography is a roentgenographic visualization of the ductal system of two of the paired major salivary glands. (Because of its multiductal anatomy, the sublingual gland does not lend itself well to this examination method.) This visualization is made possible by means of a radiographic contrast solution that is introduced into the duct.

A wide variety of contrast media is available; generally they may be classed into water-insoluble and water-soluble compounds.

A brief description of the common types follows.

Water-insoluble:
Ethiodol (Ethiodized oil) a derivative of poppyseed oil with contained iodine. Usually produces no adverse tissue reactions and is less viscid than the other water insoluble compounds.
Pantopaque (Iophendylate) a derivative of ethyl iodophenylundecanoate with 30.5

percent iodine. Is usually well tolerated by the tissues.

The above compounds are relatively viscous and essentially water insoluble; thus, they are more difficult to introduce into the gland and are slowly absorbed by tissue. These compounds may tend to "blot out" subsequent sialographic examinations because of their sustained opacity and retention.

Water-soluble:
Hypaque (Diatrizoate meglumine), *Conray* (Iothalamate sodium), *Renografin* (Diatrizoate meglumine and diatrizoate sodium) and *Cholografin* (Iodipamide meglumine) are common water soluble compounds. None maintain opacity for long periods of time or cause adverse tissue reactions. These compounds are homogeneous, miscible in body fluids and saliva, rapidly eliminated, and have low viscosities. Major criticisms of these compounds include their rapid elimination, thus requiring ready accessibility of the radiographic apparatus, and their relative lesser degree of radiopacity.

Many factors must be considered when choosing a contrast medium: the status of the gland to be examined, the possibility of adverse tissue reaction, retention duration, the solution viscosity, and the examiner's experience. No one contrast medium meets all requirements; selected situations may require different media.

Sialography, as traditionally practiced, involves the hand injection of a water-insoluble medium into the gland. The duct orifice is located and dilated if necessary with graded lacrimal probes. An injection

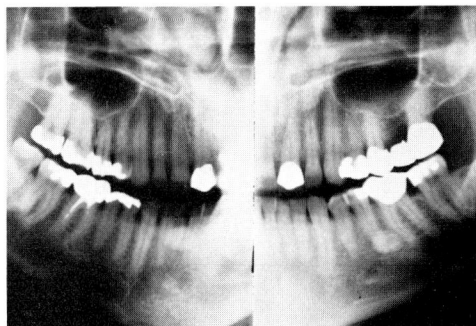

FIG. 15-16. *Calculus within the left Wharton's duct at apex of second bicuspid (same patient as shown in Fig. 15-15). (Courtesy of Dr. R. Kuba)*

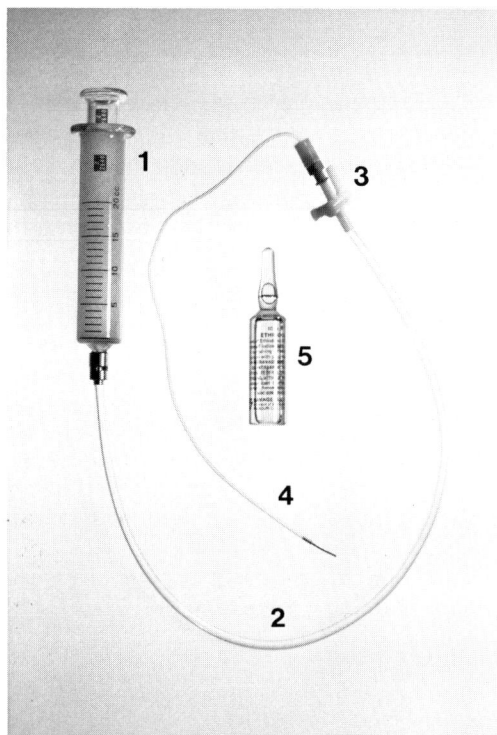

FIG. 15-17. *Instrumentation for injection sialography. (1) 20 cc glass syringe. (2) Plastic tubing approximately 20 cm in length. (3) Stopcock and adapter. (4) Sialographic catheter such as a Rabinov cannula. (5) Suitable oil base contrast medium.*

apparatus (Fig. 15-17) is assembled to include a suitably sized sialographic catheter. A stopcock is positioned between this catheter and a Luer-Lock syringe filled with a suitable contrast medium. All air is removed from the system and the terminal end of catheter is inserted 1.5 to 2 cm into the duct. The soft tissues around the ductal orifice serve as a splinter to hold the catheter in position and prevent leakage. The catheter is anchored to the patient's cheek with tape. The contrast medium is injected into the gland until the patient begins to feel pain. No preconceived or predetermined amount of dye should be injected— the amount is entirely governed by the patient's reaction. Approximate amounts to be injected may vary from 0.5 to 6 cc. At the point of the patient's pain reaction, the stopcock is closed and suitable radiographs taken.

An alternate hydrostatic sialographic technique involves the use of a water-

soluble contrast media. A similar apparatus is prepared; a sialographic catheter is attached to a 90 cm 14-18 gauge soft plastic IV catheter by means of a stopcock. The IV catheter, in turn, is attached to a syringe barrel or similar calibrated reservoir (Fig. 15-18). The contrast medium in the reservoir is positioned approximately 72 cm above the orifice of the duct, and the medium is allowed to flow until pain is felt. The stopcock is closed and a suitable radiograph taken. Proponents of this technique maintain that it gives them more control over the amount of dye introduced.

The most commonly used sialographic catheters are the Rabinov cannulas with tips ranging from .012 to .033 inches. The larger diameter cannulas are useful for parotid sialography; the smaller for the submandibular gland.

For additional detailed information the reader is directed to several articles cover-

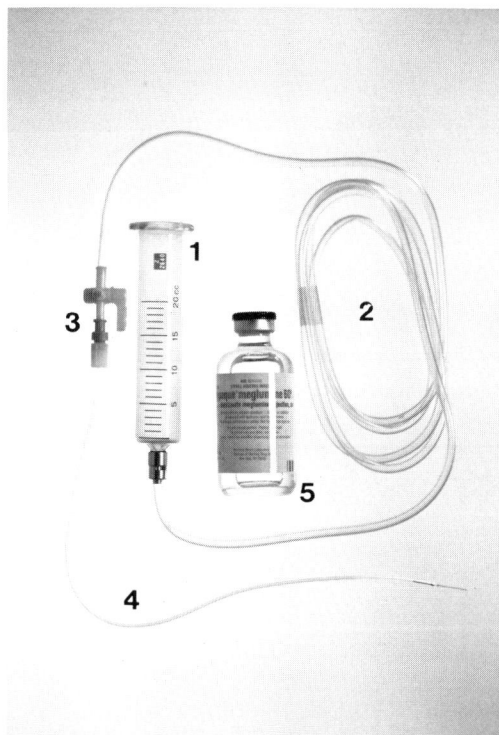

FIG. 15-18. *Instrumentation for hydrostatic sialography. (1) 20 cc glass syringe barrel. (2) Plastic tubing approximately 100 cm in length. (3) Stopcock and adapter. (4) Sialographic catheter of suitable size. (5) Suitable water-soluble contrast medium.*

ing the injection[4,5] and hydrostatic[3,6] methods of sialography.

Irrespective of the method of contrast medium introduction, the goal is the same; a completely filled ductal system. The ideally filled gland shows filling of intercalary ducts with minimal delineation of the acini (Fig. 15-19). Excessive acinar filling, the so-called "cumulus cloud effect," "cloud-like shadow," or "sialo-acinar reflux," all refer to overfilling of the gland.[4]

When the gland has been filled and suitable radiographs exposed, the catheter is removed from the duct and the patient is given a strong sialagogue such as a slice of lemon to suck. This causes an emptying of the contrast dye from the ductal system. This emptying phase has contributed as much diagnostic information as has the filling phase.[4] A normal gland shows virtually complete elimination of the dye shortly after use of this sialagogue. Postevacuation radiographic films are exposed 5 minutes and, if necessary, 24 hours following use of the sialogogue. Any dye remaining in glandular substance or ducts after 24 hours indicates an abnormality.[5]

Sialographic radiographs of the parotid gland usually include the true lateral and the anterio-posterior projections. The submandibular gland is best examined with the lateral oblique and the true lateral projections. Occlusal projections and pano-

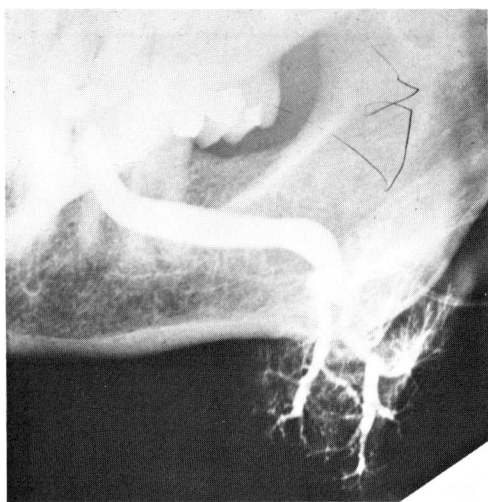

FIG. 15-20. *Submandibular sialogram showing radiolucent partial obstruction (arrow) within Wharton's duct. (Courtesy of Dr. D.E. Waite)*

ramic radiographs may also be used to advantage.[7]

Prior to the insertion of the catheter and the contrast medium, a "presialogram" or "scout film" should be taken. This film establishes a base line appearance and may be useful in comparing with the filling and postevacuation films.

Sialography illustrates the presence of ductal strictures, cysts, and fistulas; it may identify a salivary duct obstruction that may be too small or poorly calcified to be demonstrated with routine radiography (Figs. 15-20 and 15-21). Sialography may be useful in determining the status of the gland proximal to an obstruction by depicting alterations in the diffusion pattern of the radiopaque solution within the gland proper. These findings aid in the diagnosis of intra- or extraglandular neoplasms; specifics will be mentioned later when these diseases and neoplasms are discussed.

Finally, sialography may be of some therapeutic benefit. The contrast solutions may dilate the duct or break up mucous or inflammatory plugs that impede salivary flow. Some solutions may exert an antiseptic effect through the liberation of iodine from the dye itself.

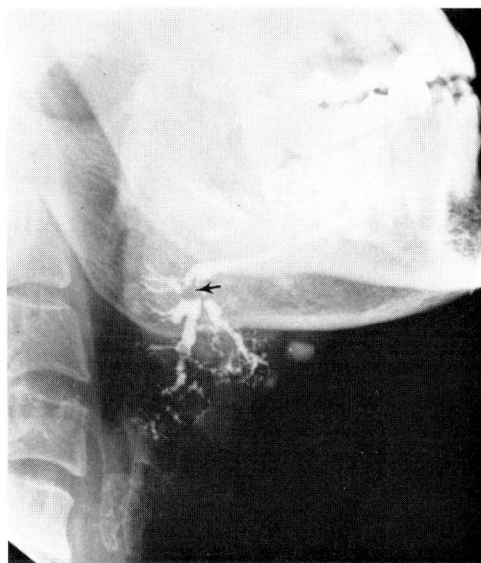

FIG. 15-19. *Submandibular sialogram. (Courtesy of Dr. D.E. Waite)*

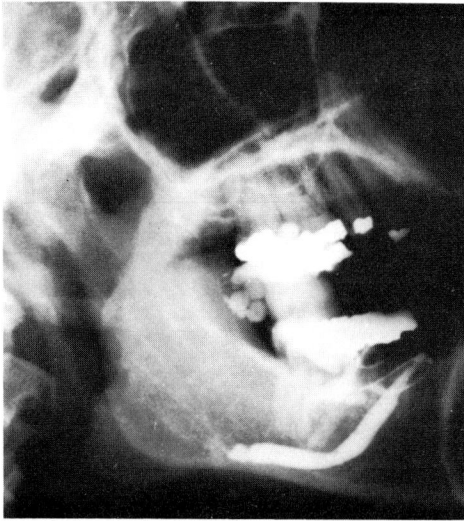

FIG. 15-21. *Submandibular sialogram showing radiolucent total obstruction of Wharton's duct. Note distal distention proximal to the obstruction and lack of glandular filling distally. (Courtesy of Drs. Vickers and Gorlin)*

Most sialographic media derive their radiopacity from the presence of iodine. Uncommonly, a patient presents a history of hypersensitivity to this element; no serious adverse effects, except this hypersensitivity, have been noted in sialography. Sialography is also contraindicated in the presence of an acute glandular or ductal inflammation; its use is superfluous if a clinical diagnosis of malignant neoplasia, radiation damage, hypersensitivity, or metabolic disease has been made.[6]

If salivary glands are not examined during periods of acute inflammation, side effects are few. Most patients exhibit some residual glandular edema for 24 hours. If this edema proves uncomfortable for the patient, a mild analgesic may be prescribed.

Adjunctive Examination Methods

Other noninvasive diagnostic methods include radionuclide scanning (scintigraphy), ultrasound, and computed tomography (CT).

Radionuclide scanning allows the physiologic imaging of the salivary glands. This procedure utilizes a radioactive isotope which, following systemic administration, is actively concentrated by the salivary glands. The artificial radioactive element technetium, administered as ^{99m} Tc pertechnetate, is most widely used in these procedures.[45] Following the intravenous administration of the technetium, the uptake concentration and excretion of the isotope is detected and recorded with scintigraphs taken at periodic intervals (Figs. 15-22 and 15-23). This examination method provides a physiologically sensitive evaluation of glandular function or lesional presence. It, however, provides no accurate structural analysis of any glandular neoplasm.

Diagnostic ultrasound permits a characterization of a known salivary gland mass through a visualization of the sonographic properties of the lesion. Masses may be characterized as solid, cystic, or intermediate. This test, however, is not sensitive enough to differentiate between different types of solid lesions and, as such, may have limited application.

Computed tomography (CT scanning) may provide the best noninvasive means to evaluate the size and extent of lesions affecting the salivary glands. Computerized tomographic scanning involves computer detection and reconstruction of the roentgenographic image produced by structures within the body. This procedure allows for radiographic imaging of selected trans-

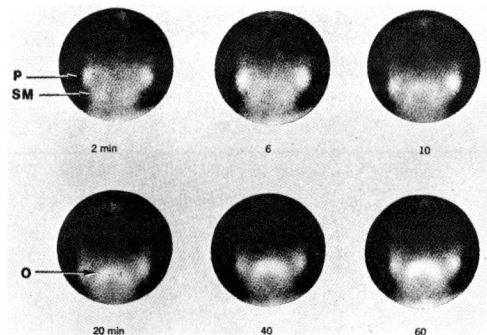

FIG. 15-22. *Scintigrams of normal salivary glands. Uptake of ^{99m} Tc pertechnetate by the parotid (P) and submandibular (SM) glands occurs immediately after administration of the technetium and shows progressive increase in concentration. Oral uptake begins at 8 to 10 min. and also increases. (Schall, G. L.: Xerostomia in Sjögren's syndrome. JAMA, 216:2109, 1971. Copyright 1971, American Medical Association, reprinted by permission)*

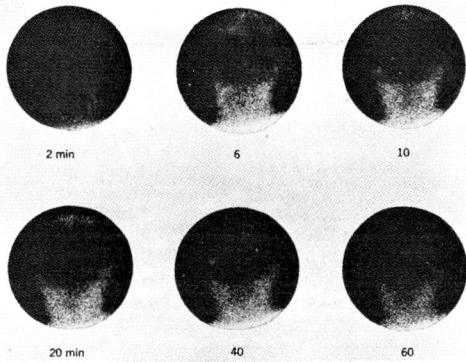

FIG. 15-23. *Scintigrams of salivary glands severely involved with Sjögren's syndrome. There is complete absence of active concentration of the* ^{99m} *Tc pertechnetate. Glandular activity is no more than background. (Schall, G.L.: Xerostomia in Sjögren's syndrome. JAMA, 216:2109, 1971. Copyright 1971, American Medical Association, reprinted by permission)*

verse planes of the body. Because of radiodensity differences between tissue types, the radiographic resolution is such that different tissue types can be distinguished from one another. While providing little or no physiologic information, CT scans do provide accurate anatomic information regarding neoplasm size and relation to adjacent structures. Certain ductal obstructions, especially sialoliths, also be diagnosed and located with this examination.

Biopsy

Surgical biopsy of salivary glands is one diagnostic procedure that may give an accurate indication of the nature of the pathologic process. Biopsy of the major salivary glands, however, may be contraindicated. The close relationship of important neurovascular structures, the creation of salivary fistulae, and the possibility of "seeding" abnormal cells must be considered when a biopsy is contemplated. In addition, tissue repair at a previous biopsy site may make subsequent biopsies or definitive surgery difficult. For these reasons, biopsy of the major salivary glands, especially the parotids, is rarely undertaken unless the lesion is superficial and a malignancy is suspected.[3]

Some work has been done in the area of aspiration biopsy of major salivary gland neoplasms in an attempt to avoid or mini-

mize the problems listed above. Eneroth and co-workers[8] reported a 92 percent positive tumor diagnosis in 1000 cases using this technique. Spiro, et al.[9] reported a somewhat lower success ratio of 62 percent and an erroneous benign diagnosis in 17 percent in 125 cases. At this time, aspiration biopsy of major salivary gland neoplasms has not gained universal acceptance.

Minor salivary gland biopsies are undertaken for two reasons: the removal of a pathologically involved gland and diagnostic purposes.

Excisional biopsies of the minor salivary glands, with few exceptions, present few of the problems noted concerning major salivary gland biopsy. This technique permits the total removal of a diseased gland and, in the case of certain systemic diseases, provides a safe and relatively easy collection of tissue to be used in laboratory studies. The operative technique used in the removal of a minor salivary gland neoplasm will be described later.

Frequently the diagnosis of systemic diseases, such as Sjögren's syndrome or sarcoidosis, is aided by a microscopic examination of salivary gland tissue. The minor salivary glands of the lower lip lend themselves readily to this procedure.

These minor glands lie immediately below the surface epithelium, above the muscle layer of the lower lip. They may be removed easily by means of an incision of 1 to 2 cm just through the epithelium on the inner surface of the lip. If an eversion of the lip over the surgeon's fingertip does not expose several glands (which clinically appear as whitish-yellow globules), blunt dissection laterally and inferiorly may be necessary. The glands thus exposed should be lightly grasped, at their base, with a cotton forceps and severed from the surrounding connective tissue with scalpel or scissors. Several glands should be thus secured, taking care that their microscopic anatomy is not distorted by the use of tissue clamps or forceps. The incision is closed with 4-0 or 3-0 black silk sutures. The sutures should be placed closely together and well tied. Because this tissue is very mobile and relatively fragile, it is not unusual for several sutures to be lost over a week's time. The patient should be supplied with a mild analgesic and instructed in methods of maintaining wound cleanliness. The salivary glands obtained should be submitted in a suitable fixative/preservative to a histopathological laboratory for diagnosis.

Laboratory Procedures

Several laboratory procedures may be helpful in the diagnosis of salivary gland disease states.

A complete blood count and a differential blood count may offer some help in determining the acuteness or chronicity of the disease. A blood examination may aid in distinguishing between several entities (mumps, infectious mononucleosis, and acute sialadenitis) that may resemble each other.

Microbiologic examinations of saliva or purulent material from an affected gland are occasionally desirable. Fluid for these studies should not be collected from the oral cavity but from the cannulated duct of the gland in question. In this fashion, oral contamination of the sample is avoided. (See section on sialography for cannulization technique.)

Disorders of the Salivary Glands

Inflammatory Disorders

Inflammation of the salivary glands, or sialadenitis, may be acute or chronic. It is due to bacterial or viral infection or other specific causes.

ACUTE BACTERIAL SIALADENITIS

Symptoms. This condition usually presents as a painful swelling of the gland accompanied by a decrease in its function. There may be low-grade fever, malaise, and headache. The overlying skin appears reddened and tense due to glandular edema. A purulent discharge may be evident from the gland's duct spontaneously or with digital expression.

Etiology. The microorganisms involved represent a wide range of normal oral bacteria: *Staphylococcus aureus, Staphylococcus pyogenes, Streptococcus viridans,* and *pneumococci.* Occasionally fungal forms may be identified. Infections involving mixed bacterial forms appear to ascend to the gland from the oral cavity; infections involving specific bacterial forms are more commonly blood borne.[10]

Diagnostic Aid. History as related by the patient, coupled with a febrile state, point to the acute nature of the problem. The blood profile may show a leukocytosis. Bacterial culture of the purulent discharge may aid in determining bacterial type and antibiotic sensitivity.

Plain radiology is valueless except when an infection of the submandibular gland must be differentiated from an infection originating within the dental alveolus. Sialography, as mentioned above, is contraindicated.

Treatment. The treatment plan involves rest, antibiotic therapy and, if necessary, surgical drainage. After the acute phase has subsided, the salivary duct may be dilated with graded salivary duct lacrimal probes to facilitate drainage. A salivary washing action should be instituted using a sialagogue such as citric acid or lemon extract. Throughout the treatment, the patient's hydration status must be maintained.

Prognosis. This condition tends to recur, in the form of a subacute or chronic form of the disease.

CHRONIC BACTERIAL SIALADENITIS

Symptoms. The symptoms of chronic sialadenitis are similar to those of the acute form, but the degree of severity may be less. Salivary flow may be reduced and a purulent discharge noted at the duct orifice. There is usually no erythema of the overlying skin.

Etiology. The etiologic agents are generally similar to those of acute bacterial sialadenitis. This condition is almost exclusively a complication to an obstruction in the duct of the submandibular gland. This obstruction in the salivary duct causes ductal dilation and salivary stasis followed by glandular atrophy and fibrosis. The gland becomes firm and hard. Bacteria move in a retrograde fashion into the duct, incubate, and form abscesses. The cause of this chronic condition in the parotid is less well known; low secretion rate is probably an important predisposing factor.

Diagnostic Aids. As with acute bacterial sialadenitis, the history is important. The patient may relate a prior episode of acute sialadenitis or glandular pain or swelling during meals. Bacterial culture of purulent material expressed from the gland aids in diagnosis. Plain radiology may show a calcified ductal obstruction.

Sialography may show a "pruned tree" appearance with lack of acinar filling (probably due to acinar edema). With a long-standing problem, there may be noted punctuate dilation of the peripheral ductules.[5] Sialography may aid in determining the status of the gland proximal to an obstruction, thereby determining optimal treatment. A diagnosis of severe chronic sialadenitis may be made from a sialogram; lesser degrees of inflammation are difficult to recognize sialographically.[11]

Treatment. Conservative treatment in the form of obstruction removal, ductual dilatation, antibiotic therapy, and therapeutic sialography may effect at least a temporary cure. Recurrence is common and surgical removal of the gland is often necessary.

CHRONIC RECURRENT PAROTITIS IN CHILDREN

The course and prognosis of chronic recurrent parotitis in children differs from that which occur in adults. This condition occurs approximately ten times less frequently in children than in adults.[3] The etiology of this condition in children is, as in the adult, uncertain. Although it can occur from the age of 1 month to 13 years, it is most common between 3 and 6 years of age.[10]

Sialography usually shows the parotid gland and ducts to be normal.[10] The course of chronic parotitis in children is characterized by spontaneous healing in the majority of the cases; a conservative approach to management and treatment is recommended.[3, 10, 11]

Differential Diagnosis. Epidemic parotitis (mumps) must be excluded in a differential diagnosis of chronic recurrent parotitis in children. Chronic parotitis is usually unilateral whereas mumps is bilateral. Purulent material is usually evident from the duct in chronic parotitis, and none is evident with mumps. Additionally, the mumps virus may be detected in saliva with the complement fixation test.

SIALECTASIA

Sialectasia, or swelling of the salivary glands, is not typical of any specific disorder. This condition probably represents the end stages of chronic, recurrent sialadenitis. Clinically, patients complain of diffuse swelling of the salivary gland, usually the parotid. This swelling may slowly increase in size over months or even years. Sialography of an involved gland produces the characteristic "bunch of grapes" appearance representing contrast medium filling of the chronically inflamed, sacculated ductal and acinar elements of the gland (Fig. 15-24).

MUMPS

Mumps, or epidemic parotitis, is a viral disease that primarily affects the salivary glands but also may affect other organs (pancreas, ovaries, testes) as well. It is the most common of all salivary gland diseases.

Symptoms. Fever, headache, and painful swelling of one or more salivary glands, most commonly the parotid, are evident. Usually one gland is affected followed by the other in 3 to 6 days. The onset of the symptoms is usually sudden. The swelling of the glands reaches a maximum within 2 days and diminishes over an additional week.[3] This clinical enlargement is due to glandular inflammation precipitated by the virus.

Etiology. Mumps is caused by a virus that can be transmitted by droplets of saliva. The incubation period is from 2 to 3 weeks.

Diagnostic Aids. Mumps is usually bilateral; it usually affects the parotids, but may also affect the submandibular glands. Purulent material cannot be expressed from the

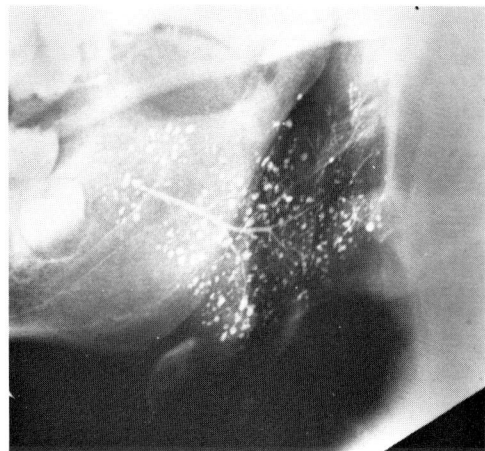

FIG. 15-24. *Parotid sialogram illustrating the "bunch of grapes" appearance. (Courtesy of Dr. D.E. Waite)*

duct. The complement fixation test is probably the best diagnostic test for mumps virus antibodies.

Treatment. The treatment of mumps is usually symptomatic. Isolation of the patient for 6 to 10 days is recommended to prevent contagion.

SALIVARY GLAND INCLUSION DISEASE

This disease results from an infection by the DNA cytomegalovirus; it may be acquired in utero or at any time postnatally. Between 50 and 80 percent of adults harbor the virus or have been exposed to it.[12]

Pathologic changes include the appearance of large intranuclear and less distinct cytoplasmic inclusion bodies in grossly enlarged cells of many organs. The organs most often affected are the salivary glands, kidneys, liver, lungs, pancreas, and thyroid. The gross tissue changes are minimal; they consist chiefly of edema and slight enlargement of the organ. Occasionally, however, areas of focal necrosis and fibrosis may occur.[12]

Infection with the cytomegalovirus may cause subclinical infection or overt illness known as cytomegalic inclusion disease (C.I.D.). Most infections are subclinical, but serious diseases characterized by prematurity, microcephaly, intracranial calcifications, hepatosplenomegaly, and thrombocytopenia may occur in the unborn infant. Acquired infection characterized by fever, rash, pneumonitis, or hepatitis may occur in immunocompromised or debilitated persons.

Diagnosis depends upon the identification of the virus in saliva, urine, blood, or tissue. It is interesting to note that the parotid gland is most often affected in the infant and child, whereas the submandibular gland is more frequently involved in adults.[10]

POSTIRRADIATION CHRONIC SIALADENITIS

Patients who have received therapeutic irradiation for malignancies of the head and neck region invariably complain of a dry mouth between 2 to 6 hours after treatment. Additionally, these patients develop pain and enlargement of the parotid and submandibular glands during the same time period. This enlargement increases for 12 to 24 hours, then rapidly subsides without treatment.

These symptoms are due to an acute inflammatory reaction within the salivary glands. From this reactive pattern, a progressive change in which continued degeneration and loss of acini, replacement of acute inflammatory cells by chronic inflammatory elements, and intralobular fibrosis may occur.[13] This degenerative process continues to complete atrophy of glandular and interstitial elements with consequent loss of function. Interestingly, no major alterations occur in the ductules within the gland.

The dry mouth, or xerostomia, following therapeutic irradiation may be transient or become permanent. Treatment for this condition is empirical at best (see xerostomia).

Obstructive Disorders

A salivary duct obstruction impedes or halts salivary excretion into the oral cavity. The gland, however, continues, at least for a time, the secretion of saliva. This damming and consequent accumulation of saliva under pressure produces pain, swelling, and if the condition is long-standing, glandular infection and atrophy.

Symptoms. A partial ductal obstruction causes acute pain and swelling in the gland region. These symptoms are especially evident immediately prior to, during, and immediately following meals due to increased stimulation of the salivary gland. The patient usually reports that the swelling slowly diminishes between meals only to recur at the next mealtime. A partial obstruction acts to cause these symptoms by allowing some saliva to leak past during periods of low salivary secretion, but by causing a saliva accumulation during periods of increased secretion.

A partial obstruction may lead to glandular infection; bacteria may ascend the duct until they reach the stagnant pool of saliva proximal to the obstruction. This condition may occur even if the degree of obstruction is not enough to cause mealtime swelling.[14]

Alternatively, the patient may be unaware of the glandular swelling, but complains of dull pain following meals. This pain may be poorly localized; it may be described as originating in the throat, molar tooth, or ear.[14]

Etiology. Ductal obstruction may be caused by mucous plugs, calculi within the duct (sialolithiasis), ductal strictures or ulcerations, or by neoplasms.

Salivary calculi (sialoliths) frequently cause ductal obstruction, particularly in Wharton's duct. Calculi are usually unilateral and may assume a wide range of size. Rauch and Gorlin[10] have presented a review of various theories on the origin and subsequent enlargement of sialoliths.

Mucous plugs may cause ductal obstruction. These may be frequently treated with the administration of a strong sialagogue. The contrast medium used in sialography may also "break up" a mucous obstruction. If both of these methods fail, these obstructions should be treated as a sialolith.

PAROTID OBSTRUCTION: *Papillary Obstruction*

Stensen's papilla and duct orifice may be traumatized by the dentition, a faulty restoration, or a dental prosthesis. Trauma to this area frequently occurs during eruption of the second and third molars.[14] The edema associated with this trauma (and possible subsequent ulceration) may cause ductal obstruction. If this trauma is of long duration, chronic fibrotic papillary stenosis occurs: a partial or total closure of the ductal orifice due to scarring.

Diagnostic Aids. Stensen's duct may resist the insertion of, or feel rigid upon the insertion of, a lacrimal probe. Following "milking" of the gland, the tissue behind the papilla may assume a bluish tone due to a pool of saliva.[14]

Sialography demonstrates a narrowing of the duct in the papillary region and a dilation of the duct proximally.[3]

Treatment. The treatment of papillary obstruction consists of removal of the cause of trauma. If stenosis has occurred, dilation of the ductal orifice with graded lacrimal probes or surgical removal of the papilla and distal duct portion may be necessary. If the surgical approach is necessary, care must be taken to suture the duct walls to the oral mucosa.

PAROTID OBSTRUCTION: *Duct Obstruction*

Parotid duct sialoliths are not as common as submandibular sialoliths; they ac-

count for only approximately 6 to 10 percent of salivary calculi.[10]

These calculi are usually smaller, but more symptomatic than Wharton's duct calculi; patients therefore seek treatment earlier.

Calculi in the parotid duct may be located in four areas; impacted at the papilla, in the submucous portion, in the extraglandular portion of the duct external to the buccinator, and in the intraglandular portion of the duct.[19]

Symptoms. The symptoms of parotid duct obstruction include acute pain and swelling associated with meals or recurrent infections of the gland.

Salivary calculi in Stensen's duct, because of their usual sharpness and pointedness, may cause pain during mastication and upon palpation.[10]

Diagnostic Aids. In some cases, the location of the calculus may be assessed by noting the area of swelling. If the accessory parotid is enlarged, the calculus lies distally in the duct; if the lower pole of the gland is involved, the calculus lies in the intraglandular duct portion.[15]

If the calculus is impacted near the ductal orifice, it may be visualized protruding from the papilla or as a hard, yellowish swelling immediately under the epithelium.

Plain radiography may be useful in establishing a diagnosis of a Stensen's duct calculus. A periapical film applied against the inner aspect of the cheek and exposed as previously described (c.f. section on plain radiology), usually demonstrates the calculus. A calculus which lies in the intraglandular portion of the duct may be difficult to demonstrate with plain radiography.

Sialography may be useful in demonstrating a mucous or poorly calcified obstruction. Care must be exercised so that calculus is not forced proximally due to contrast medium injection pressure.

CT scans may provide accurate information about the size and location of calcified obstructions and limited information about the location of uncalcified obstructions.

Treatment. If the calculus lies immediately subjacent to the ductal orifice, the orifice may be simply slit open with a surgical scissors. It may be necessary to "milk" the calculus out with salivary flow. The papilla and ductal orifice heal well without the use of sutures.

The removal of salivary calculi that lie within the buccinator portion of the duct or more proximally can be surgically difficult; the technique involved is beyond the scope of this text. For further information, the reader is referred to several reviews[3,15,16] of this technique.

SUBMANDIBULAR OBSTRUCTION

Frequently, following a surgical procedure (such as biopsy) on the anterior floor of the mouth, symptoms of submandibular gland obstruction appear. This is usually due to a ductal stricture caused by healing of the adjacent tissue.

Sialoliths are the most frequent cause of obstructions of Wharton's duct. The most common site is just distal to the body of the gland.[10] Calculi in this posterior segment of the duct may remain asymptomatic for some time due to the relatively large size and elasticity of the duct. If the stone increases in size to the point where salivary flow is slowed considerably or if infection supervenes, the patient will experience symptoms.[17]

Symptoms. Symptoms of submandibular duct obstruction include acute pain and swelling or infection.

Diagnostic Aids. Most sialoliths within at least the distal portion of Wharton's duct may be palpated. With palpation it is possible to determine the location of the obstruction and to ascertain the status of the gland proper (a fibrosed gland feels firm and inelastic, a normal gland or one with little change feels elastic).[17]

Plain radiography is usually helpful; the film should be positioned and exposed as described earlier.

Sialography should be used with caution; a sialolith may be forced proximally due to contrast medium injection pressure. Sialography may be used following the removal of the sialolith to aid in determining the status of the gland.

As with parotid obstructions, CT scans can provide accurate information regarding calcified obstructions and their relation to adjacent structures.

Treatment. If the obstructive calculus lies in the extraglandular portion of the duct and

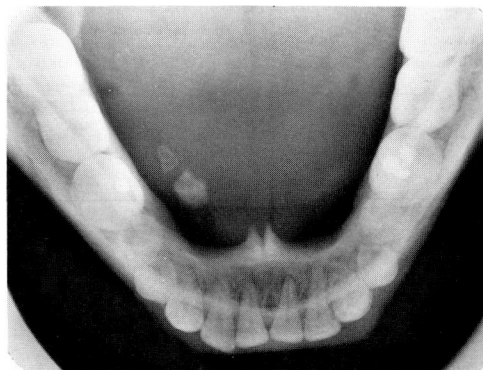

FIG. 15-25. *Preoperative radiograph of calculus within Wharton's duct.*

if the gland itself has suffered no irreparable damage, the calculus is removed surgically. If the calculus lies in the intraglandular portion of the duct or if the gland has become fibrosed due to long-standing obstruction or infection, the entire gland is removed.

The surgical removal of submandibular duct calculi that lie in the distal portion of the duct may be accomplished under local anesthesia. A brief description follows: Anesthesia is achieved via a lingual nerve block (Fig. 15-25). A suture is passed around the duct posterior to the calculus and tied gently; this prevents proximal displacement of the calculus (Fig. 15-26). Wharton's duct is identified by means of blunt dissection in the floor of the mouth

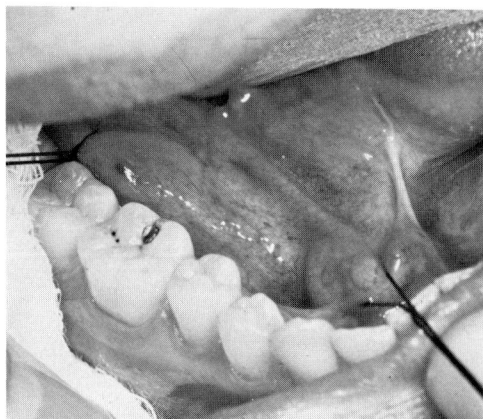

FIG. 15-26. *Removal of Wharton's duct calculus. Isolation of calculus between posterior ligature and anterior traction suture. (Courtesy of Dr. D.E. Waite)*

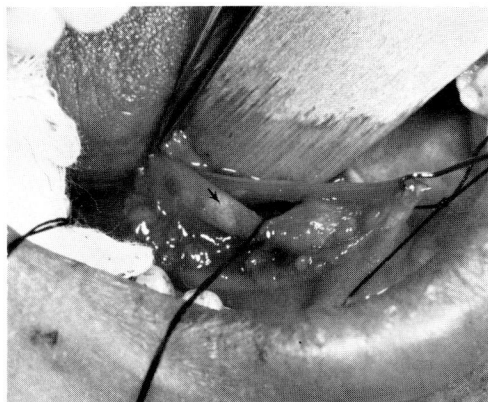

FIG. 15-27. *Removal of Wharton's duct calculus. Wharton's duct with contained sialolith (arrow) is surgically isolated with blunt dissection. (Courtesy of Dr. D.E. Waite)*

following an incision through the oral mucosa. The duct is stabilized by means of a distal suture and incised over the calculus (Fig. 15-27). The calculus is extirpated (Fig. 15-28), the duct irrigated, and the stabilization sutures removed. The mucosal incision only is sutured; attempts to suture the duct itself may lead to stricture formation (Fig. 15-29).

Submandibular calculi that lie in the proximal portion of the duct are usually removed under general anesthesia; this surgical procedure and the procedure involved in the removal of the submandibular gland proper are beyond the scope of this text. For further information regarding these procedures, the reader is referred to several articles[3,17,18,19] in the literature.

SUBLINGUAL AND MINOR GLAND
OBSTRUCTION

Obstructions of the ducts of the sublingual and minor salivary glands are not common; there have been probably fewer than 200 reported cases of minor gland sialolithiasis. The buccal mucosa and upper lip seem to be the most common sites for minor gland sialolithiasis.

Symptoms. Sublingual edema, which is localized and coupled with a small concrement near Wharton's duct, may indicate a sublingual duct sialolith.[10] Minor gland obstructions present as hard swellings.

Diagnostic Aids. Glandular palpation will aid in localizing sialoliths in these locations.

Plain radiography is useful in the diagnosis of a minor gland sialolith if located in the cheek or lip.

Treatment. If the sublingual sialolith presents at the ductal orifice, treatment is afforded by a surgical enlargement of the orifice, similar to the treatment described for a calculus impacted immediately beneath Stensen's papilla.

Treatment of minor gland sialoliths consists of removal of the entire gland and duct. The surgical technique is identical to that which will be described for the removal of a mucocele (q.v.).

SIALADENOSIS

Sialadenosis or sialosis is the noninflammatory, non-neoplastic bilateral swelling of the salivary glands. This clinical enlargement is accompanied by gland hypofunction. This disorder may affect all salivary glands, but usually only the parotids are involved.

The course of sialadenosis is chronic, undulating, recurrent, usually indolent, and afebrile. Women, especially those in the age of hormonal alterations, are often more affected.[10] The glandular hypofunction associated with this condition may lead to chronic sialadenitis since the mechanism which acts to prevent retrograde infection (salivary flow) is impaired.

Symptoms. A slowly increasing, chronic, undulating multiglandular enlargement, usually bilateral, of the salivary glands, accompanied by a systemic disorder or hor-

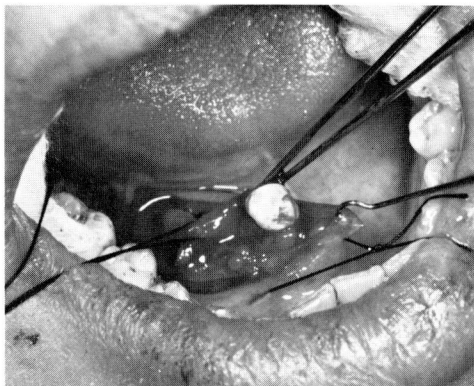

FIG. 15-28. *Removal of Wharton's duct calculus. The duct has been stabilized with traction sutures. The sialolith is removed by a longitudinal incision. (Courtesy of Dr. D.E. Waite)*

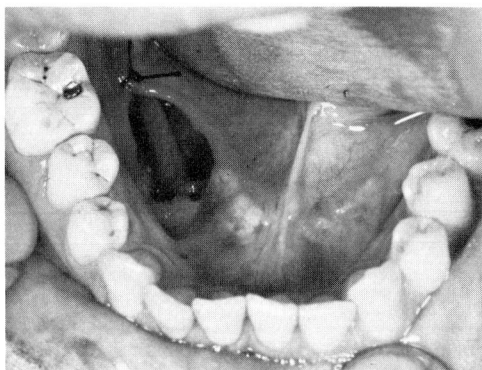

FIG. 15-29. *Removal of Wharton's duct calculus. The ductal incision is not sutured; the overlying mucosa is sutured. Note the duct traversing the surgical opening. (Courtesy of Dr. D.E. Waite)*

monal imbalance which may be undiagnosed.

Etiology. Sialadenosis may be associated with hormonal disturbances such as diabetes mellitus, hypothyroidism, menopause, Cushing's syndrome, menstruation, and pregnancy. Hepatogenic sialadenosis has been associated with alcoholism with or without cirrhosis. This condition is common in certain nutritional deficiency states, especially in hypoproteinemia. Parotid gland enlargement has been noted in association with the intake of certain drugs such as phenylbutazone, certain nonepinephrine derivatives, and catecholamine.

Diagnostic Aids. Diagnosis of this disorder may often be made by clinical history; pursuit of this diagnosis may lead to discovery of a previously unsuspected systemic condition.

Sialography reveals a normal ductal structure[3] or one exhibiting a thin, hairline architecture.[10]

Salivary secretion, upon glandular "milking," presents as a scanty, whitish, viscous flow.

Clinical palpation reveals a gland that is doughy, painless, and poorly demarcated.[10]

Biopsy of an involved gland reveals the nature of the enlargement; serous acinar cell hypertrophy, edema of the interstitial-supporting tissues, and atrophy of the striated ducts.[3]

Treatment. The treatment of the associated systemic disturbance usually affects resolution of the associated sialadenosis. This has been especially noted when the sialadenosis is associated with alcoholic cirrhosis of the liver and with malnutrition.

Glandular Atrophy

Salivary gland atrophy may be a result of disease, ductal obstruction or ligation, radiation, or the aging process.

True atrophy results from wasting diseases (disseminated carcinoma) or following radiation therapy with a decrease in both glandular and interstitial elements.

Benign atrophy shows an increase in the apparent gland size; actually this represents an increase only in the interstitial elements; the glandular component of the gland decreases. Two types of benign atrophy may be considered: (1)Fatty atrophy, the more common form, clinically presents as a uniform doughy gland without nodularity. Salivation is normal or decreased. (2) Fibrous atrophy clinically presents as a firm, finely glandular or nodular gland. Glandular atrophy following long-term ductal obstruction or radiation has been previously discussed.

Waterhouse et al.[20] noted that between childhood and old age, approximately one quarter of the active parenchymal cell volume is lost. Fat and connective tissue replace this cell volume and may even cause an increase in overall gland size. This loss of active parenchymal cell volume with senescence probably accounts for the reduction of salivary flow volume seen in some older individuals.

Developmental Anomalies

The congenital absence of salivary glands (aplasia or agenesis) or the congenital occlusion or absence of salivary ducts (atresia) is rare. These conditions may give rise to xerostomia (q.v.) and its associated increased caries rate or retention cyst formation.

Salivary gland tissue at an abnormal anatomic site is termed aberrancy. Aberrant salivary gland tissue has been reported at the base of the neck, the hypophysis, sternoclavicular joint, and middle ear.[21]

Stafne, in 1942,[22] described a series of 34 cases of bone defects near the angle of the mandible below the inferior alveolar nerve canal. Since that original report, the presence of this static bone cavity or defect has been described frequently. In most cases, these cystlike cavities have been found to contain salivary gland tissue probably representing ectopic submandibular gland nests (Fig. 15-30). Occasionally, these nests may maintain a ductal connection with the submandibular gland proper; sialography, therefore, may be helpful in the diagnosis.

This condition has been considered congenital; a premature growth of the submandibular gland causing an accommodation by the osseous structure of the mandible. Evidence has been presented, however, that indicates formation of this defect may occur after middle age.[23]

The exact method of development of these salivary tissue enclavements is open to question; a probable explanation may be surface bone resorption due to an unknown cause.

Aberrant, normal-appearing mixed salivary gland tissue has been described within bone in the incisor-premolar area of the mandible.[21] The occurrence of salivary gland inclusions in this location must be considered rare.

These examples of aberrant salivary gland tissue represent simply variations from normal and should be recognized as such; no treatment is usually necessary. It is important to note, however, that any area of aberrant salivary gland tissue may be the site of neoplastic change.

Functional Disorders

SIALORRHEA (PTYALISM)

Increased salivary flow, or sialorrhea, may result from many different causes that may be grouped into two main categories: (1) factors affecting the central nervous system, and (2) local factors which reflexly stimulate flow. Sialorrhea may occur in mentally retarded individuals; it is also associated with deteriorated schizophrenia, epilepsy, Parkinsonism, mercury poisoning, acrodynia, and other mental, psychiatric, and neurologic disturbances. The most common causes of sialorrhea are acute inflammations of the oral cavity; these cause excessive salivary secretion through reflex stimulation. Sialorrhea is common with herpetic or aphthous ulceration and acute

necrotizing gingival stomatitis. Sialorrhea may also accompany ill-fitting dentures and the eruption of teeth in young individuals.

Treatment. The underlying cause of the excessive salivary flow should be treated. Symptomatic relief may be frequently obtained with the antihistaminic drugs such as methantheline bromide (Banthine 50 mg) or atrophine sulfate (1/150 grain).

XEROSTOMIA

In 1868, A. G. Bartley wrote to the editor of London's *Medical Times and Gazette* concerning treatment of dryness of the oral mucosa and dryness and soreness of the tongue in an elderly patient. Bartley

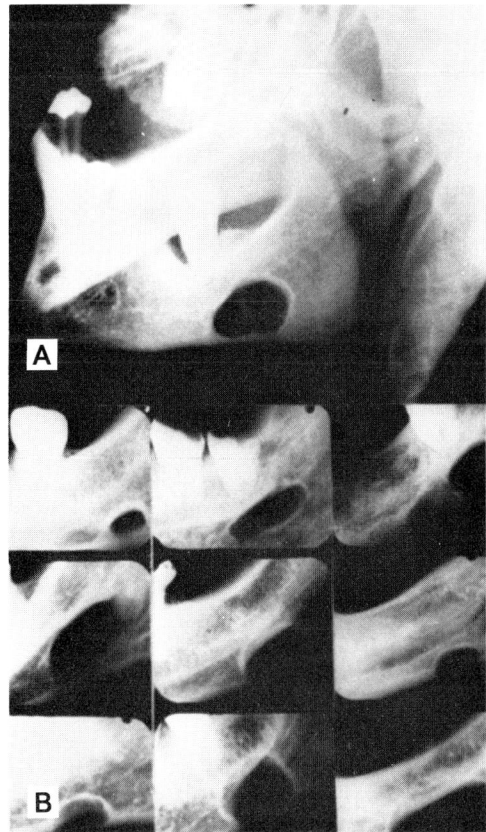

FIG. 15-30. *Static bone cavity or defect. (A) Characteristic location of defect near mandibular angle and below inferior alveolar canal. (B) Other mandibular defects that may contain salivary tissue. (A, Courtesy of Dr. E.C. Stafne. B, Stafne, E.C.: Bone cavities situated near the angle of the mandible. JADA 29: 1969, 1942. Copyright by the American Dental Association, reprinted by permission)*

became the first individual of record to describe the symptoms associated with diminished salivary flow. In 1888, Hutchinson and Hadden termed this condition xerostomia. Xerostomia may be defined as occurring when salivary secretion is equal to or less than 0 to 2 ml per 15 minutes; this flow rate is less than 4 percent of the average salivary flow rate for persons under 65 years of age.[24]

Symptoms. The patient with xerostomia often presents with a complaint of a dry mouth. Clinical examination may reveal pronounced reddening of the tongue coupled with total papillary atrophy, lobulation, or deep fissuring. Glossodynia, cheilosis of the lip commissures, dysphonia, dysphagia, taste disturbances, and denture difficulties may also be manifest. These signs and symptoms tend to increase in severity as the salivary secretion decreases.[24] Severe cases of xerostomia may be accompanied by an increased caries rate, especially in the cervical areas of the teeth. This increased caries rate is probably due to the loss of the cleansing properties of saliva.

Etiology. Xerostomia may be idiopathic or a manifestation of a local factor such as mouth breathing, inflammatory conditions of the salivary glands, irradiation, and degenerative or aging changes. Xerostomia may also be associated with systemic conditions such as anemias, certain syndromes (Sjögren's, Mikulicz's, Heerfordt's), lupus erythematosus, hormonal disturbances, drugs, emotional and anxiety states, and fluid loss.

Diagnostic Aids. The patient's medical history and clinical examination are of great importance. Approximately 80 percent of patients with xerostomia show clinical manifestations within the oral cavity.[24]

Clinical "milking" of the salivary glands may give some indication of the nature of the salivary flow.

Plain radiography, sialography, CT scans, and scintigraphy may be of assistance in the diagnosis of obstructive or systemic disorders.

Bacterial cultures and blood studies may lead to the identification of infectious or hematological disorders.

Treatment. The treatment of xerostomia is the removal of the cause. Since the majority of cases of xerostomia are due to idiopathic or obscure conditions, treatment must frequently be symptomatic.

Symptomatic treatments of xerostomia are several; none has gained universal success or acceptance. A mouthwash containing citric acid (12.5 gm), essence of lemon (20 ml) and glycerine (q.s. 1 liter) is suggested by some.[3] A newer, "saliva substitute" with viscosity and electrolyte levels adjusted to simulate whole saliva has shown clinical efficacity, at least for the relief of nocturnal discomfort.[25] Proper humidification of the ambient air and avoidance of mouth breathing are also recommended.

Whichever method of symptomatic treatment is chosen, the patient should be monitored closely to prevent a serious infection with candidal organisms, encouraged to increase fluid intake, and instructed in meticulous oral and dental hygiene.

Cysts and Cyst-Like Lesions

TRUE CYSTS

True cysts of the major salivary glands are rare if the branchiogenic cysts are not considered.[10] Cystic disorders of salivary glands may include congenital cysts, traumatic cysts, or far advanced cavitary diseases secondary to chronic sialadenitis.

Cysts of the major salivary glands occur most frequently in the parotid and represent a small percentage of surgical salivary gland problems.

MUCOCELE

The mucocele is a fluid- or semifluid-filled cavity surrounded by a capsule composed of compressed granulation tissue or epithelium. These abnormalities may be superficial or deeply located and may vary in size from a few millimeters to a centimeter or more in diameter. Superficial mucoceles have a bluish translucent color and rupture easily; those more deeply seated may assume the color of the surrounding oral mucosa.

Mucoceles may be found almost anywhere within the oral cavity; the majority occur on the lower lip. The buccal mucosa and the mouth floor may also be involved. A mucocele that involves the salivary gland tissue in the anterior ventral tongue area is

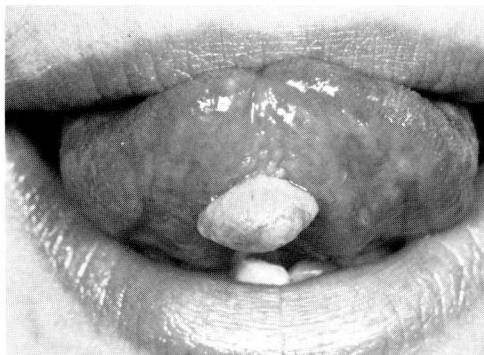

FIG. 15-31. *Mucocele of the minor salivary glands of the ventral anterior tongue, the so-called cyst of Blandin-Nuhn. (Courtesy of Dr. R. Gorlin)*

termed a cyst of Blandin-Nuhn (Fig. 15-31). Mucoceles are rarely found on the upper lip.

Mucoceles are generally considered to be of two types: extravasation or retention. The extravasation mucocele is not a true cyst since the cavity is not lined by epithelium. This type of mucocele is most frequently seen in individuals over 50 years of age.

Symptoms. Mucoceles have a rather characteristic behavior pattern. The patient reports an increase in size of an area followed usually by a spontaneous shrinkage with a subsequent enlargement. This history of alternate enlargement and shrinkage is typical, especially of lesions located superficially on the lip or buccal mucosa. The obstructed salivary gland continues to secrete saliva which escapes into the connective tissue or distends the duct. This process continues until the expanded tissue ruptures from pressure, trauma, or surgical manipulation. This rupture heals in the now collapsed lesion and the saliva again accumulates to repeat the enlargement. Occasionally, patients may report a drainage of fluid from the expanded lesion; usually, however, this drainage goes unnoticed.

Etiology. The extravasation mucocele probably occurs as a result of trauma. Trauma, chiefly mechanical, causes a rupture of the duct of a minor salivary gland resulting in secretion of saliva into the surrounding tissue. This saliva compresses the surrounding connective tissue and causes a variable degree of chronic inflammation.

The retention mucocele occurs following partial obstruction of a minor salivary gland duct. The gland continues to secrete saliva and an enlargement or ballooning of the duct results. This dilation of the duct becomes a cystic lesion lined by epithelium.

Diagnostic Aids. The clinical appearance coupled with the history should lead to the correct diagnosis. If the lesion is superficial, the contained fluid may frequently be palpated.

Treatment. Successful treatment of small mucoceles located in the labial or buccal mucosa consists of total excision of the lesion and surrounding salivary tissue.

Figure 15-32 illustrates a mucocele of moderate diameter. Anesthesia is achieved through a series of submucosal injections surrounding the lesion; a so-called "ring block" (Fig. 15-33). Anesthesia administered in this fashion does not distort the subsequent microscopic interpretation of the tissue. Stabilization without distortion of the tissue is achieved by passing a suture under the lesion; using this suture, tension may be applied to the tissue throughout the procedure (Fig. 15-34). A wedge-shaped elliptical incision is performed to include the mucocele; the tissue is separated from the underlying submucosa with sharp dissection (Fig. 15-35). Frequently, additional minor salivary glands are seen in the surgical site; these should be removed since, because of the trauma they have experienced, they may be the source of a recurrent mucocele. The surgical mar-

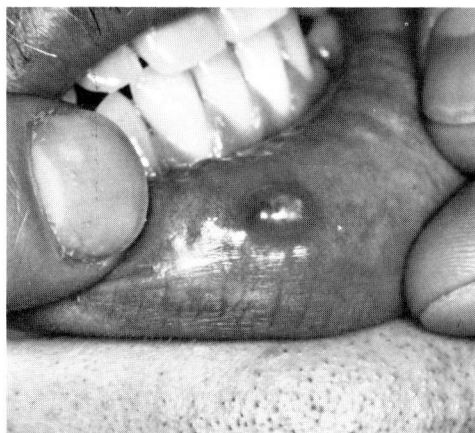

FIG. 15-32. *Preoperative appearance of superficial mucocele.*

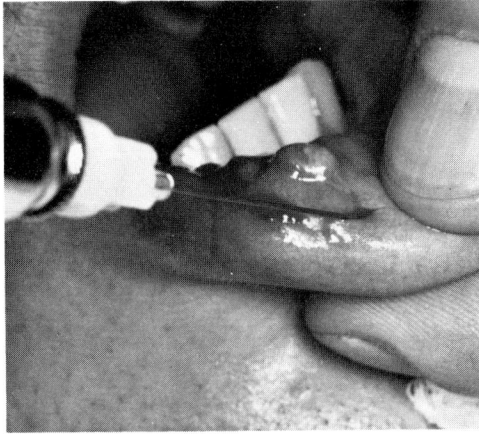

FIG. 15-33. *Ring block anesthesia for removal of superficial mucocele.*

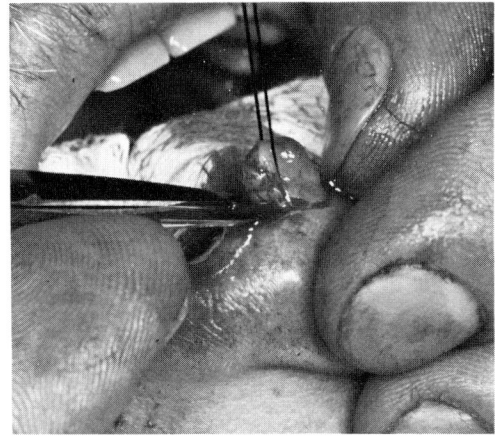

FIG. 15-35. *Removal of superficial mucocele. A V-shaped elliptical incision to include all the lesion is accomplished with a scalpel. The lesion is separated from the underlying tissue with sharp dissection. Note traction suture.*

gins are undermined with blunt dissection (Fig. 15-36) and the wound sutured through the mucosa to avoid trauma to any residual salivary tissue (Fig. 15-37). The sutures should remain in place for 5 to 7 days. The patient should be cautioned that this type of lesion may recur.

Treatment of large mucoceles (Fig. 15-38) and those lesions not located superficially involves a meticulous dissection of the mucocele from the surrounding tissue. Following complete removal, the overlying mucosa is sutured. As in the case with small mucoceles, recurrence is possible.

Surgical drainage of these lesions does not represent treatment. While this proce-

dure affects a shrinkage, healing soon occurs and the enlargement reappears.

RANULA

A mucocele occurring in the anterior floor of the mouth is rather arbitrarily termed a ranula. The name derives from its color similarity to the ventral surface of a frog (rana).

These lesions are usually unilateral and vary from 2 to 3 cm in diameter. They are soft and fluctuant and usually present a blue-violet color. The walls are thin and do

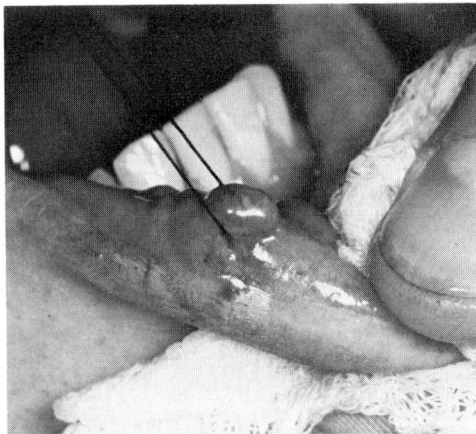

FIG. 15-34. *Removal of superficial mucocele. Traction suture passed under and outside of the lesion.*

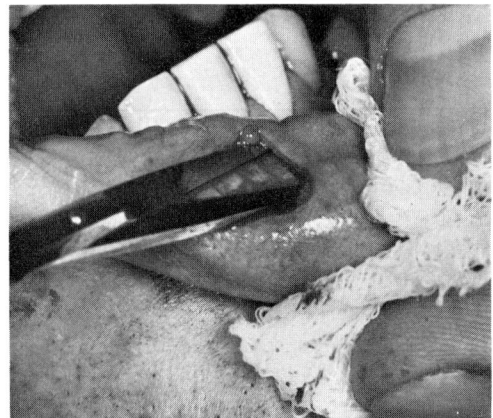

FIG. 15-36. *Removal of superficial mucocele. As a preliminary to closure, the surrounding epithelium must be undermined with blunt dissection. A surgical scissors works well.*

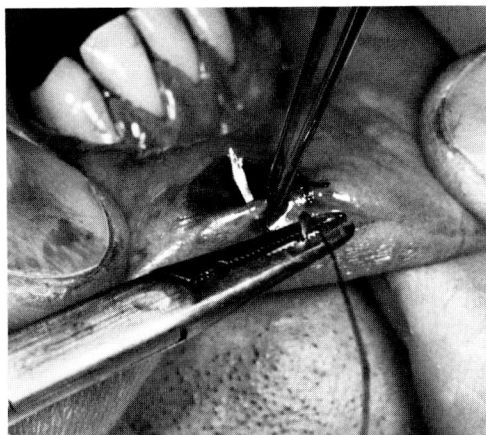

FIG. 15-37. *Removal of superficial mucocele. Closure is achieved with sutures placed through the mucosa only. Note use of tissue forceps to avoid trauma.*

not pit with pressure. They are usually associated with the sublingual gland. Ranulas are usually relatively superficial lesions lying above the mylohyoid muscles; they may extend posteriorly.

Microscopically, ranulas are generally unilocular. The lumen contains a viscous, mucoserousfluid. The wall of a ranula is composed of compressed connective tissue which contains variable numbers of chronic inflammatory elements. Rarely, ranulas may contain an epithelial lining; in these cases the lining is usually similar to that found in an excretory duct (cuboidal epithelium).

Symptoms. Ranulas are generally painless; they may interfere with speech, mastica-

tion, and deglutition due to their location or size.

Etiology. These lesions probably arise due to the partial obstruction to salivary flow; they therefore share a common etiology with mucoceles elsewhere in the oral cavity.

Diagnostic Aids. The location, clinical appearance, and history of this lesion should lead to the correct diagnosis. Clinical palpation will reveal contained fluid. As in the case of mucoceles elsewhere in the oral cavity, the patient may relate a history of periodic enlargement and shrinkage.

Treatment. Marsupialization or excision of the ranula are the treatments of choice; incision and drainage alone results in recurrence.

Marsupialization involves the removal of the superior wall of the ranula and the suturing of the remaining lining to the mucous membrane of the mouth floor. After suitable anesthesia has been established (Fig. 15-39), a tissue scissors is used to remove the overlying mucosa and ranula lining around the greatest perimeter of the lesion (Fig. 15-40). Sutures are then passed through the oral mucosa and the lesion's lining and knotted (Fig. 15-41). Recurrence is possible; the patient should be so informed.

Total excision of the ranula is a difficult procedure due to the lesion's location and thin wall but may be indicated if it is made up of multiple compartments or is deeply located.

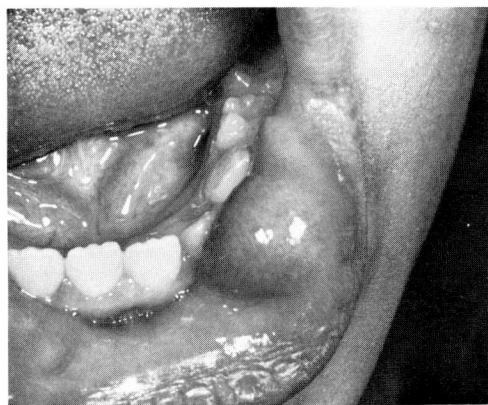

FIG. 15-38. *Large mucocele of upper lip.*

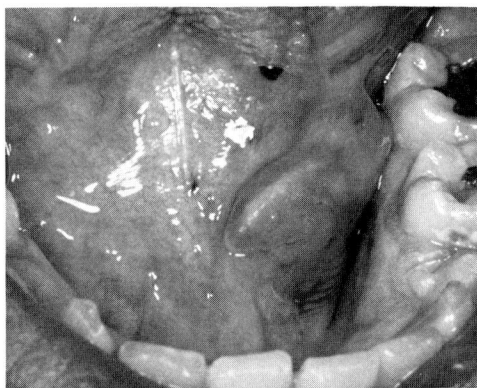

FIG. 15-39. *Preoperative appearance of ranula. Anesthesia is achieved through a block of the lingual nerve or with the ring block technique.*

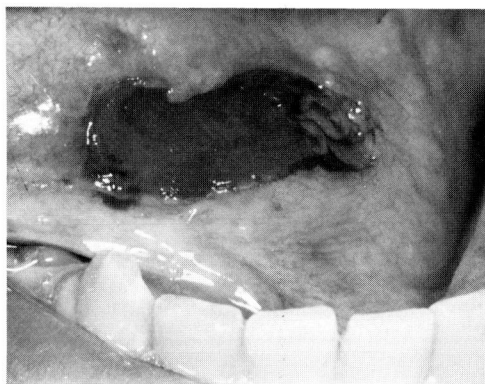

FIG. 15-40. *Following the perimeter, the ranula may be readily de-roofed with a surgical scissors.*

Salivary Gland Neoplasms

Tumors of the salivary glands are relatively rare, constituting from 1 to 4 percent of all head and neck neoplasms.[10] The following paragraphs include discussions of the most common benign and malignant salivary gland neoplasms and salivary gland problems as presented in children. For more detailed information concerning these entities, the reader should refer to a text of oral pathology or to the literature.

Benign Neoplasms

PLEOMORPHIC ADENOMA (BENIGN MIXED TUMOR)

The pleomorphic adenoma is the most common salivary gland tumor of the major or minor salivary glands. It has been estimated that this tumor accounts for approximately 90 percent of all benign tumors of all the salivary glands[26] and for over 50 percent of all tumors (benign or malignant) of all salivary glands.[27]

Clinical Features. When only the major glands are considered, this tumor most frequently involves the parotid, especially the tail of the parotid that lies below the ear lobe. The least frequently involved of the major salivary glands is the sublingual. When considering minor salivary glands, those most frequently involved are the glands of the hard palate; those least frequently involved are the glands of the lower lip.[26]

Most studies indicate that this tumor is more common in females. The majority of these neoplasms are diagnosed in the fifth and sixth decades of life.

Pleomorphic adenomas usually begin as solitary, small, painless nodules that slowly and intermittently increase in size without fixation to superficial or deeper structures. The most frequent presenting symptom is a mass that may have been present for over 5 years. Overlying skin or mucosa are seldom ulcerated even though some examples of these neoplasms are quite large.

Histologic Features. The pleomorphic adenoma is aptly named; a diverse histologic pattern is the hallmark of this group of neoplasms. Cuboidal, stellate, polyhedral, spindle, or squamous cell elements may exhibit proliferation within a connective tissue stroma. This connective tissue stroma may show a variety of mucoid, myxoid, chondroid, or hyaline patterns. Ossification foci rarely may be observed (Fig. 15-42).

The tumor is surrounded by a connective tissue "pseudo-capsule" so named because of frequent viable tumor nests within the capsule wall. An additional characteris-

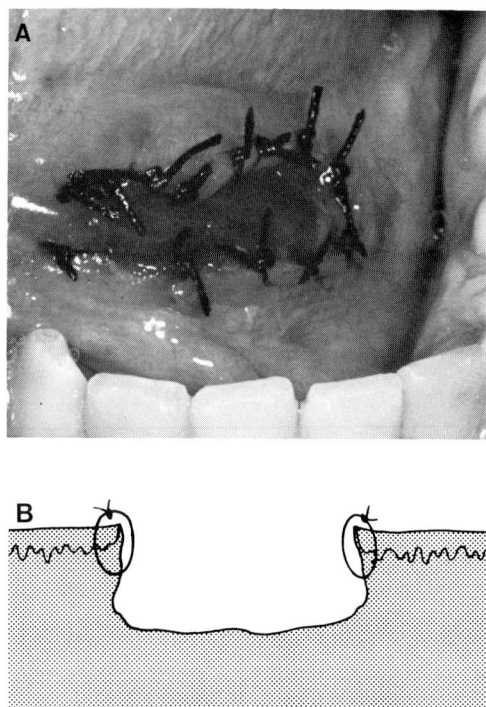

FIG. 15-41. *Marsupialization of ranula. (A) The floor of the lesion is sutured to the overlying mucosa. Upon healing, the lining of the ranula will become continuous with the oral mucosa. (B) Diagrammatic cross-sectional view of clinical view in A. Note the sutures through the epithelium and the ranula's lining.*

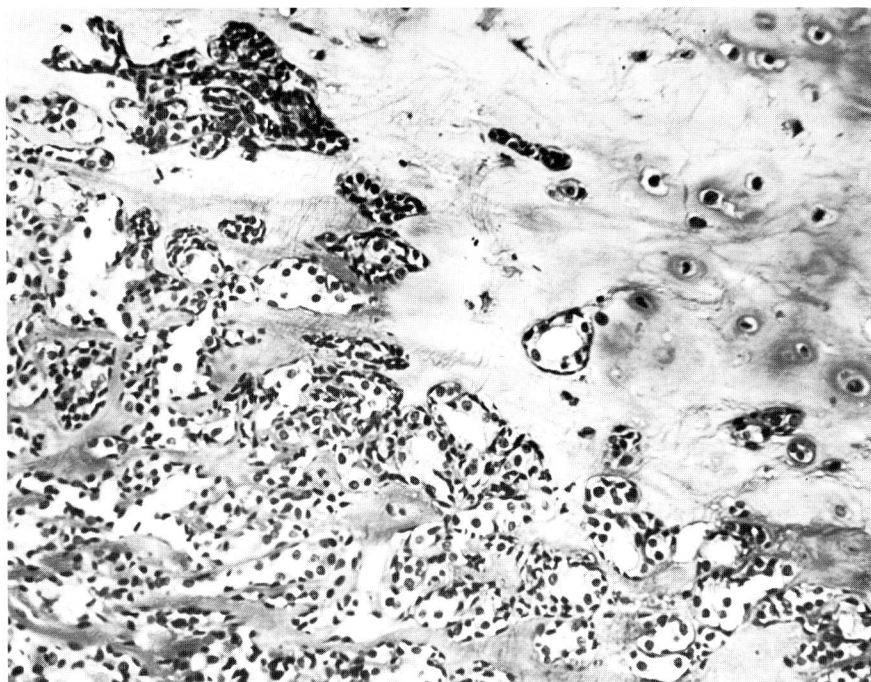

FIG. 15-42. *Photomicrograph of pleomorphic adenoma. Note the "pseudocartilaginous" relatively acellular area and the duct-like structures. (Gorlin, R.J. and Vickers, R.A.: Lips, mouth, teeth, salivary glands, and neck. In Pathology, 6th ed. W.A.D. Anderson (ed.) St. Louis, C.V. Mosby Co., 1971)*

tic of pleomorphic adenomas is their nodular outline; though most frequently rounded hummocks, the outgrowths may be pedunculated and form peninsulas with narrow necks.[28]

Treatment and Prognosis. Surgical excision is the primary treatment of pleomorphic adenomas of the parotid. The extent of the excision recommended ranges from careful local excision[3] to removal of at least the entire involved lobe.[26] Simple enucleation of these tumors cannot be recommended. There may be a well-marked plane of cleavage between the gland and tumor in most areas, but in at least some interface areas, the plane of cleavage may lie just below the surface of the tumor.[28] Additionally, the viable nests of tumor tissue within the capsule and the tumor's peninsular outgrowths may be surgically left behind.

Treatment of this neoplasm in the submandibular and sublingual glands is usually total glandular excision.

Pleomorphic adenomas of the minor salivary glands are usually treated somewhat more conservatively. The removal of the neoplasm along with a margin of surrounding normal tissue is adequate.[26,29]

In the past, recurrences following "shelling out" of the tumor were frequent. With more radical surgical procedures, the recurrence rate has dropped to less than 1 percent.[10]

Recurrences may result from incomplete initial removal. Recurrent lesions are invariably multifocal; this apparently is due to a "seeding" of some of the cells during removal or to leaving behind the nests that are contained within the capsule. These recurrences may occur as late as 47 years following initial treatment.[26] There seems to be no increased danger of malignant change with recurrence.[10]

This tumor is radio-resistant; the use of irradiation in its treatment is therefore contraindicated.

ADENOLYMPHOMA (WARTHIN'S TUMOR, CYSTADENOMA LYMPHOMATOSUM)

The adenolymphoma is the most common of the monomorphic adenomas. (Monomorphic adenomas are distinguished from pleomorphic adenomas by their uniform cell structure and pattern.) *Clinical Features.* This tumor is found most frequently in the parotid gland in a superficial location especially at the lower pole.[3] It is the only salivary gland tumor to be frequently found bilaterally, with estimates ranging from 3 to 30 percent.[10] It may also arise multifocally. This tumor has been reported in the submandibular and sublingual glands and in minor glands of the lips, buccal mucosa, palate, and maxillary sinus.

Males over middle age are most commonly affected; this represents a departure from other salivary gland tumors which more often affect females.

Adenolymphomas are generally superficial and seldom attain a size exceeding 3 to 4 cm in diameter. They are slow growing, painless, and firm to palpation; as such, they may be clinically indistinguishable from other benign salivary neoplasms.

Histologic Features. The adenolymphoma has a distinctive histologic appearance; there are two components, epithelial and lymphoid (Fig. 15-43). The epithelium usually takes the form of columnar or cuboidal cells, most often in two layers. This epithelium forms papillary projections into cystic spaces. The lymphoid component is usually abundant and is composed of mature and normally developing lymphocytes. Germinal centers are common. It

seems likely that this tumor arises from residues of salivary duct epithelium included within lymph nodes. These nodes probably become entrapped in the parotid due to the late encapsulation of the gland during development. The lymphoid component, therefore, may represent a passive element in the neoplastic process.

Treatment and Prognosis. Treatment of this neoplasm consists of surgical excision; the tumor does not tend to recur. This excision can usually be accomplished without damage to adjacent structures because of the tumor's superficial location and small size.

OXYPHILIC ADENOMA (ONCOCYTOMA)

The oxyphilic adenoma is a rare salivary gland neoplasm. It constitutes less than 1 percent of parotid gland neoplasms.[10]

Clinical Features. This neoplasm is a slow-growing, small tumor that usually occurs in the parotid. Its presence in other locations has been documented.[10] Women are more often affected with this tumor, usually within the seventh decade of life or later. It usually appears as a discrete, firm, freely mobile, small, encapsulated mass.

Histologic Features. "Oncocytoma" is derived from the resemblance of the tumor

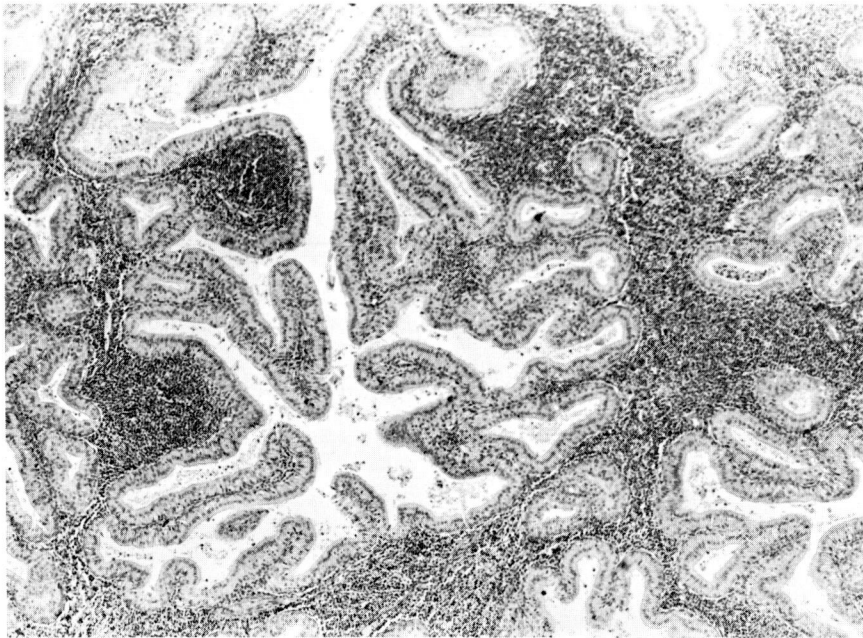

FIG. 15-43. *Photomicrograph of adenolymphoma or Warthin's tumor.*

cells to oncocytes. (Oncocytes are cells normally found within the salivary ducts of elderly persons; they may be a normal consequence of the aging process.) The cells of the oxyphilic adenoma are uniformly large eosinophilic granular cells arranged in rows, cords, sheets, or an alveolar pattern. *Treatment and Prognosis.* Treatment of oxyphilic adenoma is through complete surgical removal. The tumor has exhibited no tendency to recur.

NECROTIZING SIALOMETAPLASIA

Necrotizing sialometaplasia has been classed as a benign inflammatory condition of minor salivary glands. It is included here because of its close resemblance to more serious entities. The first report of this condition by Abrams and associates[30] appeared in 1973. Since that time, additional cases have been reported.[31] This entity must be considered unusual, but the consequences of its misdiagnosis warrant its discussion.

Clinical Features. This entity usually occurs on the posterior palate; other areas, however, such as the retromolar pad, labial glands, nasal cavity, and maxillary sinuses have been involved. Although the disease seems to be most prevalent in white middle-aged males, it has been reported in patients ranging from age 18 to old age.

This lesion usually presents as a painful ulceration which may present rolled borders and may measure up to 3 cm in diameter (Fig. 15-44).

Histologic Features. The associated epithelium exhibits hyperkeratosis and marked pseudoepitheliomatous hyperplasia. The underlying salivary gland ducts exhibit extensive squamous metaplasia. These underlying masses of squamous epithelium may be closely associated with or directly connected to the overlying epithelium, possibly giving the impression histologically of infiltration from a surface squamous cell carcinoma (Fig. 15-45). The underlying minor salivary gland regions may show areas of mucous escape and pooling with a subsequent foreign body reaction.

The cause of necrotizing sialometaplasia is unclear. The basic lesion seems to be a vascular infarction with subsequent ulceration and repair. The basis for this vascular alteration is unknown.

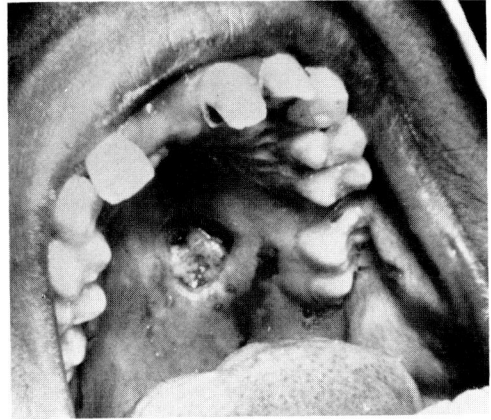

Fig. 15-44. *Necrotizing sialometaplasia may clinically appear malignant. Note the deep ulceration and rolled borders. (Courtesy of Dr. A.M. Abrams and Dr. V.J. Castaldo)*

Treatment and Prognosis. The treatment of this condition consists of recognizing its true benign nature. All reported cases have healed in 6 to 8 weeks without treatment. Recurrence has not been noted.

Malignant Neoplasms

MALIGNANT MIXED TUMOR (MALIGNANT PLEOMORPHIC ADENOMA)

This is a rather ill-defined neoplasm. Because of a lack of precise criteria for establishing a diagnosis of this neoplasm, its frequency in surveys has varied considerably.[10] Estimates suggest that it comprises approximately 3 to 5 percent of all salivary gland tumors and from 7 to 20 percent of all malignant salivary tumors.

It is uncertain whether these tumors represent originally benign neoplasms that have undergone transformation into malignant types or if they are malignant from the outset.

Clinical Features. The clinical differences between benign and malignant pleomorphic adenomas are slight. There may be fixation of the malignant tumor to overlying skin or mucosa or underlying structures. Surface ulceration and pain may be a more frequent complaint in the malignant than in the benign lesion.

Most of these neoplasms are found in the parotid; occasionally they manifest in the submandibular or minor salivary glands. Most of these tumors have been

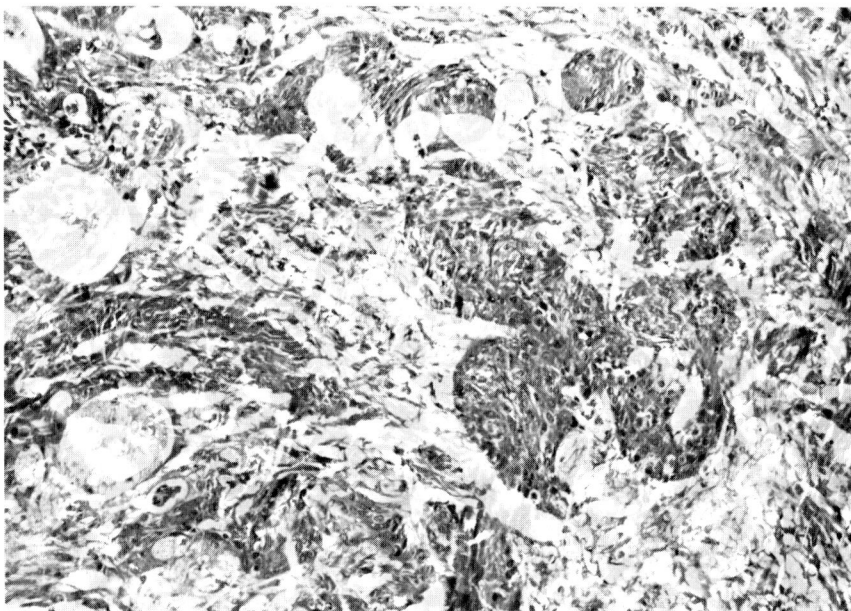

FIG. 15-45. *Photomicrograph of necrotizing sialometaplasia. Epithelial islands represent salivary gland ducts in the connective tissue that have undergone extensive squamous metaplasia. These ductal changes bear strong resemblance to squamous cell carcinoma. (Courtesy of Dr. A.M. Abrams)*

found in males between 40 and 50 years of age.

Histologic Features. The histologic variations of this tumor are numerous. In some tumors, the benign component may predominate with only a small area demonstrating evidence of malignancy (nuclear hyperchromatism and pleomorphism, increased or abnormal mitosis, increased nuclear/cytoplasmic ratio, focal necrosis, and invasion with destruction of normal tissue). In other tumors, the malignant component may almost completely overgrow the benign areas.

The microscopic criteria for malignant pleomorphic adenoma are essentially those utilized in the diagnosis of a benign pleomorphic adenoma coupled with the identification of malignant tumor regions.

Treatment and Prognosis. The treatment of malignant pleomorphic adenoma is surgical. These neoplasms exhibit a high rate of recurrence as well as regional lymph node involvement and distant metastases.

MUCOEPIDERMOID CARCINOMA

The mucoepidermoid carcinoma was originally considered a variant of pleomorphic adenoma. It has now come to be con-sidered a separate entity. This tumor represents approximately 3 to 11 percent of all salivary gland tumors.[10] Eversole,[32] in 1970, reviewed the English literature regarding this tumor. Of 815 reported cases, approximately 70 percent were found in the major glands.

The mucoepidermoid carcinoma represents the most common malignant tumor of the major salivary glands.

Clinical and histological experience have led most investigators to separate these neoplasms into those of low-grade or high-grade malignancy. These degrees of malignancy represent differences in clinical behavior, recurrence, and histology.

Clinical Features. Of the major glands, the parotid is the most commonly involved. The most commonly involved minor glands are those of the palate.

These tumors are most frequently diagnosed in persons between the third and sixth decade of life. No significant difference occurs between the sexes.

The tumor of low-grade malignancy usually presents as a soft, slowly growing, painless mass. This mass rarely exceeds 5 cm in diameter. The mass is frequently cystic, containing pools of viscid, mucoid material.

The tumor of high-grade malignancy may present a different clinical history. It grows rapidly and pain is frequently an early symptom. On palpation, the high-grade tumor feels firm; cystic spaces are less frequent.

Histologic Features. Low-grade mucoepidermoid carcinomas are characterized by mucous and epidermal cells whose architectural arrangement is characterized by duct and cyst formation (Fig. 15-46). An intermediate cell type has been described; this cell is thought to represent a transitional type.

High-grade mucoepidermoid carcinomas are characterized by epidermoid and intermediate cell types; the mucous cell is not prominent. Cysts and ductal elements are usually missing and frank histologic evidence of malignancy is present.

Neither of these variants exhibit encapsulation.

Treatment and Prognosis. Treatment of both high-grade and low-grade mucoepidermoid carcinoma is surgical excision. Local excision has proven adequate for those neoplasms of low-grade malignancy, provided that histologic confirmation of complete removal is obtained.[33] Adequate treatment of high-grade tumors includes wide excision of the tumor, overlying mucosa, and a margin of surrounding normal tissues.[29]

Generally, recurrences are much more common with tumors of high-grade malignancy.[10] Intraoral tumors (those of the accessory salivary glands) generally show a poorer prognosis than those of the parotid.[32]

Because of the differing treatments and prognosis of these tumor types, the clinician must discuss individual cases of this neoplasm with the pathologist.

ACINIC CELL CARCINOMA

The acinic cell carcinoma is a moderately malignant tumor. It constitutes approximately 2 percent of all salivary gland tumors. Prior to 1953, this tumor was considered benign; clinical experience regarding its recurrence rate and metastatic potential, however, demonstrates its malignancy.

Clinical Features. Although this tumor is almost exclusively limited to the parotid gland, it has also been reported in the sublingual gland and in the floor of the

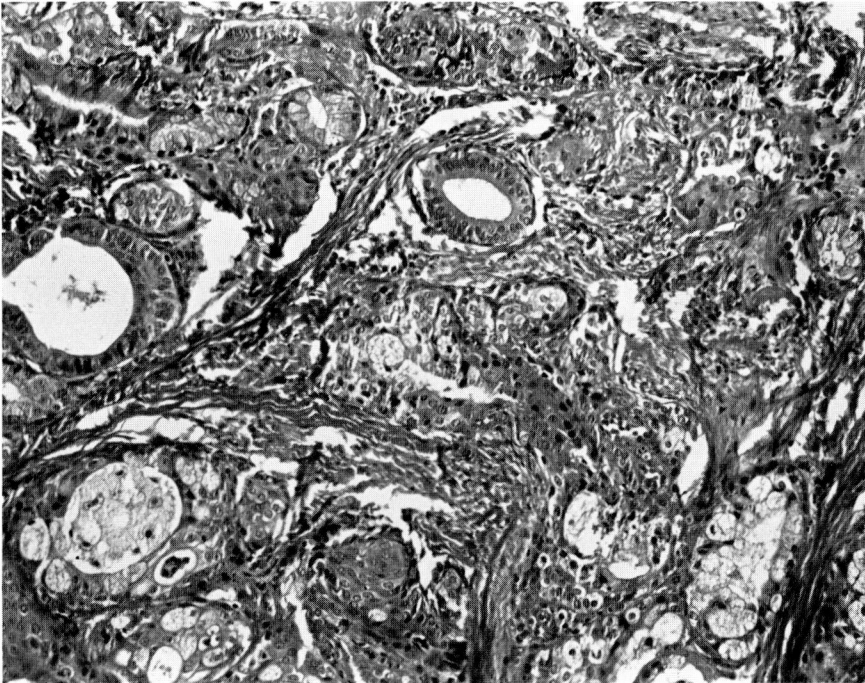

Fig. 15-46. *Photomicrograph of a low-grade mucoepidermopid carcinoma. Note the epidermoid cells, the duct formation, and the mucus accumulation.*

mouth. Usually occurring in persons at or over middle age, it has been described in children.

The clinical appearance resembles that of the pleomorphic adenoma; usually presenting as a small, round, encapsulated mass. Only rarely is there associated pain or facial nerve paralysis. On palpation, the tumor feels firm and may or may not exhibit fixation to surrounding tissue.

Histologic Features. This tumor consists essentially of solid epithelial sheets of round or polygonal cells. Glandular structures are frequently present. Cellular cytoplasm is granular and usually basophilic, thus bearing a strong resemblance to the normal serous acinar cells (Fig. 15-47).

Treatment and Prognosis. The accepted treatment of acinic cell carcinoma is surgical excision; a margin of surrounding tissue should be included. The recurrence rate of this tumor may reach as high as 50 percent.[10]

ADENOID CYSTIC CARCINOMA (CYLINDROMA)

The adenoid cystic carcinoma, first described by Billroth in 1859, represents the second most common tumor of the minor salivary glands. (The pleomorphic adenoma is the most common.) The adenoid cystic carcinoma is the most common *malignant* tumor of the minor salivary glands. Totally, this tumor represents about 2 to 4 percent of all salivary gland tumors.

Clinical Features. The adenoid cystic carcinoma is found over a wide distribution; the minor glands are involved in about 70 percent of cases and the major glands in about 28 percent.[34,35] The palate is the most frequent site of tumor formation.

This tumor occurs more frequently in women when the major glands are considered, but shows no sex predilection when minor gland frequency is considered.[34] It most frequently arises in patients between 40 and 80 years of age.

The cylindroma tends to present as a firm mass, thereby resembling the pleomorphic adenoma, but may be more adherent to surrounding tissues. Pain is a prominent feature in the early stages.[34,36] Ulceration may be present.[34] The frequent and early association with pain has been attributed to this tumor's apparent tendency to perineural or intraneural invasion.[37] Eby and associates,[36] however, found no correlation between pain and perineural extension. Paresthesia has fre-

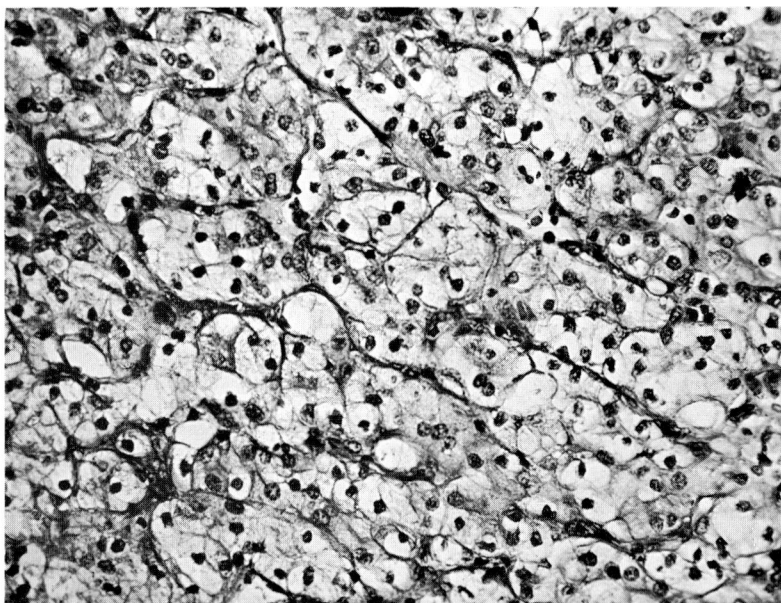

FIG. 15-47. *Photomicrograph of acinic cell carcinoma. Note tumor cells with granular cytoplasm. Mucus is not produced by this tumor. (Courtesy of Dr. D.E. Waite)*

quently been associated with this neoplasm.

Histologic Features. The adenoid cystic carcinoma is composed of small cells with darkly staining nuclei and scant cytoplasm (Fig. 15-48). These cells are usually arranged in a "swiss cheese" or cylindromatous pattern (hence the term "cylindroma"). Occasionally, the tumor cells may form solid sheets showing no cylindromatous pattern. This solid pattern may be associated with a poorer prognosis;[34,36] few pathologists, however, accept this correlation without some qualifications. The tumor cells are usually surrounded by varying amounts of connective tissue that may range from a hyaline to a myxoid composition.[35]

Treatment and Prognosis. The treatment of this tumor is surgical excision; radiation treatment has been successfully coupled with surgery. Conley and Dingman maintain that the most extensive surgical procedure that can be rationally developed is best; the inability to evaluate the perimeters of this tumor clinically dictates that a bold surgical approach should be the primary objective.[38]

This radical treatment notwithstanding, the prognosis of this tumor is poor. The adenoid cystic carcinoma exhibits a marked tendency to recur and metastasize to lymph nodes, lungs, bones, and liver. Metastasis seems to be a natural function of the neoplasm; slow in appearance and unpredictable in growth rate. Clinical experience indicates that the prognosis depends somewhat upon the location of the original tumor site; when the primary tumor is on the palate the prognosis is best, when the submandibular gland is involved primarily, the prognosis is poorest.[39,40] The late appearance of metastatic spread becomes apparent when one examines the cure rate; one study showed a 5-year cure rate of 6 percent.[35]

Salivary Gland Neoplasms in Children

Salivary gland neoplasms are more uncommon in children than adults. From 1 to 5 percent of all salivary gland tumors are found in persons under 17 years of age.[10,41]

The most frequent salivary gland neoplasm of children is the hemangioma. The pleomorphic adenoma is the most frequent

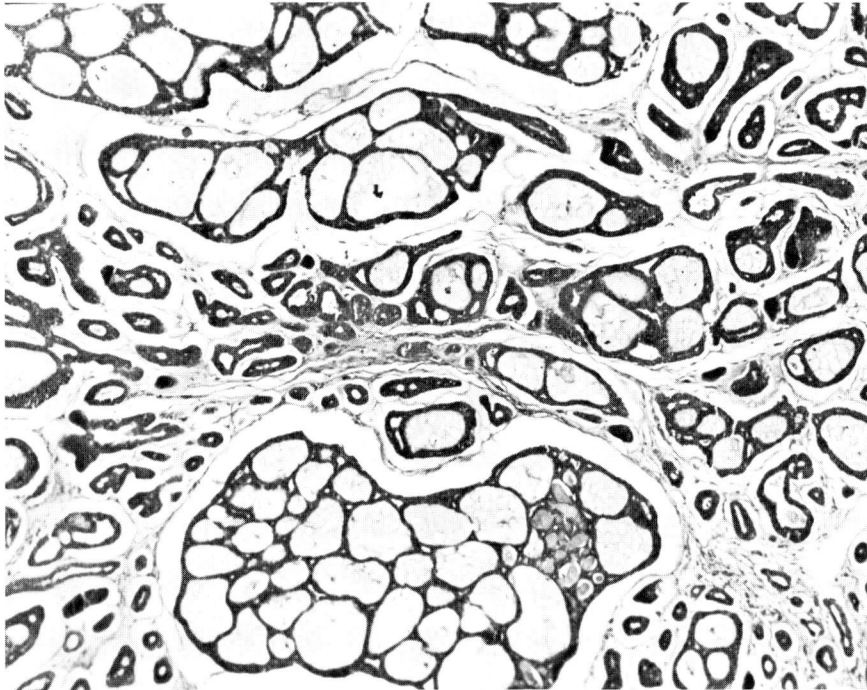

FIG. 15-48. *Photomicrograph of adenoid cystic carcinoma. (Courtesy of Dr. D.E. Waite)*

benign salivary gland tumor, while muco-epidermoid carcinoma is the most frequent malignant tumor.

HEMANGIOMA

The hemangioma usually occurs superficially in the parotid region and is usually noted within the first 6 months of life. It most commonly affects females and enlarges rapidly.

Histologic Features. As is generally the case with hemangiomas, two microscopic forms are distinguishable in children (1) the capillary type, composed of numerous small blood channels, and (2) the cavernous type, composed of large endothelial-lined, blood-filled spaces. These spaces exhibit a tendency to undergo spontaneous sclerosis and phlebolith formation. (A phlebolith is an organized coagulum which becomes calcified.)

Diagnostic Aids. Since these lesions are nearly always superficial, the diagnosis is easily made with a clinical examination and patient history. O'Riordan[42] published an article dealing with the differential diagnosis between swellings due to obstructive salivary gland disease and hemangiomas.

Plain radiology is useful in the diagnosis of hemangioma; a soft tissue mass with contained calcifications (phleboliths) may be noted. Sialography or CT scans may be useful to determine the extent of involvement of the glandular parenchyma.

Not infrequently, these phleboliths are the only residual sign in the adult of an early hemangioma; they are frequently misdiagnosed as sialoliths. Rauch and associates[10] and O'Riordan[42] listed diagnostic criteria that aid in distinguishing between residual phleboliths and sialoliths.

Treatment. The treatment of choice for these neoplasms is surgical excision if the lesion does not regress spontaneously by the age of 5 years or if the neoplasm arises late in childhood.[43]

PLEOMORPHIC ADENOMA AND

MUCOEPIDERMOID CARCINOMA

The incidence of pleomorphic adenomas in children appears to be lower than in adults. Mucoepidermoid carcinomas appear five times more frequently in children than in adults, but their course is more benign.[10] In general, salivary gland tumors

in children have a more benign course than in adults. The clinical and histologic description as well as the treatment for these neoplasms have been discussed earlier and will not be repeated here.

General Comments

As a conclusion to this section on salivary gland neoplasms, several general considerations need to be presented.

Eneroth, in his study of over 2500 salivary gland tumors, found the most common sites of occurrence to be the parotid, submandibular, and minor salivary glands of the palate; these locations account for 95 percent of all salivary gland tumors. A palpable lesion in the parotid or submandibular gland is generally a true salivary gland tumor, in the parotid, this is true in 95 percent and in the submandibular gland, 84 percent of the cases.[39,40] In the palate, only 46 percent of all tumors are true salivary gland tumors.

Of this total number of salivary gland tumors, 20 to 25 percent of parotid tumors and 40 to 60 percent of submandibular and minor gland tumors are malignant.

Malignant salivary gland neoplasms in the submandibular gland deserve special mention. They behave more aggressively than in other salivary gland systems[44] and tend to invade the parapharyngeal space and related structures, the posterior third of the tongue, and the pillars of the anterior fauces. Involvement of the soft palate and the palatal arches is also common.[2] Aggressive treatment of these neoplasms has been described; glandular resection with a frozen diagnosis—if the neoplasm proves to be malignant, an augmented local resection and composite resection is recommended.[44]

Clinically, all salivary gland neoplasms most frequently present as painless masses; ulceration is rarely present. The duration of symptoms prior to initial presentation may be lengthy; symptom duration of 3 years or more has been reported. Patients frequently present for treatment following a recent increase in size of a long-standing swelling.

Sialography has a limited use in the diagnosis of tumors of the salivary glands. This examination method may show ductal displacement or a nonopacified area in glandular parenchyma caused by a space occupying lesion. Amputation or encasement of salivary ductules may be evident with an invasive neoplasm. Intrinsic salivary gland tumors may show retention of contrast media in postevaluation films whereas extrinsic tumors near salivary glands allow complete emptying of the ductal system following gland stimulation.

Because scintigraphy provides information about the functional and pathologic state of the salivary glands, it may permit characterization of salivary gland neoplasia. Experience indicates that adenolymphomas (Wharton's tumor) tend to manifest as "hot" in that the neoplasm tends to accumulate the isotope to a greater degree than normal glandular tissue. Other neoplasms, however, tend to present as clear "cold" areas. Scintigraphy, when used to complement sialographic findings, may provide much diagnostic information.[45]

Coupled with clinical information, CT scans provide reliable differentiation between normal tissue and areas of inflammation or neoplasia. CT scans may also help to determine the anatomic relation of a lesion to the facial nerve or to other adjacent structures. Computed tomography may be the diagnostic procedure of choice in evaluating salivary gland neoplasia.

Salivary Gland Swelling— Differential Diagnosis

When a patient presents with apparent enlargement of one or more salivary glands, certain aspects of differential diagnosis must be considered. The following paragraphs discuss conditions that may mimic enlargement of the salivary glands. These conditions must be considered along with disease states such as sialadenitis, sialolithiasis, sialadenosis, neoplasms, etc., that are discussed elsewhere.

LYMPHADENOPATHY

Lymph nodes lie in close association with salivary gland tissue in several areas; enlargement of these nodes can be confused with salivary gland swellings.

The outer surface of the parotid gland is intimately associated with lymph nodes in the preauricular and lower pole areas of the gland. Inflamed preauricular nodes can be differentiated from partial parotid infection because the parotid's upper pole usually does not become infected by itself; examination should be made for sources of infection on the face or temple. The cause of lymphadenopathy of the lower pole nodes may be less obvious; these nodes drain the tonsilar regions. It should be remembered that an obstruction in the intraglandular portion of Stensen's duct may cause swelling of the lower pole only; plain radiology sialography or CT scans may be useful in this instance.[14]

Lymph nodes are also found along the lower border of the mandible on the superficial portion of the submandibular gland. Lymphadenopathy of these nodes must be distinguished from submandibular gland involvement. These lymph nodes are usually more inferior and further from the midline than the submandibular gland. These respective locations can usually be distinguished with bimanual palpation.

CELLULITIS

Sublingual cellulitis of dental origin may be confused with an infection of the submandibular gland. This cellulitis may present with swollen sublingual plica and a prominent submandibular duct papilla. If the salivary gland is involved, purulent material can be milked from the duct. If the salivary flow is clear, the possibility of a periodontal abscess or radicular infection of a mandibular tooth should be investigated.[14]

ANATOMIC ABNORMALITIES

Unilateral or bilateral masseteric hypertrophy may be confused with parotid gland enlargement. This condition (Fig. 15-49) is not uncommon; it may be inherited. Palpation reveals a soft mass with no distinct border that parallels the course and extent of the masseter muscle. This mass increases in size and hardens greatly with occlusion. This condition usually exhibits characteristic changes on the radiograph: the area of the mandibular masseteric attachment is enlarged.

Rarely, an apparent parotid mass between the mastoid process and the angle of the mandible may be caused by a prominent transverse process of the atlas. Radiographs are useful in establishing this diagnosis.[46]

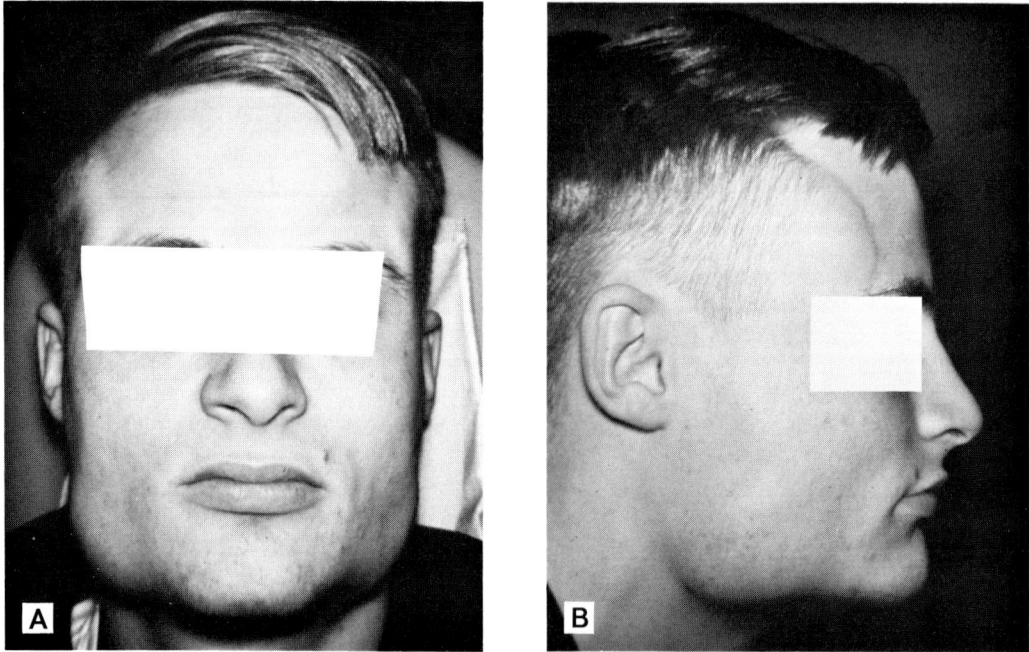

FIG. 15-49. *Bilateral masseteric hypertrophy. (A) Frontal view (compare FIG. 15-4). (B) Lateral view. Note enlargement of masseter and temporalis muscles. Radiographically, the patient's mandibular angle was enlarged.*

Complications of Salivary Gland or Associated Surgery

As has been previously noted, surgical excision is the treatment of choice for many salivary gland neoplasms and obstructions. This section deals with the most common complications of these procedures as well as those arising from surgical procedures in close proximity to salivary structures.

DUCTAL STRICTURE

Salivary duct stricture may occur following a surgical biopsy or other surgical procedure near Wharton's or Stensen's duct or their orifices. Strictures also occur following transverse incisions through a ductal wall. Clinical symptoms caused by salivary duct strictures have been discussed in the section on obstructive salivary gland problems.

Frequently, a mild stricture due to wound scarring or inflammation may be treated with the administration of a sialogogue. Strictures close to the duct opening may be treated by papillectomy, and those along the ductal course may be treated success-fully by a surgical repositioning of the ductal orifice. In this procedure, the duct is isolated, sectioned proximally to the stricture, and the distal end of the proximal section repositioned to a new surgically created opening. Ductal strictures close to the gland require gland removal. Strictures of the parotid duct can usually be treated by mechanical dilation of the duct at several day intervals over a 2-week period. This procedure, however, may afford only temporary remission.

FISTULAS

A salivary fistula is an abnormal pathway through which saliva exits to the skin or mucosal surface. These may be congenital in origin, may result from ulceration caused by ductal calculi, or from surgery on the gland or duct proper.

External fistulae present as draining tracts on the skin surface; they are obviously troublesome to the patient. Swelling may accompany the condition. Internal fistulae, since they discharge the saliva into the oral cavity, usually present no symptoms; treatment, therefore, is rarely necessary.

Treatment of salivary fistulas is usually with surgical repair, ductal ligation (with subsequent glandular atrophy), or glandular excision.

FACIAL NERVE PARESIS

Not uncommonly following a major surgical procedure on the parotid gland, temporary or permanent paresis of the facial nerve occurs.[3] This temporary paresis probably results from a decrease in the conductivity of the nerve secondary to repeated stimulation during the surgery and to postoperative edema. Permanent facial nerve paralysis produces serious results; treatment is necessary and complex.

Allied Conditions

In addition to the specific disease entities affecting the salivary glands proper such as sialolithiasis and neoplasms, certain other conditions affect the salivary glands and other organ systems. Some of these have been discussed earlier (see sialadenosis); this section discusses Sjögren's syndrome, sarcoidosis, and Mikulicz's disease.

SJÖGREN'S SYNDROME (GOUGEROT-SJÖGREN SYNDROME)

In 1933, Sjögren described a symptom complex of keratoconjunctivitis sicca, pharyngolaryngitis sicca, rhinitis sicca, polyarthritis, enlargement of the parotid glands, and xerostomia. Since the first description of Sjögren's syndrome, much investigative inquiry has taken place. It is now thought that this disease occurs in two forms—primary, which involves the exocrine glands only and secondary, associated with a definable autoimmune disease.

Primary Sjögren's syndrome consists of chronic inflammation of the lacrimal and salivary glands leading to dryness of the eye (keratoconjunctivitis sicca), dryness of the mouth (xerostomia), and in a variable number of patients, lacrimal and/or salivary enlargement. This symptom complex has been termed the "sicca syndrome." Secondary Sjögren's syndrome involves the exocrine gland changes associated with an autoimmune disease, primarily rheumatoid arthritis, and systemic lupus erythematosus.

Clinical Features. This disease is usually seen in females 50 years of age or older. It frequently presents with an insidious development of the "sicca syndrome" in a patient with a prior history of rheumatic arthritis. Patients may complain of a dryness and burning sensation of the eyes; xerostomia; and nasal, pharyngeal, vaginal, and vulvar dryness. Salivary gland enlargement is clinically variable; usually the parotid is involved bilaterally. This involvement, however, may only be clinically apparent in 15 percent of the cases.[3] Xerostomia may present with the clinical features common to this disorder as has been discussed earlier (Fig. 15-50).

Sjögren's syndrome usually manifests a remarkable prevalence of abnormal immunological features. Patients with primary Sjögren's syndrome tend to manifest nonorgan-specific autoantibodies but not antisalivary duct antibodies or rheumatoid factor. Patients with secondary Sjögren's are positive for the organ-specific antisalivary duct antibody and rheumatoid factor while manifesting few, if any, nonorgan-specific autoantibodies.

Histologic Features. Microscopically, this disease is characterized by a focal lymphocytic sialadenitis of the salivary glands in approximately 70 percent of the patients.[3]

Initially infiltration of lymphocytes and plasma cells occurs about the interlobular and centroacinar ducts. Finally, the lymphoreticular tissue overgrows the parenchyma, so that only ducts or their remnants may be found.[10] Microscopic changes may be evident in all the salivary tissue (both major and minor glands); the clinical significance of this is discussed later.

In addition to the inflammatory infiltrate in the salivary tissue, a type of epithelial proliferation may be present. This proliferation may be that of the myoepithelial cells only, or it may consist of both cell layers of the terminal salivary duct.[10]

Diagnostic Aids. A clinical examination and patient history must be accomplished to rule out other causes of salivary gland enlargement or xerostomia.

Sialography may be of use in the diagnosis of Sjögren's syndrome; the hydrostatic technique has been recommended.[3] Varying degrees of sialectasis ("bunch of grapes") appearance are consistent findings.

Scintigraphy appears to have considerable value in the assessment of salivary

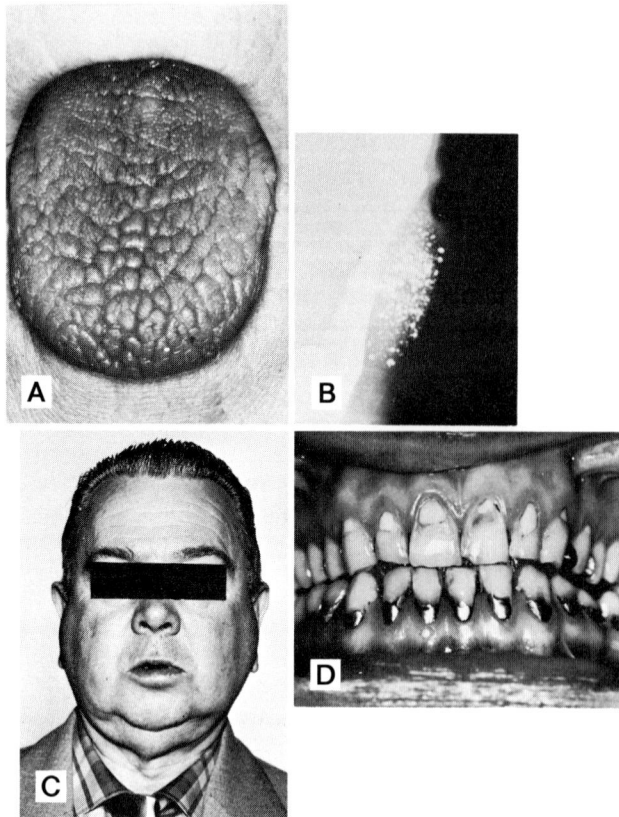

FIG. 15-50. *Sjögren's syndrome. (A) Appearance of tongue. (B) Sialogram. (C) Salivary gland enlargement. (D) Evidence of cervical caries due to xerostomia. (Bertram, U.: Xerostomia. Clinical aspects, pathology and pathogenesis. Acta Odontol. Scand. (Suppl. 49), 25: 1–126, 1967)*

gland involvement in Sjögren's syndrome. The uptake of the radioactive compound^{99m}Tc pertechnetate has been shown to be reduced in patients with Sjögren's syndrome. This method of examination may represent a safe, objective means of evaluating salivary gland involvement in this disease.

Minor salivary gland biopsy has also shown much promise in the diagnosis of Sjögren's syndrome. Focal lymphocytic sialadenitis has been demonstrated in approximately 70 percent of patients with Sjögren's syndrome. The changes manifest in the minor salivary gland tissue are reflected in the major salivary glands. This minor gland biopsy technique affords, therefore, a safe, accessible method of determining salivary gland involvement (Fig. 15-51). This minor salivary gland tissue may be taken from anywhere within the oral cavity; the inner aspect of the lower lip or the palate are common sites.

Treatment. Sjögren's syndrome has shown remarkable resistance to successful treatment. A broad, symptomatic treatment is usually employed and aimed at the multisystem symptoms of the disease. Oral treatment consists of measures to keep the oral mucous membranes moist. Sialogogues such as sour, sugarless candy work well. Patients should be encouraged to increase their fluid intake with frequent sips of water.

Because the patient with Sjögren's syndrome is especially susceptible to infections such as candidiasis, frequent patient monitoring and prompt adequate treatment of these infections are necessary.

The patient should be instructed and followed in methods of proper oral hygiene. Drugs that tend to cause xerostomia should be avoided.

Complications. Clinical and pathologic evidence seems to indicate that a patient with this disease may tend to develop extra

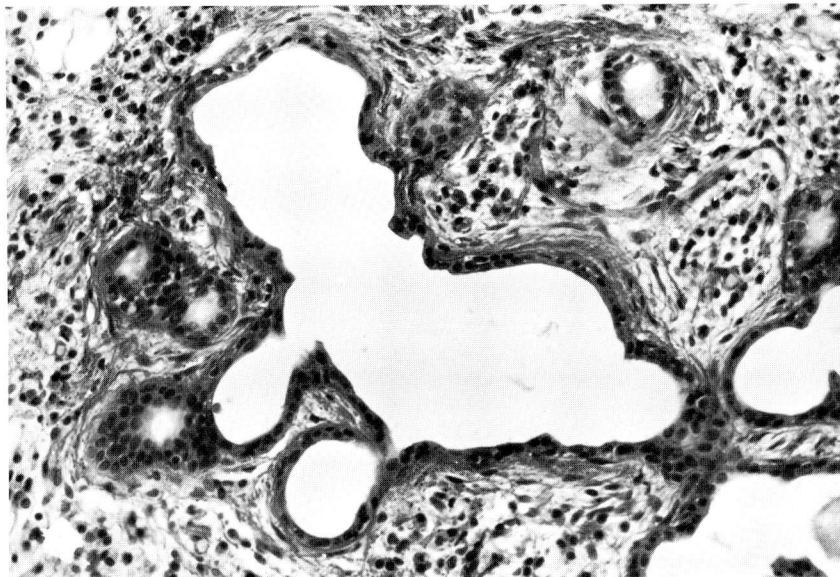

FIG. 15-51. *Photomicrograph of minor salivary glands of lip of patient with Sjögren's syndrome. Ductal dilatation with minute sacculations is apparent in addition to chronic inflammation of stromal areas. (Courtesy of Dr. D.E. Waite)*

salivary lymphoid abnormalities, including lymphoreticular malignancies such as malignant lymphomas.[10] Persons with Sjögren's syndrome, therefore, should be followed with suitable blood studies to detect early change from the benign course.

SARCOIDOSIS

This generalized disease was first described by Hutchinson in 1875. The condition was originally known as "Mortimer's Malady" after the name of Hutchinson's patient. Sarcoidosis is a systemic granulomatous disease of undetermined etiology. Lesions of sarcoidosis may involve any body site; the salivary glands are involved in from 3 to 10 percent of the cases.[47]

Clinical Features. Most patients are young and middle-aged adults; no sex difference has been observed. The most common manifestation of this disease is the cutaneous lesion. These lesions are multiple, raised red patches that occur in groups and enlarge slowly. Ulceration or crusting of these cutaneous lesions are uncommon.

Salivary gland involvement, when present, manifests as hard, painless, slow enlargement of usually the parotid glands. Involvement of other salivary tissue usually follows. Xerostomia may be present.

An acute manifestation of systemic sar-

coidosis that affects the parotid glands and uveal tracts of the eyes (uveoparotitis) is termed Heerfordt's syndrome. This manifestation occurs in only 2 to 3 percent of patients with sarcoidosis.

Histologic Features. The characteristic feature of this disease is the formation of noncaseating granulomas. These granulomas are composed of epithelioid cells, macrophages, multinucleated giant cells, and occasional eosinophils. No acid-fast organisms can be demonstrated, this being one of the few distinguishing features allowing differentiation from the granuloma of tuberculosis.

Diagnostic Aids. The diagnosis of sarcoid sialadenitis is based on the history, the presence of salivary gland symptoms such as asialia and enlargement, and positive results from other systemic tests.

Sialography may show slight changes only, since there are no gross changes in glandular ducts or parenchyma.

Minor salivary gland biopsy has been shown to be of some value in the diagnosis of sarcoidosis.[47] As in the case with Sjögren's syndrome, these minor salivary glands lend themselves to safe, uncomplicated diagnostic biopsies.

Treatment Specific treatment for sarcoidosis is unknown; cortisone therapy has been useful in the treatment of Heerfordt's syndrome.

MIKULICZ'S DISEASE (LYMPHOEPITHELIAL LESION)

In 1888, Von Mikulicz described a case of asymptomatic symmetrical enlargement of the salivary and lacrimal glands. Since that time, much confusion has existed concerning the true nature of this condition. There is increasing evidence that this disease is closely related to Sjögren's syndrome and that both are autoimmune diseases.[27]

Clinical Features. This disease manifests as a unilateral or bilateral enlargement of the parotid or submandibular glands. This glandular enlargement is diffuse and poorly outlined. Pain and xerostomia are occasionally present.

Histologic Features. This disease is characterized by lymphocytic infiltration of the salivary gland tissue. The acini are destroyed; islands of epithelial cells remain. This remaining epithelium may exhibit ductal formation or may form solid nests of poorly defined cells.

Treatment and Complications. Surgical excision and radiation treatments have been used with success in the treatment of this condition. Since this condition usually follows a benign course, conservative treatment is probably preferred.

Reports of malignant evolution of benign lymphoepithelial lesions with the formation of extrasalivary lymphoproliferative diseases and salivary carcinomas have been noted.[3,48] This would indicate that patients with this condition be reviewed on a regular basis and that irradiation as a treatment modality is contraindicated.

References

1. Schneyer, L. H., and Levin, L. K.: Rate of secretion by exogenously stimulated salivary gland pairs in man. J. Appl. Physiol., 7:609, 1955.
2. Batsakis, J. J.: Neoplasms of the minor and lesser major salivary glands. Surg. Gynecol. Obstet., 135:289, 1972.
3. Mason, D. K., and Chisholm, D. M.: Salivary Glands in Health and Disease. London, W. B. Saunders Co., Ltd., 1975.
4. Waite, D. E.: Secretory sialography of the salivary glands. Oral Surg., 27:635, 1969.
5. Yune, H. Y., and Klatte, E. C.: Current status of sialography. Am. J. Roentgenol., Radium Ther. Nucl. Med., 115:420, 1972.
6. Blair, G. S.: Hydrostatic sialography. Oral Surg., 36:116, 1973.
7. Pappas, G. C., and Wallace, W. R.: Panoramic sialography. Dent. Radiogr. Photogr., 43:27, 1970.
8. Eneroth, C. M., Franzen, S., and Zajicek, J.: Cytologic diagnosis on aspirate from 1000 salivary gland tumors. Acta Otolaryngol. (Suppl.), 224:168, 1967.
9. Spiro, R. H., Huvos, A. G., and Strong, E. W.: Cancer of the parotid gland. Am. J. Surg., 130:452, 1975.
10. Rauch, S., Gorlin, R. J., and Seifert, G.: Diseases of the salivary glands. In Thoma's Oral Pathology, 6th ed., Vol. 2. St. Louis, C. V. Mosby Co., 1970.
11. Chisholm, D. M., and Mason, D. K.: Salivary gland disease. Br. Med. Bull., 31:156, 1975.
12. Robbins, S. L., Cotran, R. S., and Kumar, V.: Pathologic Basis of Disease. 3rd Ed. Philadelphia, W. B. Saunders Co., 1984.
13. Kashima, H. K., Kirkham, W. R., and Andrews, J. R.: Postirradiation sialadenitis. Am. J. Roentgenol., Radium Ther. Nucl. Med., 94:271, 1965.
14. Seward, G. R.: Anatomic surgery for salivary calculi, Part I. Oral Surg., 25:150, 1968.
15. Seward, G. R.: Anatomic surgery for salivary calculi, Part V. Oral Surg., 25:810, 1968.
16. Seward, G. R.: Anatomic surgery for salivary calculi, Part VI. Oral Surg., 26:1, 1968.
17. Seward, G. R.: Anatomic surgery for salivary calculi, Part III. Oral Surg., 25:525, 1968.
18. Seward, G. R.: Anatomic surgery for salivary calculi, Part II. Oral Surg., 25:287, 1968.
19. Moose, S. M.: Transoral surgical removal of a sialolith in the submandibular gland. Int. J. Oral Surg., 3:318, 1974.
20. Waterhouse, J. P., et al.: Replacement of functional parenchymal cells by fat and connective tissue in human submandibular salivary glands: An age-related change. J. Oral Path., 2:16, 1973.
21. Miller, A. S., and Winnick, M: Salivary gland inclusion in the anterior mandible. Oral Surg., 31:790, 1971.
22. Stafne, E. C.: Bone cavities situated near the angle of the mandible. JADA, 29:1969, 1942.
23. Tolman, D. E., and Stafne, E. C.: Developmental bone defects of the mandible. Oral Surg., 24:488, 1967.

24. Bertram, U.: Xerostomia, Acta Odont. Scand. (Suppl. 49), *25*:11, 1967.

25. Shannon, I. L., McCrary, B. R., and Starcke, E. N.: A saliva substitute for use by xerostomic patients undergoing radiotherapy to the head and neck. Oral Surg., *44*:656, 1977.

26. Krolls, S. O., and Boyers, R. C.: Mixed tumors of salivary glands. Cancer, *30*:276, 1972.

27. Shafer, W. G., Hine, M. K., and Levy, B. M.: A Textbook of Oral Pathology. 4th ed. Philadelphia, W. B. Saunders Co., 1983.

28. Patey, D. H., and Thackray, A. C.: The treatment of parotid tumors in the light of a pathological study of parotidectomy material. Br. J. Surg., *45*:477, 1958.

29. Chandhry, A. P., Vickers, R. A., and Gorlin, R. J.: Intra-oral minor salivary gland tumors. Oral Surg., *14*:1194, 1961.

30. Abrams, A. M., Melrose, R. J., and Howell, F. V.: Necrotizing sialometaplasia, Cancer, *32*:130, 1973.

31. Gahhos, F., Enriquez, R. E., Bahn, S. L., and Ariyan, S.: Necrotizing sialometaplasia: report of five cases. Plast. Reconstr. Surg., *71*:650, 1983.

32. Eversole, L. R.: Mucoepidermoid carcinoma. J. Oral Surg., *28*:490, 1970.

33. Eversole, L. R., Rovin, S., and Sabes, W. R.: Mucoepidermoid carcinoma of minor salivary glands: Report of 17 cases with follow-up. J. Oral Surg., *30*:107, 1972.

34. Tarpley, T. M., and Giansanti, J. S.: Adenoid cystic carcinoma. Oral Surg., *41*:484, 1976.

35. Spiro, R. H., Huvos, A. G., and Strong, E. W.: Adenoid cystic carcinoma of salivary origin. Am. J. Surg., *128*:512, 1974.

36. Eby, L. S., Johnson, D. S., and Baker, H. W.: Adenoid cystic carcinoma of the head and neck. Cancer, *29*:1160, 1972.

37. Berdal, P., deBesche, A., and Mylins, E.: Cylindroma of salivary glands. Acta Otolaryngol. (Suppl.), *263*:170, 1970.

38. Couley, J., and Dingham, D. L.: Adenoid cystic carcinoma in the head and neck. Acta Otolaryngol., *100:* 81, 1974.

39. Eneroth, C. M.: Incidence and prognosis of salivary gland tumors at different sites. Acta Otolaryngol., *263*:174, 1970.

40. Eneroth, C. M.: Salivary gland tumors in the parotid gland, submandibular gland, and the palate region. Cancer, *27*:1415, 1971.

41. Krolls, S. O., Trodahl, J. N., and Boyers, R. C.: Salivary gland lesions in children. Cancer, *30*:459, 1972.

42. O'Riordan, B.: Phleboliths and salivary calculi. Br. J. Oral Surg., *12*:119, 1974.

43. Hebert, G., Ouimet-Oliva, D., and Ladouceur, J.: Vascular tumors of the salivary glands in children. Am. J. Roentgenol., *123*:815, 1975.

44. Couley, J., Myers, E., and Cole, R.: Analysis of 115 patients with tumors of the submandibular gland. Ann. Otol. Rhinol. Laryngol., *81*:323, 1972.

45. Ishikawa, H., and Ishii, Y.: Evaluation of salivary gland tumors with ^{99m}Tc-pertechnetate. J. Oral Maxillofac. Surg., *42*:429, 1984.

46. Einstein, R. A., and Katz, A. D.: Parotid area swelling caused by a prominent transverse process of atlas. Arch. Otolaryngol., *101*:558, 1975.

47. Hughes, G. R. V., and Gross, N. J.: Diagnosis of sarcoidosis by labial gland biopsy. Br. Med. J., *3*:215, 1972.

48. Batsakis, J. G., Bernacki, E. G., and Rice, D. H.: Malignancy and the benign lymphoepithelial lesion. Laryngoscope, *85*:389, 1975.

CHAPTER 16

The Maxillary Sinus

PAUL H. MCFARLAND, JR.

To exalt the present and the real,
To teach the average man the glory of his daily work or trade.
WALT WHITMAN

The maxillary sinus (antrum of Highmore) represents an anatomic hazard for the dentist. Development and expansion over many years, occupation of the greater portion of the maxilla, variation in size and shape, relative position to the posterior maxillary teeth, and unfavorable drainage patterns often pose a diagnostic dilemma and a surgical inopportunity for the unwary practitioner. For these reasons, there is no substitute for an appreciation of the growth and development, the anatomy, and the physiology of the orofacial area.

Growth and Development

The paranasal sinuses (maxillary, frontal, ethmoid, and sphenoid) develop as evaginations of the nasal mucosa on the medial side of the orbit during the third and fourth months *in utero.* In the infant, the maxillary sinus achieves considerable size and is almost totally occupied by developing teeth. Growth and development, very slow during childhood until the seventh to ninth year, progress rapidly until approximately the fifteenth year, and are followed by expansion in size in the adult (Fig. 16-1). Further expansion and pneumatization may occur into the alveolar process following premature loss of the posterior maxillary teeth (Fig. 16-2).

Anatomy

The maxillary sinus, largest of the paranasal sinuses, essentially occupies the entire body of the maxilla (Fig. 16-3).[1] Although the size and shape vary in each individual, the shape, visualized in three dimensions, is reminiscent of a pyramid. The boundaries[2] are:

Base: Lower portion of the lateral nasal wall

Apex: Projecting into the zygomatic process of the maxilla and sometimes into the body of the zygoma

Anterolateral: Facial surface of the maxilla

Posterior: Infratemporal surface of the maxilla

Superior: Orbital plate of the maxilla (the roof of the sinus is also the floor of the orbit)

Inferior: Alveolar and palatine processes of the maxilla

Other anatomic features germane to an understanding of the maxillary sinus are the blood supply, innervation, lymphatic drainage, and position of the solitary exit high in the base. The major arterial supply to the sinus is provided by the internal maxillary artery through terminal branches of the infraorbital artery via the posterior superior and anterior superior alveolar arteries. The posterior superior alveolar artery traverses the inferior portion of the infratemporal surface (posterior wall) and the anterior wall, while the anterior superior alveolar artery traverses the orbital and anterior walls.[1] Venous drainage is primarily through the anterior facial vein and the angular vein to the inferior

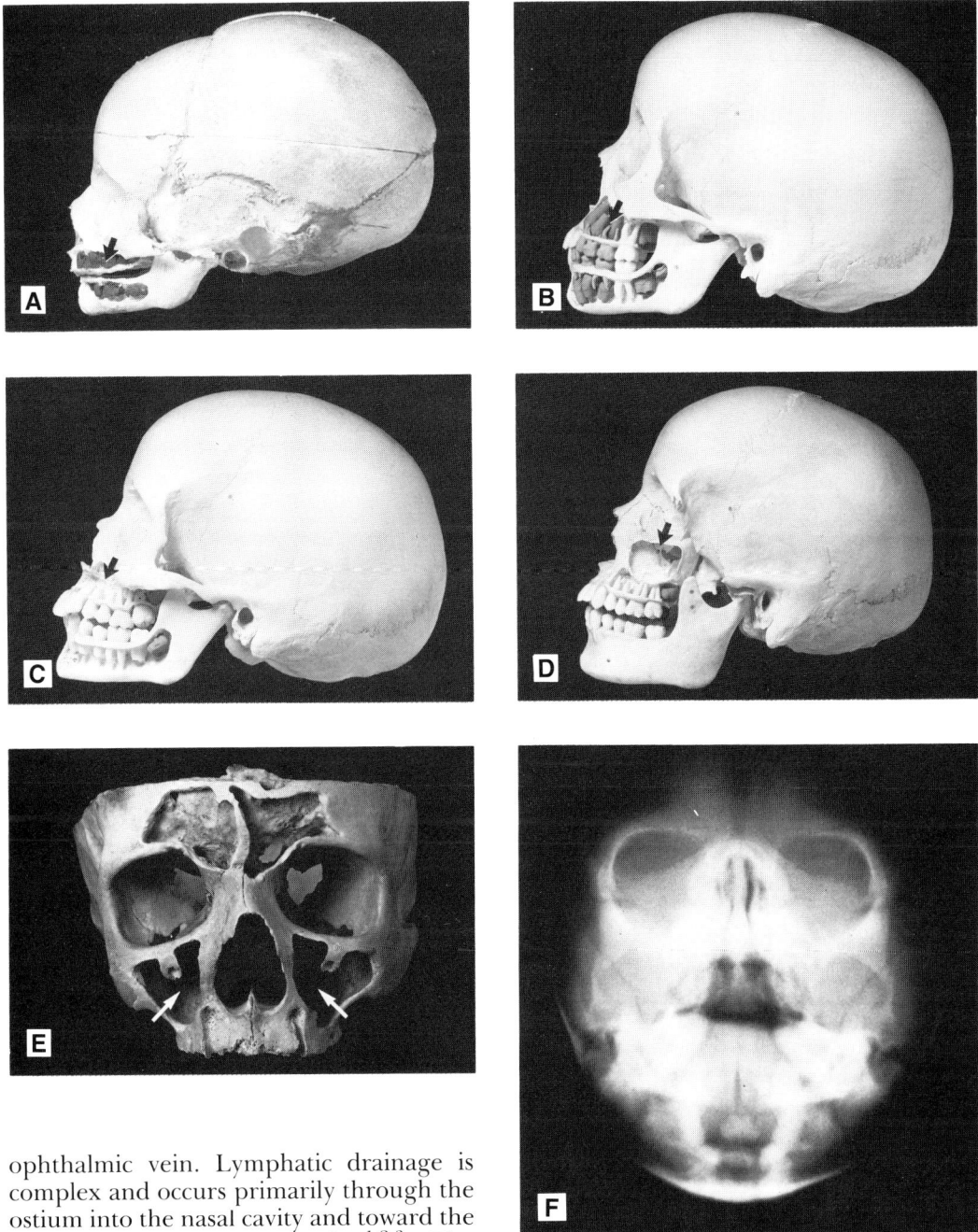

FIG. 16-1. *Sequential growth and development of the maxillary sinuses. (A) Infant. (B) Nine year old. (C) - Fifteen year old. (D) Adult—lateral view. (E) Adult— antero-posterior view (Courtesy, Department of Anatomical Sciences, The University of Texas Health Science Center at Houston, Dental Branch). (F) Radiograph of 6-day-old infant.*

ophthalmic vein. Lymphatic drainage is complex and occurs primarily through the ostium into the nasal cavity and toward the submandibular lymph nodes.[1,2,3] The nerve supply of the sinus is through terminal branches of the infraorbital nerve in company with the arterial supply. The ostium of the maxillary sinus is located in the superior part of the medial wall at the hiatus semilunaris and opens into the middle meatus of the nose. The superior location of the ostium on the medial wall of the sinus is clinically significant because it pre-

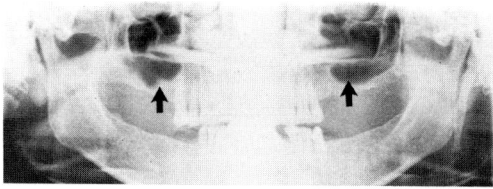

Fig. 16-2. *Expansion and pneumatization following premature loss of posterior maxillary teeth.*

disposes to an unfavorable drainage pattern.

Septa are very common in the maxillary sinus and frequently provide valleys for collection of fluid. Because of individual variations in size, shape, and prominence of ridges and septa, it is difficult to establish anatomic dimensions to the antrum. In a survey of 25 skulls from the collection of the Department of Anatomical Sciences at The University of Texas Health Science Center at Houston, Dental Branch, the average dimensions of the adult maxillary sinuses were determined to be 32 mm in height, 22 mm in width, and 33 to 34 mm in anteroposterior depth. Capacity varies remarkably because of the presence of the ubiquitous septa.

The relationship of the maxillary sinus to the teeth varies according to the degree of penetration of the sinus into the alveolar process of the maxilla. Generally, the maxillary second bicuspid and first, second, and third molars are consistently in proximity to the antrum. The roots of the second bicuspid and the first and second molars are frequently involved. Reading,[4] in a study of 138 cases of oroantral perforations, reported that 48 percent were occasioned by removal of the first molar, 26 percent with second molars, and 3 percent with bicuspids. Similarly, Killey and Kay,[5] in 250 cases, reported fistulae following extractions related to the first molar in 61 percent, the second molar in 25 percent, the bicuspids in 13 percent, and the third molar in 6 percent. In view of the anatomy of the middle face, these findings are not surprising and should serve as a warning for those who perform extractions of teeth.

Physiology

It has been suggested that the primary functions of the maxillary sinus are to decrease the weight of the craniofacial skeleton, to remove debris from inspired air, to warm inspired air, and to enhance the resonance of speech.

The maxillary sinus is lined by a mucous membrane of respiratory epithelium (pseudostratified columnar epithelium with cilia and goblet cells). The beating of the cilia tends to produce a swirl of air that transports the mucous toward the ostium in the superior medial wall of the sinus. The mucous membrane is supplied by the anterior and posterior superior alveolar

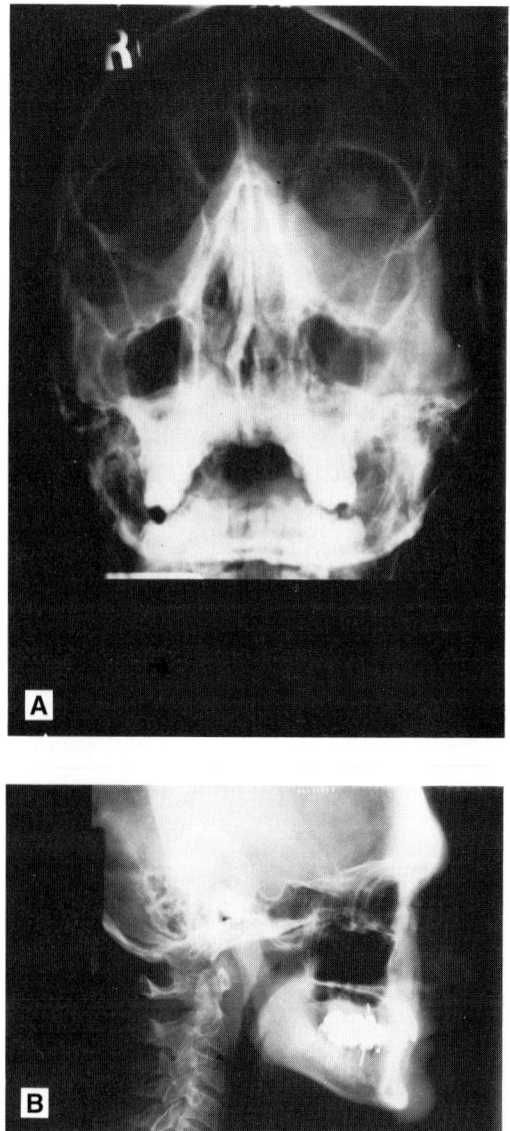

Fig. 16-3. *Radiographs of maxillary sinus. (A) Water's view. (B) Lateral view.*

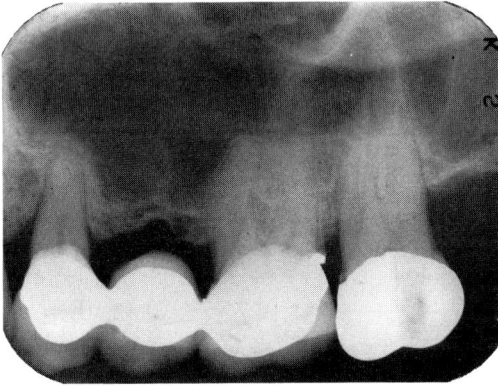

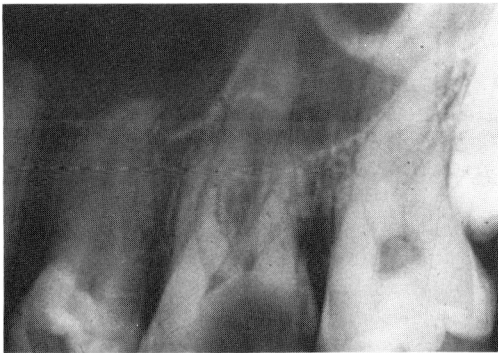

FIG. 16-4. *Periapical x-rays demonstrate variability of sinus size in relation to the roots of teeth.*

nerves together with branches from the greater palatine nerve. Often these nerves are in intimate contact with the mucous membrane, and since they also supply the posterior maxillary teeth, toothache symptoms are often associated with acute sinusitis. Similarly, with acute inflammation, fluid may collect in the sinus and exert pressure on root ends that are either not covered by bone or by a thin layer of bone. In addition, the antral membrane, an exceedingly tough and resilient structure, may increase in thickness from a normal 1 mm to approximately 15 mm during an acute or chronic inflammatory insult.

Because all paranasal sinuses drain into the nasal cavity, infection may be transmitted easily from one sinus to another. Involvement of all sinuses in an acute inflammatory process is referred to as pansinusitis.

Radiography

Radiography is an important diagnostic tool for the evaluation of maxillary sinus disorders. A number of radiographic studies may be used, but the decision to order a particular study must be based on a good history and clinical examination. Studies include (1) periapical and occlusal films, (2) panograms, (3) Water's view of maxilla (perhaps including a sinus series), (4) tomograms, and (5) CT scan.

Periapical radiographs (Fig. 16-4) are valuable to determine the relationship of the roots of the teeth to the sinus and to locate foreign bodies in and about the floor of the sinus. However, they have limited value for diagnostic purposes because they depict only an isolated area of the sinus and do not permit bilateral comparisons to be made.

Panoramic radiography (Fig. 16-5), by contrast, permits visualization and comparison of the right and left sinuses. Although this film may appear distorted and fail to demonstrate the complete outline of the sinuses, it is an excellent screening device.

The Water's view (Fig. 16-3A) is the most singularly valuable film for visualization, comparison, and evaluation of the sinuses.

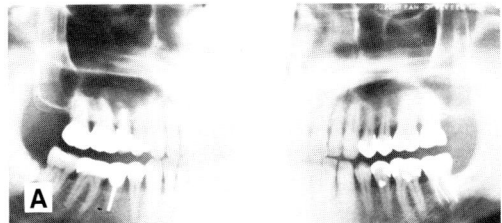

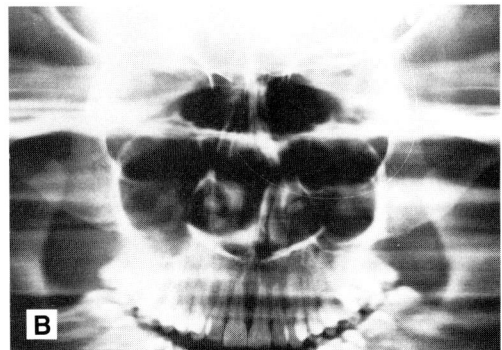

FIG. 16-5. *(A) Routine panoramic radiograph provides satisfactory view of both antra. (B) Special panoramic view of the maxillary sinuses.*

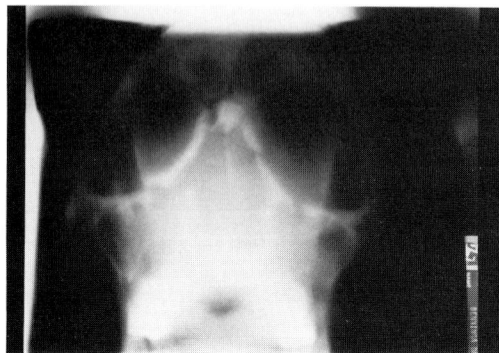

FIG. 16-6. *Tomogram.*

The tomogram (Fig. 16-6) is another desirable radiographic study that is selectively valuable to determine extent of injury or abnormality and erosion of bone. The x-rays, or "cuts," are made at specific depths to permit clear delineation of structures at the particular level and blurring of the surrounding anatomy.

A CT scan or computerized tomography (Fig. 16-7) provides enhancement of structures at predetermined levels. It is particularly useful in trauma, massive infections, and neoplastic disease.

Radiographic Interpretation

Radiographically, the maxillary sinus appears radiolucent or dark, while its boundaries are radiopaque or white. The radiolucency occurs because the sinuses are filled with air, and the radiodensity occurs because of the presence of bone.

The primary change in radiographic appearance occasioned by infection, neoplasia, or trauma is cloudiness of the antrum (Fig. 16-8). The presence of an infectious process may result in a well-defined fluid level. Retention phenomena (cysts) and polyps (Fig. 16-9) are clearly outlined structures within the sinus that are cloudy in appearance. Fractures of the middle face may result in step defects in the infraorbital and lateral orbital rims and dysharmony in the lateral antral wall (Fig. 16-10). Concurrently, the antrum appears cloudy because of bleeding into the confined space. Erosion of bony walls may be secondary to infections or neoplastic disease.

In every radiographic evaluation, comparison should be made between the right and left sides. In the Water's view, for example, a normal study should demonstrate essentially equal radiolucency of the orbits and antra, as well as bilateral symmetry of the osseous anatomy. Requests for radiographic studies should be based on a good history and an appropriate clinical examination.

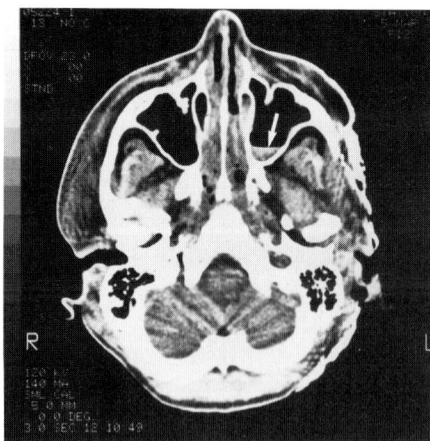

FIG. 16-7. *CT scan. Note fluid level in sinus at arrow.*

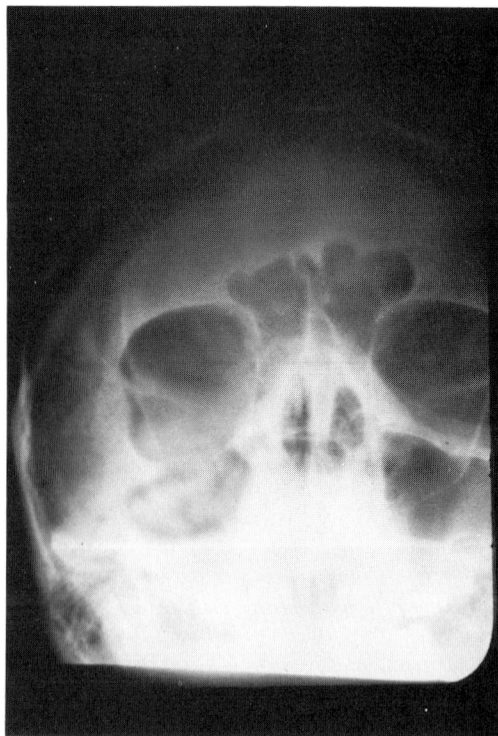

FIG. 16-8. *Water's view. Note opacity (cloudiness of one sinus and lucency or aeration of the other).*

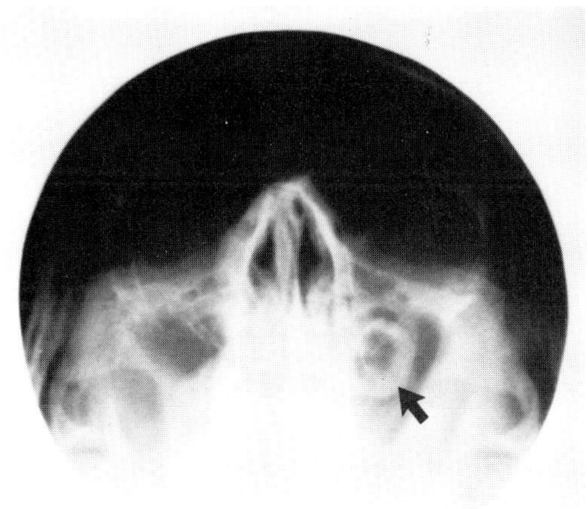

FIG. 16-9. *Water's view. Note cyst in sinus.*

Clinical Consideration

Nonsurgical

Evaluation of maxillary sinus disorders *must* be based, first and foremost, on a detailed history. There is no substitute for a sympathetic ear to the details of the problem presented by the patient and the gentle probing of the history with appropriate questions to elicit additional pertinent information. The discussion usually centers around signs, symptoms, and the course of the disease process. REMEMBER: If you listen, the patient will usually give you the diagnosis by telling you what is wrong!

The clinical examination should include inspection, palpation, percussion, and transillumination. Inspection presents evidence of symmetry or asymmetry. Palpation identifies dysharmony associated with swelling, temperature, and anatomic integrity. Percussion of the teeth may produce evidence of hypersensitivity. Transillumination may help detect changes in the sinus. It is a simple technique in which an examination is performed in a dark room. A light source (pen-light is satisfactory) is placed adjacent to the skin over the infraorbital area, and intraorally adjacent to the palate with the lips closed around the light. In the healthy state, the light transmits through the sinus and produces a brilliance on the face and palate. In the un-

healthy state, the light is not transmitted through the sinus. This procedure (an adjunctive diagnostic tool) should be employed on both sides of the face for comparison purposes.

Inflammation of the maxillary sinus may occur for many reasons, such as allergy, trauma, URI, or infection. The most common symptom is pain, which may be localized to one particular sinus or distributed over all sinuses. Other symptoms may include sensitivity to pressure, a feeling of stuffiness or fullness, headache, toothache, interference with the sense of smell, and positional discomfort of the head.

Acute and chronic infections pose diagnostic problems for the dentist. In an acute sinusitis, the patient usually notices a deep and dull ache that increases in severity over the particular sinus. Percussion to the teeth elicits tenderness, and transillumination

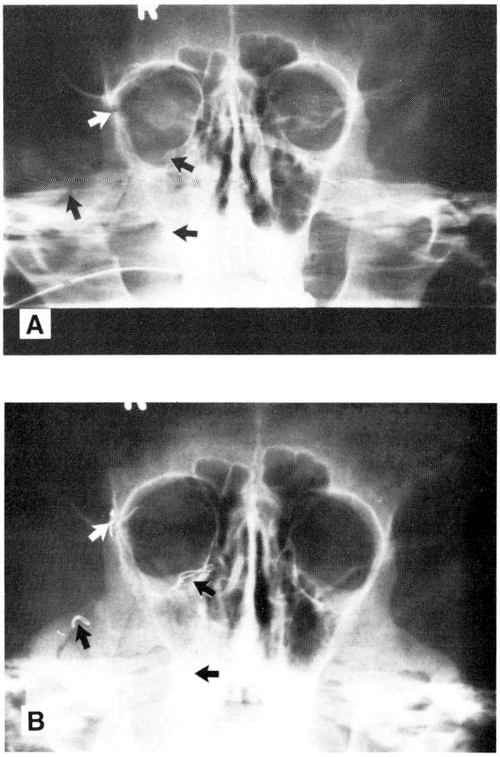

FIG. 16-10. *Special panographic views. (A) Preoperative. Note the displaced fractures at the lateral and infraorbital rims and the body of the zygoma. The sinus appears cloudy secondary to bleeding. (B) Postoperative. Note wires, sutures, and beginning aeration of sinus.*

demonstrates decreased transmission and brilliance. Increased temperature is usually present. These easy, quick, and simple procedures help to differentiate between an acute sinusitis and pulpal or periapical involvement. Appropriate radiographs demonstrate cloudiness or fluid levels in the sinus. Treatment consists of (1) humidifiers to loosen and increase the flow of secretions, (2) decongestants to reduce edema and inflammation, (3) antibiotics to reduce the bacterial flora, (4) analgesics to reduce pain, and (5) surgical intervention to establish drainage, if necessary. The normal flora of the nasal and antral cavities are staphylococci, streptococci, corynbacterium, and neisseria.[6] These organisms are usually susceptible to ampicillin—the antibiotic of choice pending culture and sensitivity reports of the exudate.

Chronic sinusitis has many causes, but it is usually characterized by episodic attacks of acute sinusitis. Radiographs demonstrate thickened sinus membranes and occasional polyps. Identification of cause is important, and treatment embraces the spectrum from the conservative management described for acute sinusitis to a sinusotomy (Caldwell-Luc) and nasal antrostomy (creation of a window for drainage in the inferior meatus).

Acute and chronic maxillary sinusitis may pose a diagnostic problem for the dentist. Referred pain from the sinus to the teeth frequently causes the patient to seek dental care. In such instances, the patient complains of a constant, dull ache in the posterior maxillary teeth and increased pain while walking or bending over. The positional change of the head causes increased pressure in the sinus and therefore increased pain in the teeth. Additionally, the teeth may "feel too long," become very sensitive to touch, and be painful when chewing. One must also be aware that periapical and periodontal lesions may perforate the sinus membrane and initiate a sinusitis without any clinical suggestion of tooth etiology.

It is apparent, then, that a detailed history, careful examination, and appropriate radiographs are desirable to diagnose the problem and to provide the proper sequential treatment.

Surgical

The normal anatomic variations of the sinus in relation to the roots of the tooth suggest that the integrity of the sinus membrane is violated during the extraction of posterior teeth far more frequently than is usually realized. In the absence of periapical and antral infection, these extraction sites heal without incident. Displaced root tips and teeth into the sinus may set the stage for antral infection and a subsequent oroantral fistula.

The presence or absence of an antral opening may be determined by gentle probing of the alveolus with a periodontal probe or by direct observation. One might also be aware of the passage of air between the antrum and the oral cavity. Under no circumstances should the patient be asked to pinch the nostrils and attempt to blow air out of the nose. This maneuver, because of increased antral pressure, may easily produce a perforation in an otherwise intact antral membrane.

Surgical closure is indicated when drainage appears from the sinus following extraction of teeth and when oroantral fistulae develop.

In all instances of surgical closure, antibiotics and decongestants are desirable, together with postoperative instructions to avoid sudden changes in head position such as bending over, sneezing, and blowing the nose. Sudden alterations in antral pressure may cause dehiscence of the wound at the suture line.

Without question, the formation and

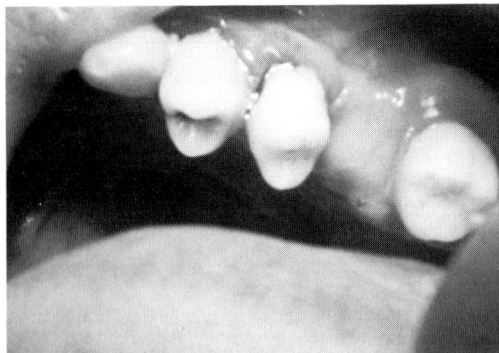

FIG. 16-11. *Final clinical appearance of closure by the mucosal relaxing incision technique.*

organization of a blood clot is imperative for uncomplicated healing. For this reason, tiny openings following extraction may be expected to heal satisfactorily if appropriate postoperative instructions and medications are provided.

Several surgical procedures have been devised to repair oroantral openings and fistulae; however, each is based on the sound principles elucidated by Waite.[7] These principles have stood the test of time and are as follows: (1) elimination and control of sinus disease, (2) adequate intranasal drainage, (3) excision of the epithelial lining of the fistula, (4) elimination of necrotic tissue, (5) broad-based flap design, (6) sharp incision and intact reflection of the flap, (7) approximation of raw surfaces, (8) minimal tension on the flaps, and (9) aseptic procedures. Adherence to these

principles should permit uncomplicated repair of the wound site.

The basic and most frequently used surgical procedures include (1) the mucosal relaxing incision technique, (2) the buccal flap technique, (3) the gold plate technique, (4) the palatal pedicle flap technique, and (5) the sinusotomy or modified Caldwell-Luc technique.

The mucosal relaxing incision technique is used primarily in the absence of sinus disease for closure of small perforations following extraction (Fig. 16-11). It embraces identification of the perforation, placement of a small amount of surgical or similar hemostatic material in the apex of the alveolus, removal of buccal and lingual alveolar crests to facilitate flap closure without tension, incision and undermining of buccal and lingual mucosae to permit edge-to-edge approximation of the mucosae over the alveolus, and closure of the

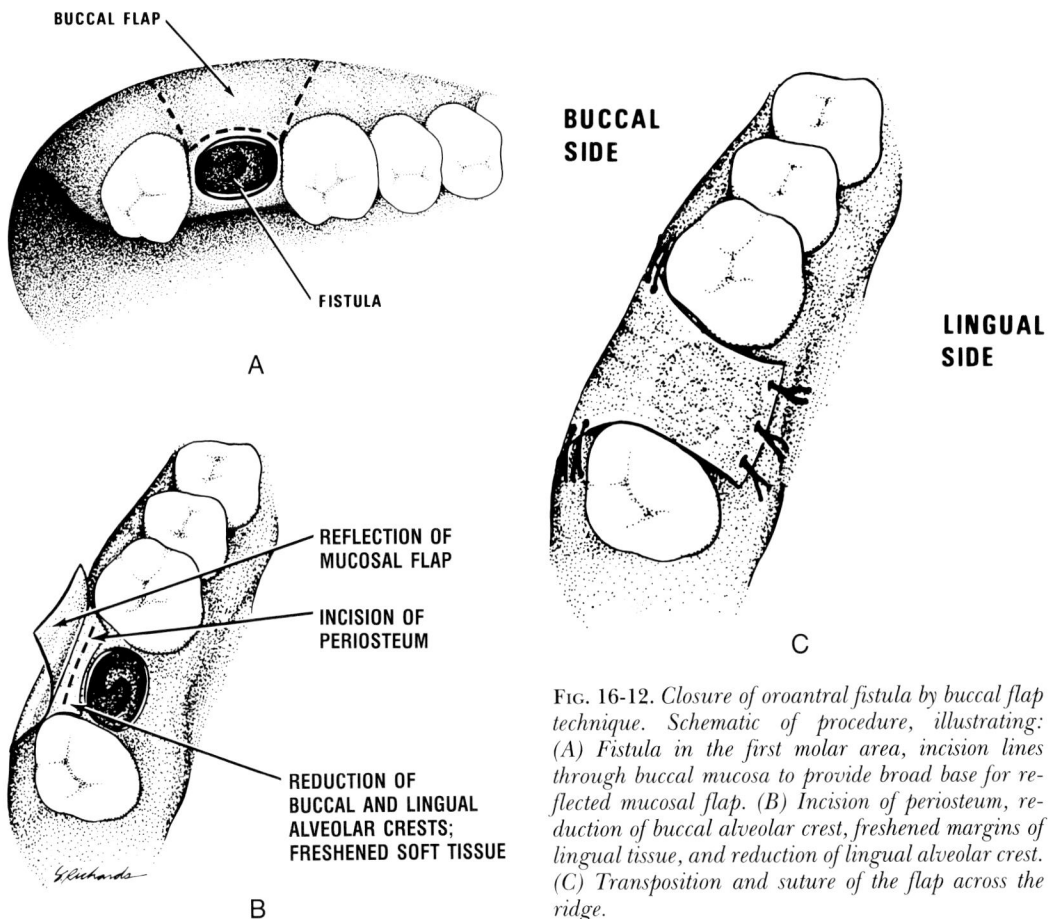

FIG. 16-12. *Closure of oroantral fistula by buccal flap technique. Schematic of procedure, illustrating: (A) Fistula in the first molar area, incision lines through buccal mucosa to provide broad base for reflected mucosal flap. (B) Incision of periosteum, reduction of buccal alveolar crest, freshened margins of lingual tissue, and reduction of lingual alveolar crest. (C) Transposition and suture of the flap across the ridge.*

A

INCISIVE FORAMEN

ANTERIOR PALATINE
NEUROVASCULAR
BUNDLE

GREATER PALATINE
FORAMEN

FISTULA

B

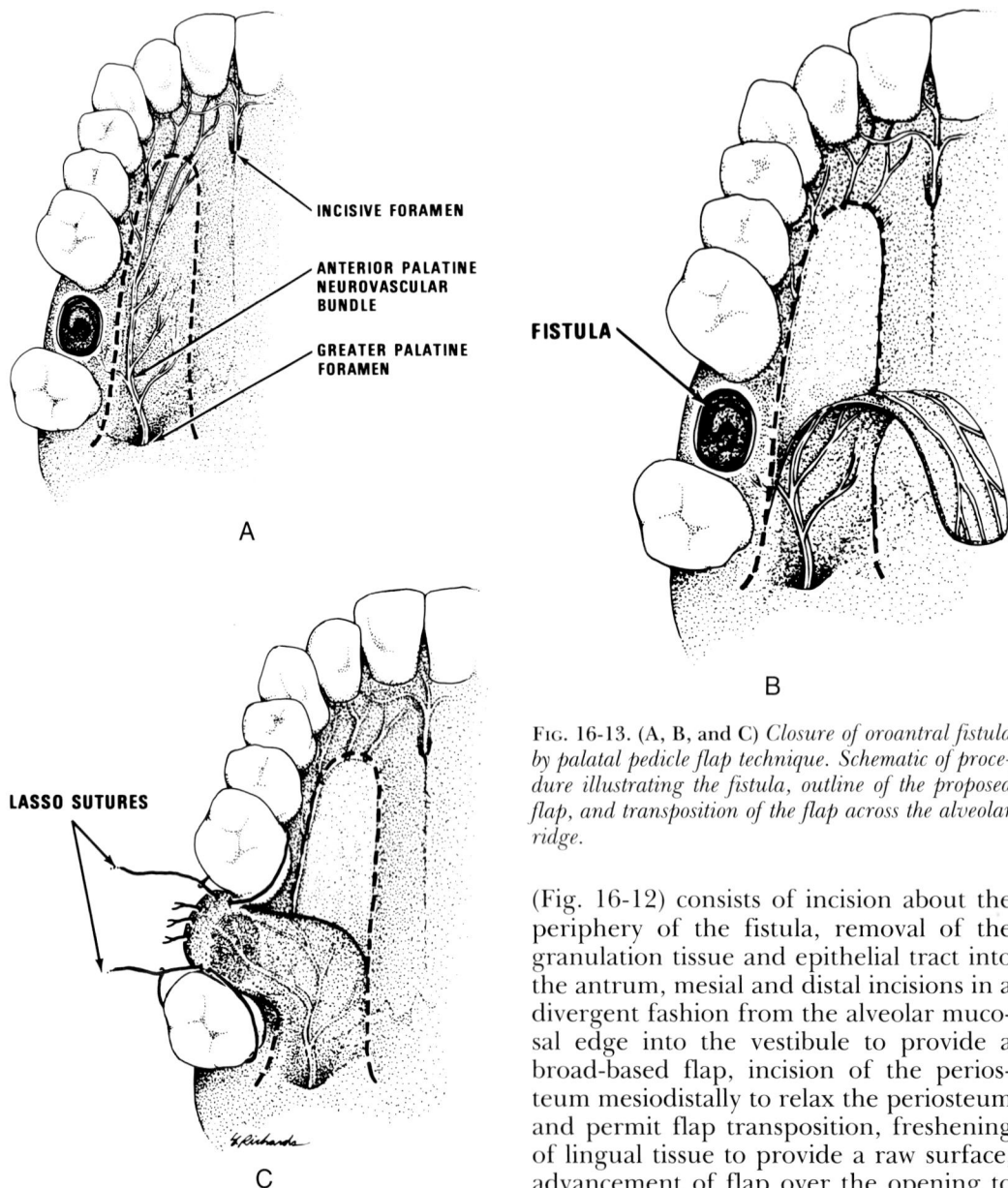

FIG. 16-13. (A, B, and C) *Closure of oroantral fistula by palatal pedicle flap technique. Schematic of procedure illustrating the fistula, outline of the proposed flap, and transposition of the flap across the alveolar ridge.*

LASSO SUTURES

C

site with multiple interrupted or mattress sutures. Periodontal packing over the site and about the adjacent teeth provides additional protection during the healing process. Sutures may be removed in 7 to 10 days.

The buccal flap technique may be used for the immediate closure of large perforations incident to removal of a tooth with attached bone and with a chronic fistula. This technique, slightly modified, was described by Berger[8] in 1939. The procedure

(Fig. 16-12) consists of incision about the periphery of the fistula, removal of the granulation tissue and epithelial tract into the antrum, mesial and distal incisions in a divergent fashion from the alveolar mucosal edge into the vestibule to provide a broad-based flap, incision of the periosteum mesiodistally to relax the periosteum and permit flap transposition, freshening of lingual tissue to provide a raw surface, advancement of flap over the opening to the lingual tissue, and closure with multiple interrupted sutures. Periodontal pack placed over the site and about the adjacent teeth provides additional protection during the initial healing process. Sutures may be removed in 7 to 10 days.

In the gold plate technique, an incision is made about the periphery of the fistula; granulation tissue and epithelial tract are removed; buccal and lingual mucoperiosteum are minimally reflected; and a 36-gauge, 24-karat gold plate is placed over the opening and the edges burnished under the periosteum over the adjacent alveolar bone. Tissue proliferates over the opening on the antral side, and in 10 to 14 days the plate becomes loose and may be gently removed.

The palatal pedicle flap or sliding palatal flap is also used to surgically correct an oroantral fistula (Fig. 16-13). An incision is made about the periphery of the fistula, the granulation tissue and epithelial tract

are excised, the sharp crestal alveolar margins are reduced, the proposed pedicle flap is outlined to ensure adequate blood supply, and the palatal mucosal flap is reflected and transposed across the ridge and sutured into place. A prepared palatal acrylic splint may be used for protection of the flap postoperatively. The donor site may granulate and epithelialize uneventfully. Clinical cases demonstrating the flexibility of the palatal pedicle or palatal sliding technique are illustrated in Figures 16-14, 16-15, and 16-16.

As mentioned previously, the anatomy of the maxillary sinuses, the anatomy of the root systems, and the relationship of the roots to the sinus suggest that violation of the antrum is not uncommon. These factors contribute to displacement of a fractured root tip beneath the antral membrane or into antrum proper. On these occasions, one should inspect the alveolus

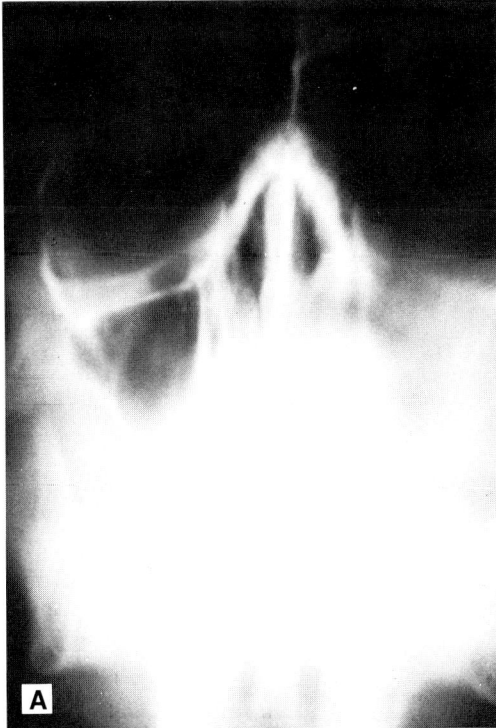

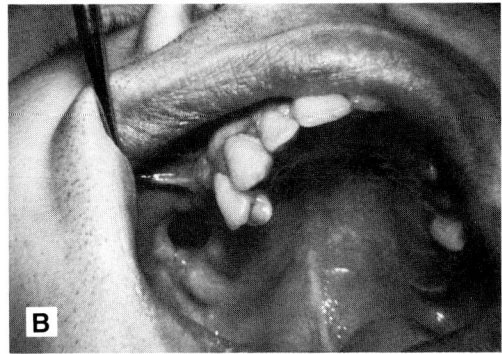

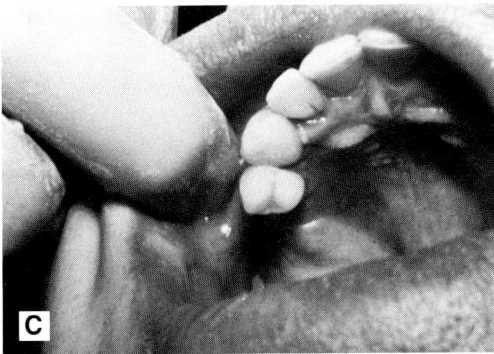

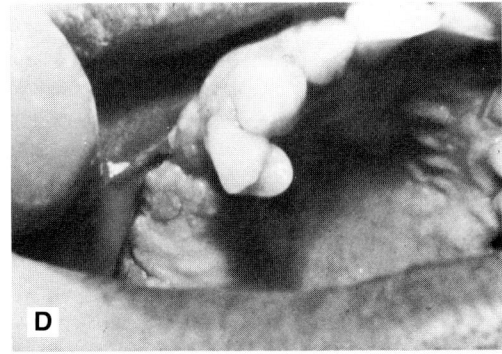

FIG. 16-14. *Clinical example of closure of an oroantral fistula that occurred secondary to infection of a primordial cyst in the third molar area. The resultant fistula was closed by the palatal slide technique. (A) Tomogram demonstrates cloudiness of the antrum; erosion of medial, lateral, and superior walls. (B) Appearance of fistula. (C) Postoperative appearance of palate. (D) Appearance of healed palate and attachment of flap.*

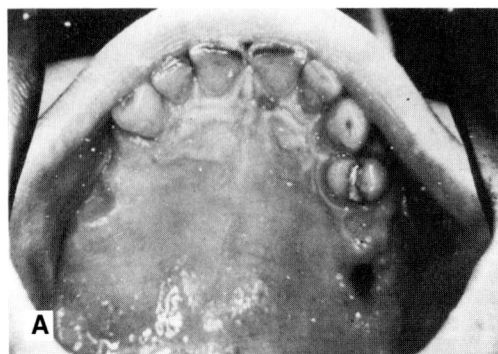

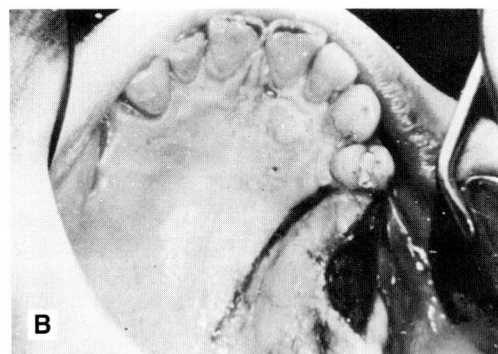

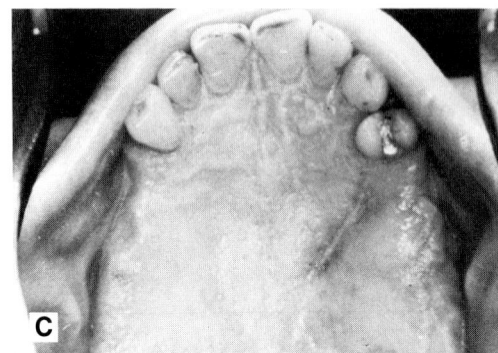

FIG. 16-15. *Clinical example of closure of an oroantral fistula that occurred secondary to extraction of a first molar. The resultant fistula was closed by the palatal slide technique. (A) Appearance of palate and fistula. (B) Debridement of the fistula and proposed incision line for palatal flap. (C) Postoperative appearance of healed site.*

with good light and good suction to determine if the root tip can be seen and if it can be retrieved through the socket by the gentle manipulation of small root picks and small suction tips. The alveolus should not be enlarged in an effort to retrieve the tip because such a maneuver will predispose toward subsequent oroantral communication.

Retrieval of a freshly fractured root tip can best be accomplished by direct surgical intervention via a modified Caldwell-Luc procedure or sinusotomy. Two basic approaches may be used in this procedure. The first is by an incision high in the vestibule by an incision through the attached mucoperiosteum which extends from approximately the second molar to the lateral incisor area, reflection of the mucoperios-

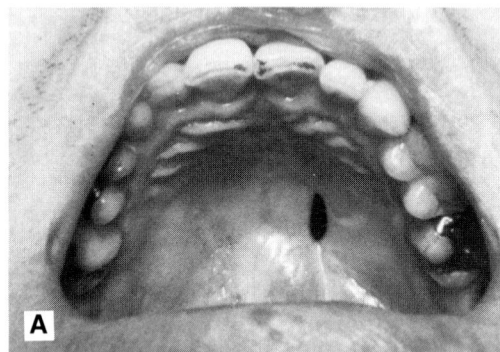

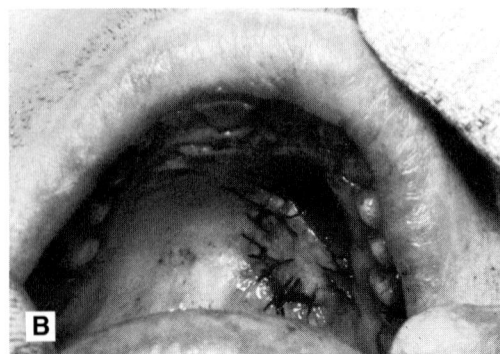

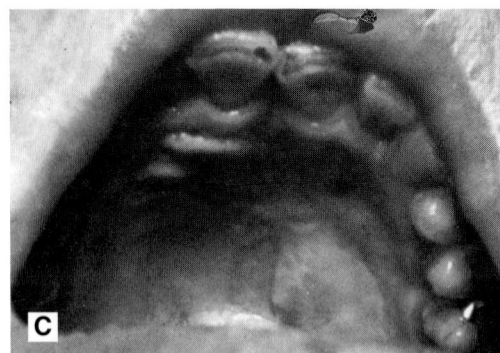

FIG. 16-16. *Clinical example of closure of an oroantral fistula that occurred secondary to severe midface trauma. (A) Appearance of palate and fistula. (B) Appearance of site at time of closure. (C) Final appearance.*

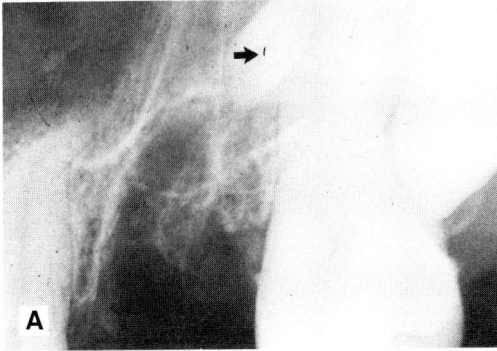

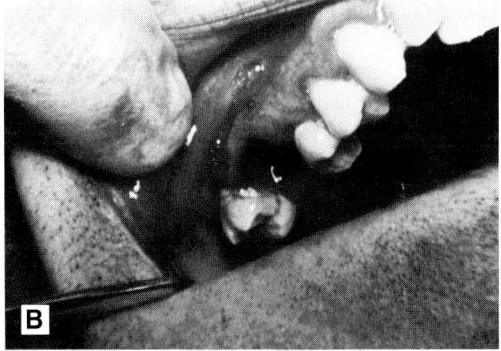

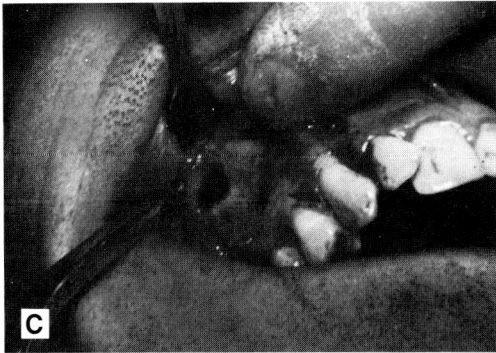

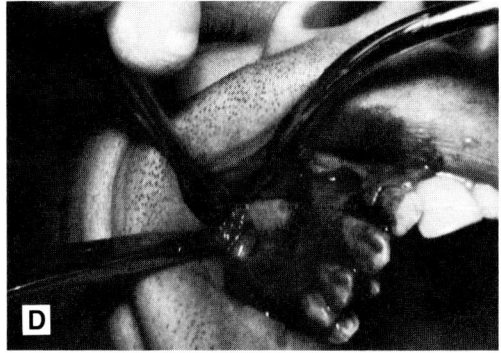

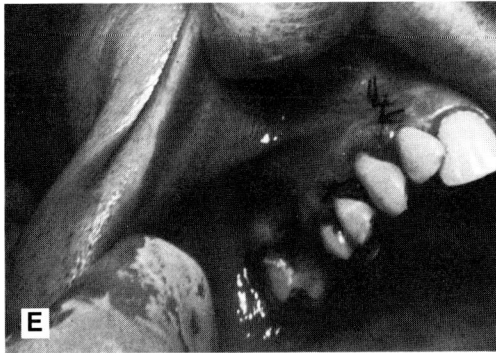

FIG. 16-17. *Clinical example of root-tip retrieval via the modified Caldwell-Luc procedure. (A) Periapical x-ray of root tip in antrum. (B) Extraction site. (C) Reflection of mucoperiosteal flap and antral window. Note the continuity of buccal cortical plate inferior to the window. (D) Retrieval of root. (E) Closure by interrupted sutures.*

teal flap, and creation of a window in the bone of the canine fossa area or the bicuspid area. This approach permits visualization into the antrum with subsequent retrieval of the root by gentle suction, irrigation with saline, and occasionally by packing with gauze to entangle the root tip. The operative site is closed by multiple interrupted sutures. This approach has several disadvantages such as increased bleeding at the incision site, difficulty in creating a window in the dense cortical bone of the canine fossa, occasional herniation of the buccal fat pad into the incision site, and increased postoperative swelling and discomfort. Nonetheless, the approach is favored by many surgeons and is completely satisfactory in experienced hands.

The second approach (Fig. 16-17) is a modified Caldwell-Luc, in which an incision is made around the necks of the posterior teeth from the second or third molar to the mesial surface of the cuspid, with a second incision in a divergent fashion from the cuspid anteriorly into the mucobuccal fold. A full-thickness mucoperiosteal flap is reflected and a window created in the thin lateral antral wall above the involved tooth. The window may be created by burs and rongeur forceps. A small opening is created in the sinus membrane, and with good light and good suction the root tip may be visualized and retrieved. Care should be exercised to create the window sufficiently high on the antral wall to preserve the integrity of the buccal cortical plate. Closure is accomplished by the placement of multiple interrupted sutures. This technique permits a broad-based flap, reduced bleeding, creation of a window in thin bone, and exposure adjacent to the root tip with enhanced ease of retrieval.

Postoperatively, as previously discussed, antibiotics, decongestants, and instructions for care are imperative.

Malignancies of the oral and maxillofacial region are often not detected early. In children and young adults, the malignancy is usually a type of sarcoma, whereas after age 40 carcinoma is most frequently encountered. Radiographs generally demonstrate cloudiness, thickened sinus membranes, and increased density. Erosion and destruction of antral walls should be considered malignant until proved otherwise by biopsy and histopathologic examination.

In summary, an appreciation of the anatomy and physiology of the maxillary sinus is a sound base on which to evaluate and diagnose antral disease. Knowledge of conservative management and familiarity with surgical approaches allows the practitioner to provide the appropriate treatment or to refer the patient to an appropriate specialist for management.

There is no substitute for a careful, detailed history, for a detailed clinical and radiographic examination, for consultation with appropriate specialists, and for selection of well-considered and time-tested techniques that permit orderly but flexible management of the disorder.

References

1. Romanes, G. J.: Cunningham's Manual of Practical Anatomy, Head & Neck & Brain. Vol. 3, 14th Ed. New York, Oxford University Press, 1979.
2. Hollinshead, W. H.: Textbook of Anatomy. 3rd Ed. Hagerstown, Harper & Row, 1974.
3. Christen, J. B., and Telford, I. A: Synopsis of Gross Anatomy. 3rd Ed. Hagerstown, Harper & Row, 1978.
4. Reading, P.: Common Diseases of the Ear, Nose, and Throat. 4th Ed. Boston, Little, Brown & Co., 1966.
5. Killey, H. C., and Kay, L. W.: An analysis of 250 cases of oro-antral fistula treated by the buccal flap operation. J. Oral Surg., 24:726, 1967.
6. Topazian, R. G., and Goldberg, M. H. (eds.): Management of Infections of the Oral and Maxillofacial Regions. Philadelphia, W. B. Saunders Co., 1981.
7. Waite, D. E.: Maxillary sinus. Dent. Clin. North Am., 15:349, 1971.
8. Berger, A.: Oroantral openings and their surgical correction. Arch. Otolaryngol., 30: 400, 1939.

Selected Reading

Ballenger, J. J.: Diseases of the Nose, Throat, and Ear. 12th Ed. Philadelphia, Lea & Febiger, 1977.

Gibilisco, J. A.: Stafne's Radiographic Diagnosis. 5th Ed. Philadelphia, W. B. Saunders Co., 1985.

Haglund, J., and Evers, H.: Local Anesthesia in Dentistry. 3rd Ed. Worcester, Hefferman Press, 1978.

Ranly, D. M.: A Synopsis of Craniofacial Growth. New York, Appleton-Century-Crofts, 1980.

Stafne, E. C., and Gibilisco, J. A.: Oral Roentgenographic Diagnosis. 4th Ed., Philadelphia, W. B. Saunders Co., 1975.

CHAPTER 17 # Infections of the Oral Cavity

Thomas R. Flynn and Richard G. Topazian

Be not the first by whom the new is tried
Nor yet the last by whom the old is cast aside.
A. POPE

More than ever before, the dental practitioner must be able to diagnose promptly, to treat appropriately, and to refer (when necessary) infections involving the teeth and supporting structures. Failure to deal effectively with infections can result in significant morbidity for the patient and professional liability for the doctor. Fewer infections occur in the usual dental practice than in an earlier era because of generally improved oral health. This, together with an overreliance on and overconfidence in the efficacy of antibiotics has created the impression that serious consequences of oral infections are a thing of the past.

Although the incidence of odontogenic infection in dental practice has declined, those infections that occur have the potential to cause great harm. Greater numbers of medically compromised patients with altered defense mechanisms, the change in oral microbial flora toward more resistant forms, and the altered efficacy of conventional antibiotic therapy have increased the potential for serious sequelae of dental infections. The literature contains many reports of significant morbidity and even mortality from odontogenic infections that have resulted in pansinusitis, orbital cellulitis, cavernous sinus thrombosis, glottal and pharyngeal edema with respiratory embarrassment, and mediastinitis following dental infection that was not effectively controlled. Therefore, an understanding of the pathogenesis and proper management of oral infections is of critical importance to the dental practitioner.

This chapter discusses host defenses, patient evaluation, oral microbiology, antibiotic and surgical therapy, and management of specific infections.

Host Resistance in Oral Infections

The Dynamic Balance Between Host and Infection

The interaction between the host and the bacteria that colonize the oral cavity can be described as a dynamic balance, a stalemated war between the host and the bacteria. Usually, the host and its resistance factors predominate. This state is synonymous with health. On the other hand, if microbes begin to predominate, infection ensues (Fig. 17-1).

Microbes use two weapons in this battle: virulence and numbers. Virulence can be defined as all the qualities of the microbe that are harmful to the host. These include invasiveness and a multitude of toxins, enzymes, and other metabolic by-products. The number of organisms in the site of infection is a critical factor in determining whether the host can neutralize and destroy the infecting bacteria. An increase in the quantity of infecting bacteria raises also the concentration of virulence factors in that site.

273

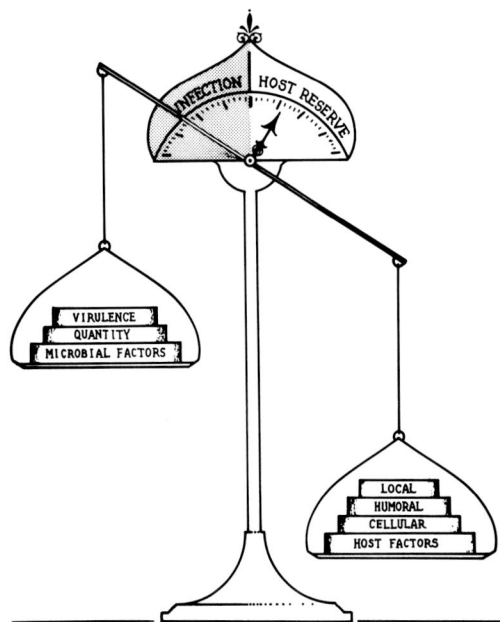

FIG. 17-1. *The dynamic balance between microbial factors that contribute to infection and host resistance factors that contribute to the host's reserve. (From: Topazian, R.G., and Goldberg, M.H., eds.: Management of Infections of the Oral and Maxillofacial Regions. Philadelphia, W.B. Saunders Co., 1981. Used with permission.)*

Host Resistance Factors

Host resistance factors, on the other side of this stalemate, can be separated into three main categories: local defenses, humoral components, and cellular components. The host's reserve is the degree to which these factors predominate over the pathogenic factors of the infecting or colonizing microbes.

LOCAL DEFENSES

The local resistance factors are the epithelial lining of the oral mucous membrane, the secretion and drainage system, the interference of one microbe with another, and the mucosal immune system. The most important of these local defenses is the epithelial lining of the mucous membrane. When it is disrupted, the host's greatest barrier to the penetration of pathogenic organisms is broken. An example of the loss of this barrier resulting in infection is a subperiosteal abscess arising after the surgical removal of several teeth. An incision has been made through the mucosa

and a mucoperiosteal flap elevated. Bacteria are then able to pass under the mucoperiosteal flap and colonize a tiny space between the elevated periosteum and the alveolar bone, where there is no blood supply. An abscess ensues.

The secretion and drainage system consists of the salivary flow, the ability to swallow salivary secretions and ingested food and fluids, and the mechanical cleansing action of the cheeks, lips, and tongue. The loss of flushing and rinsing action of the salivary flow, as a result of radiation of the salivary glands, causes a characteristic pattern of caries along the gingival margin and root surface of all of the teeth.

The normal flora that colonize the oral cavity are able to discourage the growth of new pathogenic species of bacteria. They occupy potential sites for microbial binding to epithelial cells, compete for available nutrients, and release by-products that are toxic to other microbes. The first antibiotics discovered were those synthesized by one species of bacteria, designed to kill other competing species. Bacteriocins are another microbial by-product that are protein in nature and have a narrow range of antibacterial activity. Bacteriocins are able to kill a very narrow range of competing bacterial strains similar to the producer strain.

Thus, when many of the normal colonizing flora are destroyed by the long-term administration of a broad spectrum antibiotic, the ability of the normal flora to interfere with colonization by pathogenic species is lost. Another result can be the overgrowth of normal flora usually present in much smaller proportions. An example of this is oral candidiasis following long-term administration of broad spectrum antibiotics.

The lamina propria, the connective tissue directly beneath the basement membrane of the mucosal epithelium, contains large numbers of immunocompetent cells. This is the mucosal immune system. These B-lymphocytes and plasma cells are able to synthesize antibodies that pass through the oral epithelium and are found in oral secretions, such as saliva and gingival fluid. Immunoglobulin A (IgA) is the predominant antibody in oral secretions in the normal state, and it acquires a protein secretory piece as it passes through the epithelium. This piece makes secretory IgA resistant to digestion by proteolytic enzymes that are present in saliva. In health, secretory IgA inhibits colonization of mucosal epithelial cells by occupying potential sites of attachment.

Suppression of the immune system by disease, or iatrogenically by the administration of certain drugs, can result in opportunistic infection of the oral cavity by bacteria that are normally present but not a source of infection.

HUMORAL COMPONENTS

The two humoral resistance factors found in the serum are the immunoglobulins and the complement system (Table 17-1 and Fig. 17-2). These factors work together to produce several effects: bacteriolytic activity that is important in the killing of certain microbes; the production of chemotactic factors that mobilize polymorphonuclear leukocytes (PMNs) toward the area of infection; and the formation of factors that control and enhance phagocytosis of bacteria by PMNs.

In addition, the immunoglobulins directly enhance phagocytosis of bacteria by coating the bacterial surface. These coating antibodies function like a handle, enabling the PMN to engulf the bacterium and destroy it. This process is called opsonization.

The role of the immunoglobulins and complement in enhancing phagocytosis and killing of bacteria by PMNs is illustrated in Fig. 17-3.

CELLULAR COMPONENTS

Two types of cells—the phagocytes and the lymphocytes—constitute the cellular resistance factors.

The cells responsible for phagocytosis of infecting microbes are the polymorphonuclear leukocytes (PMNs) and the mononuclear phagocytes. These latter cells are called monocytes when they are found in the blood stream and macrophages when they are found in tissue.

Phagocytosis is initiated by the attachment of a microbe to the cell membrane of the phagocyte. This attachment is greatly enhanced by opsonization, as discussed previously. Then, that portion of the cell membrane invaginates to surround the microbe, and a vacuole is formed. This phagocytic vacuole uses powerful oxidation reduction reactions, lysosomal enzymes, and nutrient depletion to kill the phagocytosed microbe.

TABLE 17-1. *Properties of the human immunoglobulin classes*

	IgG	IgA	IgM	IgD	IgE
Chemical					
Average concentration in normal serum (mg/100ml)	1000	160	100	3	0.03
Molecular weight (X 10^{-3})	152	160	950	180	200
Serum half-life (days)	22	6	5	2.8	2.3
Biologic					
Earliest antibody detected in primary immune responses			+		
Secreted on mucosal surfaces	±*	++	±	?	±
Secretory component attached		+	±		
Complement fixation	+	±†	+	−	±†
Fixes to skin and mast cells to cause anaphylaxis	?	−	−	−	+
Bonds to macrophages (cytophilic)	+	−	−	+	−

*In inflammatory conditions
†By alternate pathway
Adapted from Tomasi, T. B.: The Immune System of Secretions. Englewood Cliffs, NJ, Prentice-Hall, Inc., 1976.

CLASSIC PATHWAY
Activators, such as
immune complex

ALTERNATIVE PATHWAY
Activators, such as
endotoxin

$C1 \longrightarrow C\bar{1}$

factor D

$C4 + C2 \longrightarrow C\overline{42}$ factor Ba* + factor B(Bb) ← factor B

$C3 \longrightarrow C3b\ddagger + C3a\dagger$

$C5 \longrightarrow C5b\ddagger + C5a*\dagger$

$C6 + C7 \longrightarrow \overline{C567}*$

$C8 + C9 \longrightarrow$ Membrane lytic activity

*Chemotactic
†Anaphylatoxic
‡Phagocytosis-enhancing

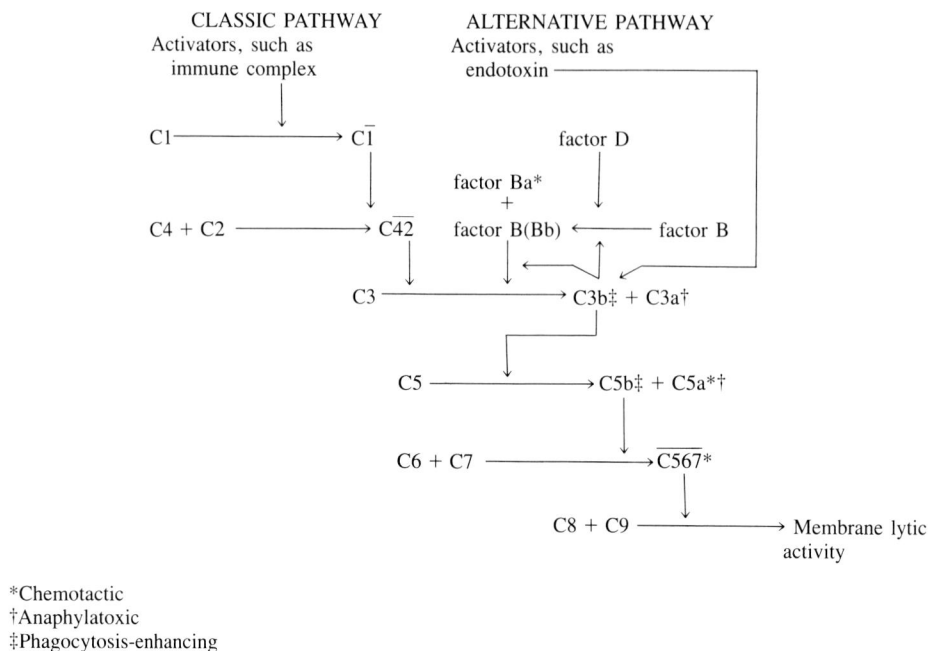

FIG. 17-2. *Complement system activation via the classic and alternative pathways. (From: Topazian, R.G., and Goldberg, M.H., eds.: Management of Infections of the Oral and Maxillofacial Regions. Philadelphia, W.B. Saunders Co., 1981. Used with permission.)*

PMNs are the first of the phagocytes to respond to the chemotactic factors which the complement system elaborates. Thus, they predominate in the acute stage of an infection, which persists for about the first week. The monocytes and macrophages respond to chemotactic factors more slowly, and therefore they do not predominate in an infection until the later chronic stages. Their function is, in essence, to "clean up the battlefield" by removing debris of dead cells and by killing bacteria that have resisted the PMNs. Macrophages respond to stimulation by and cooperate with the lymphocytes, which are the other main type of cells involved in the cellular resistance factors.

Lymphocytes consist of two types of cells: B-lymphocytes (B cells) and T-lymphocytes (T cells). Although these cells are morphologically indistinguishable, they differ considerably in their location and function. B cells predominate in the bone marrow and in the germinal centers of the lymph nodes, whereas T cells predominate in the thymus, spleen, and the deep cortex of lymph nodes.

B cells are responsible primarily for combating extracellular pathogens, particularly those bacteria that are not able to survive inside phagocytes or other cells. They differentiate to become plasma cells, which secrete specific antibodies against antigens to which the host has previously been exposed.

T cells, on the other hand, are responsible for combating the intracellular pathogens, which are primarily viruses and those bacteria that can survive within phagocytic cells. In addition, T cells are responsible for surveillance against the proliferation of tumor cells. These complex functions of the T cells are described in general as cell-mediated immunity.

Both T cells and B cells produce lymphokines—hormones that play several vital roles in resistance to infection. First, they regulate the actions of phagocytic cells. Macrophage inhibiting factor (MIF) inhibits the random movement of macrophages away from the site of infection, keeping them where they are needed. Interferon, another lymphokine, enhances lysis of bacteria by phagocytes. Mitogenic

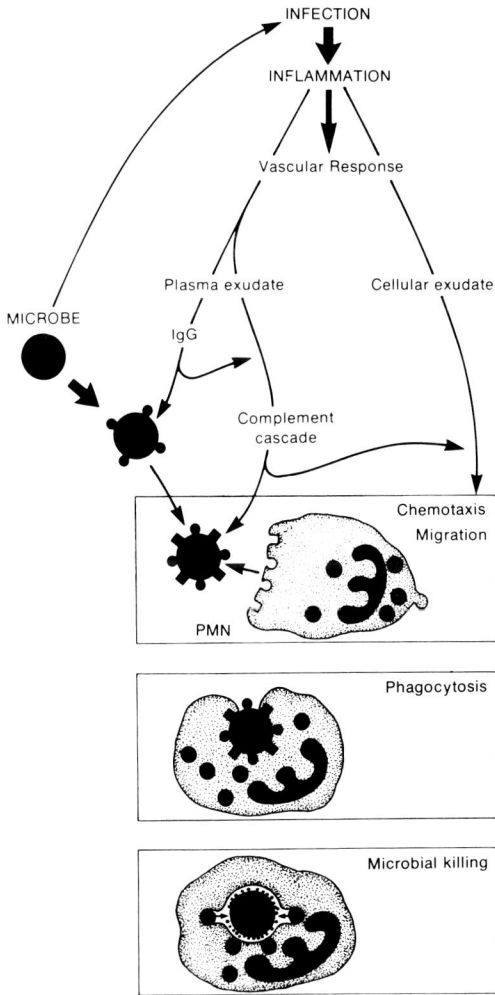

FIG. 17-3. *The interactions in the inflammatory process among the immunoglobulins, complement, and polymorphonuclear leukocytes which result in phagocytosis and killing of microbes. (From: Topazian, R.G., and Goldberg, M.H., eds.: Management of Infections of the Oral and Maxillofacial Regions. Philadelphia, W.B. Saunders Co., 1981. Used with permission.)*

factors, secreted by T cells, stimulate B cells to proliferate, enabling the body to mount an antibody response to antigenic stimulation. Thus, the lymphocytes are responsible for the modulation and control of the phagocytic cells.

Diagnosis of Infection

Signs of Infection

Galen first described the five cardinal signs of inflammation, which is the body's response to infection. They are: *rubor* (redness), *calor* (heat), *dolor* (pain), *tumor* (swelling), and *functio laesa* (loss of function).

Redness results from dilation in the blood vessels of the inflamed area and can be seen as a blush in the skin or the mucosa. It is important to compare the color of the region with the same region on the other side of the patient.

Increased heat of the infected part can best be determined by palpating the region with the dorsal surface of the fingers, where the skin is thinner and more sensitive to temperature than the palmar surface. It is also important to compare the region on the affected side with the same region on the unaffected side.

The pain associated with an infection is most consistently related to the amount of edema building up within the infected tissue spaces. Therefore, an incipient infection in the soft tissue spaces of the face and neck is much less tender than one in which a considerable inflammatory response has been mounted, and there is a great deal of redness and swelling. After the pressure has been released by incision and drainage, the amount of pain decreases markedly.

The swelling arising from a superficial infection is most often quite obvious, but it may be necessary, when examining for a deep space infection, to step back from the patient and examine the whole face and neck, comparing subtle differences of one side with the other. It is important to describe the swelling in terms of its anatomic boundaries, such as the muscles that delimit the swelling and the anatomic relationship of the swelling to the maxilla or mandible.

The loss of function is an ominous sign in infections of the head and neck. Trismus, the inability to open the mouth widely, can be the only externally visible sign of a serious pterygomandibular space infection. Trismus is caused by inflammation in the muscles of mastication and indicates that infection is spreading to deeper structures. Inability to protrude the tongue beyond the vermillion border of the upper lip and an elevated posture of the tongue are signs of a serious infection of the sublingual space. Both of these deep space infections can result in serious internal edema, which can obstruct the airway and asphyxiate the patient.

SYSTEMIC SIGNS

The development of systemic signs of infection indicates a potentially serious course of disease, requiring proper evaluation and prompt treatment.

Fever. Core body temperature is a reliable gauge of the seriousness of an infection. A normal oral temperature is 98.6° F (37° C). Elevation of the oral temperature beyond 100° F is significant. The underlying cause of the fever should be found and treated. In oral infections, it may not be possible to obtain a reliable oral temperature since reading may vary between the infected and the noninfected side. In this situation, one should not hesitate to obtain a rectal temperature, which is normally 1° F higher than the oral temperature. The axillary temperature is unreliable and should not be used in the diagnosis of infections.

Dehydration. A serious oral infection interferes with the normal intake of food and fluids. Furthermore, a serious rise in the temperature significantly increases the rate of loss of water through the skin by radiation and sweating. The normal fluid intake requirement for a 70 kg adult is 2400 cc per day. A high fever accelerates water loss by evaporation from the skin and can raise the daily fluid requirement to as much as 3600 cc per day. It is easy to imagine, then, that a significant fever of several hours' duration can fairly rapidly result in serious dehydration.

The dehydrated patient has a hot, dry skin, chapped lips, dry oral mucous membranes, and decreased salivary flow. A crying dehydrated child produces no tears.

Malaise. A very sensitive indicator of the presence of an infection is how the patient feels subjectively. Malaise can be described as a feeling of weakness, lack of energy and appetite, loss of interest in one's surroundings, and a vague, generalized discomfort. The patient who seems to be doing well for 3 days after surgery, and then develops malaise, may have an incipient postoperative infection.

Lymphadenopathy. Tender, palpable, freely mobile lymph nodes frequently accompany a significant infection. A thorough knowledge of the drainage patterns of the lymph nodes of the head and neck is indispensable in finding the source of an infection (Table 17-2). Every head and neck examination should include a thorough palpation of the lymph nodes of the face and neck.

HEMATOLOGIC SIGNS

Serious oral infections may cause an elevation of the white blood cell count. A normal white blood cell count ranges from 4000 to 10,000 cells per cubic millimeter. In infection, the white blood cell count can rise to the 12,000-20,000 cells/mm^3 range.

The differential white blood cell count can give clues as to the nature of the infectious process. This is a measure of the relative percentages of the various types of white blood cells which make up the total white blood cell count. Polymorphonuclear leukocytes (PMNs) are normally 55 to 65 percent of the white blood cell count. An increase in this percentage most often indicates an acute bacterial infection. Elevation of the lymphocyte count, which should be 25 to 35 percent of the total, indicates a chronic bacterial or viral infection. Elevation of the eosinophil count (1 to 3 percent) occurs in the common cold, asthma, allergies, and certain parasitic infections.

The erythrocyte sedimentation rate can be useful in detecting chronic inflammatory processes. This test is very sensitive to any source of inflammation, but does not specifically indicate any particular cause of inflammation. It may be useful in looking for a chronic low-grade infection, such as osteomyelitis. Normal values are 0 to 10 mm/hr in males and 0 to 20 mm/hr in females.

Laboratory Diagnosis

CULTURING TECHNIQUES

Almost any specimen can be cultured. It is not necessary to have pus available before a culture can be taken and sent to the microbiology laboratory. In fact, it is most advantageous to take a culture before a fluctuant abscess with pus has developed. Adequate samples for culture can be taken from the serosanguineous fluid in a cellulitis, soft tissue removed from an infected area, foreign bodies, and even pieces of

TABLE 17-2. *Nodal drainage of head and jaws*

Nodes	Site
Occipital	Scalp posterior to ear and occipital region
Postauricular	External ear, scalp above and behind ear
Anterior auricular (preauricular, parotid)	Skin anterior to the temple, external meatus, lateral forehead, lateral eyelids, infraorbital nodes, posterior cheek, part of outer ear, parotid gland
Inferior auricular (infraauricular)	Pre- and postauricular nodes
Accessory facial	
Infraorbital	Skin of inner corner of eye, skin of anterior face, superficial aspect of nose
Buccal	Skin over anterior face; mucous membrane of lips and cheeks; occasionally mandibular and maxillary teeth and gingiva
Mandibular (supramandibular)	Skin over mandible; mucous membrane of lips and cheeks; occasionally mandibular and maxillary teeth and gingiva
Submental	Tip of tongue, mid-portion of lower lip, chin, lower incisors and gingiva
Submandibular (submaxillary)	Upper and lower teeth and gingiva except mandibular incisors; anterior nasal cavity and palate; body of tongue, upper lip, lateral part of lower lip, angle of the mouth, medial angle of the eye, submental nodes
Superficial cervical	Pinna and adjacent skin; pre- and postauricular nodes
Deep cervical	Submandibular, submental, inferior auricular, tonsillar, and tongue nodes

From: Topazian, R. G., and Goldberg, M. H., eds.: Management of Infections of the Oral and Maxillofacial Regions. Philadelphia, W. B. Saunders Co., 1981. Used with permission.

bone, especially necrotic bone, found in an infection.

Gram stain. The ability to obtain quickly a gram stain, either in the office or in a nearby laboratory, can be most useful in determining the predominant organisms in a specimen of pus. This makes a rational choice of initial, or empiric, antibiotic therapy possible. For example, a smear consisting of gram-positive cocci in chains and gram-negative rods strongly suggests a *Peptostreptococcus* and *Bacteroides* infection, which is most likely sensitive to penicillin. A smear showing a predominance of gram-positive cocci in clumps suggests a *Staphylococcus* infection quite likely to be resistant to penicillin.

Aspiration. The most reliable technique for obtaining a culture is aspiration (Fig. 17-4). Aspiration through the skin can be accomplished by the following technique. The skin overlying the involved area is prepared with an antiseptic. Five percent tincture of iodine is ideal for this purpose because it is the most rapidly acting.

Anesthesia of the skin is attained. A large bore needle, 18 gauge or larger, is adapted to a sterile syringe and advanced through the prepared skin into the area of suspected infection. It may be necessary to probe several places within the area to find a specimen for culture. It is not a failure if pus is not obtained. Serosanguineous fluid, cystic fluid, or liquefied hematoma can also be cultured.

This same technique can be used for aspiration through the oral mucous membranes, but it is even more essential to swab the area of puncture with an antiseptic, lest the culture be contaminated with normal oral flora residing on the mucous membrane.

Once the specimen has been obtained, the needle should be thrust into a rubber stopper, and the entire stoppered syringe carried directly to the microbiology laboratory if it is readily available. Otherwise, commercially available culture tubes may be used.

Anaerobic cultures. An estimated 75 to

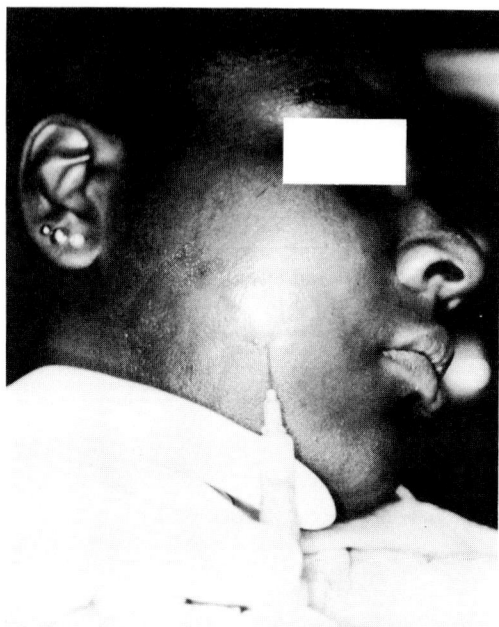

FIG. 17-4. *Aspiration of purulent material from a buccal space infection. (From: Topazian, R.G., and Goldberg, M.H., eds.: Management of Infections of the Oral and Maxillofacial Regions. Philadelphia, W.B. Saunders Co., 1981. Used with permission.)*

90 percent of the bacteria of the oral cavity are anaerobic. The role of anaerobic bacteria in the pathogenesis of oral infections is becoming increasingly apparent, as discussed subsequently. Therefore, both anaerobic and aerobic cultures should be performed on all oral specimens. The stoppered syringe is ideal for transporting the specimen to the microbiology laboratory if it is nearby, but commercially available culture tubes that establish an anaerobic environment for the specimen are acceptable when a longer holding period is necessary.

Microbiology of Oral Infections

Oral infections usually are dentoalveolar in nature, originating from an infected necrotic pulp or from periodontitis. They are caused by the organisms ordinarily found in the oral cavity. In order to select the proper antibiotic initially, especially while awaiting the results of culture and sensitivity testing, and for purposes of prophylaxis of infection, it is important to know which organisms are usually found in the oral cavity.

Table 17-3 shows the distribution of important groups of organisms found in the mouth and associated with oral infections. Both aerobic and anaerobic gram positive and gram negative rods and cocci are found.

Earlier reports of the types and distribution of oral microorganisms showed a preponderance of streptococci, staphylococci, and aerobic gram negative rods. With the development of techniques for obtaining, transferring, and culturing anaerobic specimens, anaerobic microorganisms are now reported to be predominant. In addition to the aerobes mentioned above, the anaerobes in the oral cavity are: the gram-positive cocci (*Peptostreptococcus, Peptococcus*), gram-negative cocci (*Veillonella*), gram-positive rods (*Actinomyces, Lactobacillus*) and gram-negative rods (*Bacteroides* and *Fusobacteria*).

Cultures of orofacial abscesses show that the majority are a mixture of aerobic and anaerobic species. A much smaller number are purely aerobic or purely anaerobic, whether involving a single species or several species. It is of interest to note that *Staphylococcus* and *Bacteroides fragilis,* both usually resistant to penicillin, are found infrequently in oral cultures. Therefore, empiric antibiotic therapy or prophylaxis ordinarily does not need to be directed towards those organisms.

Antibiotic Therapy

Antibiotics give the clinician a potent weapon for treating infections. It must be stressed, however, that antibiotics are not a panacea. Patients still experience serious morbidity and death from infections despite intensive antibiotic therapy. In addition, they may experience toxicity, allergy, side effects, and superinfections from the antibiotic itself.

Microbial virulence, local anatomic features, surgical and antibiotic therapy, and host defenses play a role in the outcome of an infection. Of these, host defenses are the most important in determining the outcome. Antibiotics are useful in complementing host defenses, while surgical intervention by properly timed incision and drainage (I & D) and removal of the source of infection (the infected tooth or its pulp) are essential in proper treatment. Antibiot-

TABLE 17-3. *Distribution of important groups of indigenous microorganisms in the head and neck region*

Organism	Mouth	Site Oropharynx	Skin
Gram-positive facultative cocci			
α-Streptococcus	+ + + +	+ + + +	0
β-Streptococcus	+	+ +	0
nonhemolytic Streptococcus	+ + +	+ + +	0
pneumococci	+	+ +	0
Staphylococcus epidermidis	+ + +	+	+ + + +
Staphylococcus aureus	+ + +	+ + +	0
Gram-positive anaerobic streptococcus			
Peptostreptococcus	+ + +	+ + +	0
Gram-positive facultative rods			
diphtheroids	+ + + +	+ + +	+ + + +
Lactobacillus	+ + +	0	0
Actinomyces	+ + +	+ + +	0
Gram-positive anaerobic rods			
Clostridium	+	0	0
diphtheroids	+ + +	+ + +	+ + +
Gram-negative facultative cocci			
Neisseriae	+ + +	+ + + +	0
Gram-negative anaerobic cocci			
Veillonellae	+ + + +	+ + +	0
Gram-negative rods			
Pseudomonas	+	0	0
coliform bacteria	+	+	0
Gram-negative anaerobic rods			
Fusobacterium	+ + +	+	0
Bacteroides	+ + +	+	0
Spirochetes	+ + +	+	0
Yeasts	+ + +	+ + +	+ + +

+ + + + = Generally present as major component of cultivatable flora
+ + + = Generally present as minor component of cultivatable flora
+ + = May be present as major component in carriers
+ = Often present as minor component or transient
0 = Not normally present
From: Schuster, G. S., and Burnett, G. W.: The microbiology of oral and maxillofacial infections. *In*: Management of Infections of the Oral and Maxillofacial Regions. Edited by R. G. Topazian and M. H. Goldberg. Philadelphia, W. B. Saunders Co., 1981. Used with permission.

ics alone cannot eradicate certain infections if surgical therapy is ignored. Adherence to sound principles of antibiotic therapy is essential if maximal good and minimal harm are to come from therapy.

Principles of the Use of Antibiotics

The following principles should be observed in the correct use of antibiotics.

1. Whenever possible, the identity of the organisms should be determined by culture. No single antibiotic is effective against all organisms. Therefore, identification of the responsible organism is critical if an intelligent selection of antibiotic is to be made.

2. Determine the most likely organism for the region involved. Most oral infections come from normal oral flora, e.g., *Streptococci, Peptostreptococci, Peptococci, Bacteroides,* and *Fusobacteria.*

3. Ordinarily, give a bactericidal rather than a bacteriostatic drug. This is especially important in patients with compromised defenses such as the "brittle" diabetic, immunosuppressed patients, or those on dialysis or receiving cancer chemotherapy.

4. Give the antibiotic in the proper dose, at the proper interval, and by the proper route.

5. Give the drug for a long enough period to allow the infection to be completely eradicated. Continue the drug for 3 to 5 days after symptoms have subsided. However, in cases involving actinomycosis and osteomyelitis, therapy extends for weeks or months.

6. Of the effective drugs, give the one with the least toxicity and narrowest spectrum to minimize the likelihood of unwanted side effects or superinfection.

7. Instruct the patient about the signs and symptoms of toxicity and allergy to the drug being used. Discontinue the drug if toxicity or allergy develop.

8. Be alert to the development of superinfections such as candidiasis (moniliasis, thrush).

9. Do not use an antibiotic for surgical prophylaxis when the benefit is debatable and the potential complications from not using them are minor and readily and simply treated (routine extractions and "dry-socket").

10. Be reluctant to use the newest drug in preference to the one that is well-known and of proven effectiveness. Often, side effects of newer drugs are not recognized until after several years of clinical use.

11. Consider the cost. A course of the newer antibiotics may cost as little as $40 or as much as $140 per day for equally effective drugs within the same antibiotic group, e.g., the cephalosporins. On the other hand, adequate doses of penicillin and erythromycin cost less than two dollars a day.

MECHANISMS OF ACTION

Antibiotics usually affect microorganisms by disrupting cell wall synthesis, protein synthesis, or the cell membrane.

All penicillins, the cephalosporins, and vancomycin are bactericidal and affect cell wall synthesis. Streptomycin, gentamicin, tetracycline, erythromycin, and clindamycin interfere with protein synthesis. Some are bactericidal and some bacteriostatic. Nystatin, polymyxin B, and amphotericin B are all bactericidal and act by disrupting the bacterial cytoplasmic membrane.

WHEN NOT TO GIVE ANTIBIOTICS

Antibiotics should be given only when an infection exists and there is a specific and rational expectation that they will be helpful. Giving an antibiotic with the philosophy that it can't do any harm and probably will do some good is a fallacy often held by the public as well as by some health professionals.

Antibiotic administration has several disadvantages and hazards. It may cause an allergic reaction, or it may sensitize the patient so that allergy occurs on subsequent administration of the drug. Overdose can cause toxic effects. Producing superinfections such as candidiasis, the masking of low-grade infection, and unnecessary cost are additional disadvantages. Dental patients with discomfort or pain but without systemic signs of infection, such as trismus, fever, or lymphadenopathy, usually need no antibiotics. Therefore, do not give antibiotics to otherwise healthy patients with chronically abscessed teeth, acute or chronic pulpitis, dry socket, or pericoronitis, or to those having ordinary dentoalveolar surgery such as alveoloplasty, uncomplicated extractions, routine endodontics, or periodontics.

Localized vestibular and palatal abscesses rarely require adjunctive antibiotics because localization indicates that the host is dealing effectively with the infection: only incision and drainage are indicated.

WHEN TO GIVE ANTIBIOTICS

Antibiotics are used to treat infections and to prevent infection when exposure to an infectious agent could result in serious morbidity, such as endocarditis.

Administering an antibiotic to a patient is indicated in the following situations:

1. Acute cellulitis of dental origin
2. Acute pericoronitis with elevated temperature and trismus
3. Deep fascial space infections
4. Open (compound) fractures of the mandible and maxilla
5. Extensive deep or old (more than six hours) orofacial lacerations
6. Dental infection or dental surgery in the compromised host: steroid therapy,

brittle diabetes, renal transplants or hemodialysis, cancer chemotherapy, AIDS, liver cirrhosis, and splenectomy
7. Dental infection or dental surgery in the patient who has had radiation therapy to the jaws (see section on "Osteoradionecrosis")
8. Prophylaxis for dental surgery in the patient with valvular cardiac disease, prosthetic cardiac valve replacement, or other prosthetic implants (see section on "Subacute Bacterial Endocarditis")
9. Deep surgical wounds that are clean-contaminated, contaminated, or infected

Antibiotics Useful for Oral and Maxillofacial Infections

Of the dozens of antibiotics and antibiotic products available, a limited number are particularly useful in treatment of oral infections. They are: penicillins, antistaphylococcal penicillins, erythromycins, clindamycin, tetracyclines, cephalosporins, and vancomycin. These are discussed briefly. Further information, particularly regarding pharmacology, mechanism of action, metabolism, side effects and contraindications may be found in standard textbooks of pharmacology or therapeutics. The antimicrobial spectrum of the antibiotics commonly and appropriately used for oral infections is listed in Table 17-4. Antibiotics of choice for infections caused by common oral pathogens are listed in Table 17-5. Their doses, route of administration, and major adverse effects are listed in Table 17-6.

CLINICAL COMMENTS

Penicillin. Penicillin is the first drug of choice for oral infections, based on its appropriate spectrum, effectiveness, lack of toxicity, and low cost. Allergy to penicillin is common, however, and must always be checked for.

Penicillinase-resistant penicillins. The antistaphylococcal penicillins have a relatively narrow spectrum. They should be used to treat infections caused by penicillinase-producing staphylococci. When this type of organism is found in addition to the usual flora of oral infections, an anti-staphylococcal penicillin may be added to Penicillin G or V.

Erythromycin. Erythromycin is the alternative drug for many dental infections in the penicillin-allergic patient. It is bacteriostatic to many oral anaerobic bacteria although some practitioners prefer other antibiotics, such as a tetracycline for nonserious infections and clindamycin for serious infections in the penicillin-allergic patient.

Cephalosporins. Cephalosporins are broad spectrum antibiotics affecting both gram-positive and gram-negative organisms. They are most indicated where the identity of the organism is not yet known, and thus the broad spectrum is desirable. They are divided into several "generations," or groups with varying activity. They are not the first choice for treatment of odontogenic infections since they are so broad in spectrum. Their spectrum does not coincide with the bacteria predominantly found in oral infections. They are also fairly expensive. About 15 percent of people allergic to penicillin show allergy to the cephalosporins, especially if the reaction has been anaphylactoid.

Clindamycin. Clindamycin is a good choice in the penicillin-allergic patient. It is effective against anaerobes, streptococci, and penicillinase-producing staphylococci. However, clindamycin is very expensive. Antibiotic-associated pseudomembranous colitis, a superinfection of the gut by *Clostridium difficile*, may occur when clindamycin is used. This is a serious condition diagnosed by stool culture and treated by discontinuing the drug and administering oral vancomycin. Antibiotic-associated colitis may occur with many other antibiotics as well.

Tetracyclines. The tetracyclines are bacteriostatic. They are not generally used for odontogenic infections except in penicillin-allergic patients with nonserious infections. No member of this class has clear superiority over the others.

Vancomycin. Because of its toxicity, vancomycin has limited use. However, it has value in prophylaxis for dental patients with prosthetic heart valves at risk for endocarditis (SBE), and in treatment of antibiotic-associated colitis. Because it is not absorbed by the gut, vancomycin is given

TABLE 17-4. *Antimicrobial spectrum of common antibiotics*

Antibiotic	Spectrum
Penicillins G and V	Streptococcus (except Group D enterococci) Staphylococcus (non-penicillinase-producing) Treponema Neisseria Actinomyces Most oral anaerobes
Antistaphylococcal Penicillins (Oxacillin, Dicloxacillin, Nafcillin)	Penicillinase-producing Staphylococcus (S. aureus and S. epidermidis)
Ampicillin and Amoxicillin	As for penicillin Enterococcus (Group D streptococcus) Haemophilus influenzae Escherichia coli
Erythromycin	Streptococcus Staphylococcus Haemophilus influenzae Legionella Most oral anaerobes
First generation cephalosporins (Cephalexin, Cephalothin, Cefazolin)	Streptococcus (except Group D) Staphylococcus (including penicillinase-producing) Escherichia coli Proteus mirabilis Klebsiella
Second and third generation cephalosporins (Cefamandole, Cefoxitin, Cefotaxime)	As for first generation cephalosporins Enterobacter Haemophilus influenzae Bacteroides fragilis Oral anaerobes
Tetracyclines	Streptococcus Staphylococcus Bacteroides Escherichia coli Haemophilus influenzae Shigella
Clindamycin	Streptococcus Staphylococcus Actinomyces Oral anaerobes except Eikenella corrodens Bacteroides fragilis
Metronidazole	Obligate anaerobes only Bacteroides Clostridia
Vancomycin	Streptococcus (including Group D) Staphylococcus (including penicillinase-producing) Clostridium difficile
Aminoglycosides (Streptomycin, Gentamicin, Amikacin)	Proteus Pseudomonas Escherichia coli Klebsiella Enterobacter Serratia

Adapted from Peterson, L. J.: Principles of antibiotic therapy. *In*: Management of Infections of the Oral and Maxillofacial Regions. Edited by R. G. Topazian and M. H. Goldberg. Philadelphia, W. B. Saunders Co., 1981.

TABLE 17-5. *Antibiotics of choice for common oral pathogens*

Pathogen	Type	First Choice Antibiotic	Alternative Antibiotic
Actinomyces	+,R,A	Penicillin G or V	Tetracyclines Clindamycin
Bacteroides fragilis	−,R,AN	Clindamycin	Metronidazole Cefoxitin
Bacteroides melaninogenicus	−,R,AN	Penicillin G or V	Metronidazole Clindamycin Cefoxitin
Clostridium species	+,R,A	Penicillin G or V	Metronidazole Clindamycin Tetracyclines
Eikenella corrodens	−,R,AN	Penicillin G or V	Ampicillin Erythromycin
Enterococcus (Group D streptococcus)	+,C,A	Ampicillin+ Aminoglycoside	Vancomycin+ Aminoglycoside
Fusobacterium	−,R,AN	Penicillin G or V	Metronidazole Clindamycin
Peptococcus	+,C,AN	Penicillin G or V	Clindamycin Metronidazole
Peptostreptococcus	+,C,AN	Penicillin G or V	Clindamycin Metronidazole Cefoxitin
Staphylococcus aureus	+,C,A	Penicillinase- Resistant Penicillin	Cephalosporins Vancomycin Clindamycin
Staphylococcus epidermidis	+,C,A	Penicillinase- Resistant Penicillin	Cephalosporins Vancomycin Clindamycin
Streptococcus pneumoniae (Pneumococcus)	+,C,A	Penicillin G or V	Erythromycin Cephalosporins
Streptococcus pyogenes (β-hemolytic strep.)	+,C,A	Penicillin G or V	Cephalosporins Erythromycin
Streptococcus viridans (α-hemolytic strep.)	+,C,A	Penicillin G or V	Cephalosporins Vancomycin Erythromycin

+=Gram-positive
−=Gram-negative
R = Rod
C = Coccus
A = Aerobe
AN = Anaerobe
Adapted from Peterson, L. J.: Principles of antibiotic therapy. *In*: Management of Infections of the Oral and Maxillofacial Regions. Edited by R. G. Topazian and M. H. Goldberg. Philadelphia, W. B. Saunders Co., 1981.

parenterally for SBE prophylaxis and orally for antibiotic-associated colitis.

Aminoglycosides: The best known members of this group are streptomycin and gentamicin. These drugs, which must be given parenterally, are usually reserved for patients with severe infections. They are effective against most bacteria except streptococci and anaerobes but are seldom used in oral infections.

Metronidazole: This bactericidal antibiotic has been used for many years in certain vaginal infections due to protozoa. Recently, its effectiveness against obligate anaerobic bacteria has been recognized. Its side effects include a metallic taste in the

TABLE 17-6. *Clinical pharmacology of commonly used antibiotics*

Drug	Route of Administration	Usual Adult Dose	Usual Children's Dose*	Major Adverse Effects
Penicillins				
Penicillin G	IM, IV	600,000-2 million units q 2-4 h	25,000-90,000 units/kg/day (4 doses)	allergy
Penicillin V	PO	250-500 mg qid	15-50 mg/kg/day (4 doses)	allergy
Oxacillin	IM, IV	500-1000 mg q 4-6 h	50-100 mg/kg/day (4 doses)	allergy
Dicloxacillin	PO	125-250 mg qid	12.5-25 mg/kg/day (4 doses)	allergy
Ampicillin	PO, IV	250-500 mg qid	25-100 mg/kg/day (4 doses)	allergy
Amoxicillin	PO	250-500 mg q 8 h	20-40 mg/kg/day (3 doses)	allergy
Non-Penicillins				
Erythromycin	PO, IV	250-1000 mg qid	30-50 mg/kg/day (4 doses)	GI upset
Cephalothin	IV	500 mg-1 g q 4 h	80-160 mg/kg/day (6 doses)	allergy
Cephalexin	PO	500 mg-1g qid	25-50 mg/kg/day (4 doses)	allergy
Cefamandole	IM, IV	500 mg-1g q 4-8 h	50-100 mg/kg/day (4 doses)	allergy
Tetracycline	PO	250-500 mg qid	25-50 mg/kg/day (4 doses)†	GI upset
Doxycycline	PO, IV	50-100 mg bid	2-4 mg/kg/day (2 doses)†	GI upset
Clindamycin	PO, IV	150-450 mg qid	8-16 mg/kg/day (4 doses)	diarrhea
Metronidazole	PO, IV	500 mg qid	35-50 mg/kg/day (4 doses)	nausea
Vancomycin	PO, IV	500 mg qid	44 mg/kg/day (4 doses)	phlebitis
Streptomycin	IM, IV	500 mg-1 g bid	20-40 mg/kg/day (2 doses)	renal damage

*For children weighing less than 40 kg.
†Tetracyclines should not be given before tooth development is complete (about 8 years old.)

mouth, nausea, and violent abdominal pain when combined with alcohol ingestion. It is reserved for use in serious infections caused by culture-proven obligate anaerobic bacteria like *Bacteroides*.

Pathways of Infection

Spreading of Infection Within the Tooth

Infection follows the path of least resistance. The microorganisms responsible for a deep carious lesion, once they have penetrated the pulp, stimulate the process of inflammation within the pulpal soft tissues. The fact that the dental pulp is a soft tissue enclosed by an unyielding hard tissue structure, the dentin surrounding the pulp cavity, is critical in the understanding of the spread of infection through and beyond the tooth.

As the inflammatory process within the pulp begins, vasodilatation, followed by the extravasation of tissue fluid and inflammatory cells, causes edema. Because the pulp is enclosed by unyielding tooth structure, the hydrostatic pressure within the dental pulp rises to the point where it equals or exceeds the blood pressure in the capillaries that feed the cells of the dental pulp. At this point, the circulation to the soft tissues of the pulp ceases, ischemia ensues, and eventually necrosis. Once the blood supply is cut off, access to the tissues of the pulp by the host's defenses ceases also. Parenterally administered antibiotics do not penetrate this avascular area. Therefore, the dead tissues of the dental pulp become an ideal culture medium for invading bacteria to grow in and multiply until they spread beyond the confines of the tooth itself, periodically seeding the surrounding tissues.

Spreading of Infection Within Bone

The bone of the alveolar processes is

quite similar to the dental structures in terms of its response to infection. The alveolar bone consists of interconnecting marrow spaces, delimited by unyielding calcified tissue, all of which are enclosed circumferentially by a layer of cortical bone of varying thickness. Therefore, the invasion of bacteria from the pulp canal into these marrow spaces triggers the process of inflammation, and causes the same sequence of edema, ischemia, necrosis, and isolation from the systemic circulation and the immune system. This is the process by which bacteria are able to survive within the bone of the jaws.

The path of least resistance from this point is along the medullary spaces. This explains the ability of odontogenic infections, such as osteomyelitis, to spread for great distances along the jaws before they erode through the cortical plate.

Another factor in the spread of infection within bone is the thickness of the cortical plate on either side of the bone. In the maxilla, the buccal cortical plate is thin and perforated frequently by nutrient vessels from the overlying periosteum. The palatal cortical plate, on the other hand, is much thicker and is perforated much less frequently. Therefore, it is much more common for infections from the maxillary teeth to erode through the buccal plate of the maxilla, spreading from there into the soft tissues of the face or into the oral cavity. In the posterior mandible, the opposite is true. The buccal plate of bone overlying the mandibular bicuspids and molars is much thicker than the lingual. Indeed, the mandibular second and third molars are placed quite medial to the main bulk of the body of the mandible. The thin lingual plate curves laterally toward the inferior border as it passes under the apices of these teeth. Therefore, infection arising in the mandibular posterior teeth is quite likely to erode inferiorly through the thin lingual plate, spreading into the soft tissues of the floor of the mouth.

Spreading of Infection Within Soft Tissues

Muscles, fascia, and bone function as anatomic barriers to the spread of infection within soft tissues. Because they have a tight, dense capsule surrounding them, and are well vascularized, muscles are much less susceptible to bacterial invasion than are the loose, fibrous connective tissues surrounding them. Tough condensations of this fibrous connective tissue are known as fascia. They form sheets and allow the various layers of muscle to pass over each other without friction during the functional movements of the body. Thus, the fascial layers are like the tissue paper surrounding each item of clothing within a garment box, which allows them to pass over each other without their becoming unfolded.

The Concept of Tissue Spaces

By their spatial relationships, the muscles and the fascia of the head and neck are able to define potential spaces within which invading bacteria can propagate for a while before spreading on to other spaces. These "spaces" are not empty. They contain various organs, including nerves and blood vessels, salivary glands, lymph nodes, and fat, surrounded by loose, fibrous connective tissue. The spaces of the head and neck are not perfectly enclosed. There are pathways around the muscles through which infection can spread. The surrounding fascia is perforated by blood vessels and nerves, along which infection can progress.

Infection within each space has its own particular diagnostic signs and tends to spread in an orderly, anatomic fashion from one space to another by contiguous extension. If the surgeon understands this process, he can anticipate the spread of infection into dangerous spaces and abort the process by timely incision and drainage.

Stages of Infection in Deep Fascial Spaces

Once an infection spreads beyond the alveolar bone, it enters the perialveolar soft tissues. If the point of bony perforation is on the oral side of the muscles attached to the alveolar process, such as the buccinator, it may perforate through the alveolar mucosa and drain into the oral cavity (Figure 17-5). The sinus tract thus engendered serves as a natural drain for the abscess, and the infection becomes chronic, unless treated by extraction or endodontic ther-

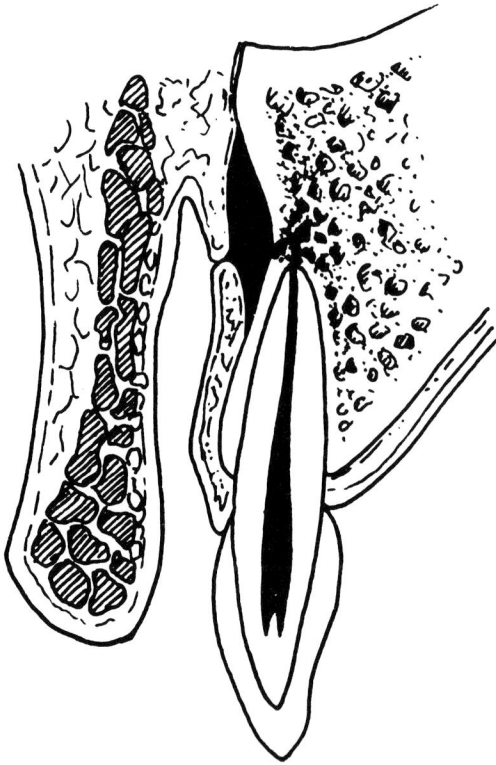

Fig. 17-5. *A chronic dentoalveolar abscess that has perforated the alveolar process and alveolar mucosa on the oral side of the muscles of facial expression.*

multiply and elaborate toxins and metabolic by-products, an intense inflammatory response is triggered. The term, cellulitis, comes from the Latin "cellula," meaning "little room." Thus, it refers to an inflammation in one of the fascial spaces of the body. It appears as a diffuse, reddened, indurated (hard), exquisitely tender swelling in the anatomic region defined by the space or spaces in question.

Antibiotic therapy should be effective for a "pure" cellulitis because there has been no tissue necrosis, and, therefore, access to all parts of the infection by the antibiotic can be obtained via the blood stream. It should be recognized, however, that by the time a cellulitis is clinically apparent, there are most often small pockets of necrotic tissue and pus with no blood supply, which are therefore isolated from the antibiotic.

Stage three: abscess. As the cellular phase of the process of inflammation progresses, inflammatory cells, consisting mainly of polymorphonuclear leukocytes, are drawn to the area of infection by various lymphokines, including leukotaxin. These phagocytes engulf bacteria and di-

apy. The course of this infection will wax and wane according to periodic release of bacteria from the infected tooth to the surrounding tissues and to periodic changes in the patient's resistance to the bacteriologic flora of the abscess.

Stage one: inoculation. If, on the other hand, the infection does not perforate the oral mucosa, it will enter one of the fascial spaces of the face and neck (Fig. 17-6). For several hours to several days after their initial entry into a soft tissue space, the bacteria grow without triggering an intense inflammatory reaction. A mild edema may be in the area, and the patient may experience some soreness. This minor swelling becomes soft and doughy to palpation. This stage of infection responds quite well to removing the dental source of the infection by either extraction or endodontic therapy. Antibiotics are usually not indicated.

Stage two: cellulitis. As the bacteria that have inoculated the soft tissue space

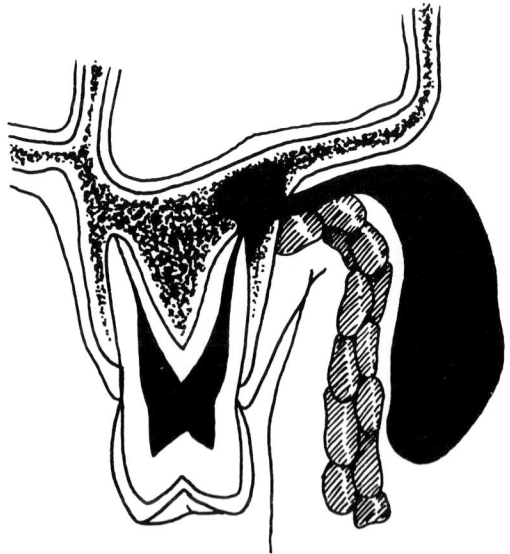

Fig. 17-6. *The attachment of the buccinator muscle coronal to the apices of this maxillary molar has allowed this infection to inoculate the buccal space. If no treatment is rendered, a buccal space abscess will result.*

gest them. Often they themselves will die in the process. Other lymphokines cause the necrosis of surrounding host tissue cells. Small pockets of this necrotic tissue form within the cellulitis, coalesce, and enlarge, compressing the surrounding fibrous connective tissue of the deep tissue space. Thus, an abscess is generated, which is a collection of pus surrounded by a wall of compressed fibrous tissue.

When palpated clinically, a superficial abscess is fluctuant. Fluctuance is determined by using the tip of one finger to press on the mass, while the other one is held over another part of the mass to detect a fluid wave caused by the distortion of the abscess. Fluctuance may be difficult to detect in deep-seated abscesses.

Stage four: resolution. One to two weeks after the beginning of the infection, the specific immune system, consisting of antibodies and activated T-lymphocytes, comes into play. This is seen histologically as a "round cell infiltrate," consisting of lymphocytes, macrophages, and plasma cells. The macrophages are highly efficient in the phagocytosis of bacteria and necrotic cellular debris, and are able over time to dispose of this material.

The process of resolution is speeded greatly by surgical drainage of the abscess cavity or by its rupture, or "pointing," through the skin or mucous membrane. Often, repair of this infected wound leaves a palpable scar (Fig. 17-7).

Surgical Treatment of Infection

Principles of the Surgical Treatment of Oral Infections

The primary treatment of acute bacterial infections of the oral cavity and the deep spaces of the head and neck is NOT the administration of antibiotics, but the establishment of dependent drainage of the infection and the removal of its cause. The following is a stepwise, orderly presentation of the correct treatment of significant infections of the oral cavity, head, and neck.

STEP ONE: OBTAIN A CULTURE

As soon as it has been determined that a patient has a significant infection, a culture should be obtained before any antibiotic

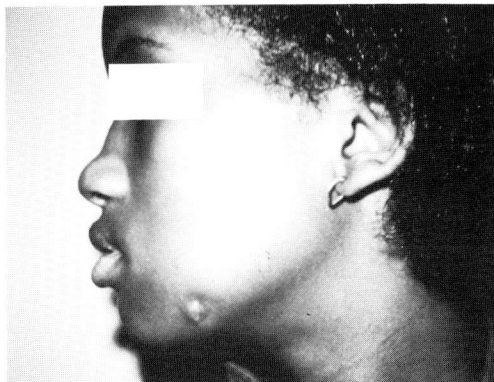

FIG. 17-7. *A puckered, contracted scar resulting from an untreated buccal space abscess that drained spontaneously through the skin.*

therapy begins. The multiplicity of organisms that can cause infections of the head and neck, as well as their varied patterns of resistance to the antibiotics one is likely to use, dictate that "shotgun therapy" for oral and head and neck infections is not acceptable. Prior antibiotic therapy can suppress the growth of a partially susceptible pathogen on subsequent culture. This distorts the true microbial picture of the infection and can lead to misdirected therapy. Therefore, a reliable culture of every significant infection must be obtained before antibiotic therapy is begun.

STEP TWO: EMPIRIC ANTIBIOTIC THERAPY

With a serious infection, it is often necessary to begin antibiotic therapy before the culture result is available. This is called empiric therapy and is directed toward the organisms most likely to cause that infection. Most often, the empiric antibiotic of choice for infections of oral origin is penicillin. For penicillin-allergic patients it is erythromycin.

Even though certain pathogens in the oral flora are becoming more resistant to penicillin and the erythromycins, these drugs remain the antibiotics of choice in empiric therapy of oral bacterial infections. Because penicillin is more effective against the oral anaerobes than erythromycin and is bactericidal to susceptible organisms, it remains the drug of first choice, except for penicillin-allergic patients.

The use of other antibiotics, such as the cephalosporins, the tetracyclines, and the aminoglycosides for empiric antibiotic therapy of oral infections is not indicated. Using these antibiotics without a specific indication based on culture and sensitivity testing increases the expense of care and the likelihood of complications without significantly adding to the effectiveness of the antibiotic therapy. These drugs should be reserved for cases in which the first-choice drugs have failed. Using them prematurely and too often can lead to the development of resistant strains, which diminishes their usefulness when they are really needed. Therefore, using second-choice antibiotics in first-choice situations can be a disservice to the patient.

STEP THREE: ESTABLISH DEPENDENT DRAINAGE

The "lancing" of an abscess is perhaps the oldest surgical procedure. It relieves pain and hastens resolution and healing. It is well known, however, that the infected wound generates more pus after the surgical drainage procedure. Therefore, it is important to allow for the gradual egress of pus and other infected drainage by gravity through a dependent incision. A surgical drain is placed to keep the wound from closing over and to provide a path for the gradual elimination of infected material from the body. The surgical technique of incision and drainage is described below.

Surgical Technique of Incision and Drainage

The surgical technique of incision and drainage is accomplished according to the following principles:

Incision in healthy skin or mucosa. Often, an abscess points through skin or mucosa by necrosis of the overlying tissues. An incision placed over underlying necrosis or through a frank perforation of the skin or mucosa heals with a puckered, contracted scar as the wound edges collapse into the abscess cavity (Fig. 17-7). Rather, an incision placed in skin or mucosa supported by healthy underlying connective tissue heals with a flat, linear scar that is much more acceptable.

Incision in a cosmetically and functionally acceptable place. One should choose the site of incision for an acceptable cosmetic result, such as under the shadow of the jaw line or in a hair-bearing area. Intraorally, the incision should avoid sites of oral function, such as the labial frenula, or the very depth of the vestibule where the flange of a denture may be expected to rest (Fig. 17-8).

Through-and-through drainage for extraoral cases. When incision and drainage is accomplished through the skin, incisions below and anterior and posterior to the site of abscess allow for the placement of the incision in healthy skin and give two paths by which pus can drain from the wound (Fig. 17-9).

One-way drains in intraoral cases. In most situations, adequate dependent drainage can be obtained from a single well-placed incision in the oral mucosa. If multiple spaces are involved, it may be necessary to pass several drains through the incision, one into each of the affected spaces.

Blunt dissection. After the initial sharp incision through skin or mucosa, blunt dissection with a hemostat is performed by gentle poking and spreading of the beaks of the instrument until the abscess cavity is encountered. Within tissue, the beaks of the hemostat should never be closed together, lest a vital structure be crushed.

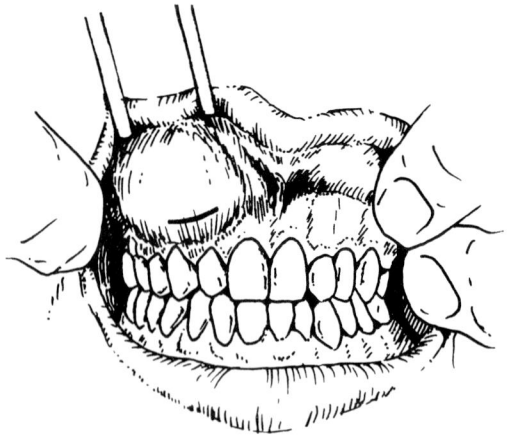

FIG. 17-8. *Intraoral incision placement on the alveolar mucosa near the mucogingival junction, which avoids the frenula and the depth of the vestibule. (Modified from Archer, W.H.: Oral and Maxillofacial Surgery. Vol. I, 5th ed., Philadelphia, W.B. Saunders Co., 1975.)*

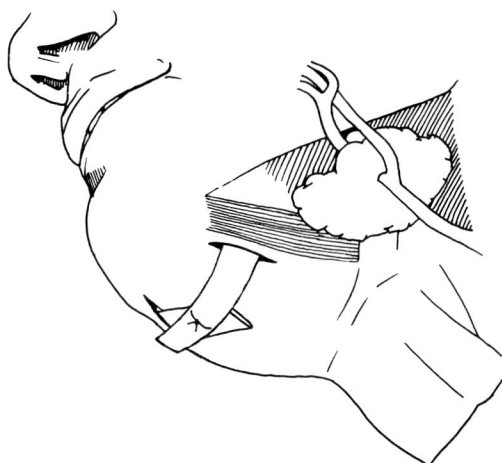

FIG. 17-9. *A through-and-through drain placed in a submental space abscess. The ends of the drain are sutured to each other to prevent its displacement.*

The direction in which the beaks of the hemostat are spread apart is important, too. This should be done parallel to the important vital structures in the region so that if encountered, they are stretched rather than torn.

Thoroughness of exploration. Detailed anatomic knowledge of the extent of the space being explored is necessary. The entire infected space must be explored with the hemostat, and in particular, dissection should extend to the alveolar process overlying the root(s) of the tooth that is the source of the infection.

Stabilization of the drain. The ends of a through-and-through drain can be sutured to each other, thus preventing its displacement (Figure 17-9). A one-way drain should be stitched with a nonresorbable suture to one lip of the incision.

Timing of Incision and Drainage

Dentists have long been taught that an abscess must be incised and drained only when it is fluctuant. The rationale for this teaching is that premature dissection into an area of cellulitis disrupts the natural resistance of the host tissues and opens further fascial planes and anatomic spaces to the infection. In the antibiotic era, however, many oral and maxillofacial surgeons note that early incision and drainage during the cellulitis stage does not spread the infection; rather, it aborts the progression from the cellulitis stage to the abscess stage, and hastens the development of suppuration and eventual resolution.

Principles in the Use of Drains

The proper use of drains follows these principles:

1. Gauze drains allow blood to clot in the interstices of their fabric. Thus, they function as plugs, not drains. They should not be used for drainage.
2. Drains should be removed when the drainage ceases or becomes minimal. After 3 to 5 days, a wound produces a small amount of exudate in response to the rubber drain material itself.
3. Drained wounds should be cleansed under sterile conditions at least twice daily to remove clots and debris. A crusted clot can plug the wound.
4. Bacteria can migrate into a wound along the drain surface. Therefore, drains should not be used in clean wounds, except in special situations.

Supportive Care in Oral Infections

Hydration and Nutrition

A significant elevation of the temperature greatly increases the maintenance fluid requirement, as discussed above. If the patient cannot maintain an adequate state of hydration by his own oral intake, hospitalization and intravenous fluid therapy are required. Similarly, fever increases the body's metabolic requirement. A 1° elevation in the temperature increases the caloric need by 13 percent. The patient should be instructed to force oral food and fluids. If oral fluid intake is inadequate, caloric intake is even more likely to suffer. Therefore, it may be necessary to establish an adequate protein, calorie, and vitamin intake with the various dietary supplement feedings available, or even enteral nutrition by a nasogastric tube.

Control of Fever

Below 103° F, fever is probably beneficial. It has been shown that phagocytosis is more efficient at mildly elevated body temperatures. The fever rises in response to endogenous pyrogen, which is composed of fragments of bacterial cell walls and is released from the host's inflammatory cells. Increasing the core body temperature increases blood flow to the infected area, raises the metabolic rate of the host tissues, and enhances the activity of enzymes, antibodies, and inflammatory cells.

Above 103° F, a fever may cease to be helpful, placing undue stress on the cardiovascular system, depleting energy stores, and hastening the dehydration process.

The best technique for controlling a fever is adequate hydration. Restoration of normal fluid status restores the volume of the extracellular fluid, which is the highway along which inflammatory cells pass from the blood stream to the site of infection.

Aspirin and the other salicylates are well known for their antipyretic effects. They should be used only in harmful fevers, above 103° F, because they can disguise a serious fever. Of themselves, they do not enhance host resistance. Aspirin, 10 grains (650 mg) is given by mouth or rectally to control serious fever in the adult patient.

A fever greater than 103° F in an adult, when accompanied by rigors and shaking chills, is a sign of bacteremia, the presence of bacteria in the blood stream. This is an indication for the taking of blood cultures, a specific technique that should be accomplished by hospital-trained personnel.

Control of the Airway

Airway occlusion by infection is one of the most frequent causes of the death of an otherwise healthy dental patient. Many oral and maxillofacial surgeons are familiar with cases of patients who died because of an infection that involved the airway. Soft tissue swelling in the airway caused by infection of the parapharyngeal spaces is first detected by the patient as dysphagia, or difficulty swallowing. The patient may also feel a lump in the throat. These ominous signs should be evaluated thoroughly by a person experienced in serious infections of the head and neck.

Correct positioning is an important emergency measure in the patient with a significant infection involving the airway. The supine position causes the soft tissues of the tongue to fall against the swollen tissues of the oropharynx. This, of course, worsens the impending airway obstruction. The patient should be placed in the prone position, on his side, or leaning forward to

separate these tissues, thus clearing the airway. The patient should be taken directly to a hospital, where definitive control of the airway must be established as soon as possible.

Airway control is established by endotracheal intubation or tracheostomy. A hazard of intubation in cases of parapharyngeal infection is the rupture of an abscess into the pharynx, which can precipitate aspiration of infected material into the lungs. If the patient survives the immediate airway obstruction this would cause, he may succumb to the severe pneumonitis that would ensue.

Sometimes, therefore, it is advisable not to risk this disastrous event by performing prompt and orderly tracheostomy. One must never delay in ensuring the patency of the airway. "The time to do a tracheostomy is when you first think that one may be necessary."

Specific Oral Infections

Pericoronitis (Fig. 17-10)
Causes. Pericoronitis is an infection surrounding a partially erupted tooth. Usually, the offending tooth is a mandibular third molar. This infection is essentially

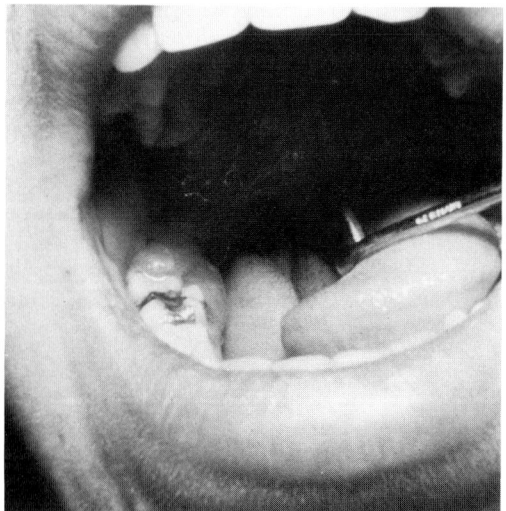

FIG. 17-10. *Pericoronitis of a partially impacted mandibular third molar. (From: Topazian, R.G., and Goldberg, M.H., eds.: Management of Infections of the Oral and Maxillofacial Regions. Philadelphia, W.B. Saunders Co., 1981. Used with permission.)*

a periodontal abscess and has the same microbial flora.

Diagnosis. The patient with pericoronitis is usually an adolescent undergoing stress. The patient presents with pain in the third molar region, intraoral and extraoral swelling, cervical lymphadenopathy, and often trismus. When trismus is present, it is important to evaluate for a pterygomandibular space infection (see "Pterygomandibular Space Abscess" on page 299). Frequently, pus exudes from underneath an operculum, which is a flap of soft tissue overlying the partially impacted tooth. Culturing this material initially can prove helpful if a serious infection is present.

Treatment. The first treatment for someone with pericoronitis is to irrigate, under local anesthesia if necessary, underneath the operculum after a culture has been obtained. This treatment decreases the bacteria in the area, and if further surgical treatment is not instituted immediately, it may allow for some resolution of the infection prior to definitive care. Next, empiric antibiotic therapy, usually penicillin, is begun, and a decision made as to whether further definitive care should be accomplished immediately or in a few days, after antibiotic therapy has afforded the patient some resolution of the infection. This patient should be referred to an oral and maxillofacial surgeon for definitive care.

Dentoalveolar Abscess (Fig. 17-11)

Causes. A dentoalveolar abscess is most often caused by a carious tooth in which bacterial invasion has progressed beyond the root canal and into the surrounding alveolar bone. Often, the bacteria involved are a mixed flora, related to the organisms that caused the carious lesion. Typically, there is a combination of a facultative streptococcus of the *Viridans* group and an anaerobic bacterium such as *Fusobacterium nucleatum* or *Bacteroides melaninogenicus*. Penicillin is still the drug of choice for these organisms.

Diagnosis. Most often, the carious tooth that has caused the dentoalveolar abscess is obvious. Sometimes, however, the redness, tenderness, and edema of the alveolar mucosa do not lie directly over the in-

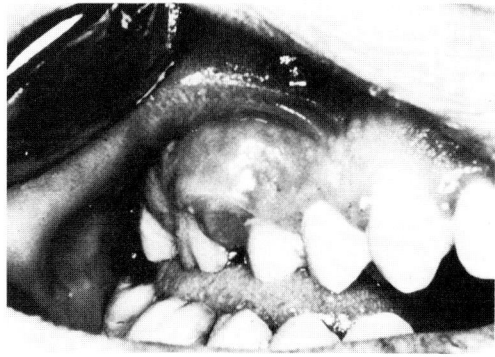

FIG. 17-11. *A dentoalveolar abscess causing a swelling on the attached gingiva and alveolar mucosa. (From: Topazian, R.G., and Goldberg, M.H., eds.: Management of Infections of the Oral and Maxillofacial Regions. Philadelphia, W.B. Saunders Co., 1981. Used with permission.)*

volved tooth because the infectious process can burrow through alveolar bone for some distance before it ruptures the cortical plate and inoculates the overlying soft tissues. In cases of a chronic dentoalveolar abscess, there may be a draining sinus tract in the alveolar mucosa (Fig. 17-5). It may be helpful to probe this sinus tract with a gutta purcha point if doubt exists as to which tooth is causing the infection. An x-ray with the gutta purcha point in place often indicates the apex of the offending tooth. The periapical x-ray also demonstrates a periapical radiolucency when the dentoalveolar abscess has been present for several weeks. An acute dentoalveolar abscess will not have had the time necessary to resorb the mineralized component of the bone structure, and therefore the x-ray of the area may not disclose any bony abnormality. The pulp of the offending tooth usually tests nonvital. Occasionally, however, the tooth may be hypersensitive.

Treatment. Extraction or root canal therapy is indicated for treatment of the pulpal infection. For the infection that has progressed beyond the tooth, gentle curettage of the apical portion of the socket is indicated if the infected soft tissue cannot be found at the end of the extracted root. In an uncomplicated dentoalveolar abscess, antibiotic treatment is usually not necessary.

Follow-up. One can expect loss of cortical bone overlying the apex of a tooth involved in a dentoalveolar abscess. Sometimes this bone loss extends up the buccal surface of the root and may cause an esthetic and periodontal defect for later reconstruction. Further infection, if it has progressed beyond the alveolar process, may continue in the soft tissue spaces surrounding the alveolar process once the tooth has been extracted or root canal therapy has been completed.

Subperiosteal Abscess

Causes. A subperiosteal abscess is caused by the spread of a dentoalveolar abscess. If the infective process perforates the cortical plate of bone without perforating through the overlying periosteal envelope, pus can collect between the periosteum and the bone. The hydrostatic pressure of this pus can dissect the periosteum from the bone, which is an acutely painful process.

A subperiosteal abscess can also arise after a mucoperiosteal flap has been raised from the bone, as during surgical extraction of teeth. When this occurs, often a small piece of necrotic bone or foreign body has been left underneath the flap and acts as a nidus for bacterial growth. The incidence of postsurgical subperiosteal abscesses can be reduced markedly by copious irrigation underneath mucoperiosteal flaps prior to their closure.

Diagnosis. A subperiosteal abscess usually presents as a rounded swelling overly-

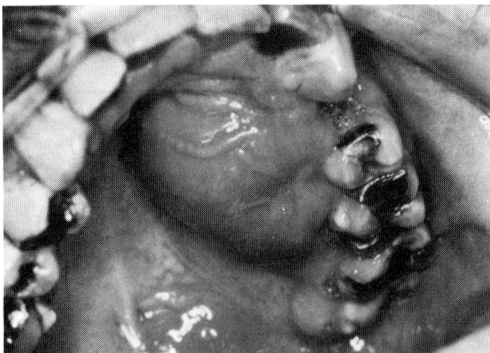

FIG. 17-12. *A subperiosteal palatal abscess arising from a maxillary bicuspid periapical infection. (From: Topazian, R.G., and Goldberg, M.H., eds.: Management of Infections of the Oral and Maxillofacial Regions. Philadelphia, W.B. Saunders Co., 1981. Used with permission.)*

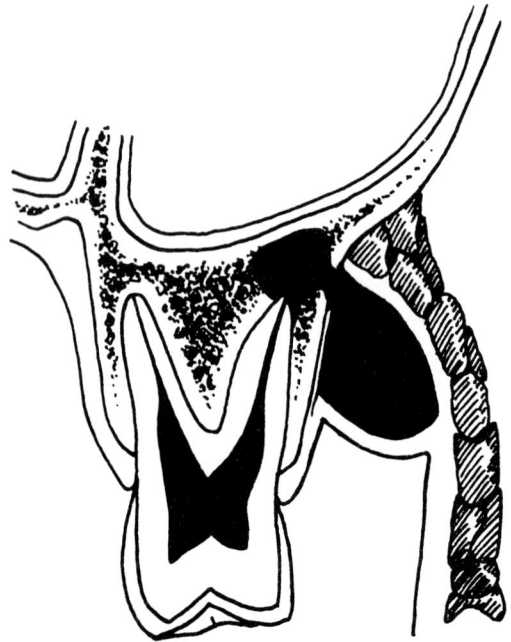

FIG. 17-13. *The attachment of the buccinator muscle superior to the apices of this maxillary molar has directed the spread of the infectious process into the oral vestibule, causing a vestibular space abscess.*

ing the cortical surface of the maxilla or mandible. It is often quite firm on palpation because of the pressure of the underlying fluid, but it is extremely painful. The palatal abscess is a good example of a subperiosteal abscess. It often results from an infection arising from the palatally inclined apex of a maxillary lateral incisor, or from the maxillary bicuspids or molars (Fig. 17-12).

Treatment. Incision with dependent drainage is the treatment of choice for a subperiosteal abscess. In the postsurgical subperiosteal abscess, it will be necessary to re-elevate the mucoperiosteal flap, remove any visible debris, and irrigate copiously the cortical bone and the undersurface of the mucoperiosteal flap.

Vestibular Abscess (Fig. 17-13)

Cause. A vestibular abscess is caused by the extension of a dentoalveolar abscess through the buccal cortical plate of bone and its overlying periosteum into the vestibular space. The vestibular space is the potential space lying between the alveolar, buccal, or labial mucosa and the buccinator or other muscles of facial expression. Entry of an infectious process into this space is determined by the level of the root apex of the infected tooth in relation to the attachment of the buccinator or labial musculature. If the root is short and the apex of the tooth lies coronal to this muscle attachment, the infectious process perforates the cortical plate on the oral side of this musculature, thereby infiltrating the vestibular space.

Diagnosis. The most important sign of a vestibular space abscess is obliteration of the mucobuccal fold. The swelling in this area may be discolored yellow by the underlying pus. The mucosa may be tense due to the hydrostatic pressure of the underlying fluid. A diffuse swelling may be seen extraorally.

Treatment. Intraoral incision and drainage is the primary treatment for the vestibular abscess. In the maxilla, dependent drainage can be readily obtained. In the mandible, however, the principle of dependent drainage is often violated; therefore, it is important to coach the patient thoroughly in expressing pus superiorly along the drain into the oral cavity during the recuperative phase.

A simple stab incision down to bone is adequate for obtaining access to most vestibular abscesses. On the other hand, vital structures that should be avoided by using blunt dissection are the mental nerve in the mandibular bicuspid region, and the labial and buccal frenula. It is also advisable to avoid placing a scar at the depth of the mucobuccal fold which may compromise denture retention in the future (Fig. 17-8). The drain should be placed in the depth of the abscess cavity and sutured to one lip of the incision to ensure its stability.

Deep Space Infections of Odontogenic Origin

Classification of the spaces that odontogenic infections are likely to occupy serves to identify the location of pus and to guide surgical therapy (Figs. 17-14 and 17-15). Each deep space infection has its own characteristic presentation and its own propensity to spread to neighboring spaces. Therefore, it is important to know thoroughly the anatomy and presenting signs of each deep space infection (Tables 17-7

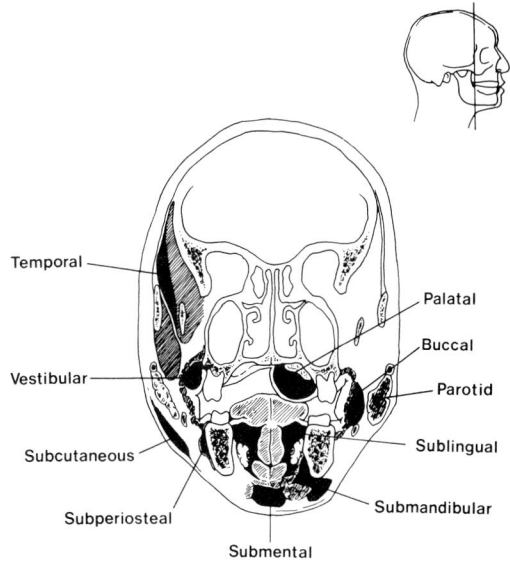

FIG. 17-14. *A coronal section of the face through the region of the maxillary first molar, illustrating the anatomic relations of various deep space infections of odontogenic origin. (Modified from Tiecke, R.W., ed.: Oral Pathology. New York, McGraw-Hill Book Co. Inc., 1965.)*

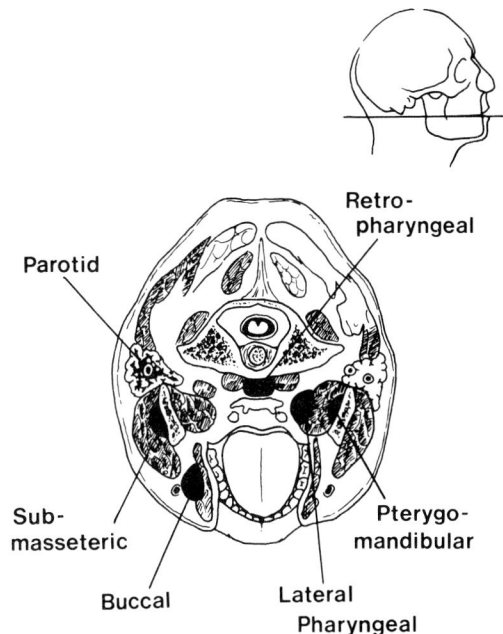

FIG. 17-15. *A horizontal section of the face and neck at the oral commissure, illustrating the anatomic relations of various deep space abscesses of odontogenic origin. (Modified from Tiecke, R.W., ed.: Oral Pathology. New York, McGraw-Hill Book Co., Inc., 1965.)*

TABLE 17-7. *Borders of the deep spaces of the head and neck*

SPACE	BORDERS							
	Anterior	Posterior	Superior	Inferior	Superficial	Deep	Medial	Lateral
Buccal	Corner of mouth	Masseter m. Pterygomandibular sp.	Maxilla Infraorbital space	Mandible	Subcutaneous tissue and skin	Buccinator m.		
Infraorbital		Buccal space	Quadratus labii superioris m.	Levator anguli oris muscle	Subcutaneous tissue and skin	Maxilla	Nasal cartilages	
Submandibular	Anterior belly digastric m.	Post. belly digastric m. Stylohyoid m. Stylopharyngeus muscle	Inf. and medial surfaces of mandible	Digastric tendon	Platysma m. Investing fascia	Mylohyoid, Hyoglossus, Sup. constrictor muscles		
Submental	Inf. border of mandible	Hyoid bone	Mylohyoid m.	Investing fascia				Anterior bellies digastric mm.
Sublingual	Lingual surface of mandible	Submandibular space	Oral mucosa	Mylohyoid m.			Muscles of tongue	Lingual surface of mandible
Pterygomandibular	Buccal space	Parotid gland	Lateral pterygoid m.	Inf. border of mandible			Medial pterygoid m.	Ascending ramus of mandible
Submasseteric	Buccal space	Parotid gland	Zygomatic arch	Inf. border of mandible			Ascending ramus of mandible	Masseter muscle

m. = muscle
sp. = space
Inf. = inferior
Sup. = superior
Post. = posterior

and 17-8) so that the patient can receive prompt and appropriate treatment. These serious infections are best treated by an oral and maxillofacial surgeon.

Principles of Treatment

Benjamin J. Gans, in his *Atlas of Oral Surgery*, articulated these principles:

1. Drain all significant deep space infections. A deep space infection is significant when it has evoked a systemic response by the patient, such as fever, dehydration, and leukocytosis. Further, a deep space infection is significant when it threatens vital structures such as the airway.
2. Do not wait for fluctuance. In deep space infection, fluctuance is a late sign. It occurs only after the suppurative process has burrowed close to the surface. Far more important in the decision to drain a deep space are the duration and nature of the swelling, as well as the systemic status of the patient.
3. Determine incision placement. Incisions for drainage of deep space infections should be designed to avoid important anatomic structures, provide dependent drainage, and leave a cosmetically acceptable scar. Incisions should be placed intraorally whenever possible, but the surgeon should not hesitate to incise extraorally to ensure the patient's well-being.
4. Institute definitive treatment as soon as possible. The offending teeth should be removed as soon as possible unless root canal therapy is planned, or if their removal would be so complicated that it would significantly increase the morbidity of an already sick patient.
5. Check for systemic disease. The patient with a deep space infection of odontogenic origin may have a compromise of his natural defenses. Therefore, a thorough medical history and physical examination are necessary to detect systemic compromise. The compromised host may require significant alterations in therapy, ranging from control of the systemic disease to the use of bactericidal antibiotics and more aggressive surgical therapy.

TABLE 17-8. *Odontogenic deep space abscesses*

Space	Likely Causes	Contents	Neighboring Spaces	Approach for I&D
Buccal	Upper bicuspids Upper molars Lower bicuspids	Parotid duct Ant. facial a. & v. Transverse facial artery & vein Buccal fat pad	Infraorbital Pterygomandibular Infratemporal*	Intraoral (small) Extraoral (large)
Infraorbital	Upper cuspid	Angular a. & v. Infraorbital n.	Buccal	Intraoral
Submandibular	Lower molars	Submandibular gland Facial a. & v. Lymph nodes	Sublingual Submental Lateral Pharyngeal Buccal	Extraoral

Submental	Lower anteriors
	Fracture of
	  symphysis
		Ant. jugular v.
		Lymph nodes
			Submandibular
			  (on either side)
				Extraoral

Sublingual	Lower bicuspids Lower molars Direct trauma	Sublingual glands Wharton's ducts Lingual n. Sublingual aa.	Submandibular Lateral Pharyngeal Visceral (trachea and esophagus)*	Intraoral Intraoral-Extraoral

Pterygo-
mandibular
	Lower 3rd molars	Mandibular div. of
		  Trigeminal n.
		Inf. alveolar
		  a. & v.
			Buccal
			Lateral Pharyngeal
			Submasseteric
			Deep temporal*
			Parotid*
			Peritonsillar*
				Intraoral
				Intraoral-Extraoral

Submasseteric	Lower 3rd molars Fracture of angle	Masseteric a. & v.	Buccal Pterygomandibular Superficial temporal* Parotid*	Intraoral Intraoral-Extraoral

Lateral
Pharyngeal
	Lower 3rd molars
	Tonsils
	Infection in
	  neighboring
	  spaces
		Carotid a.
		Internal jugular v.
		Vagus n.
			Pterygomandibular
			Submandibular
			Sublingual
			Peritonsillar
			Retropharyngeal
				Intraoral
				Intraoral-Extraoral

*For more information on these spaces, see section of Selected Reading on "Odontogenic and Deep Space Infections."

Clinical Comments on Deep Space Abscesses

BUCCAL SPACE ABSCESS (Fig. 17-16)

The attachment of the buccinator muscle relative to the apices of the posterior teeth determines whether an infection arising in a particular tooth will enter the vestibular or the buccal space. For example, if the buccinator attaches inferior to the apex of a maxillary first molar, an infection arising in that tooth will enter the buccal space. The infection will pass out of the bone on the external side of the buccinator muscle as it curves around the mucobuccal fold to attach on the alveolar process of the maxilla. Note that the buccal space is also a subcutaneous space, and therefore abscesses in this region cause necrosis of the overlying skin before they rupture and drain out onto the skin surface. This would leave an unsightly scar on a prominent portion of the face (Fig. 17-7). Therefore, prompt definitive treatment of a buccal space abscess is indicated.

INFRAORBITAL SPACE ABSCESS

The maxillary cuspid tooth is most likely to cause an infraorbital space abscess (Fig. 17-17) because its long root often places its apex superior to the attachment of the levator anguli oris (caninus) muscle. The le-

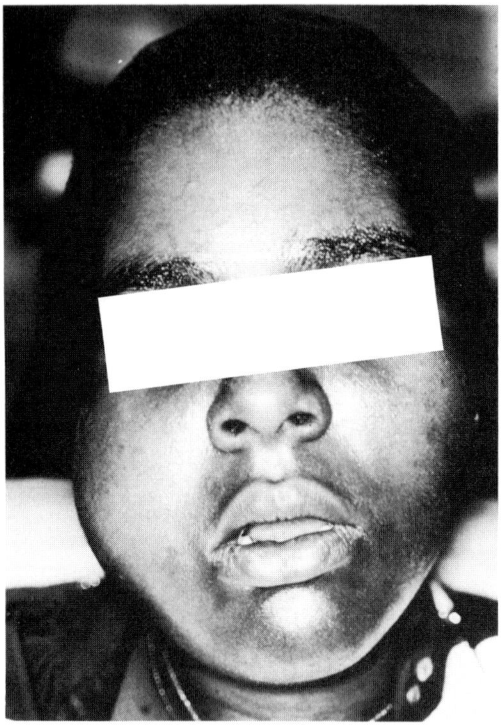

FIG. 17-16. *Clinical appearance of a buccal space abscess. Note how distensible the buccal space is. (From: Topazian, R.G., and Goldberg, M.H., eds.: Management of Infections of the Oral and Maxillofacial Regions. Philadelphia, W.B. Saunders Co., 1981. Used with permission.)*

vator labii superioris muscle, part of the quadratus labii superioris, attaches to the infraorbital rim and acts as a barrier to the pointing of an infraorbital space abscess in the middle of the lower eyelid. An abscess in this space is therefore likely to rupture through the skin of the lower eyelid, either medial to this muscle near the medial canthus (Fig. 17-18), or lateral to this muscle about 1 cm medial to the lateral canthus. The unsightly scar resulting from the external rupture of an abscess in the lower eyelid can be prevented by the timely establishment of dependent drainage using an intraoral drain in the bottom of the infraorbital space (Fig. 17-19).

An infection in the infraorbital space is especially dangerous because of the presence of the angular vein. If an infection erodes into this vein, it can ascend into the orbit through this vein and into the cavernous sinus (see "Cavernous Sinus Thrombosis" on page 301).

SUBMANDIBULAR SPACE ABSCESS (Fig. 17-20)

On the lingual surface of the mandible, the mylohyoid muscle functions like the buccinator muscle on the lateral surface of the maxilla and mandible. The mylohyoid muscle attaches to the medial surface of the mandible on the mylohyoid ridge that runs from close to the inferior border anteriorly to a point high on the alveolar process of the mandible in the second molar region. Therefore, an infection arising from the relatively long roots of the molars is likely to rupture the thin lingual plate inferior to the mylohyoid muscle, thus entering the submandibular space. On the other hand, an infection arising from the shorter roots of the anterior teeth is more likely to rupture the lingual plate of the mandible superior to the mylohyoid muscle, thus entering the sublingual space (see "Sublingual Space Abscess").

The submandibular space is continuous with the sublingual space around the posterior edge of the mylohyoid muscle. An infection can spread readily from either space to the other by this route. Infections in the submandibular space can also enter

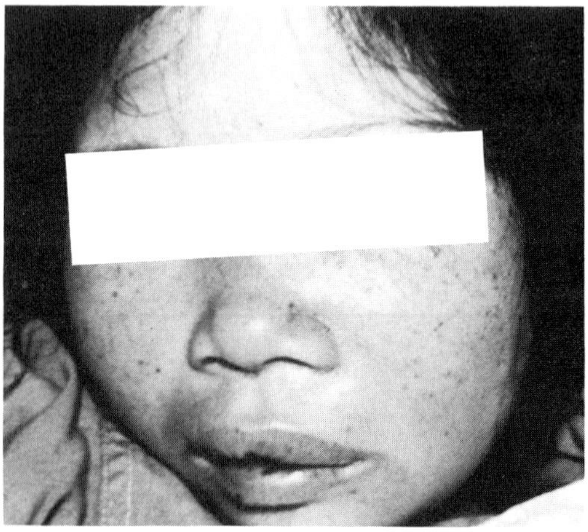

FIG. 17-17. *Clinical appearance of an infraorbital space abscess. Note the periorbital swelling, the edema of the upper lip, and the lifting of the ala of the nose. This abscess is about to point medial to the levator labii superioris muscle, near the medial canthus. (From: Topazian, R.G., and Goldberg, M.H., eds.: Management of Infections of the Oral and Maxillofacial Regions. Philadelphia, W.B. Saunders Co., 1981. Used with permission.)*

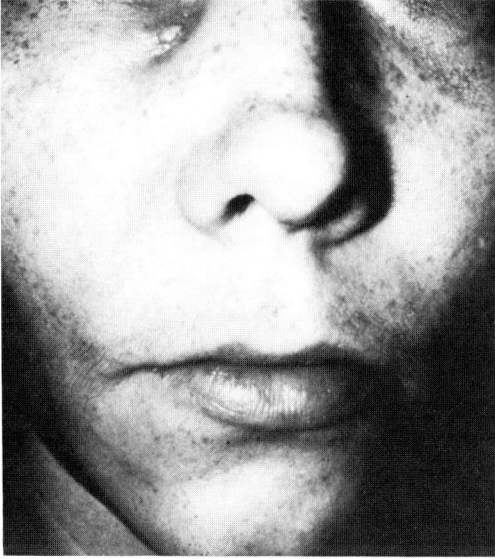

FIG. 17-18. *A chronic infraorbital space infection that has ruptured the skin medial to the levator labii superioris muscle, leaving a draining sinus tract in the lower eye lid. (From: Topazian, R.G., and Goldberg, M.H., eds.: Management of Infections of the Oral and Maxillofacial Regions. Philadelphia, W.B. Saunders Co., 1981. Used with permission.)*

the submental space merely by passing around the digastric muscle. Infections that pierce through the cervical investing fascia enter the subcutaneous space, which is also continuous with the buccal space. Since the posterosuperior border of the submandibular space is the superior constrictor muscle of the pharynx, infection can pass along this muscle to enter the lateral pharyngeal space. Lateral pharyngeal space abscesses can be a serious threat to life (see "Parapharyngeal Space Abscess" on page 302).

SUBMENTAL SPACE ABSCESS (Fig. 17-9)

No midline septum is in the submental space; therefore, an infection entering this space extends rapidly across the midline, delimited by the anterior belly of a digastric muscle on either side. This space often becomes involved by direct extension of an infection from the submandibular space. Lower anterior teeth may also cause a submental space abscess.

SUBLINGUAL SPACE ABSCESS (Fig. 17-21)

No midline septum is in the sublingual space. Therefore, an infection arising in

part of this space rapidly becomes bilateral. Infections also are likely to occur in this space as a result of extension from the neighboring submandibular spaces. Occasionally, a sublingual space infection results from direct trauma, as from an uncontrolled dental handpiece or exodontia elevator.

Swelling in the sublingual space elevates the tongue against the roof of the mouth and prevents the patient from extending the tongue beyond the vermilion border of the upper lip. Further, infection in this space can dissect very rapidly through the base of the tongue to the epiglottis, causing significant edema in the airway. Infections in the sublingual space are a threat to the airway and must receive prompt definitive management.

PTERYGOMANDIBULAR SPACE ABSCESS (Fig. 17-22)

Infection in the pterygomandibular space causes inflammation in the medial

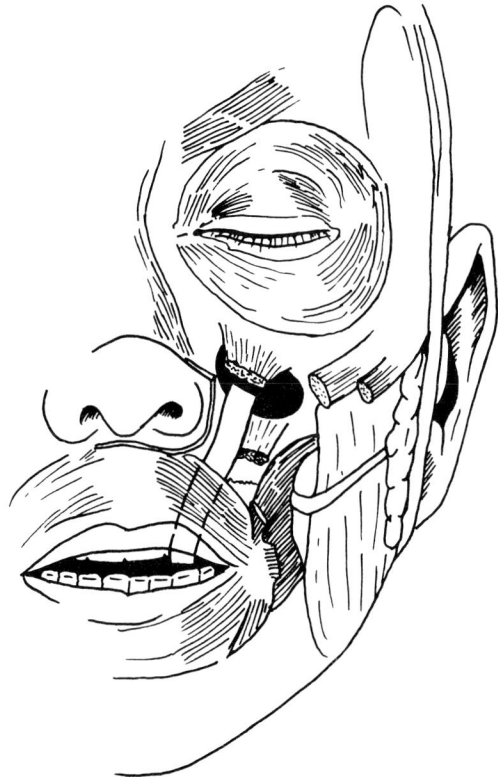

FIG. 17-19. *Intraoral placement of a drain into the infraorbital space.*

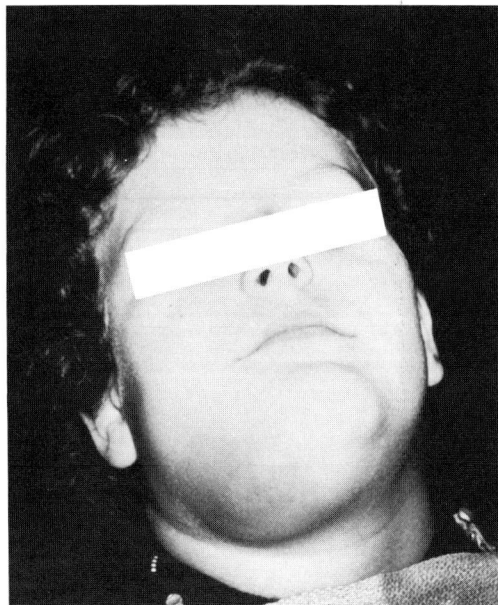

FIG. 17-20. Clinical appearance of a submandibular space abscess. Note the swelling below the inferior border of the mandible which is defined by the two bellies of the digastric muscle. (From: Topazian, R.G., and Goldberg, M.H., eds.: Management of Infections of the Oral and Maxillofacial Regions. Philadelphia, W.B. Saunders Co., 1981. Used with permission.)

pterygoid muscle, resulting in muscle spasm and trismus. A pterygomandibular space infection is difficult to detect because no external swelling may be visible. The clinician must rely upon a history of dysphagia (difficulty in swallowing and sore

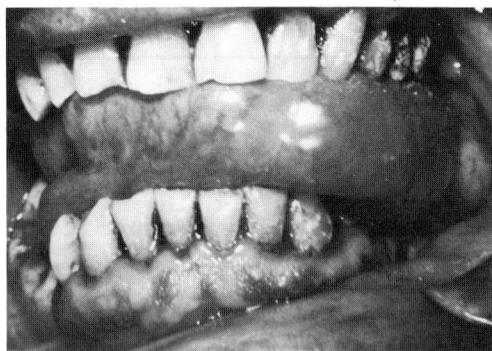

FIG. 17-22. Clinical appearance of a pterygomandibular space abscess. It is difficult to examine this patient because of trismus. Note the bulging of the soft palate and tonsillar pillar, with displacement of the uvula away from the infected side.

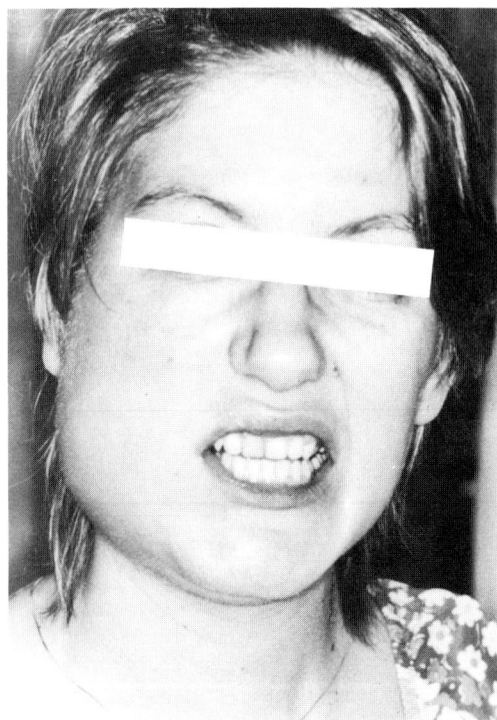

FIG. 17-21. Clinical appearance of a sublingual space abscess. Note that the tongue is raised by the swelling in the floor of the mouth. This patient cannot protrude his tongue, which is indurated and tender to palpation.

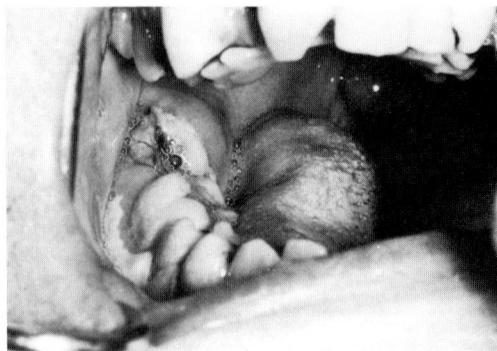

FIG. 17-23. Clinical appearance of a submasseteric space abscess. Note the severe trismus and the delineation of the swelling by the inferior and posterior borders of the mandible and the zygomatic arch. (From: Topazian, R.G., and Goldberg, M.H., eds.: Management of Infections of the Oral and Maxillofacial Regions. Philadelphia, W.B. Saunders Co., 1981. Used with permission.)

throat) in addition to trismus. Often, the examiner must gently pry open the mandible a bit to observe marked swelling and redness of the pterygomandibular raphe and anterior tonsillar pillar region. The uvula will be deviated away from the affected side.

Pterygomandibular space infections can spread very easily around either the anterior or the posterior edge of the internal pterygoid muscle to enter the lateral pharyngeal space. These are a serious threat to life (see "Parapharyngeal Space Abscess"). Therefore, prompt, definitive management of the pterygomandibular space abscess is mandatory.

SUBMASSETERIC SPACE ABSCESS (Fig. 17-23)

The tight adhesion of the masseter muscle to the lateral surface of the ascending ramus of the mandible usually inhibits the spread of infection into this area, except where it has been violated by trauma or surgery.

The masticator space consists of the submasseteric space and the pterygomandibular space. Infection in these spaces can cause trismus due to spasm of the elevator muscles of the mandible, including the internal pterygoid, temporal, and masseter muscles.

Other Serious Deep Space Infections

CAVERNOUS SINUS THROMBOSIS (Fig. 17-24)

Odontogenic infections arising in the face can enter the venous system of the head and neck, and travel against the flow of blood into the cranial cavity. This process is aided by the fact that no valves exist in most veins of the head and neck.

Odontogenic infection can reach the cavernous sinus by two routes. The anterior route commonly involves the infraorbital space and the angular vein which it contains. An abscess that erodes into the angular vein can cause thrombosis and phlebitis extending superiorly along the

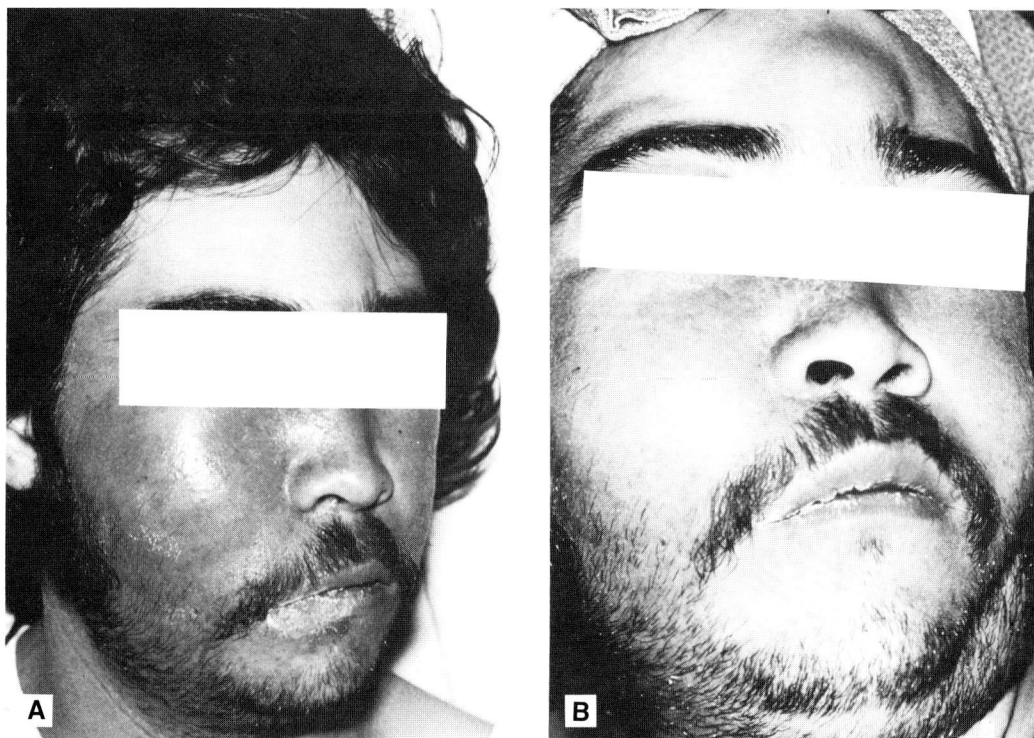

FIG. 17-24. (A) A patient with an infraorbital space abscess which has extended into the buccal, periorbital, and orbital spaces. (B) The same patient, 4 hours later. The infection has spread to involve the infratemporal and temporal spaces and has caused cavernous sinus thrombosis.

course of the angular vein and into the ophthalmic veins. The ophthalmic veins then course posteriorly in the orbit to enter the cranium via the superior orbital fissure. Soon thereafter, they enter the cavernous sinus, which contains many vital structures, including the internal carotid artery and the third, fourth, fifth, and sixth cranial nerves.

The posterior route to the cavernous sinus involves infections that arise in the buccal, pterygomandibular, or temporal spaces, and pass into the infratemporal space, where they erode into the pterygoid plexus of veins. The pterygoid plexus of veins sends emissary veins through the foramina ovale and lacerum, as well as the foramen of Vesalius. These emissary veins then communicate intracranially with the cavernous sinus.

Full-blown infections and thrombosis of the cavernous sinus are most often fatal, constituting a severe meningitis. Rarely does cavernous sinus thrombosis resolve without severe and permanent morbidity, such as blindness or brain damage. Cavernous sinus thrombosis can be prevented by prompt and definitive treatment of odontogenic infections, especially those arising in the maxilla.

LUDWIG'S ANGINA (Fig. 17-25)

Ludwig's angina is classically described as a brawny, board-like induration of the submandibular spaces bilaterally and the sublingual and submental spaces. The cellulitis described here often progresses quite rapidly to involve swelling and obstruction of the larynx and possible death by asphyxiation. Streptococci were once cited as the causative organisms in this infection; however, many organisms, including anaerobes, have been identified.

The treatment for Ludwig's angina includes prompt and definitive management of the airway by tracheostomy, and incision with thorough drainage of the spaces involved in the infection. Intensive antibiotic therapy is also used.

PARAPHARYNGEAL SPACE ABSCESS

The parapharyngeal space consists of three spaces—the lateral pharyngeal space on either side (see Table 17-8) and the retropharyngeal space (Fig. 17-15). A para-

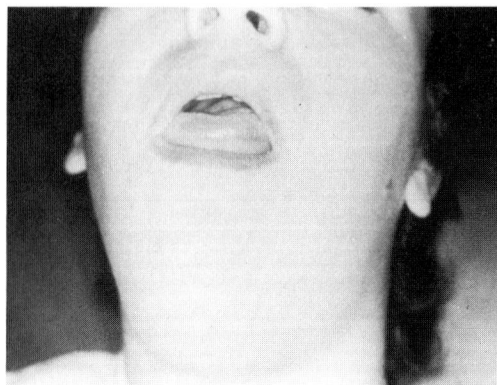

FIG. 17-25. *Clinical appearance of Ludwig's angina. Note the large swelling under the mandible extending from the posterior belly of the digastric muscle on one side to the posterior belly of the digastric muscle on the other side. The floor of the mouth is edematous, elevating the tongue. Typically, the patient has to open the mouth and lean forward to breathe.*

pharyngeal space abscess is caused most often by an infection from a mandibular third molar spreading through the pterygomandibular space into the lateral pharyngeal space. Infection from the tonsils, the parotid gland, or a traumatic wound may also involve the parapharyngeal space.

Abscesses of the parapharyngeal space can cause mortality in two ways. The first is by airway obstruction due to swelling involving the pharynx. The second is by overwhelming infection, since an abscess in the retropharyngeal space can dissect inferiorly to involve the mediastinum. A mediastinal abscess can severely compromise and erode into the great vessels, the esophagus, or the main stem bronchi. A mediastinal abscess can even encircle and compress the heart, causing cardiac tamponade.

SUMMARY

Early recognition and prompt definitive treatment are essential in preventing serious morbidity and possible mortality from deep space odontogenic infections. Never ignore, put off, or dismiss lightly the patient who may be developing such an infection. Deep space infections of the face, head, and neck should be referred to an oral and maxillofacial surgeon for definitive care.

Osteomyelitis of the Jaws

The majority of dental infections are effectively localized by host defenses. Aided by incision and drainage and antibiotics when indicated, they usually resolve without complications. Occasionally, however, the infection becomes established within the mandible (and less frequently in the maxilla), causing osteomyelitis. Osteomyelitis is a bone infection that begins within the medullary portion and spreads to the cortical bone and periosteum with resulting bone necrosis. Osteomyelitis may be either suppurative, i.e., pus producing, or nonsuppurative.

Suppurative Osteomyelitis (Figure 17-26)

The suppurative form of osteomyelitis may be acute or chronic. Host factors play an important role in establishing the condition. It occurs primarily in individuals with marked malnutrition, such as chronic alcoholics and drug abusers, but is also seen in diabetics and patients with agranulocytosis, leukemia, and other conditions affecting host resistance.

The infection usually begins as a periapical infection from a carious tooth or from a secondarily infected mandibular fracture. It spreads according to the process described previously in "Spreading of Infection Within Bone."

Predominant organisms are: *Staphylococcus aureus*, the anaerobic *Bacteriodes* and *Fusobacteria*, and anaerobic and facultative streptococci.

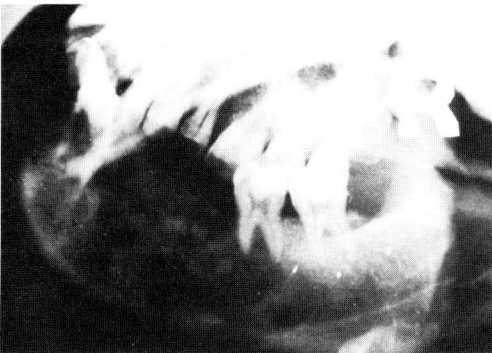

FIG. 17-26. *Lateral oblique radiograph showing destructive changes with formation of sequestra in a patient with osteomyelitis.*

Diagnosis. Typically, the patient presents with pain and loose teeth from around which pus may be expressed. Mucosal fistulas and diffuse firm enlargement of the bone and surrounding soft tissues are seen. In the acute phase, the temperature is elevated; local tenderness and lymphadenopathy are found.

Radiographically, areas of radiolucency are seen early, representing destruction of bone. Segments of nonvital bone of variable sizes (sequestra) are seen later.

Treatment. Prompt recognition and aggressive treatment are necessary to localize the process and to preserve teeth and bone. Initial management consists of intravenous antibiotics, hospitalization, repeated taking of cultures, and surgical debridement. Once osteomyelitis is recognized, referral to an oral and maxillofacial surgeon is wise.

Effective antibiotics are penicillin combined with an antistaphylococcal penicillin, or clindamycin if the patient is allergic to penicillin. The antibiotic selected is based on the results of sensitivity testing.

Depending on the course of the disease, definitive care may consist of sequestrectomy, saucerization, decortication, or occasionally, segmental resection and reconstruction of the chronically infected bone. Treatment with hyperbaric oxygen (HBO) has also been found to be useful in conjunction with antibiotics and surgical treatment.

Nonsuppurative Osteomyelitis

In several forms of osteomyelitis pus is not produced. Of special interest are Garré's sclerosing osteomyelitis and radiation osteomyelitis and necrosis (osteoradionecrosis).

GARRÉ'S OSTEOMYELITIS.

Garré's osteomyelitis is a chronic, nonsuppurative, sclerosing osteomyelitis seen most often in individuals under the age of 20. It is characterized by a localized, hard, nontender swelling of the mandible. Fever, pain, and lymph node enlargement are not found. Usually there is an associated deeply carious first molar tooth.

It has been suggested that in highly resistant individuals, the response to the products of the infection may be a proliferation of bone under the periosteum in the involved area. Radiographs show a localized smooth enlargement of bone with a laminated or onion peel appearance (Fig. 17-27). Treatment consists of extraction or endodontic treatment of the tooth. Antibiotics are not indicated. If the bone has not remodeled by 6 months after extraction or endodontic therapy, or if no likely dental cause has been found, biopsy should be performed to rule out a bone tumor.

OSTEORADIONECROSIS OF THE JAWS.

Patients with a history of radiation therapy involving the jaw have a high potential for developing necrosis of the bone with ensuing loss of a considerable segment of the bone, along with marked pain and discomfort (Fig. 17-28). Cancericidal doses of radiation cause a decreased vascular supply to soft tissue and bone, with localized tissue hypoxia, and cell death. These tissues are unable to transport humoral and cellular resistance factors and antibiotics through the blood stream to the infected area. When a subsequent tooth extraction or denture ulceration exposes the underlying bone, an infection ensues, because of the diminished capacity to combat and localize the infection. Ultimately the bone often must be resected. Reconstruction is

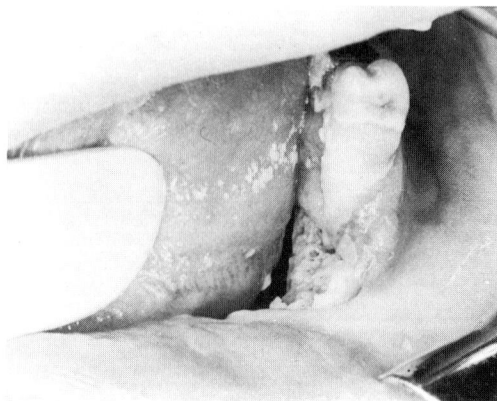

FIG. 17-28. *Exposed bone in a patient with osteoradionecrosis. Note the loss of overlying soft tissue. This painful condition often results from tooth extraction in previously irradiated bone. (Courtesy Dr. Arie Shteyer) (From: Topazian, R.G., and Goldberg, M.H., eds.: Management of Infections of the Oral and Maxillofacial Regions. Philadelphia, W.B. Saunders Co., 1981. Used with permission.)*

difficult because of the compromised blood supply to the adjacent bone and soft tissues.

The dentist can play a major role in preventing osteoradionecrosis. Two aspects of care should be considered:

1. For all patients about to receive radiation therapy in which the jaws will be traversed by the beam, the following steps should be taken:
   a. All nonrestorable teeth in the direct line of radiation should be extracted. If there is marked periodontal disease with poor oral hygiene and motivation, all remaining teeth should be extracted. Alveoloplasty should be performed with careful approximation of the mucoperiosteum. Radiation therapy should be delayed for 10 to 14 days to allow for initial healing.
   b. All remaining teeth should be restored and periodontal therapy completed. Fluoride gel should be applied daily thereafter in a customized tray.
2. If a patient presents for extraction who has previously received radiation therapy to the jaws, extractions should be avoided, if at all possible, utilizing endodontics instead. If the tooth is nonrestorable, antibiotic coverage and careful

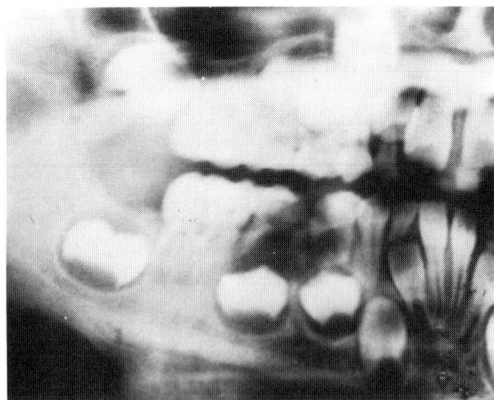

FIG. 17-27. *Panoramic radiograph showing onion peel lamination at the inferior border, typical of Garre's osteomyelitis. (Courtesy Dr. L.J. Peterson) (From: Topazian, R.G., and Goldberg, M.H., eds.: Management of Infections of the Oral and Maxillofacial Regions. Philadelphia, W.B. Saunders Co., 1981. Used with permission.)*

extraction is carried out. Hyperbaric oxygen therapy prior to extraction may prevent or minimize subsequent osteoradionecrosis. Consultation with an oral and maxillofacial surgeon is advisable.

Subacute Bacterial Endocarditis

Subacute bacterial endocarditis (SBE) is an uncommon but devastating complication of dental treatment. Prior to the antibiotic era, dental treatment was the most common precipitating cause of this disease. At present, parenteral drug addiction and prior cardiac surgery are the leading precipitating causes of SBE. Nonetheless, dentists must remain vigilant in identifying those patients at risk for SBE, and in correctly using the most recent recommendations of the American Heart Association for prophylaxis of SBE. Conditions requiring antibiotic prophylaxis for bacteremia caused by dental procedures are listed in Table 17-9.

Any oral procedure likely to stimulate bleeding may cause a bacteremia, the entry of bacteria into the blood stream. Dental extractions, periodontal procedures including prophylaxis, and even the placement of a matrix band, can cause a bacteremia. Home care procedures (brushing, flossing, or using a water-irrigating device) and chewing food can precipitate a bacteremia in patients with significant periodontal disease.

Bacteremia is not normally a danger to the patient without preexisting cardiac disease. In fact, bacteremias probably occur on a daily basis in most people.

The dental patient with a preexisting cardiac defect or valvular lesion is, however, at risk should a bacteremia occur. Bacteria entering the blood stream during an oral manipulation may settle on the irregular surface of a congenital heart defect, or in the interstices of a thrombus that becomes attached to the irregular surface of a damaged heart valve. These bacteria may then find a place to grow, sheltered from the body's resistance factors, yet surrounded by ample sources of nutrition.

Acute bacterial endocarditis is a uniformly disastrous infection that usually results in death in less than 8 weeks from the onset of the disease. *Staphylococcus aureus* is the most common infecting organism in

TABLE 17-9. *When to use endocarditis prophylaxis†*

Endocarditis Prophylaxis Recommended:

> Prosthetic cardiac valves (including biosynthetic valves)
> Most congenital cardiac malformations
> Surgically constructed systemic-pulmonary shunts
> Rheumatic and other acquired valvular dysfunction
> Idiopathic hypertrophic subaortic stenosis (IHSS)
> Previous history of bacterial endocarditis
> Mitral valve prolapse with insufficiency*
> Parenteral drug addiction §
> Synthetic vascular grafts or patches ¶
> Orthopedic prosthetic implants ¶

Endocarditis Prophylaxis Not Recommended:

> Isolated secundum atrial septal defect
> Secundum atrial septal defect repaired without a patch six months or more after surgery
> Patent ductus arteriosus ligated and divided six months or more after surgery
> Postoperative coronary artery bypass graft
> "Functional" heart murmur of mitral insufficiency

---

†This table is not all-inclusive. Medical consultation is indicated in cases that are not clear-cut.

*Patients with mitral valve prolapse are at low risk of development of endocarditis, but the risk-to-benefit ratio of prophylaxis in these cases is uncertain.

§Patients with a history of parenteral drug addiction have a high incidence of valvular lesions on the right side of the heart due to septic emboli from unsterile hypodermic equipment.

¶Antibiotic prophylaxis for surgical implants may be indicated in certain cases. Medical consultation is advisable.

Adapted from Shulman, S. T., et. al.: Prevention of bacterial endocarditis, a statement for health professionals by the Committee on Rheumatic Fever and Infective Endocarditis of the Council on Cardiovascular Disease in the Young (American Heart Association). Circulation *70:*, 1123A, 1984.

this disease. It is not a member of the normal oral flora, and is, therefore, not frequently a result of dental procedures.

On the other hand, SBE is the diagnostic term applied to those patients who have survived the onset of their disease by 8 weeks or more. In the preantibiotic era, more than 90 percent of cases of SBE were caused by streptococcus species of the *Viridans* group. These bacteria are normal residents of the oral cavity. Currently, *S. viridans* species are thought to be responsible for only 35 to 50 percent of cases, and have been surpassed by staphylococci as the most common causative microorganism.

The prophylactic administration of an antibiotic likely to be effective against the *Streptococcus viridans* species may prevent bacteremia caused by dental procedures. Specific recommendations for this procedure are issued periodically by the American Heart Association's Committee on Prevention of Rheumatic Fever and Bacterial Endocarditis. Recent recommendations, based on the best scientific data available to date, are summarized in Table 17-10.

Since a bacteremia can be caused even by chewing in a patient with significant periodontal disease, it is important to establish and maintain a high degree of oral health in patients with any of the conditions discussed above that would predispose to SBE.

Hepatitis B and AIDS

Hepatitis B

Hepatitis B, also known as serum hepatitis and viral hepatitis, develops in approximately 200,000 people in the United States each year and several thousand die hepatitis-related deaths. The significance of hepatitis B in dental treatment is that it can be communicated by contact of a patient's blood or saliva, carrying the hepatitis B virus, with the blood or mucous membrane of a dentist treating that patient. Thereafter, the infected dentist can communicate this disease with his other patients in the same manner, or by infected office equipment or instruments.

Oral and maxillofacial surgeons have a 5 percent annual risk of hepatitis. It is estimated that approximately 30 percent of oral and maxillofacial surgeons will develop hepatitis B infection during their careers. A chronic carrier state can follow acute hepatitis B infection, involving an estimated 2 percent of oral and maxillofacial surgeons. The incidence of hepatitis B after accidental needle stick exposure is 10 to 19 percent. Therefore, dentists and, in particular, oral and maxillofacial surgeons, must take special precautions to prevent acquiring or transmitting Hepatitis B.

AIDS

Acquired immunodeficiency syndrome (AIDS) is an almost uniformly fatal disease that was first recognized in 1981. Approximately 50 percent of the cases reported have had a fatal outcome. Recently, a novel retrovirus, the human T-lymphotropic virus type III (HTLV-III), has been shown to be the likely etiologic agent for AIDS.

This disease, and a group of signs and symptoms that may be prodromal for AIDS, called AIDS-related complex (ARC), has its greatest incidence in certain populations. These are homosexuals, intravenous drug abusers, hemophiliacs, Haitians, Central Africans, and recipients of random blood products. Even more recently, the HTLV-III virus has been found in the saliva, semen, and blood of people with ARC and healthy homosexual men at risk for AIDS.

This prevalence seems to indicate a method of transmission of AIDS similar to that of hepatitis B, and that AIDS may be caused by a virus transmitted either by repeated mucosal contact or serum contact between individuals.

It is not yet known whether significant risk of infection with the HTLV-III virus occurs among health care workers. A recent study of 33 victims of needle stick or blood exposure of hospital employees to AIDS victims or AIDS specimens has disclosed not a single HTLV-III seroconversion after a follow-up of up to 20 months. The incubation period for the virus, however, may be as long as 14 years.

Preventing Hepatitis B and AIDS Infection

Other ways in which hepatitis B (and possibly AIDS) may be transmitted are: direct contact of hands with infectious saliva or blood, aerosol droplets of saliva generated by sneezing, entry of infected spray from dental handpieces into the conjunctiva or mouths of dental health care workers, blood transfusion, laboratory contact with infected specimens (such as impressions and models), and contact with infected instruments during cleaning procedures.

Therefore, it is reasonable to establish infection control guidelines for the dental treatment of patients with hepatitis B, AIDS, or ARC.

INFECTION CONTROL GUIDELINES FOR PATIENTS WITH HEPATITIS B, AIDS, AND ARC

The Task Force on the Acquired Immunodeficiency Syndrome has developed in-

TABLE 17-10. *Summary of recommended antibiotic regimens for dental/respiratory tract procedures*

Standard regimen	
For dental procedures that cause gingival bleeding, and oral/respiratory tract surgery	Penicillin V 2.0 g orally 1 hour before, then 1.0 g 6 hours later. For patients unable to take oral medications, 2 million units of aqueous penicillin G intravenously or intramuscularly 30-60 minutes before a procedure and 1 million units 6 hours later may be substituted
Special regimens	
Parenteral regimen for use when maximal protection desired (for example, for patients with prosthetic valves)	Ampicillin 1.0-2.0 g intramuscularly or intravenously, plus gentamicin 1.5 mg/kg intramuscularly or intravenously, one-half hour before procedure, followed by 1.0 g oral penicillin V 6 hours later. Alternatively, the parenteral regimen may be repeated once 8 hours later
Oral regimen for penicillin-allergic patients	Erythromycin 1.0 g orally 1 hour before, then 500 mg 6 hours later
Parenteral regimen for penicillin-allergic patients	Vancomycin 1.0 g intravenously slowly over 1 hour, starting 1 hour before. No repeat dose is necessary

Note: Pediatric doses: Ampicillin 50 mg/kg per dose; erythromycin 20 mg/kg for first dose, then 10 mg/kg; gentamicin 2.0 mg/kg per dose; penicillin V full adult dose if greater than 60 lb (27 kg), one-half adult dose if less than 60 lb (27 kg); aqueous penicillin G 50,000 units/kg (25,000 units/kg for follow-up); vancomycin 20 mg/kg per dose. The intervals between doses are the same as for adults. Total doses should not exceed adult doses.

From: Council on Dental Therapeutics: Prevention of bacterial endocarditis: A committee report of the American Heart Association. JADA, 110:98, 1985. Used with permission.

fection control guidelines for patients with AIDS. The guidelines were developed to address two main concerns: the transmissibility of the HTLV-III virus, and the transmissibility of opportunistic pathogens from health care providers to affected patients. In general, they are consistent with those suggested for the prevention of hepatitis B, and can be used for hepatitis B patients as well.

1. These precautions should be taken for persons with: opportunistic infections that are not associated with other underlying immunosuppressive disease or therapy; Kaposi's sarcoma in patients under age 60; chronic generalized lymphadenopathy, unexplained weight loss, and/or prolonged unexplained fever in persons who belong to groups with apparently increased risk of AIDS; and patients under evaluation for possible AIDS.

2. Specimens from these patients should have a warning label of the biohazard type and should be placed in a waterproof bag or container for transport.

3. Gloves, gowns, and masks should be worn by persons who are in contact with blood, blood specimens, tissue, or any body fluids, excretions, or articles potentially contaminated by these patients.

4. Protective eyewear should be worn to protect against any splattering of blood, bloody secretions, or body fluids.

5. Thorough hand washing is mandatory before and after contact with these patients.

6. Environmental surfaces contaminated with blood or other body fluids should be cleaned immediately with a disinfectant such as a 1:10 dilution of 5.25% sodium hypochloride solution (household bleach).

7. Needles and syringes should be disposed of in rigid wall puncture-resistant containers and should *not* be resheathed after use. Disposable equipment should be used wherever possible.

8. All contaminated disposable items should be considered infectious waste and identified as such. Contaminated linen should be double-bagged.

9. Any instrument that comes into contact with blood, secretions, excretions, or tissue must be sterilized before reuse. This includes dental handpieces. It may be necessary to use ethylene oxide or other means of sterilization for those instruments which cannot be autoclaved.

Accidental Exposure to Hepatitis B or AIDS

The protocol in Table 17-11 has been suggested for the management of accidental exposure of a health care worker to the blood or secretions of a patient with hepatitis B. No similar protocol has been proposed for the management of accidental exposures occurring during the care of patients with AIDS. If such an accident occurs, contact a physician familiar with AIDS immediately for advice.

Two thirds of accidental needle stick exposures to AIDS patients take place during the process of needle resheathing. Therefore, it is reasonable to suggest that future accidents may be minimized by not resheathing needles, but by immediate destruction and disposal of those needles after their use.

Vaccination for Hepatitis B

Recently, a vaccine for prevention of hepatitis B infection has been developed (Heptavax: Merck Sharp and Dohme). The efficacy of this vaccine in preventing infection is 80 to 95 percent, depending upon several variables, including the number of vaccination injections that have been received. This vaccine is widely available and can be administered simply and effectively at reasonable cost.

The current epidemic of AIDS and fear that its causative agent contaminates the currently available hepatitis B vaccine may have deterred vaccine use. This fear has arisen because the vaccine is synthesized from specimens derived from homosexual patients at high risk for the development of both hepatitis B and AIDS. Among the 500,000 vaccine recipients to date, however, no case of AIDS has occurred in individuals who do not have other risk factors.

Recently, Merck Sharp and Dohme announced test results that apparently prove that the process used to inactivate the hepatitis B virus in the vaccine also inactivates any HTLV-III present in the donor specimen.

In summary, currently available knowledge indicates that the risk of acquiring or transmitting hepatitis B or AIDS can be minimized by:

1. Hepatitis B vaccination
2. Strict isolation procedures when treating patients with hepatitis B or AIDS
3. Prompt diagnosis and treatment, should an accidental exposure occur

Selected Reading

Host Resistance

Maderazo, E.G., and Ward, P.A.: Infections and the host. In Oral and Maxillofacial Infections, 2nd ed. Edited by R.G. Topazian and M.H. Goldberg. Philadelphia, W.B. Saunders Co., 1987.

McElroy, T.H.: Infection in the patient receiving chemotherapy for cancer: Oral considerations. JADA, 109:454, 1984.

Diagnosis of Infection

Bartlett, R.C.: Laboratory diagnostic techniques. In Oral and Maxillofacial Infections, 2nd ed. Edited by R.G. Topazian and M.H. Goldberg. Philadelphia, W.B. Saunders Co., 1987.

Quintiliani, R., and Maderazo, E.G.: Infections in the compromised patient. In Oral and Maxillofacial Infections, 2nd ed. Edited by R.G. Topazian and M.H. Goldberg. Philadelphia, W.B. Saunders Co., 1987.

Schuster, G.S., and Burnett, G.W.: Oral manifestations of systemic infectious diseases. In Oral and Maxillofacial Infections, 2nd ed. Edited by R.G. Topazian and M.H. Goldberg. Philadelphia, W.B. Saunders Co., 1987.

Microbiology of Oral Infections

Bartlett, J.G., and O'Keefe, P.: The bacteriology of perimandibular space infections. J. Oral Surg., 37: 407, 1979.

Hunt, D.E., and Meyer, R.A.: Continued evolution of the microbiology of oral infections. JADA, 107:52, 1983.

Kannangara, D. W., Thadepalli, H., and McQuirter, J.L.: Bacteriology and treatment of dental infections. Oral Surg., 50:103, 1980.

Labriola, J.D., Mascaro, J., and Alpert, B.: The microbiologic flora of orofacial abscesses. J. Oral Maxillofac. Surg., 41: 711, 1983.

Schuster, G.S., and Burnett, G.W.: Microbiology of oral and maxillofacial infections. In Oral and Maxillofacial Infections, 2nd ed. Edited by

TABLE 17-11. *Protocol for accidental exposure to blood or saliva*

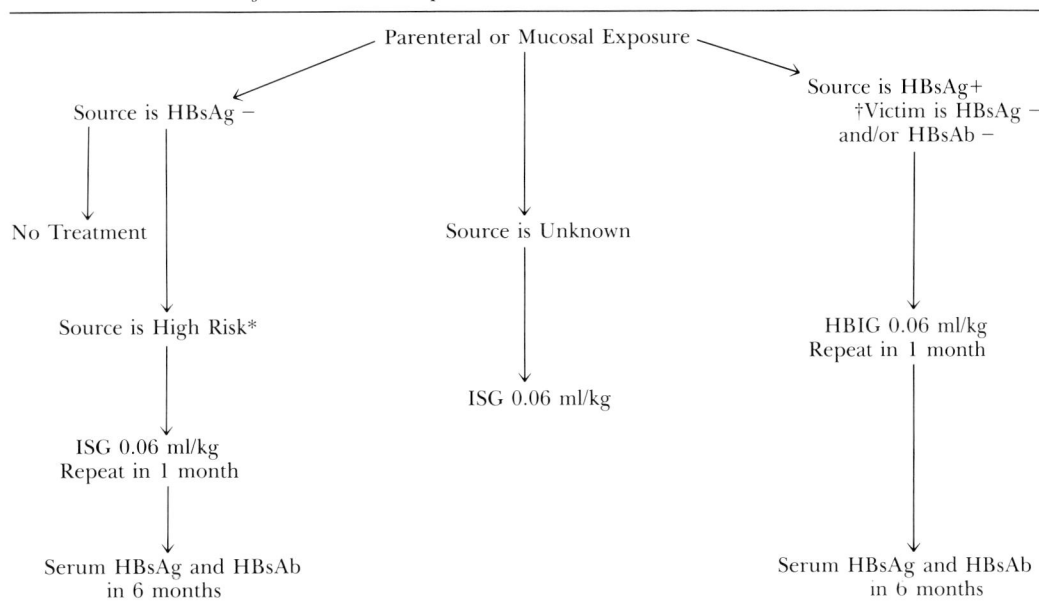

Parenteral or Mucosal Exposure

Source is HBsAg −

No Treatment

Source is High Risk*

ISG 0.06 ml/kg
Repeat in 1 month

Serum HBsAg and HBsAb
in 6 months

Source is Unknown

ISG 0.06 ml/kg

Source is HBsAg+
†Victim is HBsAg −
and/or HBsAb −

HBIG 0.06 ml/kg
Repeat in 1 month

Serum HBsAg and HBsAb
in 6 months

*Known case of non-A, non-B Hepatitis
History of multiple blood transfusions
History of parenteral drug abuse
Hemodialysis patient
†If the victim is HBsAg+ or HBsAb+, no treatment is needed.
Developed by the Cook County Hospital Infection Control Committee, Dr. Charles A. Kallick, Chairman.

ISG = Immune Serum Globulin
HBIG = Hepatitis B Immune Globulin
HBsAg = Hepatitis B Surface Antigen
HBsAb = Antibody to Hepatitis B Surface Antigen

R.G. Topazian and M.H. Goldberg. Philadelphia, W.B. Saunders Co., 1987.

Antibiotic Therapy

Greenberg, R.N., et al.: Microbiologic and antibiotic aspects of infections in the oral and maxillofacial region. J. Oral Surg., *37*:873, 1979.

Hunt, D.E., King, T.J., and Fuller, G.E.: Antibiotic susceptibility of bacteria isolated from oral infections. J. Oral Surg., *36*:527, 1978.

The Medical Letter, 21 (Issue 545):97, 1979.

The Medical Letter, 26 (Issue 656):19, 1984.

Peterson, L.J.: Principles of antibiotic therapy. *In* Oral and Maxillofacial Infections, 2nd ed. Edited by R.G. Topazian and M.H. Goldberg. Philadelphia, W.B. Saunders Co., 1987.

Odontogenic and Deep Space Infections

Chow, A.W., Roser, S.M., and Brady, F.A.: Orofacial odontogenic infections. Ann. Intern. Med., *88*:392, 1978.

Conover, M.A., and Donoff, R.B.: Facial infections: A review of 175 admissions. American Association of Oral and Maxillofacial Surgeons, Scientific Abstracts, Las Vegas, Sept. 1983, p. 1.

Dzyak, W.R., and Zide, M.F.: Diagnosis and treatment of lateral pharyngeal space infec-

tions. J. Oral Maxillofac. Surg., *42*:243, 1984.

Flynn, T.R., Hoekstra, C.W., and Lawrence, F.R.: The use of drains in oral and maxillofacial surgery: A review and a new approach. J. Oral Maxillofac. Surg., *41*: 508, 1983.

Gans, B.J.: Atlas of Oral Surgery. St. Louis, C.V. Mosby Co., 1972.

Goldberg, M.H., and Topazian, R.G.: Odontogenic infections and deep fascial space infections of dental origin. *In* Oral and Maxillofacial Infections, 2nd ed. Edited by R.G. Topazian and M.H. Goldberg. Philadelphia, W.B. Saunders Co., 1987.

Granite, E.L.: Anatomic considerations in infections of the face and neck: Review of the literature. J. Oral Surg., *34*:34, 1976.

Laskin, D.M.: Anatomic considerations in diagnosis and treatment of odontogenic infections. JADA, *69*:54, 1964.

Palmersheim, L.A., and Hamilton, M.K.: Fatal cavernous sinus thrombosis secondary to third molar removal. J. Oral Maxillofac. Surg., *40*:371, 1982.

Strauss, H.R., Tilghman, D.M., and Hankins, J.: Ludwig angina, empyema, pulmonary infiltration, and pericarditis secondary to extraction of a tooth. J. Oral Surg., *38*:223, 1980.

Osteomyelitis of the Jaws

Topazian, R.G.: Osteomyelitis of the jaws. *In* Oral and Maxillofacial Infections, 2nd ed. Edited by R.G. Topazian and M.H. Goldberg. Philadelphia, W.B. Saunders Co., 1987.

SBE

Council on Dental Therapeutics: Prevention of bacterial endocarditis: A committee report of the American Heart Association. JADA, *110*:98, 1985.

Durack, D.T., Kaplan, E.L., and Bisno, A.L.: Apparent failures of endocarditis prophylaxis. JAMA, *250*:2318, 1983.

Gregoratos, G., and Karliner, J.S.: Infective endocarditis: Diagnosis and management. Med. Clin. N. Amer., *63*:173, 1979.

Jacobsen, P.L., and Murray, W.: Prophylactic coverage of dental patients with artificial joints: A retrospective analysis of thirty-three infections in hip prostheses. Oral Surg., *50*:130, 1980.

Shulman, S.T., et al.: Prevention of bacterial endocarditis: A statement for health professionals by the Committee on Rheumatic Fever and Infective Endocarditis of the Council on Cardiovascular Disease in the Young. Circulation, *70*:1123A, 1984.

Thornton, J.B., and Alves, J.C.M.: Bacterial endocarditis: A retrospective study of cases admitted to the University of Alabama Hospitals from 1969 to 1979. Oral Surg., *52*:379, 1981.

Hepatitis B and AIDS

Brun-Vezinet, F., et al.: HTLV-III in saliva of people with AIDS-related complex and healthy homosexual men at risk for AIDS. Science, *226*:447, 1984.

Conte, J.E., et al.: Special report: Infection-control guidelines for patients with the acquired immunodeficiency syndrome (AIDS). N. Engl. J. Med., *309*:740, 1983.

Hirsch, M.S., et al.: Risk of nosocomial infection with human T-cell lymphotropic virus III (HTLV-III). N. Engl. J. Med., *312*:1, 1985.

Sacks, H.S., Rose, D.N., and Chalmers, T.C.: Should the risk of acquired immunodeficiency syndrome deter hepatitis B vaccination? JAMA, *252*:3375, 1984.

Safeguarding the physical well-being of dentists. JADA, *110*:17, 1985.

Sarngadharan, M.G., et al.: Antibodies reactive with human T-lymphotropic retroviruses (HTLV-III) in the serum of patients with AIDS. Science, *224*:506, 1984.

Wormser, G.P., Joline, C., and Duncanson, F.: Letter to the Editor: Needle-stick injuries during the care of patients with AIDS. N. Engl. J. Med., *310*:1461, 1984.

CHAPTER 18
Hospital Dental Practice

KENNETH K. KEMPF

The cautious seldom err. CONFUCIUS

The Dentist's Role in the Hospital

The role of dentistry in a hospital is well established. Hospital inpatient dental services are an indispensable part of the total health care of the patient. Over 40,000 dentists in the United States have appointments to medical staffs in acute care hospitals, and approximately 73 percent of those hospitals have at least one dentist on their medical staff.[1] The hospital has a responsibility to the community to provide comprehensive care for its patients. Like other health care professionals, the dentist must share in that responsibility by providing dental care for hospitalized patients. The level of dental care in the hospital varies from on the ward consultation visits by a dentist, to acute dental care provided in an emergency room and comprehensive dentistry provided by a clinical hospital dental service with complete facilities and a full time staff.[2] The oral and maxillofacial surgeon, through training and experience, understands hospital protocol and feels comfortable in the hospital environment.[3] The pedodontist and periodontist are also well trained to treat the hospital patient. General dental practitioners who can extend their treatment capabilities into the hospital can provide a broader scope of service for their patients and should find the hospital experience most rewarding.

Certain dental patients are best treated in the hospital environment. This group includes:
1. The medically compromised patient
2. Very young or very old patients who cannot be managed in the office
3. Severe mentally or emotionally handicapped patients
4. Financially and educationally disadvantaged patients
5. Patients requiring extensive surgical and/or restorative treatment that is best managed under a general anesthetic.

Hospital Protocol

Medical Staff Membership

To admit patients to a hospital, the dentist must be a member of its medical staff.[4] Requirements for medical staff membership may vary from one hospital to the next but usually include: graduation from a recognized dental school, licensure to practice dentistry, and membership in an appropriate dental association. Licensed dentists may apply for staff membership through the secretary of the hospital membership committee. Documented evidence of training, experience, current competence, professional ethics, and health status is usually required. The credentials committee reviews the application, grants

311

membership status, and defines clinical privileges. If the hospital has a clinical dentistry service, the head of that service sits on the credentials committee and aids in certifying dental applicants.

Admission History and Physical Examination

A qualified oral and maxillofacial surgeon who admits a dental patient without medical problems may complete an admission history and physical examination and assess the medical risks of the procedure to the patient. Patients admitted to the hospital by a dentist who is not a qualified oral surgeon must have an admission history and physical examination performed and recorded in the medical record by a physician who is a member of the hospital's medical staff.[5] When a significant medical abnormality is present, the final decision to proceed with dental treatment must be a joint responsibility of the dentist and physician. The admitting dentist should arrange for the patient's family physician or another physician, preferably an internist or family practitioner who is a medical staff member, to perform the admission history and physical examination.

Preadmission Preparation

In addition to arranging for the admission physical examination, the following should be accomplished prior to admission day to avoid inconvenience and delay for the patient.

1. Call the hospital to reserve a bed for the patient.
2. Call the operating room supervisor and anesthesia service to reserve operating room time.
3. Inform the O.R. supervisor about special equipment needed in the O.R. (e.g., instrument packs, handpieces, head lights) and extra equipment that will be brought to the O.R. Operating room nurses may not be familiar with dental instruments and procedures. It is helpful to have instrument lists or photographs and procedure outlines on file with the O.R. supervisor. This helps the case proceed smoothly and educates the O.R. personnel.
4. Inform the O.R. supervisor if an outside assistant is to be used.

5. Inform anesthesia service about the patient's special medical problems as well as medications being taken that could influence the conduct of anesthesia. Also, give a preference for patient position, whether oral or nasal intubation is to be used, and estimate the length of time for the procedure. Open communication and close cooperation with the anesthesia service adds greatly to the smooth delivery of care to the patient. The anesthesiologist not only cares for the patient in the O.R. but also follows him during recovery from the anesthesia and makes postoperative rounds later in the day.
6. Counsel the patient about professional fees and estimated hospital costs. The patient may want to contact the hospital business office to make financial arrangements prior to admission. Some insurance companies require the dentist to complete preauthorization forms before treatment.

In the hospital, the dentist may be called upon to function as a diagnostician, consultant, restorative dentist, or dental surgeon. Since patients are often admitted for multiple dental extractions, this chapter describes in detail the steps the dentist should follow when admitting a patient for dental extractions.

Admitting the Patient

The patient is admitted to the hospital on the day before surgery to allow ample time for the admission process, completion of the medical record, laboratory tests, preoperative counseling, and a visit by the anesthesiologist. Except for patients admitted through the emergency room, elective surgical patients are admitted through the admissions office. The following information should be provided to the admissions office: patient's name and age, admitting dentist's name, admitting diagnosis, date of admission, type of room requested (private, semiprivate), and name of physician responsible for the patient's physical examination and medical care.

The Medical Record

The medical record or hospital chart is a complete and accurate account of the pa-

TABLE 18-1. *Abbreviations commonly used on orders and reports*

ABBREVIATION	DEFINITION	ABBREVIATION	DEFINITION
a.c.	before meals	mal	malposed
ad lib.	at pleasure	mg.	milligram
alvcty	alveolectomy	NAD	no apparent distress
AMB	ambulatory	neg.	negative
Ant.	anterior	NKA	no known allergies
A.P.	anteroposterior	NL	normal
apico	apicoectomy	NPO	nothing by mouth
ASA	aspirin	NS	normal saline
ASAP	as soon as possible	N/V	nausea and vomiting
ASHD	arteriosclerotic heart disease	#	number
b.i.d.	twice daily	OPD	outpatient dept.
B.M.	bowel movement	O.R.	operating room
B.M.R.	basal metabolic rate	OMFS	oral & maxillofacial surgery
B.P.	blood pressure	P.A.	posteroanterior
B.S.S.	black silk sutures	para	number of births
			(para I, para II, etc.)
c	with	Path	pathology
C.C.	chief complaint	p.c.	after meals
CBC	complete blood count	Pdcl	periodontoclasia
C.H.D.	congenital heart disease	PE	physical exam
C.N.S.	central nervous system	P.H.	past history
C.O.D.	cause of death	P.M.H.	previous (past) medical history
COPD	chronic obstructive		
	pulmonary disease	P.O.	per os (by mouth)
CV	cardiovascular	POD	postoperative day
CVA	cardiovascular accident	post.,	posterior
CVD	cardiovascular disease	post-op	postoperative
D5W	dextrose 5% in water	POT	postoperative treatment
DSG	dressing	P.R.	pulse rate
EBL	estimated blood loss	p.r.n.	as occasion requires
ECG, EKG	electrocardiogram	Pt.	patient
E.N.T.	ear, nose, throat dept.	q3h	every 3 hours
E.S.R.	erythrocyte sedimentation rate	q.i.d.	4 times a day
F.H.	family history	q.s.	quantity sufficient
FME	full-mouth extractions	q.n.s.	quantity not sufficient
FMTE	full-mouth tooth extractions	RBC	red blood cell
FMS	full-mouth series of radiographs	r/c	root canal
Fx	fracture	R.H.D.	rheumatic heart disease
G.A.	general anesthesia	ROS	review of systems
G.I.	gastrointestinal	Rt.	right
gr.	grains	RTC	return to clinic
gravida	pregnancies	s	without
G.U.	genitourinary	S.O.B.	shortness of breath
Hb	hemoglobin	Sub Q, S.C.	subcutaneous
HCT	hematocrit	RT	surgical removal
H.P.I.	history of present illness	TE	tooth extraction
hs	at bedtime	Temp	temperature
Hx	history	t.i.d.	3 times a day
I & D	incision and drainage	T&A	tonsillectomy and
			adenoidectomy
I.M.	intramuscular	UAL	Up Ad Lib
Imp	impaction, impressions	UCHD	usual childhood diseases
I.V.	intravenous	VS	vital signs
L > R	left greater than right	WBC	white blood cell
LDDS	local dentist	W/D	well-developed
L.&W	living and well	WNL	within normal limits
LMD	local medical doctor	w/o	without
Lt.	left	W/F (W)	White female
M	male	W/M (or W)	white male
MM	murmur	N/F	black female
		N/M	black male

tient's treatment from admission to discharge. It is the joint responsibility of the dentist and physician to ensure the record is filled out properly and signed within 24 hours of admission and prior to any surgical procedure.[6] To save time and space, abbreviations are commonly used when making entries into the medical record (Table 18-1). The format of the record may vary with each hospital but must contain the following basic components:

Cover Sheet. This page of the record contains the patient's personal data, name of the admitting dentist/physician, principal admitting diagnosis with code, and procedures performed with code. The dentist must ensure that the principal diagnosis and code are correct.

Admission Orders. The newly admitted patient receives no care without admission orders signed by the admitting dentist. (Fig. 18-1). The admission order is the first entry on the doctor's orders form and contains the ward and service to which the patient is being admitted, diet desired, laboratory tests and x-rays requested, orders for medications the patient is currently taking, and request for history and physical examination by a staff physician.

Medical History. The components of the medical history (Fig. 18-2) include: chief complaint (CC), history of present illness (HPI), past medical history (PMH), and review of systems (ROS).[7]

The chief complaint is recorded in the patient's own words. It usually relates to the disease or problem that prompts the admission.

The history of present illness describes briefly the events leading to the chief complaint as well as duration, degree, and disability of the illness.

The past medical history reviews previous state of health, diseases, operations, family and social histories, and known allergies.

The review of systems is a detailed description of present conditions, abnormalities, or diseases within each body system.

The dentist is responsible for recording the chief complaint, history of present illness, and the dental portion of the past medical history and review of systems. The dentist and physician sign the medical history.

Physical Examination. The physician is responsible for recording the findings of the physical examination (Fig. 18-3). The dentist, however, completes that part of the physical examination concerned with dentistry—namely, the head, neck, oral, and dental examinations. Both physician and dentist sign the physical examination record.

Preoperative Orders. Preoperative orders (Fig. 18-1) are written on the evening before the day of surgery and become the second entry on the doctor's orders form. The orders list NPO precautions, surgical site preparation, preanesthetic medications, the patient's existing medications, and medication prescribed for sleep. The dentist signs the preoperative orders.

Patient Consent Form. The patient must be counselled by the dentist on all potential complications resulting from the planned surgery and anesthesia, as well as alternative treatment choices, expected results, and potential problems if treatment is not rendered. The patient must fully understand the information given concerning the operation and sign the consent form (Fig. 18-4) in the presence of a witness, who is not a member of the surgical team. The dentist signs the consent form. This is an extremely important document and must be completed properly. If the patient is under age, a parent or legal guardian must sign for him.

Progress Notes. The progress notes (Fig. 18-5), written by the dentist, describe the patient's daily care and progress. They include the admission, preoperative, operative, postoperative, and discharge notes. The dentist must date and sign each entry. Daily entries must be made as long as the patient remains in the hospital. The "S.O.A.P." method, referred to in Chapter 4, can be used to organize each note: Subjective (S), Objective (O), Assessment (A), Plan (P).

Operation Report. The operation report (Fig. 18-6) is dictated as soon after surgery as possible. The typed copy must be signed by the dentist before it can be included in the record. The description of the procedure should be complete but not wordy.

Laboratory and Radiographic Reports. One section of the record usually contains

Exception to Standard Form 508
Approved by OMB

MEDICAL RECORD		DOCTOR'S ORDERS			

NOTE: *Physician's signature must accompany each entry including standing orders. Date and time for instituting and discontinuing the orders must be recorded.*

DATE AND TIME	PROB. NO.	ORDERS *(Another brand, equal in quality, of the same basic drug may be dispensed, UNLESS checked.)* ▶	√	NURSE'S SIGNATURE
7/6/85				
10:00 AM		Admission orders		
		1) Admit to ward 7W, Dental Service		
		DX = multiple dental caries and		
		periodontitis		
		2) Labs: CBC c diff., U-A, P.T., P.T.T.,		
		E.K.G.		
		3) CXR: P-A & lat.		
		4) Hospital privileges		
		5) Regular diet		
		6) Vital signs - routine		
		7) Physical exam by staff M.D.		
		D.C. Prime, D.D.S.		
7/6/85				
7:00 PM		Preoperative Orders		
		1) NPO after midnight		
		2) Dalmane 30 mg Cap. h.s. prn sleep		
		(continued)		

Enter in space below: PATIENT IDENTIFICATION – TREATING FACILITY –WARD NO. – DATE

Jones, Joseph A.   SS# 000-00-0000

7/6/85

University Hospitals and Clinics

MEDICAL RECORD

DOCTOR'S ORDERS

VA FORM
OCT 1975 10-1158

EXISTING STOCK OF
VA FORM 10-1158, MAY 1973
AND VA FORM 10-1158c, NOV 1972,
WILL BE USED.

FIG. 18-1. *Example of doctor's orders form.*

Exception to Standard Form 508
Approved by OMB

MEDICAL RECORD	DOCTOR'S ORDERS

NOTE: *Physician's signature must accompany each entry including standing orders. Date and time for instituting and discontinuing the orders must be recorded.*

DATE AND TIME	PROB. NO.	ORDERS *(Another brand, equal in quality, of the same basic drug may be dispensed, UNLESS checked.)* ▶	√	NURSE'S SIGNATURE
		3) Void, shower and shave in AM on call from O.R.		
		4) Chart with labs to O.R. c̄ patient		
		5) Pre-anesthesia meds:		
		Demerol 50 mg		
		Valium 20 mg ⎫ I.M. on call		
		Atropine 0.4 mg ⎭ from O.R.		
		6) Consent - signed		
		D.C. Prime, D.D.S.		
7/7/85		Postoperative Orders		
		1) V.S. q15 min. until stable, then q1h x 4, then routine		
		2) I.V. fluids: complete present I.V. at 120 cc/h then D5W in ½ N.S. at 100 cc/h.		
		3) Diet: clear liq. as tolerated		
		4) Elevated head of bed 30°		
		5) Ice to face		
		(continued)		

Enter in space below: PATIENT IDENTIFICATION – TREATING FACILITY – WARD NO. – DATE

Jones, Joseph A. SS# 000-00-0000

7/6/85

University Hospitals and Clinics

MEDICAL RECORD

DOCTOR'S ORDERS

VA FORM OCT 1975 10-1158

EXISTING STOCK OF VA FORM 10-1158, MAY 1973 AND VA FORM 10-1158c, NOV 1972, WILL BE USED.

Exception to Standard Form 508
Approved by OMB

MEDICAL RECORD	DOCTOR'S ORDERS

NOTE: Physician's signature must accompany each entry including standing orders. Date and time for instituting and discontinuing the orders must be recorded.

DATE AND TIME	PROB. NO.	ORDERS (Another brand, equal in quality, of the same basic drug may be dispensed, UNLESS checked.) ▶	√	NURSE'S SIGNATURE
		6) Meds: Demerol 50 mg IM q4h prn pain		
		Tigan 200 mg IM q6h prn nausea		
		7) Gauze packs to stay in mouth until		
		12 noon, then prn for hemostasis		
		8) BRP with assistance		
		9) Petroleum jelly to lips		
		10) Dr. Prime's beeper #765		
		D.C. Prime, D.D.S.		

Enter in space below: PATIENT IDENTIFICATION – TREATING FACILITY – WARD NO. – DATE

Jones, Joseph A.   SS# 000-00-0000

7/7/85

University Hospitals & Clinics

MEDICAL RECORD

DOCTOR'S ORDERS

VA FORM
OCT 1975 **10-1158**

EXISTING STOCK OF
VA FORM 10-1158, MAY 1973
AND VA FORM 10-1158c, NOV 1972,
WILL BE USED.

Standard Form 504
Rev. August 1954
Bureau of the Budget
Circular A-32

✿ U.S. GPO: 1974—528-657/5079

CLINICAL RECORD	HISTORY—Part I

NATURE AND DURATION OF COMPLAINTS (*Include circumstance of admission*)

CC: "painful, broken teeth, gums bleed easily."

Admitted for removal of all remaining teeth under general anesthesia.

HISTORY OF PRESENT ILLNESSES

Mr. Jones is a 34-year-old male who admits to a long history of dental neglect. For the past six months he has experienced increased dental pain and bleeding gingiva when he attempts to brush. A complete clinical and x-ray exam revealed severe alveolar bone loss in both arches and non-restorable caries in all remaining teeth.

The patient is extremely apprehensive, has a strong gag reflex, and prefers to be "put to sleep" for dental extractions.

He is being admitted to the hospital for treatment under general anesthesia.

D.C. Prime, D.D.S.

(Continue on reverse side)

PATIENT'S IDENTIFICATION (*For typed or written entries give: Name—last, first, middle; grade; date; hospital or medical facility*)	REGISTER NO. 84-0003-1	WARD NO. 7W

Jones, Joseph A.   SS# 000-00-0000

7/6/85

University Hospitals and Clinics

HISTORY—Part 1
Standard Form 504
504-105

FIG. 18-2. *Example of medical history form.*

Standard Form 505
Rev. August 1957
Bureau of the Budget
Circular A—32 (Rev.)

CLINICAL RECORD	HISTORY—Part 2

PAST HISTORY

INSTRUCTIONS.—*Include (1) OCCUPATION (Civilian and military), (2) MILITARY HISTORY (Include geographic locations and dates), (3) HABITS (Alcohol, tobacco, and drugs), (4) FAMILY HISTORY, (5) CHILDHOOD ILLNESSES, (6) ADULT ILLNESSES, (7) OPERATIONS, (8) INJURIES, and (9) DRUG SENSITIVITIES AND ALLERGIC REACTIONS.*

1) Occupation: truck driver for A.C. Van Lines, this city.

2) N/A

3) Habits: drinks 1 or 2 beers daily, cigarettes 1 pkg/d x 15 yrs.

   Denies use of nonprescription drugs.

4) Family history: father--age 59 L & W, mild hypertension
   mother--died age 50 "heart attack"
   1 brother--age 28 L & W
   2 sisters--age 30 & 36 both L & W

   Married, no children

5) Was sensitive to dust and pollens as child, had usual childhood illnesses without sequelae.

6) Hepatitis age 19 while in Army, antibody negative.

7) T & A age 6 w/o complications
   Open-reduction right femur age 19--blood transfusion hepatitis.

8) Fractured right femur--fell from ladder, no present limitations.

9) No known drug allergies.

J.T. Fine, M.D.   D.C. Prime, D.D.S.

(Continue on reverse side)

PATIENT'S IDENTIFICATION (For typed or written entries give: Name—last, first, middle; grade; date; hospital or medical facility)	REGISTER NO. 84-0003-1	WARD NO. 7W

Jones, Joseph A.   SS# 000-00-0000

7/6/85

University Hospitals and Clinics

HISTORY (Parts 2 and 3)
Standard Form 505
505–105

HISTORY—Part 3

SYSTEM REVIEW

INSTRUCTIONS.—*Include (1) GENERAL, (2) HEAD [Including (3) EYE, (4) EAR, (5) NOSE and (6) THROAT], (7) NECK, (8) RESPIRATORY, (9) CARDIOVASCULAR, (10) GASTROINTESTINAL, (11) GENITO-URINARY [and (12) GYNECOLOGICAL], (13) HEMOPOIETIC, (14) LYMPHATIC, (15) MUSCULO-SKELETAL and (16) NEURO-PSYCHIATRIC SYSTEMS.*

1) GENERAL: good general health, obese, no recent weight change.

2) HEAD: no headaches, no previous head trauma.

3) EYES: no glasses, no loss of vision or blurring.

4) EARS: no hearing loss, vertigo or tinnitis.

5) NOSE: seasonal nasal congestion, denies epistaxis.

6) THROAT: no recent voice change, no persistant hoarseness.

7) NECK: no cervical tenderness, no lumps or masses.

8) RESPIRATORY: chronic upper respiratory congestion in A.M.

9) CARDIOVASCULAR: negative for murmur, RF, RHD, hypertension or dyspnea.

10) GASTROINTESTINAL: noncontributory

11) GENITO-URINARY: noncontributory

12) GYNECOLOGICAL: N/A

13) HEMOPOIETIC: whole blood transfusions age 19--hepatitis B.

14) LYMPHATIC: noncontributory

15) MUSCULOSKELETAL: no joint pain.

16) NEUROPSYCHIATRIC: well-adjusted, no history of drug/alcohol abuse.

SIGNATURE OF PHYSICIAN	DATE
D.C. Prime, D.D.S. J.T. Fine, M.D.	7/6/85

☆ GPO: 1972 474-062

Standard Form 506

CLINICAL RECORD	PHYSICAL EXAMINATION

DATE OF EXAM.	HEIGHT	WEIGHT			TEMPERATURE	PULSE	BLOOD PRESSURE
		AVERAGE	MAXIMUM	PRESENT			
7/6/85	178 cm			97 Kg	36/8°C	80	136/85

INSTRUCTIONS.—Describe (1) General Appearance and Mental Status; (2) Head and Neck (General); (3) Eyes; (4) Ears; (5) Nose; (6) Mouth; (7) Throat; (8) Teeth; (9) Chest (General); (10) Lungs; (11) Cardiovascular; (12) Abdomen; (13) Hernia; (14) Genitalia; (15) Rectum; (16) Prostate; (17) Back; (18) Extremities; (19) Neurological; (20) Skin; (21) Lymphatics.

1) GENERAL: pleasant, cooperative, moderately obese white male in NAD.

2) HEAD & NECK: normocephalic, neck supple, no masses or tenderness, thyroid normal.

3) EYES: PERRLA, fundi benign, EOM's intact, sclera & conjunctiva normal.

4) EARS: TM's intact and mobile, EAC's clear, hearing grossly intact.

5) NOSE: normal mucosa, septum midline, nasal airway patent.

6) MOUTH: mucosa and saliva normal, hyperplastic gingiva.

7) THROAT: normal

8) TEETH: 18 teeth all carious, chronic fistula tooth #3.

9) CHEST: no deformity, increased A-P diameter.

10) LUNGS: clear

11) HEART: RSR, no murmur, PMI at 5th ICS, MCL.

12) ABDOMEN: obese, nontender, no organomegally, active bowel sounds.

13) HERNIA: negative

14) GENITALIA: normal male

15) RECTUM: no hemorrhoids

16) PROSTATE: nontender, no enlargement.

17) BACK: slight scoliosis, no CVA tenderness.

(Continue on reverse side)

PATIENT'S IDENTIFICATION (For typed or written entries give: Name—last, first, middle; grade; date; hospital or medical facility)	REGISTER NO.	WARD NO.
	84-0003-1	7W

Jones, Joseph A. SS# 000-00-0000

7/6/85

University Hospitals & Clinics

PHYSICAL EXAMINATION
Standard Form 506

General Services Administration and
Interagency Committee on Medical Records
FPMR 101-11.806-8
October 1975   506-105

FIG. 18-3. *Example of physical examination form.*

PHYSICAL EXAMINATION

18) EXTREMITIES: full range of motion, surgical scar R lat. thigh
                  peripheral pulses strong and equal bilaterally.

19) NEURO: cranial nerves II-XII intact, motor and sensory intact,
            normal gait and speech, DTR's

20) SKIN: dry, tattoo right forearm

21) LYMPHATICS: no lymphadenopathy

IMPRESSION: 1) Obese 35 y/o male in good general health.

             2) Advanced, non-restorable caries and generalized
                 periodontal disease.

D.C. Prime, D.D.S.   J.T. Fine, M.D.

INITIAL IMPRESSION

SIGNATURE OF PHYSICIAN

MEDICAL RECORD	REQUEST FOR ADMINISTRATION OF ANESTHESIA AND FOR PERFORMANCE OF OPERATIONS AND OTHER PROCEDURES

A. IDENTIFICATION

1. OPERATION OR PROCEDURE

Multiple dental extractions and alveoloplasty under general anesthesia.

B. STATEMENT OF REQUEST

1. The nature and purpose of the operation or procedure, possible alternative methods of treatment, the risks involved, and the possibility of complications have been fully explained to me. I acknowledge that no guarantees have been made to me concerning the results of the operation or procedure. I understand the nature of the operation or procedure to be_____
(Description of operation or procedure in layman's language)

Remove all my remaining teeth while under a general anesthetic.

which is to be performed by or under the direction of Dr. Prime, D.D.S.

2. I request the performance of the above-named operation or procedure and of such additional operations or procedures as are found to be necessary or desirable, in the judgment of the professional staff of the below-named medical facility, during the course of the above-named operation or procedure.

3. I request the administration of such anesthesia as may be considered necessary or advisable in the judgment of the professional staff of the below-named medical facility.

4. Exceptions to surgery or anesthesia, if any, are: _____none_____
(If "none", so state)

5. I request the disposal by authorities of the below-named medical facility of any tissues or parts which it may be necessary to remove.

6. I understand that photographs and movies may be taken of this operation, and that they may be viewed by various personnel undergoing training or indoctrination at this or other facilities. I consent to the taking of such pictures and observation of the operation by authorized personnel, subject to the following conditions:

    a. The name of the patient and his/her family is not used to identify said pictures.

    b. Said pictures be used only for purposes of medical/dental study or research.

(Cross out any parts above which are not appropriate)

C. SIGNATURES   *(Appropriate items in Parts A and B must be completed before signing)*

1. COUNSELING PHYSICIAN/DENTIST: I have counseled this patient as to the nature of the proposed procedure(s), attendant risks involved, and expected results, as described above.

D.C. Prime, D.D.S.
(Signature of Counseling Physician/Dentist)

2. PATIENT: I understand the nature of the proposed procedure(s), attendant risks involved, and expected results, as described above, and hereby request such procedure(s) be performed.

Jane Doe, R.N.	Joseph A. Jones	July 6, 1985
(Signature of Witness, excluding members of operating team)	(Signature of Patient)	(Date and Time)

3. SPONSOR OR GUARDIAN: (When patient is a minor or unable to give consent) I,_____
sponsor/guardian of _____ understand the nature of the proposed procedure(s), attendant risks involved, and expected results, as described above, and hereby request such procedure(s) be performed.

(Signature of Witness, excluding members of operating team)	(Signature of Sponsor/Legal Guardian)	(Date and Time)

PATIENT'S IDENTIFICATION *(For typed or written entries give: Name—last, first, middle; grade; date; hospital or medical facility)*	REGISTER NO. 84-0003-1	WARD NO. 7W

Jones, Joseph A.

7/6/85

University Hospitals and Clinics

STANDARD FORM 522 (Rev. 10-76)
General Services Administration &
Interagency Comm. on Medical Records
FPMR 101-11.806-8
522-109

☆U.S. GOVERNMENT PRINTING OFFICE 1983 381-488/2995

FIG. 18-4. *Example of patient consent form.*

MEDICAL RECORD	PROGRESS NOTES
DATE	
7/6/85	Admission note:
8 A.M.	34 y/o male admitted for removal of all teeth under
	general anesthesia tomorrow A.M.
	Plan: 1) physical exam by staff M.D.
	2) routine admission workup
	3) removal of 18 teeth & alveoloplasty in O.R.
	D.C. Prime, D.D.S.
7 P.M.	Preoperative note:
	Labs normal, chest x-ray clear. Physical exam completed
	and signed, no abnormalities noted.
	Patient counseled, operative permit signed and in chart,
	patient ready for surgery.
	D.C. Prime, D.D.S.

(Continue on reverse side)

PATIENT'S IDENTIFICATION *(For typed or written entries give: Name—last, first, middle; grade; rank; rate; hospital or medical facility)*	REGISTER NO. 84-0003-1	WARD NO. 7W
Jones, Joseph A. S.S. #000-00-0000	**PROGRESS NOTES**	
7/6/85	STANDARD FORM 509 (Rev. 11-77) Prescribed by GSA/ICMR, FPMR (41 CFR) 101-11.806-8 509-110	
University Hospitals & Clinics		

FIG. 18-5. *Example of progress notes form.*

PROGRESS NOTES

DATE	
7/7/85	Operative Note:
10:30 AM	1) Pre and post-op dx: dental caries and periodontitis
	2) Surgeon: D.C. Prime, D.D.S.
	3) Scrub nurse: J. Long, R.N.
	4) Anesthesia: general, nasoendotracheal, Forane,
	nitrous oxide=oxygen
	5) Procedure: extraction teeth #2, 3, 4, 5, 6, 7, 8, 9,
	10, 11, 14, 15, 20, 21, 25, 27, 30, 31
	Alveoloplasty, 3=0 black silk sutures.
	6) E.B.L.: 200 cc
	7) Fluid replacement: 800 cc D5W in R.L.
	8) Complications: none
	Pt. tolerated procedure well, returned to recovery
	ward, extubated, awake and stable.
	D.C. Prime, D.D.S.
3:45 PM	Postoperative note:
	Multiple dental extractions
	S -- mild discomfort
	O -- chest clear to ausc., BP 120/70, P=70, resp 20,
	temp 36°C, minimal oozing from wound.
	(continued)

STANDARD FORM 509 BACK (Rev. 11-77)

MEDICAL RECORD	PROGRESS NOTES
DATE	

Voided at 3 P.M. (500 cc), sipping water (300 cc)

I.V. infusing well.

A - normal post-op progress

P - 1) Start on clear liq. diet

2) Ambulate

3) Plan for discharge tomorrow A.M.

D.C. Prime, D.D.S.

7/8/85

9:00 AM

Had a restful night, complete hemostasis at extraction sites, vital signs are normal, afebrile, good p.o. intake, voiding q.s., lungs clear, ready for discharge.

Discharge orders:

1) Discharge today

2) Medications: Tylenol #3 tabs x 15, one or two q6h PRN pain.

3) full liquid diet

4) rinse mouth p.s. c̄ warm salt water

5) R.T.C.: outpatient dental clinic

7/14/85 @ 1:00 P.M.

D.C. Prime, D.D.S.

PATIENT'S IDENTIFICATION *(For typed or written entries give: Name—last, first, middle; grade; rank; rate; hospital or medical facility)*

Jones, Joseph A.   SS# 000-00-0000

7/6/85

University Hospitals & Clinics

REGISTER NO.
84-0003-1

WARD NO.
7W

PROGRESS NOTES
STANDARD FORM 509 (Rev. 11-77)
Prescribed by GSA/ICMR,
FPMR (41 CFR) 101-11.806-8
509-110

Standard Form 516
Rev. August 1954
Bureau of the Budget
Circular A—32

16 GPO 16 - 77658 - 1

CLINICAL RECORD	OPERATION REPORT

PREOPERATIVE DIAGNOSIS

Non-restorable dental caries and advanced periodontitis

SURGEON	FIRST ASSISTANT	SECOND ASSISTANT	
D.C. Prime, D.D.S.			
ANESTHETIST T. Smith, M.D.	**ANESTHETIC** Forane, N_2O-O_2, nasoendo	**TIME BEGAN** 8:00 AM **TIME ENDED** 10:00 AM	
SURGICAL NURSE J. Long, R.N.	**INSTRUMENT NURSE**	**TIME OPERATION BEGAN** 8:20 AM	**TIME OPERATION COMPLETED** 9:45 AM
OPERATIVE DIAGNOSES	**DRAINS** (*Kind and number*) none	**SPONGE COUNT VERIFIED** yes	

same as preoperative

MATERIAL FORWARDED TO LABORATORY FOR EXAMINATION

18 teeth

OPERATION PERFORMED

Multiple dental extractions teeth #'s 2, 3, 4, 5, 6, 7, 8, 9, 10, 11, 14, 15, 20, 21, 25, 27, 30, 31.

Alveoloplasty x 4 quadrants

DESCRIPTION OF OPERATION (*Type(s) of suture used, gross findings, etc.*)	**MAJOR** X	**MINOR**	**DATE OF OPERATION** 7/7/85

After induction of satisfactory general anesthesia via nasoendotracheal route, the patient was prepped and draped in the usual manner for an intraoral surgical procedure. A moist oral-pharyngeal gauze pack was placed and the four quadrants were infiltrated with a total of 10 cc of 2% Xylocaine with 1:100,000 epi. The gingiva in the maxilla was sharply excised from around the teeth, a mucoperiosteal flap was then elevated buccally. Teeth #2, 3, 4, 5, 6, 7, 8, 9, 10, 11, 12, 14, 15 were elevated and extracted with a dental elevator and forceps. A minimal alveoloplasty was performed and the sockets were irrigated with copious amounts of normal saline. The mucoperiosteal flap was reapproximated and closed with a continuous 3-0 black silk suture. Attention was then turned to the mandible where teeth #'s 20, 21, 25, 27, 30 and 31 were similarly extracted and alveoloplasty performed. Following the procedure, the oral cavity was irrigated and suctioned, the oral-pharyngeal pack removed and oral gauze packs placed for hemostasis. Estimated blood loss was 200 cc, none replaced. The patient tolerated the procedure well, was extubated on the table and taken to Recovery Room awake and in good condition.

SIGNATURE OF SURGEON D.C. Prime, D.D.S.	**DATE** 7/8/85
PATIENT'S IDENTIFICATION (*For typed or written entries give: Name—last, first, middle; grade; date; hospital or medical facility*)	**REGISTER NO.** 84-0003-1	**WARD NO.** 7W

Jones, Joseph A.   SS# 000-00-0000

7/6/85

University Hospitals and Clinics

OPERATION REPORT
Standard Form 516
516-104

FIG. 18-6. *Example of operation report.*

DISCHARGE SUMMARY	DATE 7/8/85

DISCHARGE SUMMARY

Admission Date: 7/6/85   Discharge Date: 7/8/85

Service: Dental

●File in B section of appropriate admission●

DATE 7/8/85
HOSP. NO. 84-0003-1
NAME Jones, Joseph A.
BIRTHDATE 3/26/51
ADDRESS 1509 1st St.
Hometown, USA
IF NOT IMPRINTED, PLEASE PRINT HOSP. NO., NAME AND LOCATION

REASON FOR HOSPITALIZATION AND PRINCIPAL DIAGNOSIS (no abbreviations or symbols):

Advanced dental caries and periodontal disease

ADDITIONAL DIAGNOSES:

None

SIGNIFICANT FINDINGS (pertinent lab, x-ray, physical findings):

Non-restorable dental caries in all remaining teeth and generalized periodontitis.

OPERATIONS AND/OR PROCEDURES (Including dates):

7/7/85 - Odontectomy (18 teeth)
7/7/85 - Alveoloplasty (4 quadrants)

MEDICAL/OPERATIVE COMPLICATIONS (including nosocomial infections):
none [X]

TREATMENT RENDERED:

Removal of all remaining teeth.

CONDITION ON DISCHARGE (Indicate changes from admission in specific terms):

Afebrile, taking liquid diet well, comfortable.

Overall condition good.

INSTRUCTIONS TO PATIENT OR FAMILY:

Medications	Tylenol #3 tabs x 15, i=ii q4h PRN pain	☐ none indicated
Physical Activity	Light activity x 5 days	☐ none indicated
Diet	Full liquid x 7 days, then soft diet	☐ none indicated
Follow-up	Return to dental clinic 7/14/85 at 1:00 PM	☐ none indicated
Other		

WERE ANY PREPRINTED INSTRUCTIONS GIVEN THE PATIENT? TYPE OF INSTRUCTIONS?*_____
_____ Diet instructions and wound care instructions _____

_____

*Copies must be on file in Medical Records Department

Signatures: _____ D.C. Prime, D.D.S.
Resident Physician   Staff Physician

FIG. 18-7. *Example of discharge summary.*

all results of laboratory tests and reports of radiographic exams. The dentist should initial the reports to indicate that he has read them. The results of all lab tests and radiographs must be in the record before the patient enters the O.R.

Consultation Reports. A request for medical consultation may be initiated by the admitting dentist or physician when a medical problem exists on admission or develops during hospitalization. The completed report describes any precautions or recommendations for the medical management of the patient.

Discharge Summary. The discharge summary (Fig. 18-7), completed at the time of discharge, summarizes all care the patient received during the hospital stay. It includes admission and discharge dates, diagnosis, treatment, post-treatment recommendations, and the arrangements made for follow-up care.

Preoperative Rounds

The preoperative visit on the evening before surgery is a most important aspect of patient care. The chart is checked for completeness to include all necessary signatures. The laboratory results and x-rays are reviewed for any abnormalities. Details of the surgery as well as postoperative management are reviewed carefully with the patient so that he understands fully what is going to happen. A close relative or friend may be included in the discussion. The consent form is reviewed for completeness and accuracy and signed by both patient and surgeon. NPO precautions are reviewed, and the patient is advised to ask for a sleeping pill if still awake by 11:00 P.M.

Day of Operation

Plan to arrive at the hospital at least an hour before the scheduled surgery. First check on the patient to be sure nothing has occurred overnight which might cause a cancellation of the surgery. After putting on scrub clothes the dentist should go directly to the operating room to be sure all needed personnel, equipment, and instruments are there. The patient will not be anesthetized until the dentist is present in the operating suite. It is very comforting to the patient to know his doctor is there before he is anesthetized.

O.R. nursing personnel may not be familiar with dental surgical instruments. As the instruments are placed on the instrument table, discussing the names and use of each instrument with the nurse helps the nurse to be of greater assistance during the procedure. All unnecessary talking should cease and the O.R. kept quiet during the induction phase of anesthesia. Every effort should be made to employ the same surgical techniques that are used in the office. Any last minute changes in technique usually result in delay and increased operating time.

After the surgery is completed and the patient is extubated, the dentist must accompany the patient and anesthesiologist to the recovery area and stay by the patient's bed until vital signs have been taken and it is obvious that the patient is stable and has a good airway. While in the recovery area postoperative orders are written. Since surgery cancels all preoperative orders, the postoperative orders must also include any medication that the patient was taking before surgery.

Postoperative orders should include the following: (Fig. 18-1)
1. Frequency of vital signs monitoring
2. Position of patient in bed
3. I.V. fluid plan for next 24 hours
4. Pain medication
5. Medication for nausea/vomiting
6. Wound care plan
7. Diet
8. Orders for ambulation and bathroom privileges

The postoperative orders must be dated and signed by the dentist. Before leaving the hospital it is good practice to visit briefly with any waiting relatives or friends of the patient to explain how the surgery went, how the patient is doing, and when they can expect the patient to return to his or her room.

Postoperative Care

The dentist must see the patient on the evening of surgery. During this early postoperative phase the patient is most in need of good nursing care and follow-up by the dentist. Before seeing the patient, the following should be checked at the nurse's desk:
1. Vital signs: blood pressure, pulse, tem-

perature and respirations

2. Intake and output (I & O): do total fluid losses match up with intake? A quick calculation determines if the patient is adequately hydrated.

AVERAGE DAILY FLUID LOSSES
FOR 70 KG PATIENT
urine: 1200 cc (50 cc/hr)
lungs and skin: 1000 cc
stool: 150 cc

total losses: 2350 cc/day without fever

Anticipated daily losses + blood loss
= amount of fluids the patient needs
for the first day after surgery.
Example: 2350 cc + 350 cc (blood loss)
= 2700 cc.

If the patient is taking nothing by mouth then all fluid must come from intravenous replacement, which means he would need an I.V. flow of about 120 cc per hour. If there is oral intake, the I.V. rate can be reduced to 100 cc per hour. Remember the kidneys must be producing at least 50 cc of urine an hour to maintain fluid and electrolyte balance.

3. Check the nursing notes for any comments made on the patient's progress, or consult with the nurse personally. Next, visit the patient at bedside. A pocket light and disposable dental mirror or tongue blade aid in the oral examination. The bedside visit should include an examination and appraisal sufficient to answer the following questions:

Is the patient alert and recovered from anesthesia?
Is the patient comfortable?
Are the lungs clear?
Is the I.V. flowing at the proper rate?
Is the surgical site being properly managed?
Has the patient voided?
Are orders being correctly carried out by the nursing staff?

If the answer to these questions is "yes," the postoperative course is satisfactory. If there are "no" answers, adjustments in postoperative orders should be made.

The patient should be visited twice daily until discharged. Whenever the patient is seen on the ward an entry must be made in the progress notes, which is dated and signed. The S.O.A.P. method can be used to organize the notes.

After the patient has recovered sufficiently from the operation and further hospitalization is considered unnecessary, a discharge order may be written. Before the patient is discharged, the following conditions must be satisfied:

1. Afebrile
2. Complete hemostasis at surgery site
3. Adequate oral intake (>1500 cc)
4. Adequate urine output
5. Comfortable on oral analgesics

A discharge note is made in the progress notes and a discharge summary is dictated. A definite appointment should be made for the patient's follow-up visit to the office. Be sure to enter the properly worded diagnosis, operation, and codes on the cover sheet of the medical record.

Operating Room Procedure

Asepsis—the absence of infected matter or freedom from infection—may be the single-most significant advance in the history of surgery. In 1847, Ignaz Semmelweis of Vienna demonstrated that handwashing significantly reduced the incidence of wound infection. This finding was later corroborated by Oliver Wendell Holmes in Boston. However, because of bitter opposition, Semmelweis' findings were not accepted until Joseph Lister published, between 1865 and 1891, his studies on the prevention of wound infection. Lister applied dilute carbolic acid (phenol) to infected wounds and later nebulized it to disinfect the operating room and equipment.[8]

Modern aseptic technique prevents the access of microorganisms into the surgical wound through observance of strict operating room protocol that must be observed by all who enter and work within the operating room area.

The dentist who brings his patient into the operating room must be thoroughly familiar with the principles and technique of sterile procedure so he is not the weak link in the chain of sterility. He may not maintain the same level of aseptic technique in the office that is practiced in the operating room of the hospital. Nevertheless, he owes it to his patients to provide such measures within the office or clinic to eliminate the possibility of cross-contamination. At first, the operating room aseptic technique may seem cumbersome and time-consuming, but by learning the principles well, gaining practice and experience, and developing a routine, the dentist soon becomes quite familiar and comfortable with the procedures.

Operating Room Suite

The operating room suite includes locker rooms for doctors and other personnel, a nursing supervisor's office where the day's operating schedule is posted, an anesthesia office and work room, an instrument cleaning and sterilization area, a nonsterile and sterile storage area, scrub rooms, operating rooms (Fig. 18-8), and a recovery room (Fig. 18-9). The suite is designed to provide the following advantages:

1. Geographic isolation. Operating rooms are located in an area of the hospital offering limited, controlled access from the outside.
2. Bacterial isolation. All personnel working within this area must wear special clothing and footwear. Filtered air is continually circulated within the O.R. Patients with known infections are further isolated in special operating rooms.
3. Centralization of equipment. The suite is an integrated unit, its sole function being to provide an atmosphere for safe and effective surgery. It maintains its own equipment and supplies and can function on a daily basis without relying on outside assistance.
4. Centralization of trained personnel. The combined talents of many groups of trained personnel form the O.R. staff. By working together day in and day out, the staff acquires a great deal of efficiency, cooperation, and skill.

Within such an environment it is possible to provide a patient with the best possible surgical care.

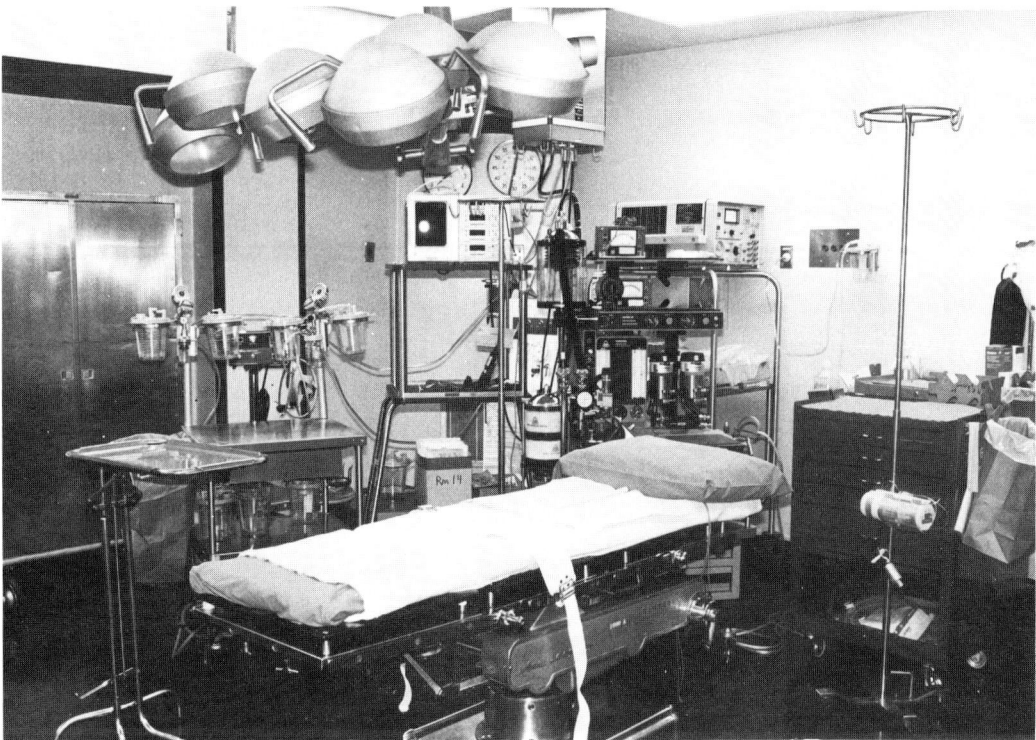

FIG. 18-8. *A modern operating room.*

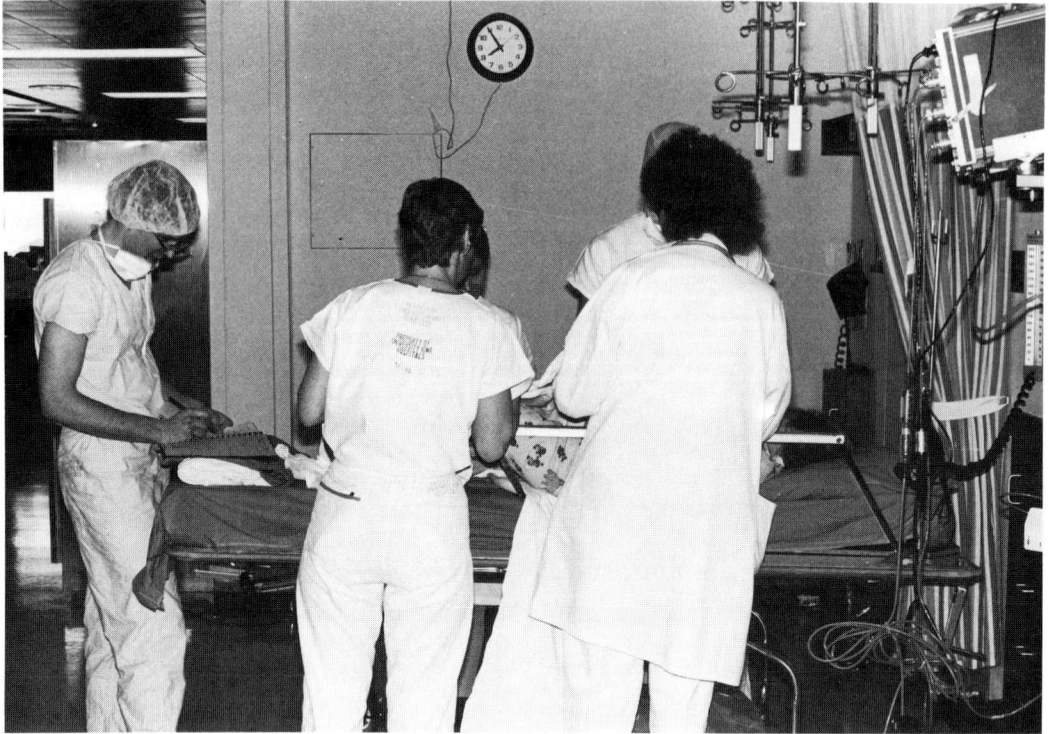

FIG. 18-9. *The recovery room. Recovery room staff assists patient; dental surgeon stays at the bed until vital signs are taken.*

Operating Room Personnel

The dentist should get to know each of the O.R. personnel individually as well as their specific duties.

The *nursing supervisor* supervises all nursing and ancillary personnel working in the O.R., oversees activities in the operating room, and enforces proper aseptic technique. The supervisor's office often establishes the O.R. schedule.

The *surgical nurse* (scrub nurse) is a member of the surgical team who is fully gowned and gloved. The surgical nurse assists the surgeon to gown and glove himself, and drape the patient, places the sterile instruments on the instrument trays, and assists by suctioning and passing instruments. In the absence of a second surgeon, the surgical nurse becomes the first assistant.

The *circulating nurse* does not gown and glove but remains free to move about the O.R., getting sutures or other materials for the surgeon. The circulating nurse assists in setting up the power equipment and suction, keeps a sponge count, and acts as intermediary between the scrubbed surgical team and the rest of the operating room suite.

The *anesthesiologist* assumes responsibility for the anesthetic, medical, and fluid management of the patient during the operation, keeping account of blood loss and informing the surgeon of any deviation from a normal course during anesthesia. The anesthesiologist also keeps an accurate record of the anesthesia and surgical procedure. This record becomes a permanent part of the patient's hospital medical record. Finally, he supervises the immediate postoperative care and recovery of the patient.

Operating Room Conduct

The introduction of pathogens into the operating area must be reduced to a minimum. All personnel entering the operating room suite must therefore be properly dressed. A sign on a door usually denotes the area in which street clothing cannot be worn.

Operating Room Attire

The dentist removes rings, watches, other jewelry, and all street clothing except underwear and socks. The scrub suit consists of cotton pants and a shirt that should be tucked into the pants. A disposable cap covers the hair; a cap with a hood should be worn to cover long hair. Shoes dedicated only to O.R. use are to be worn and covered with disposable shoe covers. Since flammable and explosive gases are seldom used for anesthesia, conductive shoes or covers are not routinely required. Check with the head nurse on this point. Before entering the O.R. a cap and mask must be in place. The mask must be snug and well adapted to the face. Masks are often found in the scrub room. Before scrubbing, the dentist enters the O.R., greets the O.R. personnel and introduces himself, confers with the anesthesiologist on anesthetic techniques, positioning of the patient, and estimated length of the procedure, and offers reassurance to the patient. Once the I.V. and induction of anesthesia begin, the dentist leaves the O.R. and begins the surgical scrub.

Scrubbing

Scrubbing is done in the scrub room adjoining the operating room. One scrub room often serves two operating rooms. If a headlight is worn, it must be adjusted before starting the scrub. The scrub procedure, usually posted above each sink, should be strictly followed. The first scrub of the day takes 10 minutes to complete, between cases it takes 5 minutes, and after an infected case 10 minutes.[9] It has been shown that 20 to 30 percent of surgeon's gloves are punctured at the end of an average operation. This is certainly the case when working in the oral cavity with complicated instrumentation, jagged teeth and bone and, at times, orthodontic appliances. It is imperative, therefore, that an adequate mechanical scrubbing be done in conjunction with the use of an antiseptic scrubbing solution. A number of prepackaged brushes contain a scrubbing solution such as iodophor. The presence of the iodophor greatly enhances the effectiveness of the scrub in reducing surface bacterial counts.

The following is a typical scrub procedure:[10]

1. Wash hands and arms to above the elbow for 1 minute to remove gross dirt.
2. Open a scrub packet and use the enclosed plastic nail cleaner to clean under nails with running water (Fig. 18-10A). The nail cleaner is then discarded.
3. Moisten the sponge/brush, forming a lather, and complete the 10-minute scrub as follows:
   a. Start with the fingertips. Think of each finger as having four surfaces and scrub each surface down to the interfinger web. (Fig. 18-10B)
   b. Scrub the hands in a circular motion—both ventral and dorsal surfaces—with special attention to the wrist area.
   c. Divide the arm into four surfaces and scrub each surface to several inches above the elbows. (Fig. 18-10C) The following number of scrub strokes are used:

   Fingernails—20 strokes each
   Finger and hand surfaces—10 strokes each surface
   Arms—6 strokes each surface to above elbows

4. Rinse: fingers first, then hands, arms, and elbows, keeping hands held above the elbows.
5. Scrub the other hand and arm in the above manner.
6. Rinse the second arm.
7. Rinse the brush, work up more lather, and repeat the above scrub procedure. Stop the scrub just below the elbow.
8. Rinse well and again allow the water to flow from the fingers toward the elbows (Fig. 18-10D). Do not contaminate the clean hands on the faucet or sink edges. Should contamination occur, rescrub the hand or arm with the number of scrub strokes described previously. Hold hands above elbows, keep hands and arms toward the front so they can be seen, and enter the O.R. by backing through the door.

Gowning and Gloving

Upon entering the O.R., the dentist is given a towel by the scrub nurse. The hands and forearms are dried using one surface of the towel for each arm. (Fig. 18-11) Do not dry above the elbows. Discard the towel and proceed with gowning.

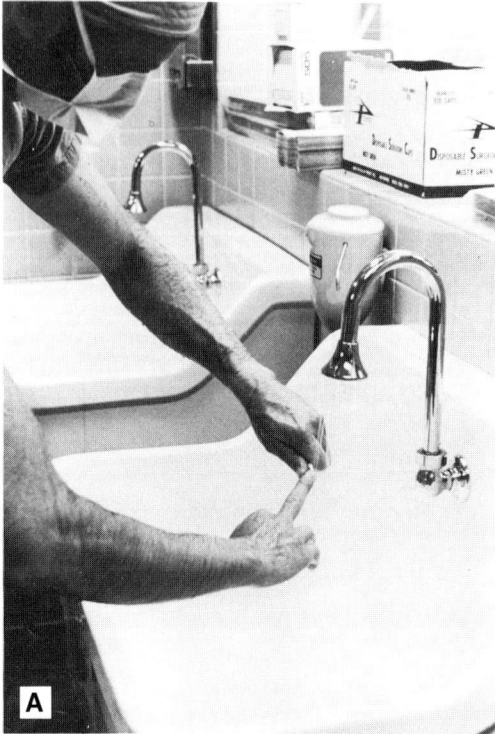

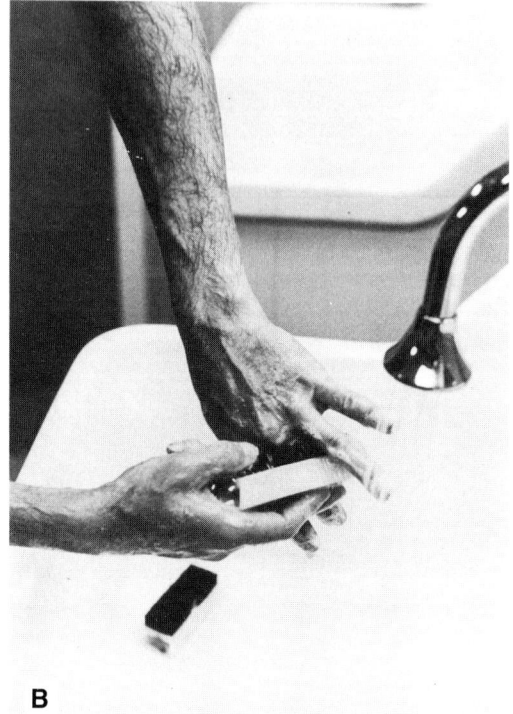

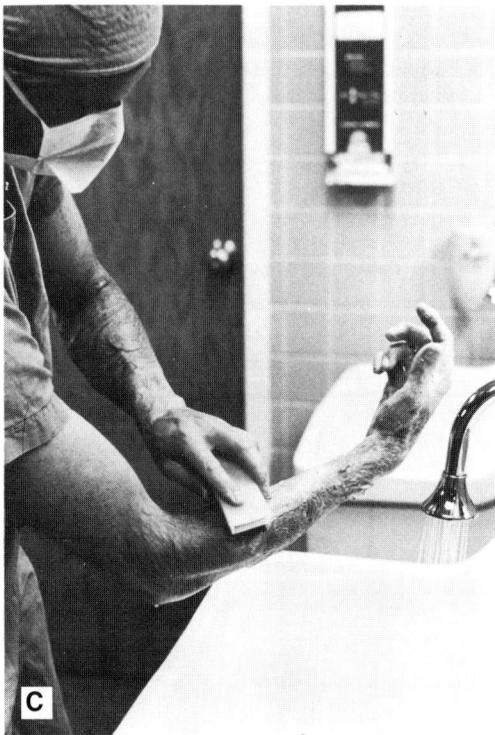

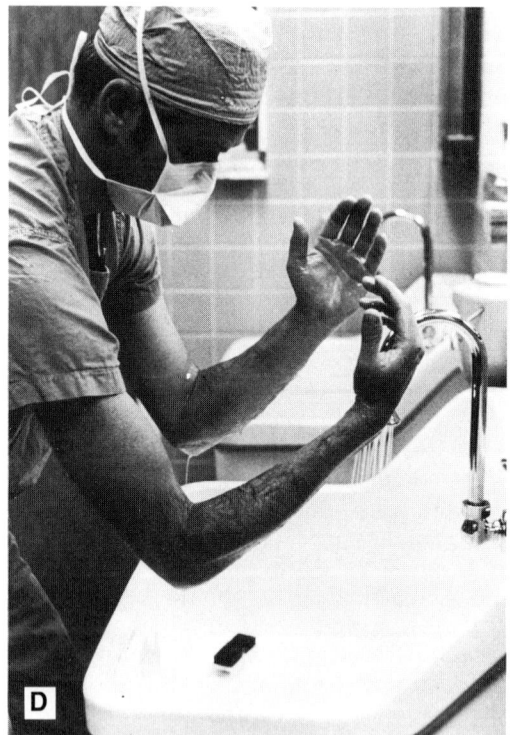

FIG. 18-10. (A) The surgical scrub begins with nail cleaning under running water. (B) Each finger surface is scrubbed with special attention given to interfinger web. (C) Each surface of the arm is scrubbed to several inches above the elbow. (D) The hands are held above the elbows while rinsing.

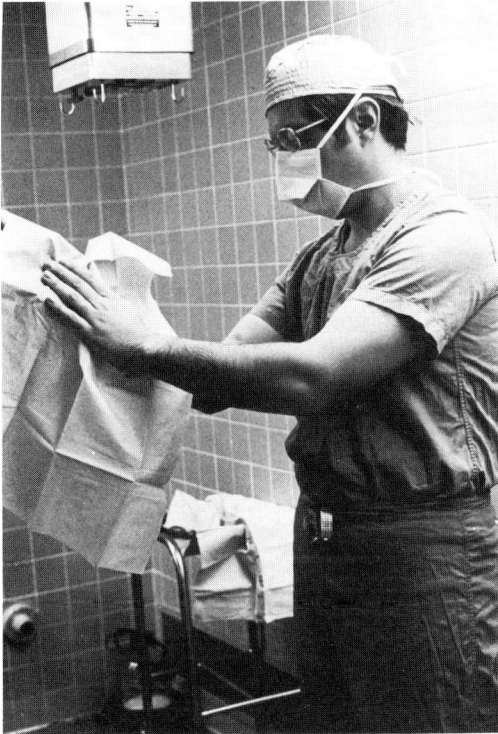

Fig. 18-11. *The hands and forearms are dried with a sterile towel.*

GOWNING AND GLOVING WITH ASSISTANCE

1. A sterile gown and towel pack is opened by the circulating nurse. (Fig. 18-12A)
2. The nurse unfolds the sterile gown and holds it in position. The dentist inserts his arms, being careful not to touch the nurse's gown, gloves or the exterior of his own gown (Fig. 18-12B).
3. The circulating nurse pulls the gown into position and ties the back (the back side of the gown is not sterile).
4. The scrub nurse holds the right glove with the rolled cuff stretched widely, the dentist inserts his hand firmly into the glove and the nurse unfolds the cuff over the sleeve (Fig. 18-12C). The left glove is put on in like manner except the dentist assists by placing the first and index finger of the gloved hand under the cuff of the left glove and pulls the cuff over the left sleeve.

GOWNING WITHOUT ASSISTANCE (CLOSED GLOVING TECHNIQUE)

Under some conditions the scrub nurse may not be available because of other duties and the dentist must gown and glove unassisted.

1. A sterile gown and towel pack is opened by the circulating nurse.
2. The dentist grasps the towel at a corner with one hand, unfolds the towel, and dries in the usual manner.
3. The gown that has been folded with the inner surface outward is grasped by the dentist and unfolded being careful not to touch the outer surface or drag the gown across the unsterile surface. The arms are inserted into the sleeves and the gown is pulled on and tied by the circulating nurse.
4. The gloves are opened with the thumbs facing upward. The dentist grasps the right glove by the cuff with the left hand, inserting the right hand and pulling the glove into place (Fig. 18-13). The cuff is returned and not rolled over the sleeve at this point.
5. The gloved fingers of the right hand are placed under the cuff of the left glove, the left hand is inserted, and the glove is pulled into correct position (Fig. 18-14). Both cuffs are then carefully rolled over the sleeves. At no time do bare fingers touch the outside of either glove.

Preparing ("Prepping") the Operative Site

"Prepping" the patient is done just before draping. It is usually done by a surgical assistant while the dentist is scrubbing, but should not be delegated to someone without the proper training. If an intraoral procedure is planned, the oral and perioral areas must be prepped. If an extraoral procedure is planned, only the skin need be prepped. Female patients should be advised not to wear any makeup to the O.R., and male patients should be clean shaven.

Before beginning the prep, place the patient's head in the proper position for surgery (Fig. 18-15). Pull back the hair and cover it with a surgical cap. Remove earrings and pull the sheet covering the patient down to the clavicles. Place waterproof plastic-coated paper towels on either side of the head to prevent the operating table from getting wet. The prep package is opened by the circulator and prep solu-

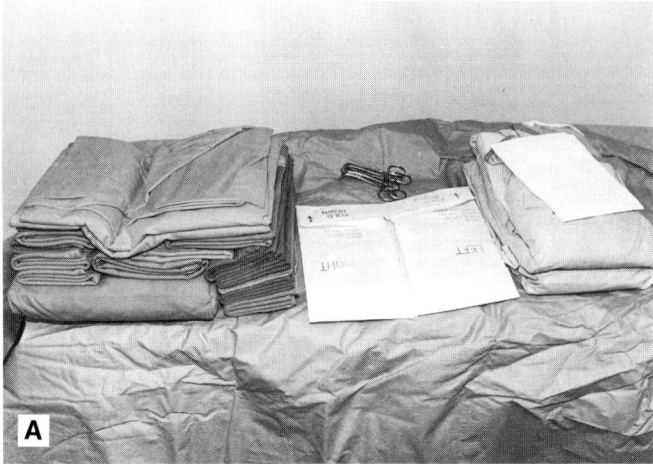

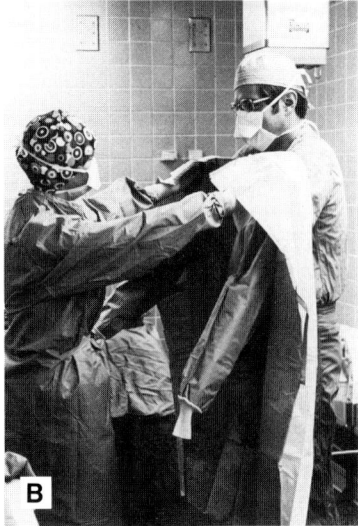

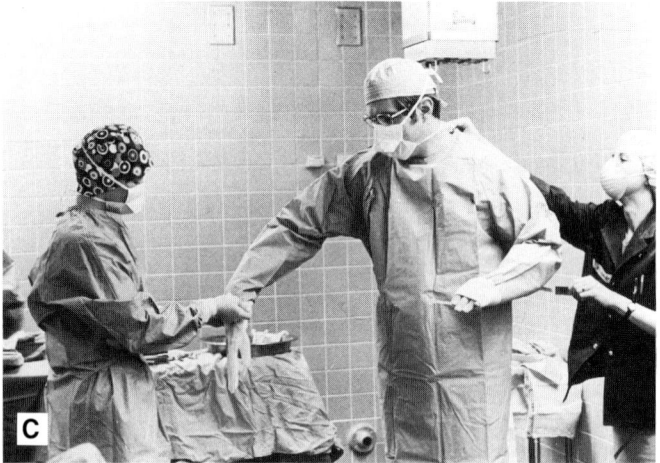

FIG. 18-12. *(A) Sterile gown and towel pack. (B) Surgical nurse gowns surgeon. (C) Surgical nurse gloves surgeon while circulating nurse ties back of gown.*

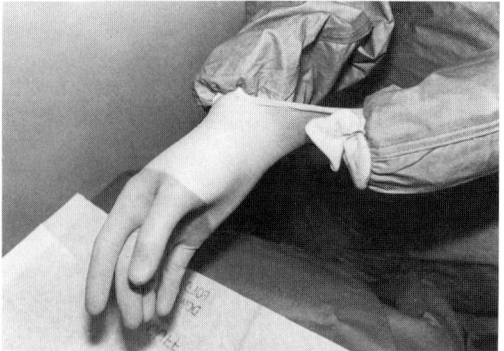

FIG. 18-13. *Self-gloving technique. Bare hands never touch the outer surface of the glove.*

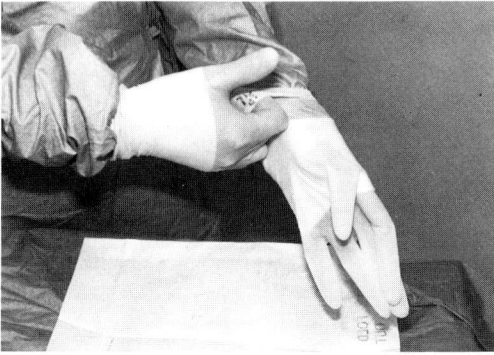

FIG. 18-14. *Self-gloving technique. Second hand is gloved by the first hand. Cuffs are rolled over the sleeves.*

tion is poured into a sterile cup on the prep tray. The person doing the prep dons sterile gloves and crosses two sterile towels over the patient's lower neck. A third towel covers the upper face and head.

SKIN PREP USING POVIDONE-IODINE SOLUTION

1. Saturate the sponge stick with the prep-ping solution and scrub the area for five minutes (Fig. 18-16). Start at the point of incision and extend it gradually to a larger area, being careful not to return to the initial point with the same sponge. Be especially careful not to allow the solution to run into the eyes. When prepping near the eyes, hold a dry sterile sponge over each eye. Should the solution enter the eye, immediately retract the eyelids and rinse with sterile water.

2. Using a fresh sponge, repeat the above scrub sequence. The scrub solution is not removed but allowed to dry.

The oral cavity cannot be disinfected as readily as the skin; however, a circumoral prep is indicated to prevent the transfer of skin microorganisms to the mouth. An oral prep is needed to cleanse the mouth of accumulated oral debris; this will lower the bacterial count significantly and reduce the incidence of bacteremia during tooth extraction. This is particularly important for patients with histories of rheumatic heart disease, prosthetic heart valves, organ

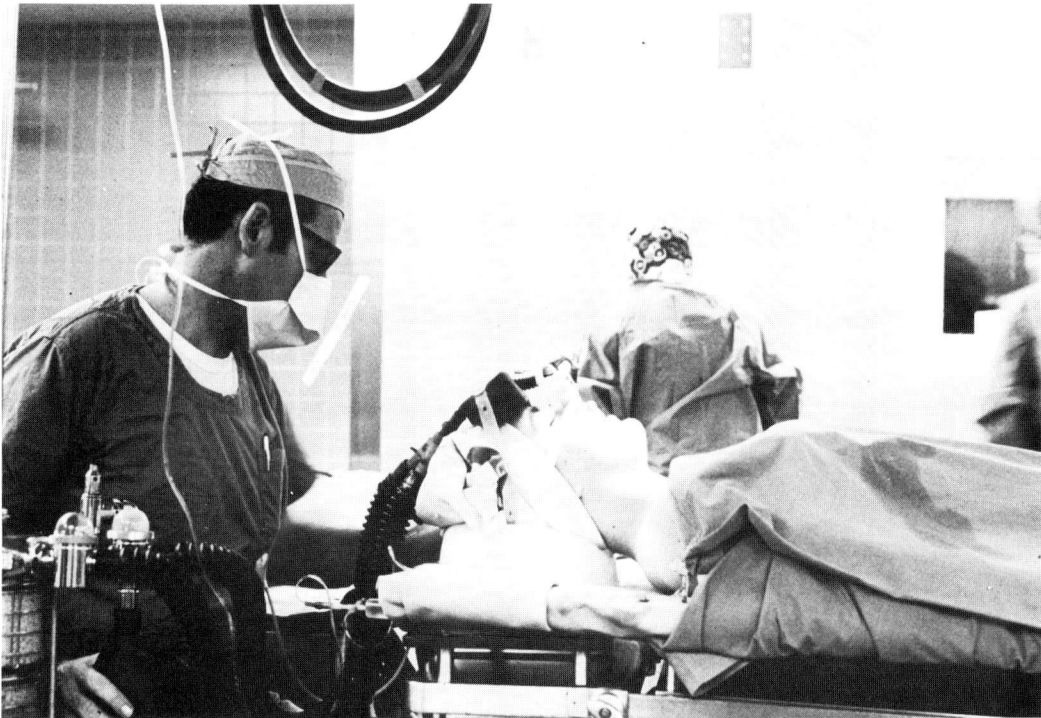

FIG. 18-15. *Patient positioned ready for prepping. The hair is covered and an anesthetic tube and monitors are secured with tape.*

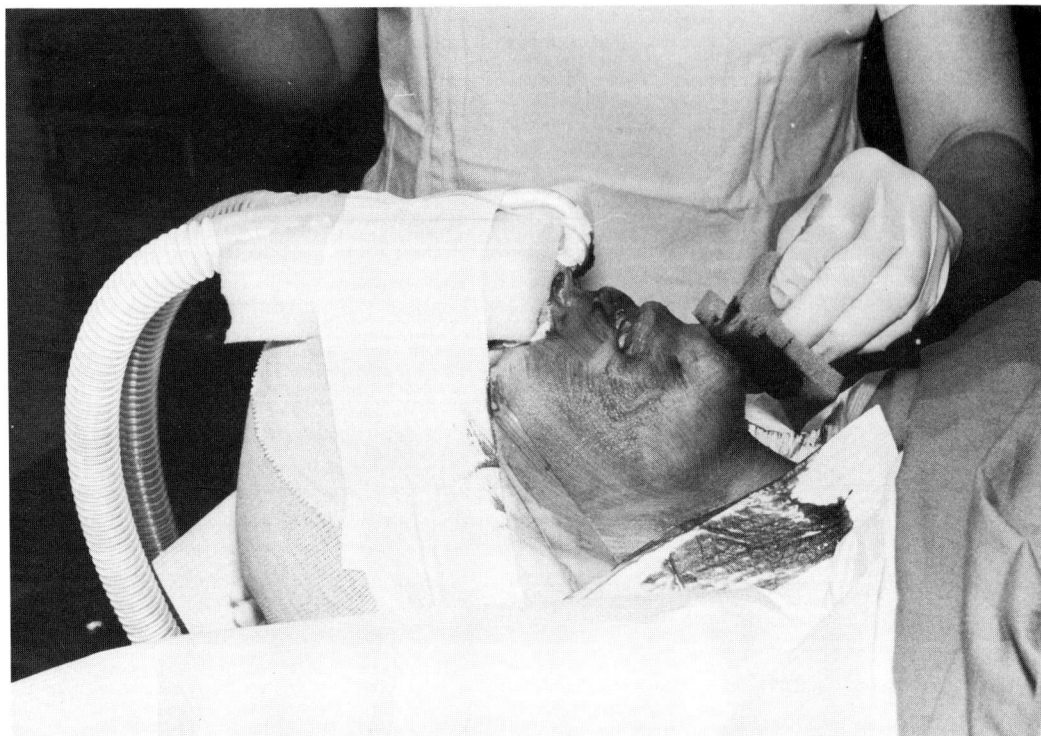

FIG. 18-16. *Skin preparation with povidone-iodine solution.*

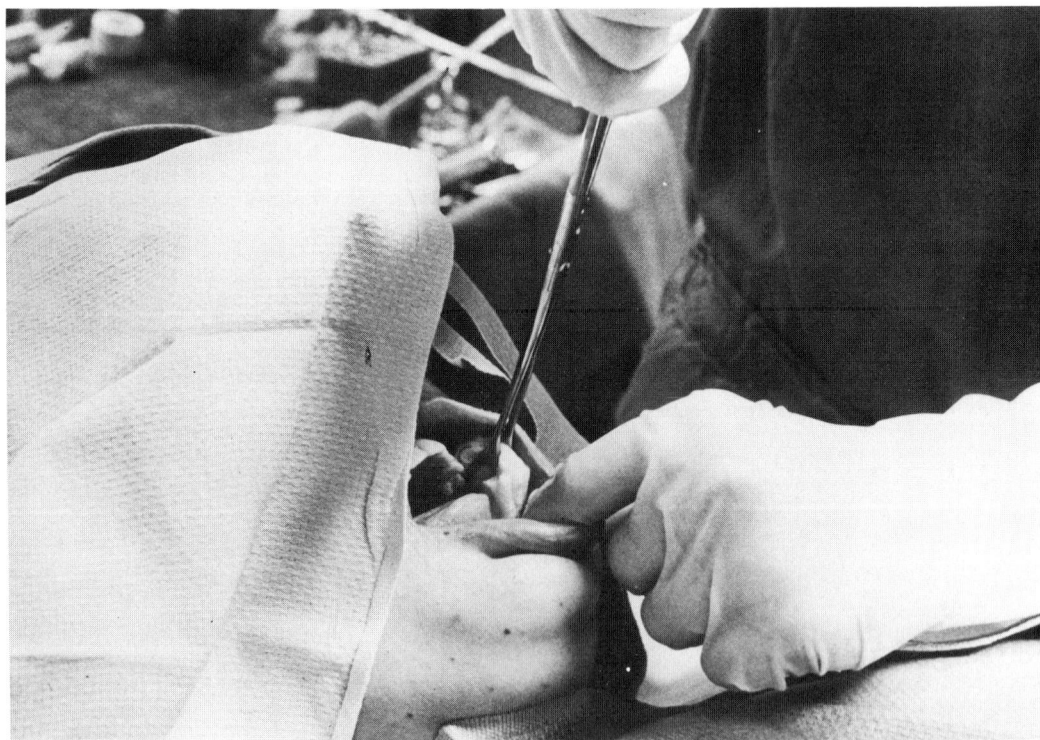

FIG. 18-17. *Intraoral preparation with sponge stick and saline.*

transplants, total hip prosthesis, and im-munosuppression.[11]

INTRAORAL PREPARATION

1. Place a moistened gauze pack to isolate the oral cavity from the pharynx.
2. Scrub the gingiva, tongue, and palate with a stick sponge or a gas-sterilized toothbrush; rinse with copious amounts of saline and suction well. Discard the brush, and remove the gauze pack (Fig. 18-17).
3. Scrub the circumoral skin with a sponge or gauze soaked in povidone-iodine for 5 minutes.

Draping the Patient

The drape isolates the prepared area from the nonprepared areas of the body and assures that during the operation no contact occurs between the operative site and nonsterile equipment and personnel in the operating room. Before draping be sure the patient is positioned in the center of the table, legs are uncrossed, and arms are tucked at his side. Also check with the anesthesiologist to assure all monitoring devices are in place and secure. Draping is usually performed by the dentist or the first assistant and the scrub nurse.

The following method is recommended for draping the head in preparation for an oral procedure. (Fig. 18-18A through C)

1. Make a head drape by placing two towels one on top of the other and place these on top of a half sheet. The patient's head is elevated by an assistant and the head drape is placed under the patient's head. The half sheet beneath the towels covers the head of the table.
2. Cross the opposite ends of the two towels over the patient's face near the bridge of the nose and secure with a towel clip.
3. Place another towel over the nose and endotracheal tube and secure to the head towel with two or three towel clips.
4. Then cross the two towels over the neck and secure in the middle and to the head towel with towel clips.
5. Use a full drape sheet, laparotomy drape, or thyroid drape to cover the remainder of the body. The laparotomy and thyroid drapes have a hole in them, which can be conveniently centered over the mouth.
6. A half sheet is placed between the anesthesiologist and the patient by suspending it between two I.V. poles. The lower end of the sheet is clipped to the body sheet. (Fig. 18-19A).

Once the draping is complete, members of the surgical team position themselves around the operating table (Fig. 18-19B). The surgeon must remember that the drapes below waist level of the surgical team are considered unsterile and must not be touched by hands or instruments.

This draping method can be easily modified for an extraoral procedure by placing an additional towel to cover the mouth and lower lip. The towel is sutured to the skin below the lower lip with 3-0 silk sutures and fastened to the head towel with several towel clips.

A clean plastic drape with an adhesive side effectively isolates the oral cavity from the surgical site. The adhesive side is pressed down over the lower lip, and the rest of the plastic sheet drapes over the mouth, nose, and endotracheal tube.

An oral pharyngeal pack must be placed for all oral procedures even if a rubber dam is being used for restorative procedures. Approximately 18 inches of vaginal packing, which has been moistened, makes an excellent pack. The tongue is retracted inferiorly with a Weider retractor, and the throat pack is layered from the base of the tongue to the soft palate with special care to pack completely around the oralendotracheal tube. Since there is often incomplete skeletal muscle relaxation during general anesthesia, a rubber mouth prop is usually necessary. Upon completion of the procedure the oral cavity should be vigorously rinsed with saline, suctioned, and the throat pack and mouth prop removed.

Sterilization Methods

Sterilization is the process by which all microbial forms are destroyed. Proteins and other polymolecular structures can serve as a protecting layer for microorganisms and prevent penetration of the sterilizing medium. Therefore, surgical instruments must be scrupulously cleaned of debris including blood, saliva, and necrotic material to allow penetration of the sterilizing agents. Soiled instruments are hand

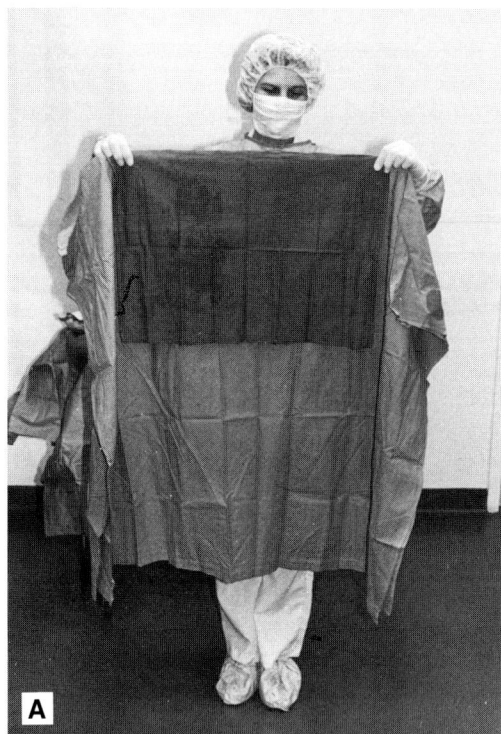

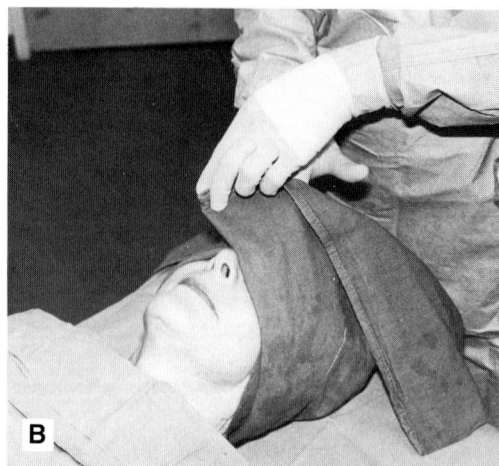

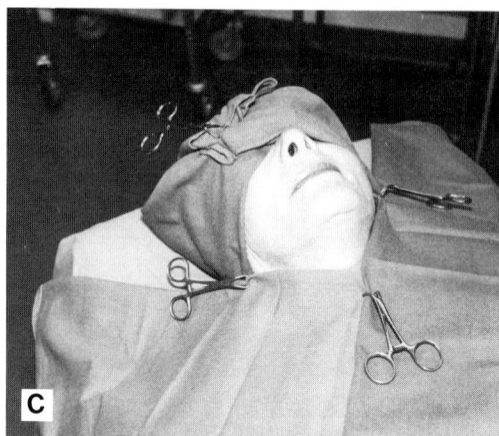

FIG. 18-18. *(A) Head drape made with a hand towel and half sheet. (B) Half sheet covers end of table and towel covers patient's head and eyes. (C) Towels crossed over neck and clipped to head drape.*

washed to remove gross debris and placed in ultrasonic cleaning devices before being dried, packaged, and sterilized (Fig. 18-20).

Methods of sterilization for instruments and supplies used in oral surgery include:

A. Physical Agents
    1. Steam heat
    1. Dry heat
B. Chemical Agents
    1. Glutaraldehyde (Cidex)
    2. Ethylene oxide
    3. Radiation

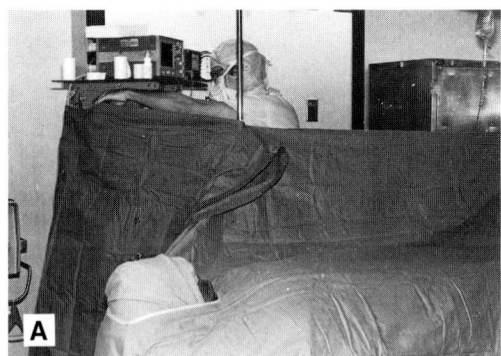

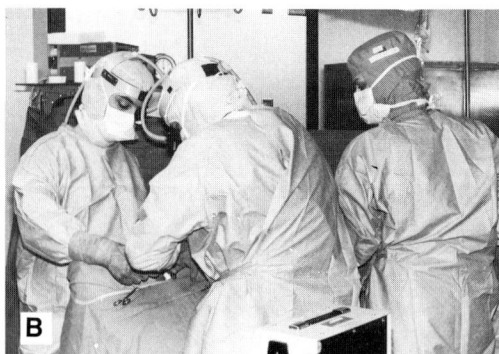

FIG. 18-19. *(A) Sheets separate anesthesiologist from the sterile area. (B) Surgical team positioned around operating table.*

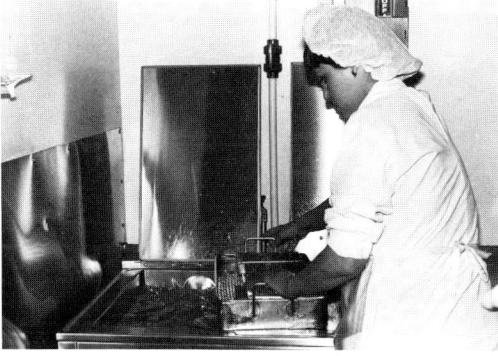

Fig. 18-20. *Instruments are cleansed in an ultrasonic cleaner before sterilization.*

Steam Heat

Steam under pressure is the most effective and practical method of sterilization (Fig. 18-21). Steam at a temperature of 121.5°C under 15 p.s.i. pressure requires only 12 minutes to kill all living organisms. The instrument wrap slows the process of sterilization; therefore, sterilizing for 20 to 30 minutes provides a margin of safety.

Instrument packs are secured with a thermosensitive tape that changes in color when sterilization is adequate (Fig. 18-22). Metal instruments and glass containers are ideally sterilized by steam. Because rubber goods and plastic may melt, they are best treated by other means. Steam corrodes and dulls cutting edges of metal instruments. The Harvey autoclave is a small table-top unit that uses vaporized alcohol under pressure rather than steam. This type of sterilization does not dull or corrode instruments (Fig. 18-23).

Dry Heat

Dry heat has poor penetration properties and is not well conducted by air. A temperature of 160°C for 2 hours is necessary to obtain sterility. Dry heat kills by dehydration and oxydation. It does not cause corrosion of the cutting edges of metal instruments.

Glutaraldehyde (Cidex)

Glutaraldehyde kills vegetative bacteria, spores, fungi, and viruses by alkylation on

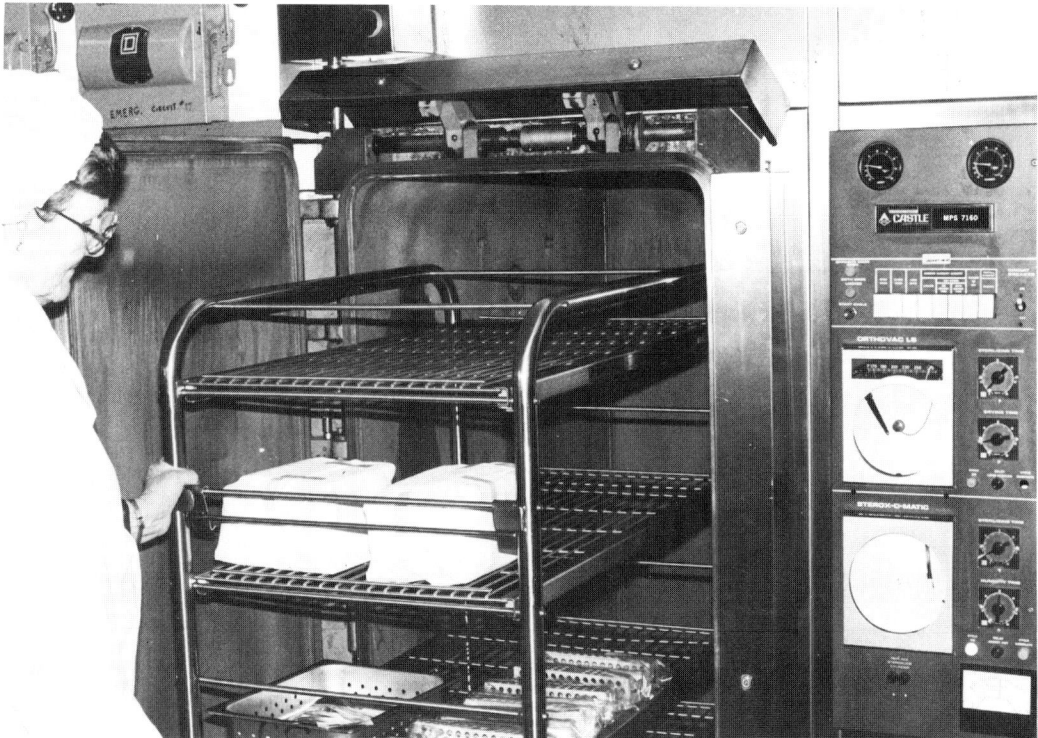

Fig. 18-21. *Steam autoclave in sterilization room.*

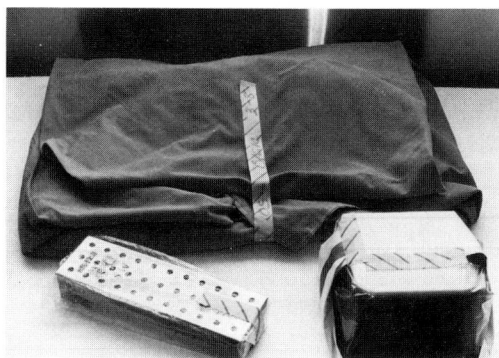

FIG. 18-22. *Dark lines appear on thermosensitive tape after autoclaving.*

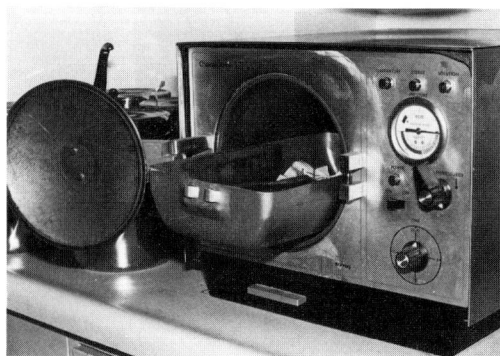

FIG. 18-23. *The Harvey autoclave uses vaporized alcohol under pressure to sterilize. It will not dull or corrode instruments.*

10-hour contact with the item to be sterilized. It is toxic and irritating and therefore must be removed thoroughly with sterile water or alcohol before the instrument is used. Porous objects should not be sterilized with glutaraldehyde.

Ethylene Oxide

Gas sterilization with ethylene oxide offers an excellent method for sterilizing items that cannot be readily steam-sterilized. The gas at temperatures above 10.8°C destroys organisms by alkylation. Sterilization takes 4 to 12 hours. Porous materials, to include the wrapping materials, readily absorb the gas and considerable time is required for elution of the gas from these items. Some plastics, for example, take 1 to 7 days to de-gas. Despite these limitations, ethylene oxide is a highly effective means of sterilization and especially suited for cutting and delicate instruments.

Radiation

Ionizing radiation—such as x-rays, gamma rays, and nonionizing ultraviolet light—can be used to kill or inactivate microorganisms. It is used primarily by industry to sterilize disposable materials such as suture, needles, and drugs sensitive to heat. Ultraviolet light is most commonly used for air purification in the operating room.

References

1. American Dental Association, Bureau of Economic Research and Statistics. The 1983 Survey of Hospital Dental Practice. Chicago, American Dental Association, 1984.
2. Sulley, J. J., Van Ostenberg, P. R., and Gump, M. L.: Dentistry and its future in the hospital environment. JADA, *101*:236, 1980.
3. Smith, B. W.: Dentistry in the hospital setting. Spec. Care Dent., *4*:56, 1984.
4. Donohue, M. P., and Gift, H. C.: Dental practice in hospitals. New Dent., *11*:29, 1980.
5. Accreditation Manual for Hospitals, Chicago, Joint Committee on Accreditation of Hospitals, 1984.
6. Weed, L. L.: Medical records that guide and teach. N. Engl. J. Med., *278*: 593, 1968.
7. Hillman, R. S., et al.: Clinical Skills. New York, McGraw-Hill Book Co., 1981.
8. Laskin, D. M.: Oral and Maxillofacial Surgery, Vol. I. St. Louis, C. V. Mosby Co., 1970.
9. Hooley, J. R.: Hospital Dentistry. Philadelphia, Lea & Febiger, 1970.
10. Douglas, B. L.: Introduction to Hospital Dentistry, 2nd ed. St. Louis, C. V. Mosby Co., 1970.
11. Autcher, J. L., et al.: Control of bacteremia associated with extractions of teeth. Oral Surg. *31*:602, 1971.

CHAPTER 19

Trauma of the Soft and Hard Tissues

Edward L. Mosby

Extraordinary results follow only extraordinary effort.

The management of injuries to the maxillofacial regions is a common surgical responsibility of the oral surgeon. As a specialty of the dental profession, oral surgery has greatly improved knowledge of and surgical capabilities in diagnosis and management of trauma to the face and jaws. The more significant advancements in the diagnosis and treatment of maxillofacial injuries occur during periods of man's conflicts. The increased incidence of such injuries and the interprofessional cooperation needed for the management of these patients are the reasons for improved total patient care in this area.

Facial structures are frequently affected by all types of trauma including motor vehicle accidents, interpersonal violence, sporting injuries, and falls. The resultant injury may interfere with daily activities such as eating, speaking, and drinking. More severe facial injuries, such as LeFort-type fractures and some mandibular fractures, can lead to a compromised airway and may be associated with other serious injuries of the head and thoracic and intra-abdominal regions.

The total patient must be evaluated carefully before any local or minor treatment is begun. Management of severe facial injuries must follow a systematic approach. Emergency treatment, such as establishing an airway, hemorrhage control, and management of shock, requires immediate attention. Serious concomitant injuries, such

as head, thoracic, and intra-abdominal injuries, must be addressed before any treatment of facial injuries is begun.

Soft tissue lacerations of the head and neck are best treated as soon after injury as possible. When the patient's condition is stable, facial fractures should be treated definitively. Treatment should always be from the "inside out and bottom up"; that is, placing the teeth in occlusion, starting with the mandible, and proceeding superiorly to the most stable bone, while anatomically reducing all bones in between. Bony treatment should be accomplished prior to closure of skin and mucosal lacerations. This regimen allows support to soft tissues and minimizes or eliminates surgical reentry through lacerations for osseous repair. Debridement should be thorough yet conservative to prevent loss of tissues vital to the desired result.

Adequate antibiotic coverage instituted early helps prevent infection. Tetanus antitoxin should be given to patients with contaminated wounds. If primary closure of lacerations is not possible initially, the tissues should be approximated with holding sutures. The wound edges may be freshened and closed later. If soft tissue has been avulsed, bone and other vital structures should be covered until surgical flaps can be mobilized to contour and protect the area. Typing and cross-matching of blood and complete laboratory evaluation should be accomplished as soon as possible

343

to help in patient management and possibly reveal occult disease; underlying disease should be treated and controlled to ensure healing of the injuries.

Examination

The general principles of management of maxillofacial injuries are divided into five phases:

1. Resuscitation and emergency procedures
   a. establish and maintain a clear airway
   b. control hemorrhage
   c. treat shock
   d. primary care of the wounds
      It is important at this stage that manipulation be avoided, so as not to exacerbate the original injury; for example, manipulation of an unstable cervical spine injury.
2. General and local examination
   a. patient is stabilized and vital signs are monitored
   b. general physical examination is made
   c. a good history is obtained
   d. other specialists' opinions are requested as necessary
3. Investigations
   a. hematology
   b. biochemistry
   c. radiology
4. Definitive treatment
   a. patient is appraised of findings
   b. injuries are treated as appropriate
   c. postoperative care begins
5. Rehabilitation
   a. patient is followed during the recovery period
   b. complications are treated
   c. rehabilitation is instituted

Care of the Traumatized Patient

The precedence for the care of the traumatized patient must be given the proper sequencing so that treatment procedures accomplish the most good in the best time frame. They are categorized as follows: lifesaving measures, medical evaluation and triage, care and treatment of the injuries, and postoperative care.

Lifesaving Measures

AIRWAY MAINTENANCE

Of great importance for any injured patient, maintenance of an airway is particularly important for a patient with a maxillofacial injury. The tongue may fall back and occlude the oropharynx if there are fractures of the jaws or if the patient is unconscious. Care must be taken to evaluate the patient—the examiner must utilize patient positioning and suction to ascertain that mucous, blood, or other foreign material is cleared and not occluding the airway. Debris such as broken teeth, broken dentures, alveolar bone segments, and other foreign bodies should be removed from the oral cavity and pharynx. Other prosthetic appliances should be removed unless they are being left in place for fixation or for advantageous use in administering basic or advanced cardiac life support. The tongue should be checked for bleeding and/or edema.

Even though the need for an emergency tracheotomy occurs infrequently, opening the airway through the crycothyroid membrane (coniotomy) should be part of the treatment regimen available to all practitioners. The crycothyroid membrane lies between the thyroid cartilage and the cricoid cartilage, and once it is located, a transverse incision can be made through the overlying skin and through the crycothyroid membrane. Bleeding with the procedure is minimal. The opening must be maintained.

The following maxillofacial injuries may require tracheostomy:

1. Gunshot wounds of the face
2. Crush injuries of the face
3. Bilateral mandibular fractures associated with LeFort fractures of the maxilla
4. Mandibular fractures associated with extensive laceration of the tongue and floor of the mouth
5. Grossly posteriorly displaced maxillary fractures with palate split and profuse bleeding from the nasopharynx
6. Fractures of the facial skeleton associated with cranial, thoracic or spinal injuries
7. Extensive burns of the face or neck

Several immediate complications that may result from tracheostomies include hemorrhage, subcutaneous emphysema, pneumo- or hemothorax, and recurrent laryngeal nerve paralysis. Delayed complications may include massive arterial hemorrhage, tracheal stenosis, tracheoesophageal fistula, and infection.

HEMORRHAGE CONTROL

Profuse bleeding that is life-threatening is usually not a problem with maxillofacial injuries, unless a major vessel is involved. Local pressure or hemostats may be utilized to control hemorrhage in the facial area. Hemostats or clamps should be left in place in larger vessels until proper lighting and instrumentation are available to allow the vessels to be tied off or hemorrhage to be controlled with vascular clips. Pressure bandages may be applied but must be monitored constantly to ensure that they have not obstructed the airway. Determine the amount of blood loss. CBC, HCT, and differentials should be done as soon as possible, and where appropriate, type cross-match of blood for transfusion.

SHOCK MANAGEMENT

Shock does not routinely accompany maxillofacial injuries. However, if a patient with maxillofacial injuries is in shock, a total medical evaluation is necessary, as shock is probably presenting secondary to some other injury.

The significant event surrounding shock is a reduction in the circulating blood volume and, therefore, a reduction in the oxygen-carrying potential. If shock results from hemorrhage, whole blood should be given. If little or no red cell loss has occurred, plasma or some other substitute may be administered. If whole blood or blood components are to be utilized, type and cross-match must be done. In severe emergencies, type O-negative blood may be administered. Oxygen should be administered when appropriate. The patient may be placed in Trendelenburg position to increase cerebral blood flow and reduce pooling in the extremities. Attempts should be made to maintain body temperature, making certain that the patient is not hyperpyretic. Vasopressors may be utilized cautiously.

INFECTION CONTROL

Infections likely to follow maxillofacial injuries could include tetanus and wound and bone infection. Prophylaxis against tetanus infection is accomplished by administration of tetanus toxoid, if the patient is known to have been previously immunized. If not, tetanus antitoxin should be given. Antibiotics should be given as appropriate for the injury. Penicillin is the drug of choice for maxillofacial injuries and fractures of the facial bones. Additions or changes should be made to this regime, depending upon the patient's other accompanying injuries and/or allergies. The neurosurgeon may suggest using different antibiotics in patients with open or closed head injuries, as may the orthopedic or general surgeon in patients with injuries related to his specialty. Therefore, the treatment of patients with antibiotics may be multidisciplinary treatment and should be thoroughly coordinated.

PAIN CONTROL

Analgesics, whether narcotic or non-narcotic, should be administered minimally and with care. Administration of narcotics prior to a definitive diagnosis may hinder and delay patient evaluation. Narcotics given to a patient with a probable head injury (1) stimulate the oculomotor nucleus, causing miosis that masks the development of neurologic eye signs vital to recognition of cerebral hemorrhage; (2) may depress respirations; and (3) may stimulate nausea and vomiting.

Medical Evaluation of the Patient

Following the completion of all lifesaving treatment, the patient must receive a medical evaluation and triage to determine how rapidly definitive care can be rendered. The patient must be thoroughly evaluated so that treatment may be given by appropriate specialists in a proper sequence. Consultation with a neurosurgeon should be sought if any questions arise regarding the patient's neurologic status. The neurologic status can be readily evaluated by comparing contralateral reflexes. The presence of a positive Babinski's sign, Battle's sign, and comparing eye responses and pupil size, along with the presence of cerebral spinal fluid rhinorrhea or otorrhea should be noted. An open or closed head injury or neurologic change should be evaluated and followed by a neurosurgeon.

The evaluation, treatment planning, and subsequent management of maxillofacial

injury require a basic knowledge of anatomy. The practitioner must be familiar
with bony and dental architecture, as well
as the soft tissue anatomy in the contiguous
areas. Accurate diagnosis plays an important role in management of both the emergency and definitive treatment phases. An
improper diagnosis can result in misman-
agement that produces an inability to function properly.

Occlusion. A detailed knowledge of occlusion is paramount in establishing an
accurate diagnosis. The clinician must be
aware that approximately 10 percent of the
population has a malocclusion and, therefore, 10 percent of fracture patients have a
preexisting malocclusion prior to the traumatic incident. Utilization of the occlusion
also enables accurate alignment of maxillary and/or mandibular fractures, encouraging proper bone healing and avoiding a
malocclusion that may require corrective
orthodontics and/or orthognathic surgery.
Proper function of the jaws is one of the
goals of fracture treatment and is based on
an aligned and balanced occlusion.

Anesthesia or Hypesthesia. Numbness
or hypesthesia may aid the diagnostician in
determining the anatomic site of trauma
and possible fracture (see Chapter 11). It
should be kept in mind that interruption of
the function of a sensory nerve only indicates that a fracture may be present.
Trauma and the resultant edema can interrupt nerve function without bony fracture
being present. If nerve function is altered,
the clinician should rule out fractures that
could produce this change in sensation.

Facial Deformities. Certain types of
fractures are recognized by the facial appearance following displacement of the
fractured part; for example, a "dished out"
appearance occurs in posteriorly displaced
maxillary fracture (Fig. 19-1).

Ecchymosis. Bleeding into the soft tissues indicates certain areas of trauma; for
example, a subconjunctival and infraorbital ecchymosis may indicate injury to the

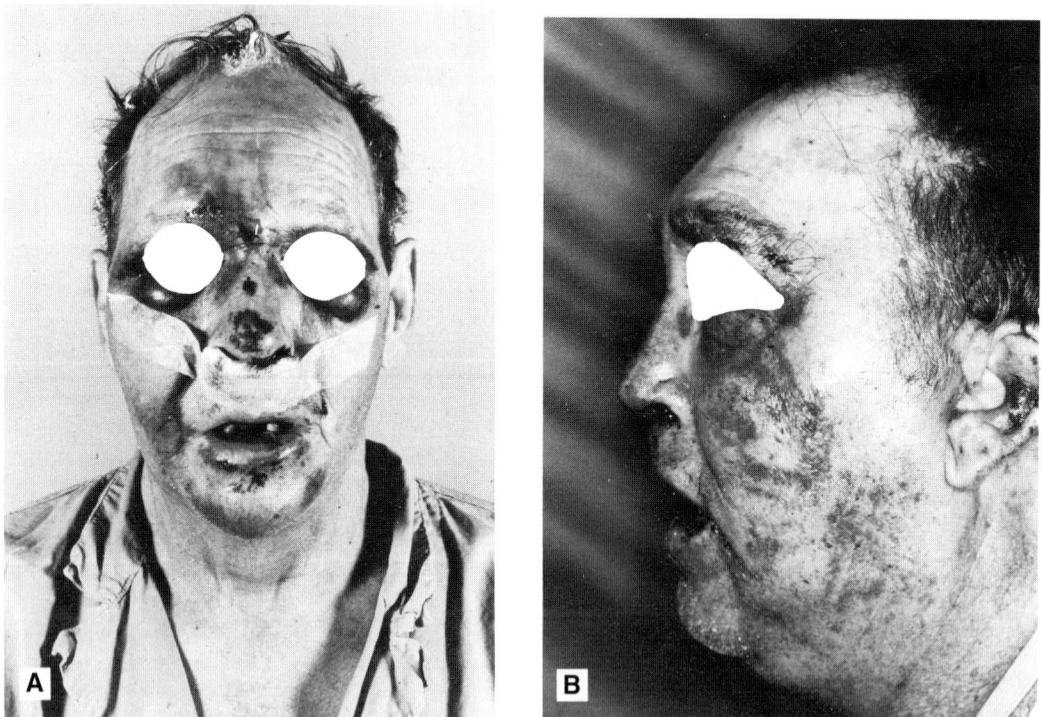

FIG. 19-1. (A) Facial appearance of patient having LeFort III-type facial injuries. Note the facial elongation and bilateral orbital ecchymosis. (B) Lateral facial profile of a patient with a LeFort III-type injury. Note the elongation of the face, as well as the "dishpan" facial concavity.

maxillary zygomatic complex, maxilla, or nasal bones. Ecchymosis of the floor of the mouth is a classic sign of a mandibular symphysis or mandibular body fracture; however, trauma to the soft tissues alone may produce a similar picture.

Crepitus. A grating or grinding of the fractured segments against each other is indicative of an underlying facial fracture.

Bleeding from a Cavity. Bleeding from the mouth, nose, or ears should lead to an evaluation of the facial bones associated with those areas for trauma and possibly fracture.

Mobility or Movement of the Maxilla or Mandible. Movement of the maxilla or segments of the mandible, as well as movement of the teeth or alveolar segments, indicates fractures and areas requiring treatment.

Pain. Pain may or may not be present either at rest or in effecting maximum occlusion. Pain may also be present at rest or on palpation.

X-ray Evaluation of Facial Trauma. Recent advances in high resolution CT and MRI imaging have provided marked improvement in bone imaging. Complex facial fractures, especially those associated with craniocerebral or spinal injuries, are better and more safely assessed by computerized tomography. Degrees of comminution previously grossly underestimated by conventional radiography are more accurately assessed by CT or MRI. The transaxial axis remains a dominant modality and superbly demonstrates displacement. Complications of soft tissue structures (orbit, brain) are diagnosed at the time of study and provide information often obtainable by other modalities. High resolution CT or MRI has become a definitive study of complex facial fractures involving the mid or upper third of the facial skeleton and has become a tremendous aid in diagnosis.

Care must be taken when evaluating x-ray films of the head and face because of superimposition of overlying structures. Special care should be used to determine if bony fragments or segments overlap and if foreign body objects are present. Suture lines should not be confused with fractures. Some x-rays that should be utilized in fracture diagnosis include: Water's/stereo Water's, Caldwell, submental vertex, right and left lateral oblique of the mandible, Towne's view, posterior-anterior (PA) and lateral of the mandible, PA and lateral of the skull, panorex, and maxillary occlusal of the maxilla and mandible.

Tomograms of the area may also be useful as a means of isolating an area so that a better x-ray can be obtained, enabling the clinician to make a more accurate diagnosis.

Clinical Judgment. The accurate diagnosis and effective management of maxillofacial trauma depend totally on the clinician's ability to utilize all the diagnostic aids as well as the clinical examination in making a diagnosis. No diagnostic aids (x-rays, lab studies, etc.) are 100 percent accurate in diagnosis of maxillofacial trauma. The clinical interpretation remains the most significant means towards an understanding of the nature of the fracture. Evaluation of diagnostic aids and clinical findings enables the clinician to be as accurate as possible in determining the extent of the patient's injury, the locations of the specific bony fracture sites, and the displacement or distraction at the fracture sites. An accurate diagnosis is of utmost importance to devise a treatment plan coincident with the patient's injuries. The treatment plan is based on the correlation of all data obtained in the examination and evaluation, with a thorough understanding of treatment modalities to be utilized. Without a treatment plan, based on a logical, scientific, sequential data base, the correct treatment cannot evolve.

Considerations in Treatment

The immediate life-sustaining considerations have already been covered; namely, shock, cardiorespiratory (including basic cardiac life support, advanced cardiac life support, airway management), bleeding and blood loss. Secondary considerations, although not lifesaving in nature, are equally important to primary considerations in that failure to consider them or to demean their importance would adversely affect the final treatment result.

Cerebrospinal Fluid. Drainage from the nose, ears, or eyes should be evaluated for the presence of cerebrospinal fluid. Neurologic damage and/or deficiency may be coupled with many facial fractures, and specialist consultation should be sought for these abnormalities. CSF leaks are most often sealed with adequate reduction, fixation, and immobilization of the facial fractures; therefore, every attempt should be made to attain definitive treatment as soon as possible.

Lacerations, Abrasions, and Contusions. These conditions should be completely and thoroughly debrided, sutured, and/or drained as soon as the patient is stable. Many materials such as road tar and gunpowder cause tattooing and must be removed with scrub brushes, dental curettes, etc. If primary closure is not possible, stay mattress sutures should be placed to approximate all skin edges. Since the laceration provides a treatment avenue during fracture reduction and fixation that must be delayed, skin edges should be freshened as little as possible, only removing damaged and nonvital tissue. All contaminated wounds should be drained with advancement removal of the drains over the first 72 hours.

Antibiotics. The patient should begin receiving antibiotics immediately. The coverage depends on and relates to the multiplicity of wounds. Penicillin is the ideal antibiotic utilized in the treatment of facial fractures. Coordination of antibiotic therapy must be made with all consulting specialists and should include coverage for all injuries.

Tetanus Prophylaxis. Patients with compound and/or contaminated wounds should receive tetanus prophylaxis. Tetanus human immune globulin is preferred to tetanus equine antitoxin for passive immunization, and is used if the patient has received less than two immunizing doses of tetanus toxoid, if the wound is unattended for more than 24 hours, or if the history of immunization is uncertain. Active immunization with tetanus toxoid for the unimmunized should be initiated concomitantly and at a different site with a different syringe used for the injection. Appropriate antibiotics have already been discussed.

Diet. Adequate and appropriate diet should be prescribed for the trauma patient. It may initially eliminate feeding by mouth, thus necessitating a balanced IV fluid regimen. Diet post-treatment may begin with clear liquids and progress to full liquid and mechanical soft before returning to a regular diet. During all phases, adequate caloric intake, as well as a balance of protein, carbohydrate, fat, vitamins, and essential elements must be maintained for a post-trauma patient. This must be coordinated with the medications taken by the patient, and consultation with a dietitian may be desired.

Temporary Immobilization. If definitive care is not possible immediately following the injury, temporary immobilization should be utilized for improved esthetics and comfort of the patient. Accomplishment of this type of immobilization requires innovation by the clinician using various devices such as Barton bandages, temporary splints of compound or acrylic, arch bars, wires to stabilize teeth or bones, or various inventions that fit the situation.

Treatment Planning.

A philosophy for treatment planning involves following a logical and rational sequence of events. The principle of treating from the inside out requires that intraoral injuries—such as luxated and/or avulsed teeth, the fractured and/or displaced alveolar bone, gingiva and mucosal lacerations—as well as *all* of the facial fractures, be definitively treated prior to closure of the skin. It is equally essential that facial fractures be treated from the bottom up. One goal in the management of maxillofacial trauma is the restoration of a functional occlusion. When teeth and alveolar segments are aligned and fixated, the remainder of the face follows. Therefore, the patient must be treated from the *inside out* and the *bottom up!*

Injuries and Treatment

Maxillofacial Fractures (Figs. 19-2 through 19-5)
LeFort I
LeFort II
LeFort III
Maxillary zygomatic complex
Zygomatic arch
Nasal fracture
Nasal, orbital, ethmoid fractures
Mandibular condyle fractures

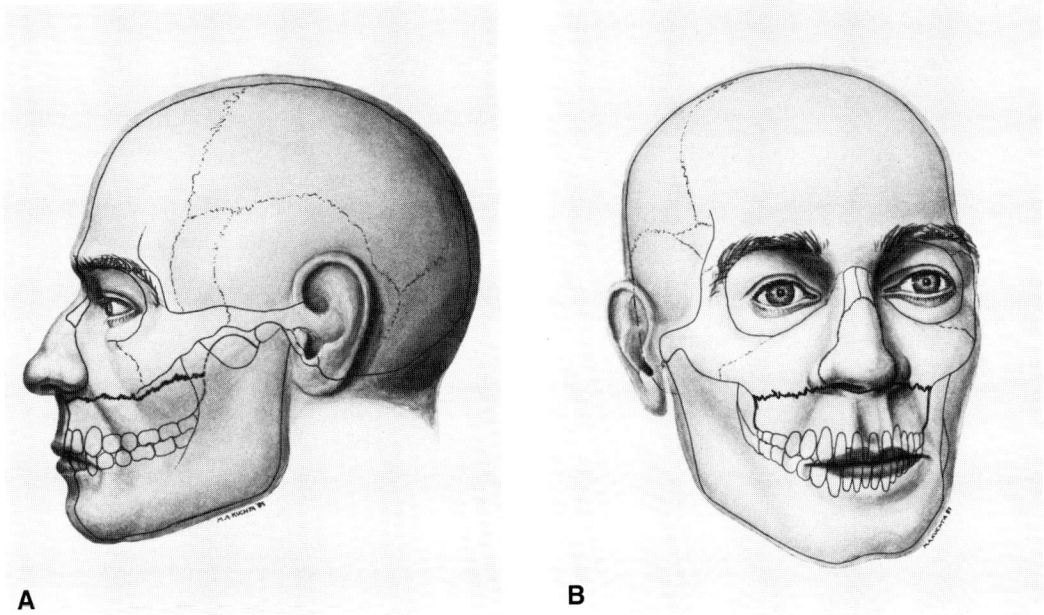

FIG. 19-2. *(A) LeFort I fracture (lateral view). (B) LeFort I (horizontal) fracture.*

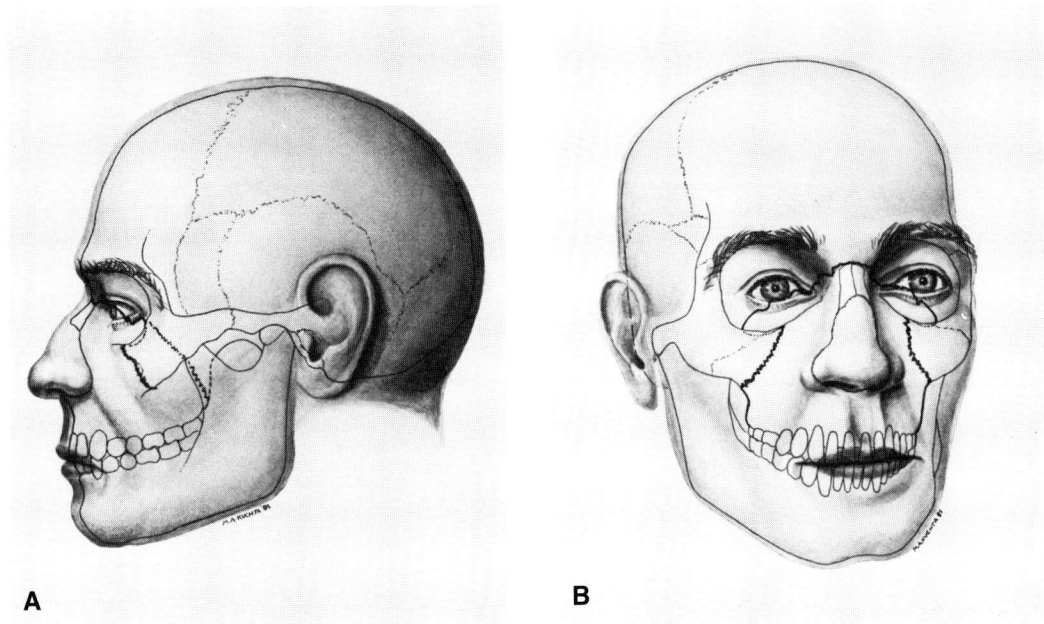

FIG. 19-3. *(A) LeFort II fracture (lateral view). (B) LeFort II (pyramidal) fracture.*

Mandibular ramus fractures
Mandibular body fractures
Mandibular symphysis fracture
Alveolar fractures
Tooth fractures
    The patient's diagnosis should begin with the most complex fracture and be expanded and elaborated upon as the fractures and/or injuries become less severe. Facial fractures rarely occur exactly as described. Fractures should be described anatomically; for example, a LeFort I fracture

A

B

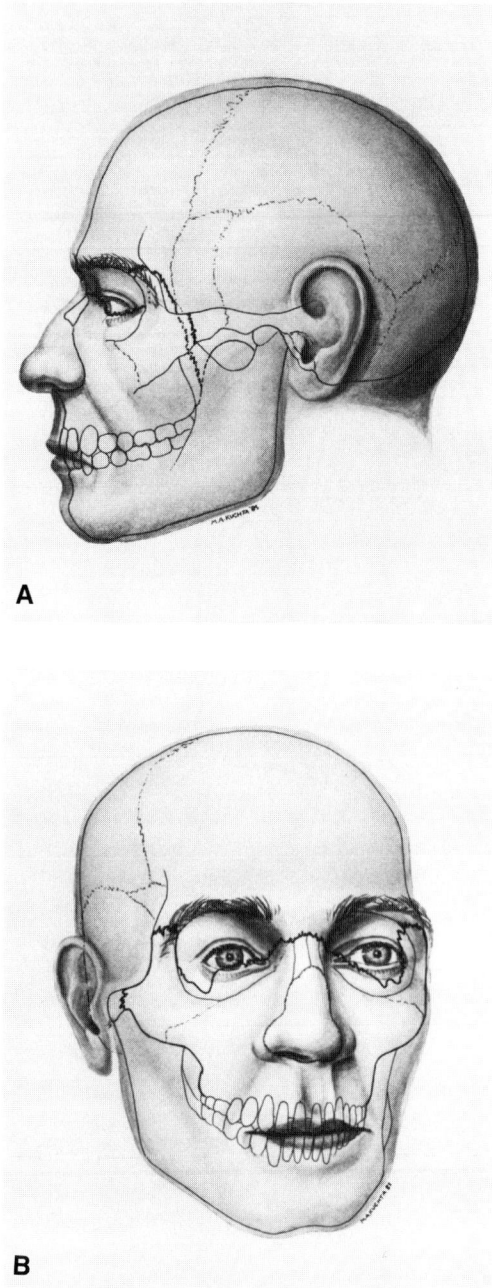

FIG. 19-4. *(A) Lateral view of LeFort III fracture. (B) LeFort III (cranial facial disjuncture) fracture.*

combined with a left Zygomatic Maxillary Complex (ZMC) fracture is not a left-sided or unilateral LeFort II—it is a LeFort I and left ZMC fracture.

Injuries and Treatment of Teeth

INJURIES

A traumatized or a fractured permanent or deciduous tooth (or teeth) is a common maxillofacial injury. The clinician must prevent loss of these injured teeth, so that they may become an integral part of reconstruction. Trauma to a tooth may result in fracture of the tooth, loosening or avulsion, and/or damage leading to death of the pulp. Fracture of the enamel and/or dentin, causing no serious damage to the pulp and not causing pulpal exposure, can be treated by smoothing off the involved area and covering it with a protective agent or temporary crown. Fracture of the crown involving the pulp requires extirpation of the pulp and endodontic therapy. Fracture of the root portion (that portion completely embedded in bone) may heal by formation of new cementum over the defect and may or may not require intervention with endodontic therapy, but intra-arch stabilization of the tooth is required. Incompletely formed teeth occasionally retain vitality regardless of trauma. Stabilization of the traumatized tooth is almost always advisable with a splinting or stabilizing device. Appropriate antibiotic coverage is necessary. Replantation is utilized occasionally and is successful in most instances, when the avulsed tooth can be root canal treated and replaced soon after the accident. Care must be taken with loosened and/or avulsed teeth to attempt to maintain all of their supporting alveolar bone when designing treatment plans.

Injuries to the teeth can be classified as follows:

1. Crown cracked or crazed
2. Crown fracture
   Enamel only
   Enamel and dentin involved
   Enamel, dentin, and pulp involved
3. Root fracture
4. Crown root fracture
5. Concussion (sensitivity)
6. Subluxation (mobile)
7. Tooth displacement
8. Evulsion
9. Compression of the alveolar socket
10. Alveolar socket wall fracture
11. Alveolar process fracture

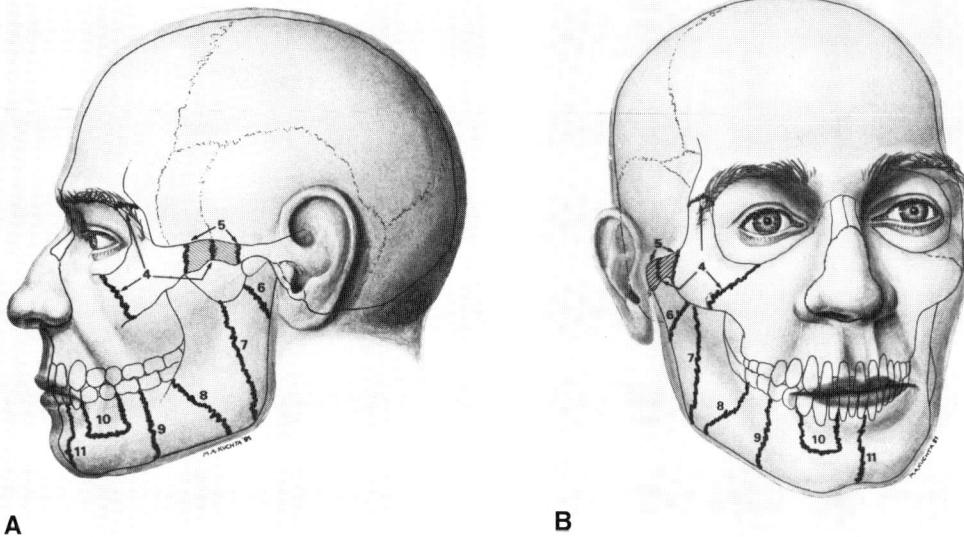

FIG. 19-5. (A) Lateral view. (B) Frontal view. 1. Zygoma (ZMC) fracture. 2. Zygomatic arch fracture. 3. Condylar fracture. 4. Subcondylar (ramus) fracture. 5. Angle fracture. 6. Bony fracture. 7. Alveolar fracture. 8. Symphysis (or parasymphysis) fracture.

Complications of dental injuries to primary and/or permanent teeth include:

1. Primary
   - Failure to continue eruption
   - Color change
   - Infection/abscess
   - Loss of space in the dental arch
   - Ankylosis
   - Injury to the developing permanent tooth
   - Abnormal exfoliation
   - Financial cost for maintaining dental arch space and restoration
2. Permanent
   - Color change
   - Infection or abscess
   - Loss of space in the dental arch
   - Loss of alveolar bone support
   - Ankylosis
   - Resorption of the root structure
   - Financial cost of potential root canal therapy, periodontal therapy, and restorative and prosthetic therapy
   - Abnormal root development

TREATMENT

Treatment of *enamel fracture* is limited to smoothing the tooth and soothing the irritation. *Crown fractures* involving dentin or dentin and pulp frequently exhibit sensitivity to thermal or direct stimuli. Exposed dentin may result in pulp inflammation, necrosis of the pulp, and/or abscess. In crown fractures involving dentin, the immediate dental therapy is directed toward preserving the integrity of the pulp. When a crown fracture involves the pulp, the patient should receive dental evaluation and therapy as soon as possible, to include root canal therapy. Crown and root fractures frequently require extraction.

Sensitive teeth should be reduced to eliminate functional contacts and followed closely to be evaluated for the need for root canal therapy. Mobile teeth should be splinted and maintained in a stable position. Displaced teeth should be cleaned in saline or tap water and the tooth replanted as soon as possible. If the tooth cannot be replanted within the first few minutes, a root canal therapy should be instituted.

Fractures of the alveolar process usually contain teeth; however, if they do not, the alveolar process should be placed in proper alignment manually and may require no further stabilization. The alveolar process containing teeth should be evaluated to determine if the teeth remaining in the segment are firm or if they have been avulsed from their sockets. Fractured segments should be placed manually in their proper relationship and evaluated by assessing the occlusion. Segments may be held in place by bonding orthodontic brackets or heavy gauze wires with arch bars applied to adjacent stable teeth. Then the fractured alveolar process segment is stabilized to the arch bar or wire with wires applied to the teeth in the segment or fractured alveolar segments stabilized to the wire with acid etch composite materials and wire mesh. Care must be taken in stabilizing the teeth and alveolar process fractures so that the stabilizing or fixating device does not cause supraeruption of either stable or unstable teeth. These fractures usually take from 4 to 12 weeks to heal sufficiently before their supporting appliances can be totally removed. Once the supporting appliances have been removed, the fracture segment should be supported by a retainer or splint as appropriate.

Mandibular Fractures

The mandible is the most commonly fractured facial bone. The body of the mandible is predominantly cortical bone, as contrasted to the tooth-bearing alveolar ridge, which is predominantly cancellous and easily resorbed following loss of teeth. The ovoid-shaped condyle joins the ramus by a thin condylar neck. The ramus joins the body of the mandible at the mandibular angle, and the anterior-superior portion of the ramus terminates with the coronoid process. The mandibular foramen is located at the medial portion of the ramus at the lingula where the inferior alveolar neuro-vascular bundle enters the mandibular ramus. Fractures occurring in the mandibular ramus and body from the lingula to the mental foramen frequently cause damage to the inferior alveolar nerve, resulting in loss of sensation within the area of distribution of that nerve. The symphysis is in the anatomic midline, and that portion of the mandible containing the central lateral and canine teeth is termed the parasymphysis. The muscles attaching to the mandible play an important role in the displacement of mandibular fractures.

The location and direction of the fracture line in its relation to the elevator and depressor muscles create either a favorable or unfavorable muscle pull at the fracture line. If the pull of muscles tends to reduce the fracture, it is termed favorable muscle pull; if the pull tends to distract the fractured segments, it is termed unfavorable muscle pull. Bilateral mandibular fractures, at or distal to the angle, allow the depressor muscles to create a badly displaced fracture. Other factors that can influence the treatment of a mandibular fracture include the soft tissue injury, bony comminution, and absence or presence of viable teeth. The sites of mandible fracture are grouped anatomically; i.e., condyle, condylar neck, coronoid, ramus, angle, body, parasymphysis, and symphysis.

A stable mandible with both condyles correctly positioned in the glenoid fossa serves as a guideline and orientation for treatment of fractures of the remainder of the face. If the only facial fracture is a mandibular fracture, its treatment is related to the occlusion. In fractures of the midface involving the maxilla, the mandible must be stabilized and placed in the proper relationship to the cranial base, prior to reduction of maxillary fractures. Fractures solely of the midface must first be related by placing the maxillary teeth in occlusion with the mandibular teeth. The successful treatment of facial fractures is judged primarily by the restoration of functional occlusion rather than esthetics alone. Function and esthetics are inextricably intertwined. As in all facial fractures, reduction, fixation, and immobilization must be accomplished as soon as possible. The risk of nonunion or fibrous union is enhanced by delayed treatment, as is the risk of bone infection or osteomyelitis. Early reduction, fixation, and immobilization decrease the patient's pain, discomfort, and edema. As stated previously, the reduction of facial fractures is accomplished from the bottom up and from the inside out; therefore, reduction of mandibular fractures and establishment of mandibular continuity is of prime importance.

CONDYLAR FRACTURES

The condyle and condylar neck are frequently fractured. The condylar head may remain in the articular fossa, may be dislocated or, on rare occasions, may be driven into the middle cranial fossa. The diagnosing of a condylar fracture is enhanced by pain in the area of the temporomandibular joint and/or a loss of maximum occlusion. Treatment, in most cases, is accomplished by placing and maintaining the teeth in proper occlusion. Functional elastics that allow the patient to open and close but overcome the freeway space in the rest position, maintaining the teeth in proper occlusion, may provide adequate reduction of the fractured segments. If proper occlusion cannot be maintained with functional elastics, and/or if pain is not relieved, rigid intermaxillary fixation with wires may be required. Rarely is open reduction of the mandibular condyle required, especially intracapsular fracture. Open reductions of mandibular condyle fractures may be indicated to establish a stable mandible and facial height as a base for reduction of midfacial fractures (Fig. 19-6).

Research by Durkin, Healy, and Irving and Petrovic, Stutzman, and Oudet has provided information that counteracts the old theories of condylar growth and condylar growth guidance. This group feels that an intramembranous condition exists throughout nearly all parts of the mandible that are sensitive to pressures, allowing for adjustive and adaptive growth within the entire

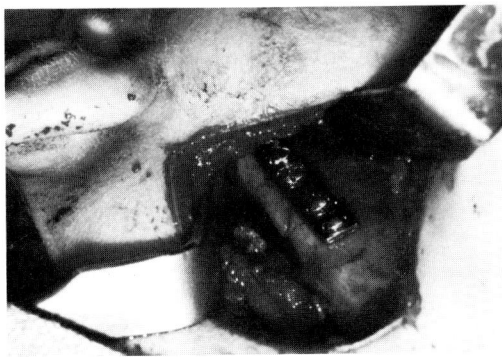

FIG. 19-6. *A mini-compression plate on a subcondylar fracture, providing osteosynthesis of the fractured segments.*

mandible. Thus, the indications for open reduction of condylar fractures, or the reduction and pinning of condylar fractures, might have an increased application.

Rapid function of fractures of the mandibular condyle decreases the propensity for fibrosis or ankylosis within the temporomandibular joint. The utilization of rigid fixation in fractures of the mandibular ramus body and symphysis facilitates this early mobilization.

LOWER FRACTURES OF THE ASCENDING RAMUS AND ANGLE

Fractures of the regions of the mandible from the depth of the sigmoid notch to the anterior aspect of the attachment of the masseter muscle are considered mandibular angle fractures. They are often displaced by the pull of the elevator muscles of the mandible and frequently involve the erupted or impacted third molar tooth. These fractures are optimally managed by the removal of the third molar tooth and open reduction with internal wire or compression plate fixation, in most cases, intraorally (Fig. 19-7). Immobilization of the mandible may be accomplished by arch bars and intermaxillary wires. Utilization of mandibular compression plates allows for early, if not immediate, mobilization.

MANDIBULAR BODY FRACTURES

The body of the mandible is that portion of the mandible anterior to the attachment of the masseter muscle and posterior to the canine tooth. Fractures in this portion of the mandible in a dentate patient are considered compound, being open to the oral cavity by the periodontal ligament. These fractures, in most instances, involve the inferior alveolar nerve and may produce altered sensation. Teeth that can provide function should be maintained, where possible, even if pulpal therapy may be indicated. The treatment of mandibular body fractures is optimally accomplished by open reduction and internal fixation with wires and/or compression plates (Fig. 19-8). Immobilization of the mandible is accomplished by arch bars and intermaxillary wires.

FRACTURES OF THE SYMPHYSIS

Symphysis and parasymphyseal frac-

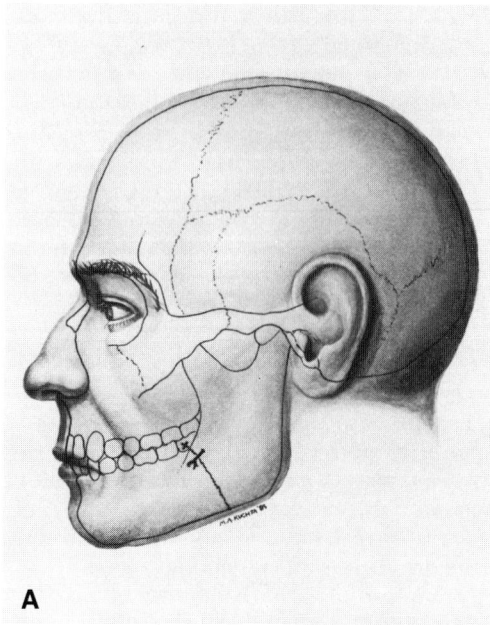

A

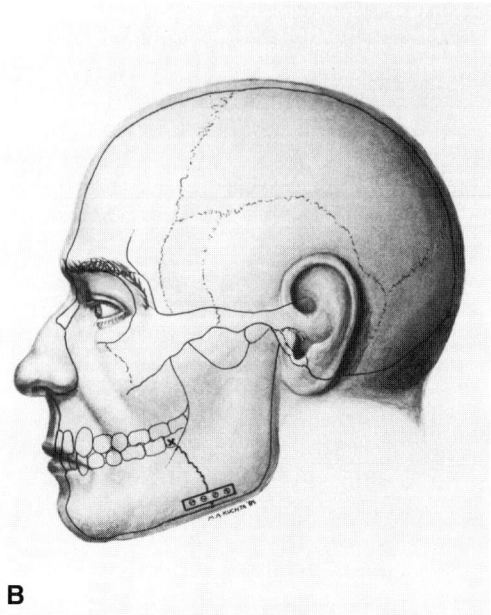

B

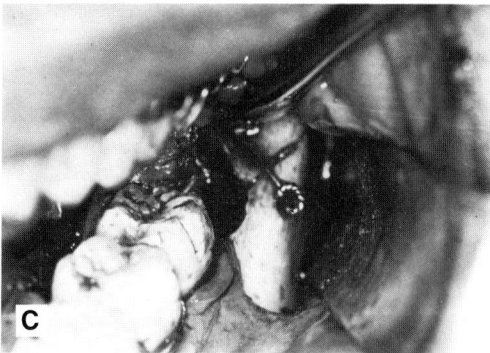

C

Fig. 19-7. *(A) Transoral open reduction of the mandibular angle fracture, showing removal of the third molar and para-alveolar wiring of the fracture. (B) Open reduction and internal fixation of a mandibular angle fracture, with removal of the third molar and osteosynthesis of the fracture with a compression bone plate. (C) Transoral open reduction of a mandible angle fracture, showing tooth socket of the removed third molar and a para-alveolar wire reducing and fixing the fractured segments.*

tures generally cause bleeding into the floor of the mouth, resulting in ecchymosis or hematoma of that area, with splaying of the inferior border and frequent comminution. Open reduction and internal fixation with wire and/or compression plates can most often be accomplished intraorally (Fig. 19-9). Previously applied maxillary and mandibular arch bars and intermaxillary fixation and immobilization complete the treatment.

METHOD OF FRACTURE REDUCTION AND IMMOBILIZATION

The most common techniques utilized to obtain fixation and stabilization of mandibular fractures consist of:

Intraosseous Wiring. This is the most popular and standard wiring, with 24-gauge stainless steel wire, applied in either a staple and/or "figure 8" fashion. A figure 8 wire over the inferior border stabilizes the inferior border from splaying, while a staple wire in the body of the mandible prevents alveolar ridge splaying (Fig. 19-10).

Intramedullary Pin. The passage of a pin or wire through the fractured segments is practiced by few but is not felt to be the method of choice in most mandibular fractures. This method may have an increased application for the pinning of mandibular condylar or subcondylar fractures.

Biphasic Pin Appliance. This external appliance is utilized by placing screws into the mandible proximal and distal to the fracture, reducing the fracture using rods that lock and then incorporating the screws

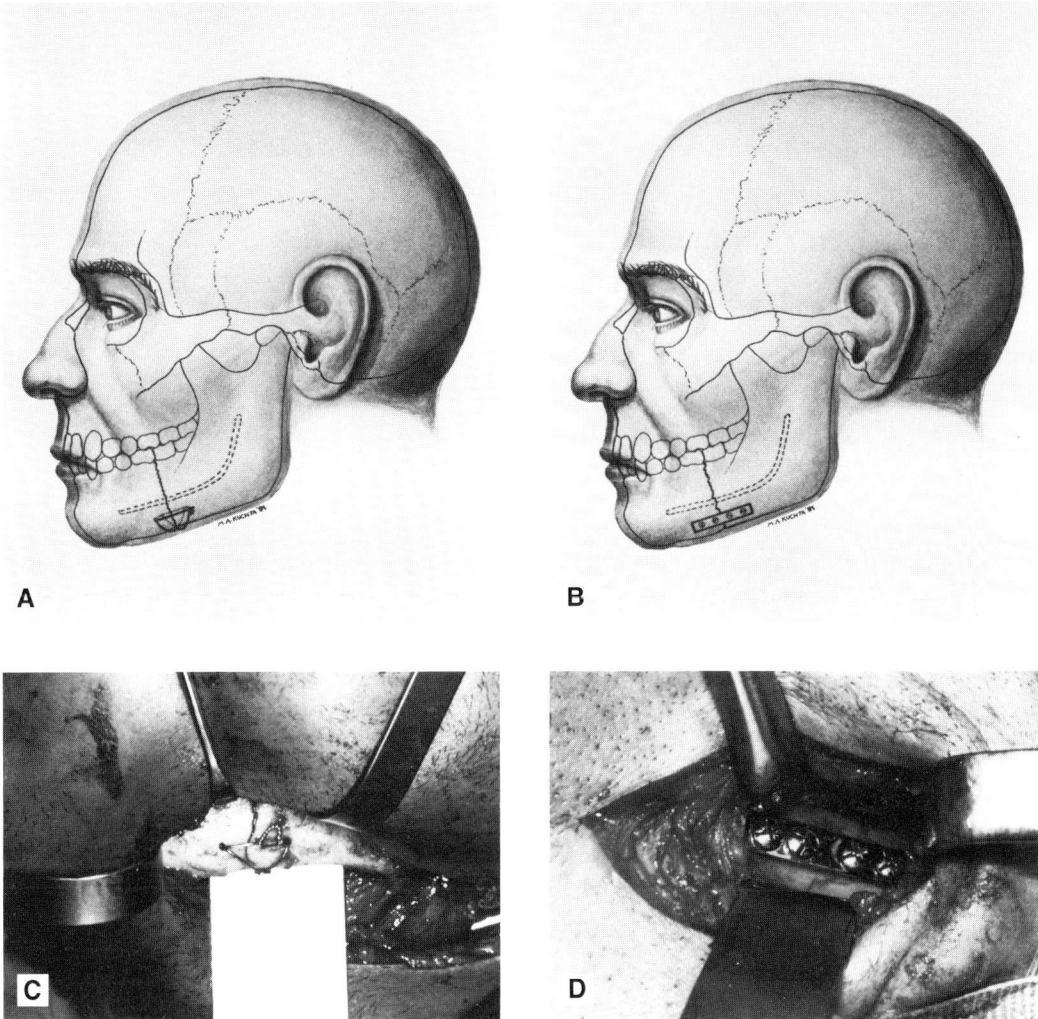

FIG. 19-8. *Mandibular body fracture. (A) Extra-oral reduction and fixation of the body fracture with a staple and figure 8 wire. (B) Reduction and fixation; the mandibular body fracture with osteosynthesis with a compression bone plate. (C) Extra-oral open reduction with a mandibular body fracture, showing the use of a figure 8 and staple wiring technique. The figure of 8 wire draws the segments together at the inferior border; the staple wire keeps the superior alveolar crest section from distracting. (D) A mini-compression plate, a mandibular body fracture, providing stability and osteosynthesis of the fractured segments.*

into an acrylic bar, providing long-term stability. The advantages of this appliance include: (1) the ability to span comminuted fractures, thus allowing molding of the segments without periosteal stripping; (2) early function of the temporomandibular joint; (3) good stability of the fracture without direct open reduction over the fracture line.

Compression Plates. The use of compression plates for treating facial fractures has not gained universal acceptance in the

United States. The advantages of compression plates are that they provide a rigid and stable fixation and either reduce the time or eliminate the need for intermaxillary fixation and immobilization. The disadvantages include the necessity for open reduction, considerable periosteal stripping to allow for placement, the inability to make minor occlusal adjustments, and the possible eventual requirement for removal of the compression plate. Some clinicians feel that the majority of mandibular frac-

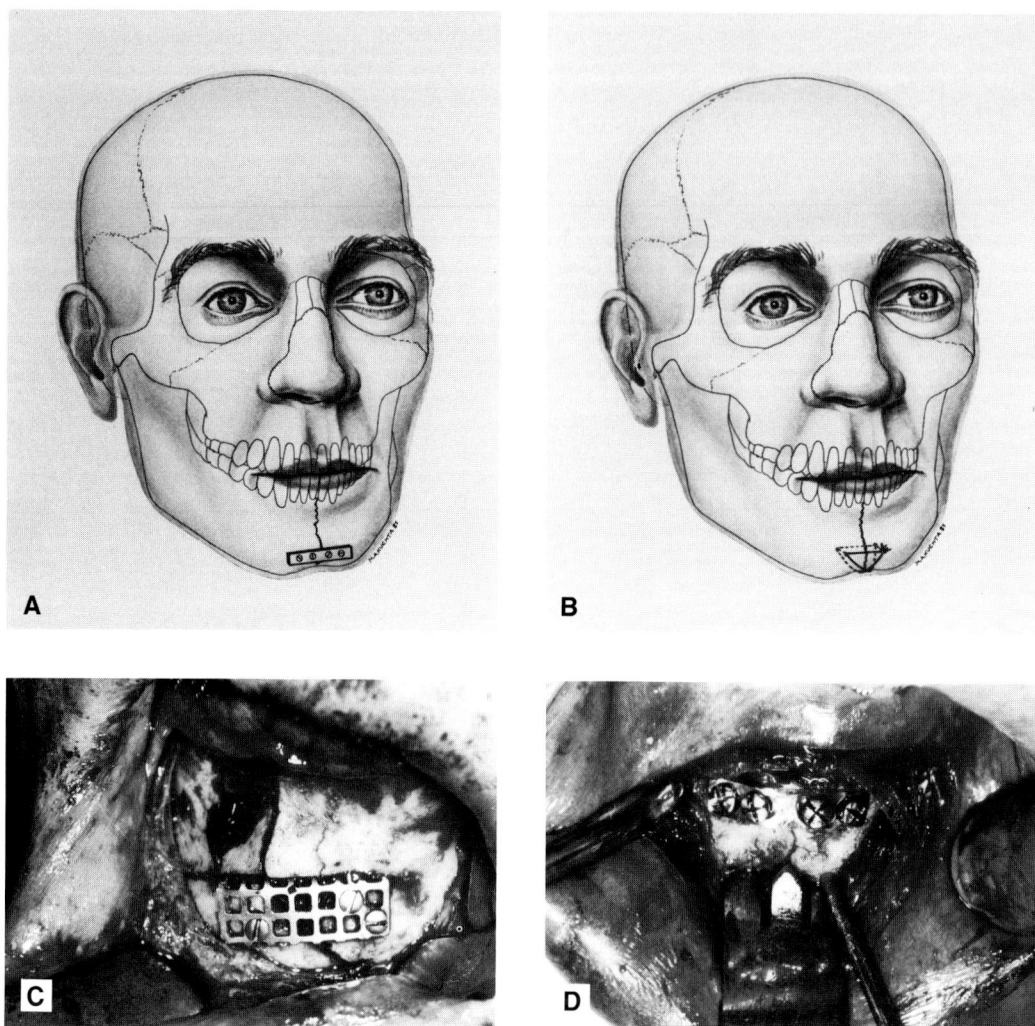

FIG. 19-9. (A) The reduction and fixation of a symphysis fracture with osteosynthesis from a compression bone plate. (B) An open reduction, either transorally or extra-orally, of a symphysis fracture reduced and fixed with a staple and figure 8 wire. (C) A titanium mesh L plate is secured in place with screws to prevent distraction or motion of the segments. (D) A mini-compression plate placed transorally, a mandibular symphysis fracture, offering stability and osteosynthesis of the fractured segments.

tures can be managed with application of arch bars and intermaxillary fixation and immobilization only, while others believe that open reductions and internal fixation are not indicated. The author believes that the utilization of open reduction and internal fixation *makes* things happen, rather than treating the fracture with a closed reduction and *hoping* that things happen.

ANTIBIOTICS

All compound mandibular fractures demand the use of therapeutic antibiotics (this includes *all* mandibular fractures in the area of erupted teeth, or impacted teeth that have the potential to communicate with the mouth). Closed mandibular fractures, accompanied by hematoma formation, should also receive antibiotic therapy. If circummandibular wires, intraosseous wires, or compression plates are to be removed after healing of mandibular fractures, antibiotic therapy would again be initiated.

Staple Wire

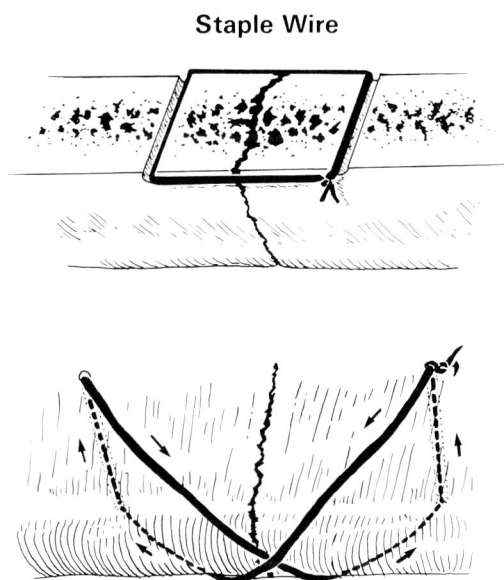

Figure 8 Wire

FIG. 19-10. *Placement of a staple and figure 8 wire.*

INTERMAXILLARY FIXATION AND IMMOBILIZATION

Immobilization time is variable, depending on the patient's medical status and the location and the method of reduction and fixation of the fracture. Condylar fractures should be immobilized for a minimal amount of time (7 to 28 days, with optimum time being 7 to 10 days). Once function is initiated in the treatment of these fractures, the maintenance of proper occlusion must be observed with frequent postoperative visits. Mandibular angle fractures should be kept immobilized for approximately 3 to 4 weeks; body fractures, 4 to 6 weeks; symphysis and parasymphysis fractures, 8 to 12 weeks. These immobilization periods can be reduced or eliminated with the utilization of compression plates. The amount of time of the mobilization listed is for healthy adults under 40 years of age. Patients in compromised health and/or over 40 must have adjusted intermaxillary fixation and immobilization periods. The immobilization period is not scientific and must be adjusted for each patient.

ARCH BAR APPLICATION

Arch bars are applied to the maxillary and mandibular teeth in the following manner: the arch bar is contoured and cut so that it may be ligated to all erupted and stable teeth required for fixation. Single wires of 24 gauge (.020 inches in diameter) should be passed around each tooth. The mesial wire should be apical to the arch bar, and the distal wire should be occlusal to it. As the wire is twisted and tightened, it should be tightened on a corner of the arch bar and not on its flat portion. Individual wires should be tightened around secure and stable teeth, thus effecting a stable arch bar. Unstable teeth and/or alveolar processes should be secured to the stable arch bar in proper alignment.

Maxillary Fractures

In 1901, LeFort determined the areas of structural weakness of the maxilla, proving accurate and valuable in the assessment and classifications of midface fractures. The LeFort I occurs above the level of the apices of the teeth and includes the alveolar process, the vault of the palate, and pterygoid processes in a single block. The LeFort II or pyramidal fracture begins in the nasal bones and frontal process of the maxilla, extending laterally through the lacrimal bone and inferior rim of the orbit and transversing the orbital rim at or near the zygomaticomaxillary suture line. The fracture then extends laterally and backward along the lateral wall of the maxilla through the pterygoid plates. The LeFort III fracture, or craniofacial disjunction, occurs through the zygomaticofrontal, maxillofrontal, and nasalfrontal suture lines, through the orbital floors, and through the ethmoid and sphenoid sinuses. This fracture produces complete separation of the facial bones from the cranium. Rarely do fractures of the midface fall into one of these categories in a pure fashion.

Cases involving patients who sustain midface fractures are remarkably similar. The face is usually markedly edematous with multiple ecchymoses and hematoma formation. Although displacement of bones from the midface is generally posterior and downward, the classic dish face elongation of the middle third of the face is seldom apparent on initial examination. This appearance is probably a consequence of the mobility of the fractured bones and the marked edema of the surrounding soft tissues. The classic appearance of the elongated, depressed middle third of the face is most often seen several days to weeks after injury in untreated patients (Fig. 19-1).

In all midface fractures, a thorough ophthalmologic examination should be performed prior to any manipulation or treatment to rule out any injury to the eye. The exact nature of a midface fracture can best be determined by gentle, but firm, bimanual manipulation of the injured bones. The anterior portion of the maxilla is grasped between the thumb and the index finger; the other hand then palpates various areas in the midface and skull to determine the level of the fracture. The patient with a LeFort I fracture, with a free-floating inferior segment, demonstrates mobility of the palate, but stability of the nasal pyramid and inferior orbital rims. The patient with a LeFort II fracture demonstrates movement of the nasal dorsum with the mobile palate. Palpation of the infraorbital rims demonstrates the mobile medial segment of the infraorbital rim. Manipulation of a patient with a LeFort III demonstrates mobility of the entire facial skeleton. Palpation at the frontozygomatic suture should demonstrate a mobile, inferior segment and a stable superior segment, except when there are unstable fractures of the cranial vault.

TREATMENT

Since the advent of treatment of midface fractures with open reduction and internal fixation (Fig. 19-11), indications for the use of extraskeletal fixation devices are limited. Indications include: (1) severely comminuted fractures in which stable reduction and normal position cannot be achieved by standard techniques; (2) impacted or partially healed malunited fractures requiring constant traction for adequate reduction; (3) LeFort fractures associated with maxillary discontinuity defects. The most commonly used method of immobilization of maxillary or midface fractures, besides internal wire fixation at the fracture sites, is suspension wiring to proximal stable bones. Suspension wires should be dropped from the zygomatic processes of the frontal bones, from stable points on the

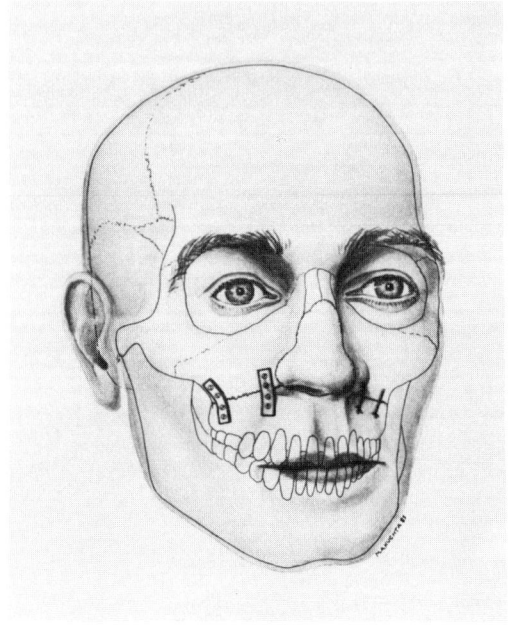

FIG. 19-11. *LeFort I fracture (reduced and fixed). The right side shows fixation and immobilization with osteosynthesis and compression bone plates. The left side shows reduction and fixation with transosseous wires.*

zygomatic arch, from a stable infraorbital rim, or a stable pyriform aperture (Fig. 19-12). A pull out wire may be used and passed around the suspension wire at the level of the frontozygomatic suture for easy retrieval of the suspension wire. The suspension wires can usually be removed at 4 to 6 weeks after surgery. Great care must be used with suspension wires because they can produce retrodisplacement of the maxilla and a subsequent open-bite malocclusion.

The three basic steps of treatment are: reduction, fixation, and immobilization. Many fractures of the maxilla are free floating and can be reduced easily by manipulation. In rare instances, the fractured segments may be firmly impacted and disimpaction forceps may be required to reduce the fracture. After the fractured bones are reduced and appropriate intermaxillary fixation attained, fixation of fracture sites should be accomplished. This should preferably be obtained by open reduction and a direct interosseous wire or plate fixation. Sites for wire fixation include the frontozygomatic suture, the in-

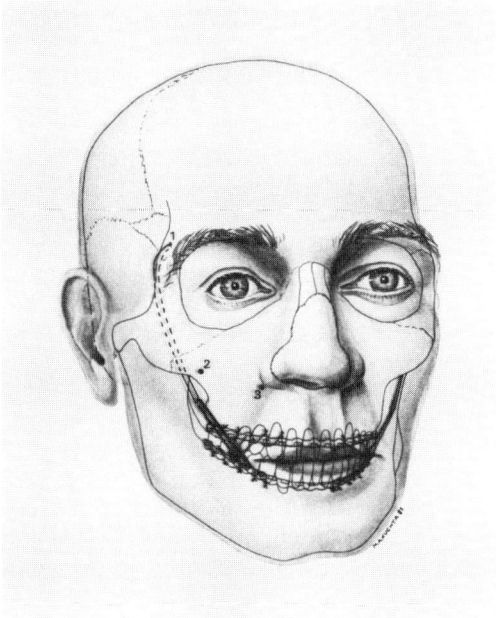

FIG. 19-12. *Placement of suspension wires: (1) wire placed from the frontal bone, just superior to the frontal zygomatic suture, the wire dropping behind the zygoma and coming down to the mandibular arch bar via an intermediate wire. This wire may also be placed, depending upon stability, at (2) the buttress of zygoma, or (3) the lateral border of the pyriform rim.*

fraorbital rim, and the piriform aperture. The third and final step in the treatment of these fractures is immobilization.

Midface Maxillofacial Fractures

INJURY

Fights resulting in trauma to the cheek or body of the zygoma from fists or other objects are the most frequent cause of isolated fractures of the maxillary zygomatic complex. These fractures are generally found to be displaced medially and inferiorly with a bodily rotation according to the direction of the injuring force. Fractures accompanying this injury generally occur at the following sites: there is usually a separation at the frontozygomatic suture, and one or more fractures with or without depression along the zygomatic arch. There is usually step deformity in the infraorbital rim with accompanying comminuted fracturing of the orbital floor. This fracture occurs most frequently along the infraorbital canal and through the infraorbital foramen, thereby producing altered sensation in the infraorbital nerve. The zygomatic buttress is usually caved in to the maxillary sinus with single or comminuted fractures of the lateral wall of the sinus. The maxillary sinus is almost always filled with blood, and there is frequently herniation of the contents of the orbit through the comminuted fracture in the orbital floor. This can cause downward displacement of the globe with enophthalmia. Loss of integrity of the orbital floor is possibly one of the more debilitating complications of this injury if it has not been recognized and treated. These patients should be examined by an ophthalmologist prior to treatment.

The signs and symptoms of orbital floor involvement can include swelling and discoloration, usually occurring in the lower eyelid within the first 24 hours following injury. It is usually accompanied by edema. There may or may not be visible or palpable deformities of the orbital rim, even in the presence of a step deformity that may be masked by edema. If infraorbital nerve anesthesia persists for more than 24 hours, it indicates damage to the nerve by shearing, tearing, or pressure within its canal. Diplopia may be present early and then disappear as the developing edema subsides. If loss of fat tissue support occurs within the orbit due to herniation, the diplopia is likely to return 6 to 8 weeks following injury. Frequently, the defect in the orbital floor does not develop totally until the zygoma has been reduced and positioned in its proper anatomical place, leaving behind a deficit in the orbital floor. This must be explored and treated if present.

TREATMENT

Treatment of fractures of the maxillary zygomatic complex is adequately managed by (1) exposing the infraorbital rim and entire orbital floor; (2) manipulating the principal fragments; (3) wire fixation of the fragments; (4) exposing the frontozygomatic suture; (5) reconstructing the bony floor; (6) repairing periorbital tears. The orbital floor is exposed posteriorly for 3.5 to 4.0 cm, carefully freeing the infraorbital nerve vascular bundle, and any hematoma in the maxillary sinus is evacuated.

The frontozygomatic suture is explored and fixed with a wire suture. If laceration of the periorbital periosteum has occurred, herniation of fat may necessitate retrieval of the fat and repair of the torn periorbita. Immediate repair of the orbital floor defect is indicated. Many different materials have been used successfully for reconstruction of orbital floor defects. These materials may include autotransplants such as split rib, and alloplastic materials such as silastic or teflon-coated proplast.

Ocular Injury

Approximately 25 percent of the patients with head injury have associated orbital and/or ocular injury. Examination of the injured eye should include visual acuity, visual field, responsiveness of the pupil, extraocular motility, and external examination of the eyelids for lacerations. The globes should be examined for exophthalmos or enophthalmos. A slit lamp examination should be accomplished whenever possible to identify potential foreign bodies, corneal or scleral lacerations, hyphema, and lens and iris injuries. Intraocular pressure should be measured and a funduscopic examination should assess retinal damage. Radiograph examination can include plain x-ray views, Water's view, Caldwell view, and CT scans.

TREATMENT OF LID, ORBITAL, AND OCULAR INJURIES

Lid Hematoma. Bleeding into the upper and/or lower lids (black eye) is usually an innocuous problem. Treatment consists of application of ice packs to reduce the swelling. This event should alert the astute clinician to evaluate for fractures.

Eyelid Lacerations. Eyelid lacerations require reapproximation and apposition. Canalicular lacerations—when the lower canaliculus has been lacerated, patency of the nasal lacrimal duct apparatus must be reestablished through the use of sutures or stint left in position for 6 to 12 weeks.

Orbital Hematoma. Retrobulbar bleeding following orbital injuries usually has a benign course and spontaneously regresses in 2 to 3 weeks. However, it should be ascertained as to whether the volume of blood filling the retrobulbar space is signif-

icant enough to result in an increased orbital and ocular pressure that may occlude the central retinal artery. If so, this should be drained anteriorly through the conjunctiva and Tenon's capsule.

Orbital Foreign Bodies. Nonorganic intraorbital foreign bodies, such as metal and buckshot, are usually inert and may be left safely in the orbit if they are not sharp. Organic objects, such as thorns, splinters, pencils, etc., cause intraorbital abscess formation and must be removed.

Anterior Chamber Hyphema. A concussive blow often causes bleeding into the anterior chamber resulting in a blockage of the egress of the aurous humur from the trabecular meshwork that, in turn, causes a rise in intraocular pressure. The current treatment for hyphema consists of bed rest and patching of both eyes until the anterior chamber is clear. The intraocular pressure should be checked twice daily. The patient should be followed to be sure that acute glaucoma does not develop.

Retinal Detachment. Concussive injuries to the eye may produce a retinal detachment days or even weeks following the injury and require persistent follow-up. The patient who has sustained ocular injury should be advised about the necessity of future follow-up care. The three principal last sequelae of concussive ocular injuries are angle recession glaucoma, cataract, and retinal detachment.

A wound cleanser that is nonirritant and nontoxic to the eye should be used to clean lacerations of the periorbital region.

TREATMENT COMPLICATIONS

Of all the complications, ocular displacement is one of the most distressing. It is impossible to overstress the importance of early recognition and treatment of the factors producing it. The downward displacement of the globe can be corrected by a variety of implant materials. The presence of loss of integrity of the orbital floor in a great number of zygomaticomaxillary and maxillary fractures has been proven by exploration. Typically, a fracture line extends through the infraorbital canal and foramen, with or without comminution of the maxilla and/or zygoma, and with or without separation of the frontozygomatic suture. The floor is fractured along the fissure with accessory lines radiating laterally and medially. Displaced fragments may lie upended, telescoped posteriorly, or may have dropped into the antrum. The defect is often largest immediately posterior to the rim margin.

DIAGNOSIS OF ORBITAL FLOOR INVOLVEMENT

The signs and symptoms of orbital floor involvement are: (1) Swelling and discoloration. Typically, the ecchymosis would appear in the lower eyelid, accompanied by edema, which frequently results from shearing the infraorbital vessels within the bony fissure or canal. Coming from within the orbit, the discoloration is limited to the eyelid by the palpebral fascia. (2) Visible or palpable deformities of the orbital rim where irregularities in the infraorbital rim and separation of the frontozygomatic suture exist, a major posterior movement of the fragment may have occurred and disruption of the floor must be ruled out. (3) When infraorbital nerve anesthesia persists for more than 24 hours, injury within the bony canal by shifting fragments is indicated. (4) Diplopia may be present early and disappear as developing edema and hemorrhage camouflage the loss of fat tissue support. Unfortunately, such a history is not available frequently enough to be generally reliable. Diplopia is usually a late finding. The first sign that all is not well occurs after 6 or 8 weeks. It is quite probable that, in some instances, the fracture reduction itself is responsible because the deficit in the floor did not develop until the main body of the fragment was brought forward, leaving behind an unstable collection of telescoped, displaced, bony fragments unable to support the orbital contents, prevent herniation of fat, or later resist the pull of the contracting scar tissue. X-rays provide further aid in this diagnosis. Water's, Caldwell views, tomograms, and CT scans often provide the diagnostic acumen that is needed.

EXOPHTHALMOMETRY

In most instances, the patient is not seen by the surgeon charged with his definitive care for several hours. By this time, orbital edema has compensated for the disturbed volumetric relationship and has restored the globe to a near normal position. This limits the value of exophthalmometry. These methods require the external rim as a point of reference and would be inaccurate were that part displaced. It is apparent that this method of examination is valuable at least during the period when accurate diagnosis and treatment are most urgent. In the final analysis, a complete, accurate diagnosis is rarely possible except by surgical exploration of the orbital floor.

Selected Reading

Abou-Rass, M.: The status of endodontics 1985: Concepts, materials and methods. Canad. Dent. Assoc. J., 50:24, 1984.

Adams, G.L.: Mandibular reconstruction: External fixation. Otolaryngol. Head Neck Surg., 90:583, 1982.

Born, C.P.: Ocular injuries—treat or refer? Postgrad. Med., 73:311, 1983.

Bowers, S.A., and Marshall, L.F.: Severe head injury: Current treatment and research. J. Neurosurg. Nurs., 14(5):210, 1982.

Budassi, S.A.: Ophthalmic examinations. J. Emerg. Nurs., 10(2):112, 1984.

Clark, W.D.: Nasal and nasal septal fractures. Ear Nose Throat J., 62:25, 1983.

Close, L.G.: Fractures of the maxilla. Ear Nose Throat J., 62:44, 1983.

Cooper, D.L.: This sporting life. Emerg. Med., 11:287, 1979.

Culbertson, W.W.: Diagnosis and management of ocular injuries. Otolaryngol. Clin. North Am., 16:563, 1983.

DeFries, H.O.: Management of maxillofacial injuries: Medical viewpoint. Milit. Med., 136:558, 1971.

Frensilli, J.A., Kornblut, A.D., and Tenen, C.: Reconstruction of a mandible after shotgun trauma; report of case. JADA, 110:49, 1985.

Frost, D.E., El-Attar, A., and Moos, K.F.: Evaluation of metacarpal bone plates in the mandibular fracture. Br. J. Oral Surg., 21:214, 1983.

Hargis, H.W.: Trauma to permanent anterior teeth and alveolar processes. Dent. Clin. North Am., 17(3):505, 1973.

Hildebrandt, J.R.: Dental and maxillofacial injuries. Clin. Sports Med., 1:449, 1982.

Josell, S.D., and Abrams, R.G.: Traumatic injuries to the dentition and its supporting structures. Pediatr. Clin. North Am., 29:717, 1982.

Kelly, J.F.: Bone graft rehabilitation of maxillofacial battle casualties. Milit. Med., 136:562, 1971.

Langdon, J.D., and Rapidis, A.D.: Maxillofacial injuries. Br. J. Hosp. Med., 28(6):589, 1982.

Luce, E.A.: Maxillofacial Trauma. Chicago, Year Book Medical Publishers, 1984. pp. 6–68.

McCoy, F.J., et al.: An analysis of facial fractures and their complications. Plast. Reconstr. Surg., *29:*381, 1962.

Maniglia, A.J., and Kline, S.N.: Maxillofacial trauma in the pediatric age group. Otolaryngol. Clin. North Am. *16*(3):717, 1983.

Molyneux-Luick, M.: The ABCs of multiple trauma. Nursing, *7:*30, 1977.

Morris, J.: Biphase connector, external skeletal splint for reduction and fixation of mandibular fractures. J. Oral Surg., *2:*1382, 1949.

Norris, J.W., Chirls, I., Allen, L., and Paul, A.: Initial management of eye trauma. J. Med. Soc. N.J., *80:*29, 1983.

Packer, A.J.: Ocular trauma. Primary Care, *9:*777, 1982.

Rees, A.M., and Weinberg, S.: Fractures of the mandibular condyle: Review of the literature and presentation of five cases with late complications. Oral Health, *73:*37, 1983.

Sazima, H.J.: Diagnosis and treatment of fractures of the malar eminence. Milit. Med., *136:*888, 1971.

Spiessel, B.: Maxillofacial injuries in polytrauma. World J. Surg., *7:*96, 1983.

Weinberg, S.: Surgical correction of facial fractures. Dent. Clin. North Am., *26:*631, 1982.

Zachariades, N., et al.: The significance of tracheostomy in the management of fractures of the facial skeleton. J. Maxillofac. Surg., *11:*180, 1983.

Zide, M.F., and Kent, J.N.: Indications for open reduction of mandibular condyle fractures. J. Oral Maxillofac. Surg., *41:*89, 1983.

CHAPTER 20

Reconstructive Preprosthetic Surgery

John F. Helfrick
Daniel E. Waite

You have to see well what you do in order to do well what you see.   G.C. INGHAM

The field of reconstructive preprosthetic surgery has undergone tremendous progress in the past 20 years. In 1967 MacIntosh and Obwegeser's article stimulated oral and maxillofacial surgeons in the United States to reassess their approach to preprosthetic surgery.[1] Since that time, clinicians have accepted the reconstructive challenge of the edentulous patient. It is no longer necessary or acceptable for a patient to experience pain and dysfunction because of an oral deformity. The soft and hard tissue procedures described in this chapter, alone or in combination with endosteal or transosteal implants, are designed to reconstruct the oral cavity so that esthetic, masticatory, and speech functions are maximized.

Soft Tissue Surgery

The oral surgeon performs soft tissue surgery to correct and adjust soft tissue problems such as frenulum attachments, gingival hyperplasia and hypertrophy, and fibromatoses. It may also be necessary to reposition soft tissue structures to create an acceptable ridge for a prosthesis. Surgical manipulation of these soft tissue attachments to attain the desired U-shaped ridge should be considered only when the anatomy and physiology of the particular soft tissue and the underlying osseous structures are clearly understood. The maxillary sinus, the inferior alveolar canal, the mental foramen, muscle insertions and origins, the salivary ducts, and lingual nerves are important structures to consider when planning a reconstructive surgical procedure.

Anatomy[2]

The dentist should clearly understand the basic anatomy of the desired edentulous ridge contour. Bulbous and knife-edge ridges are encountered regularly and dealt with accordingly. However, when no vestibular depth exists because of alveolar bone atrophy, trauma, or other causes, surgical intervention may become necessary for prosthodontic purposes. An awareness of the attachment of the muscles of facial expression to the surface of the mandible and maxilla is necessary in the execution of these surgical procedures (Fig. 20-1). The buccal and labial folds of the upper vestibule are determined by the bony origins of certain facial muscles.

363

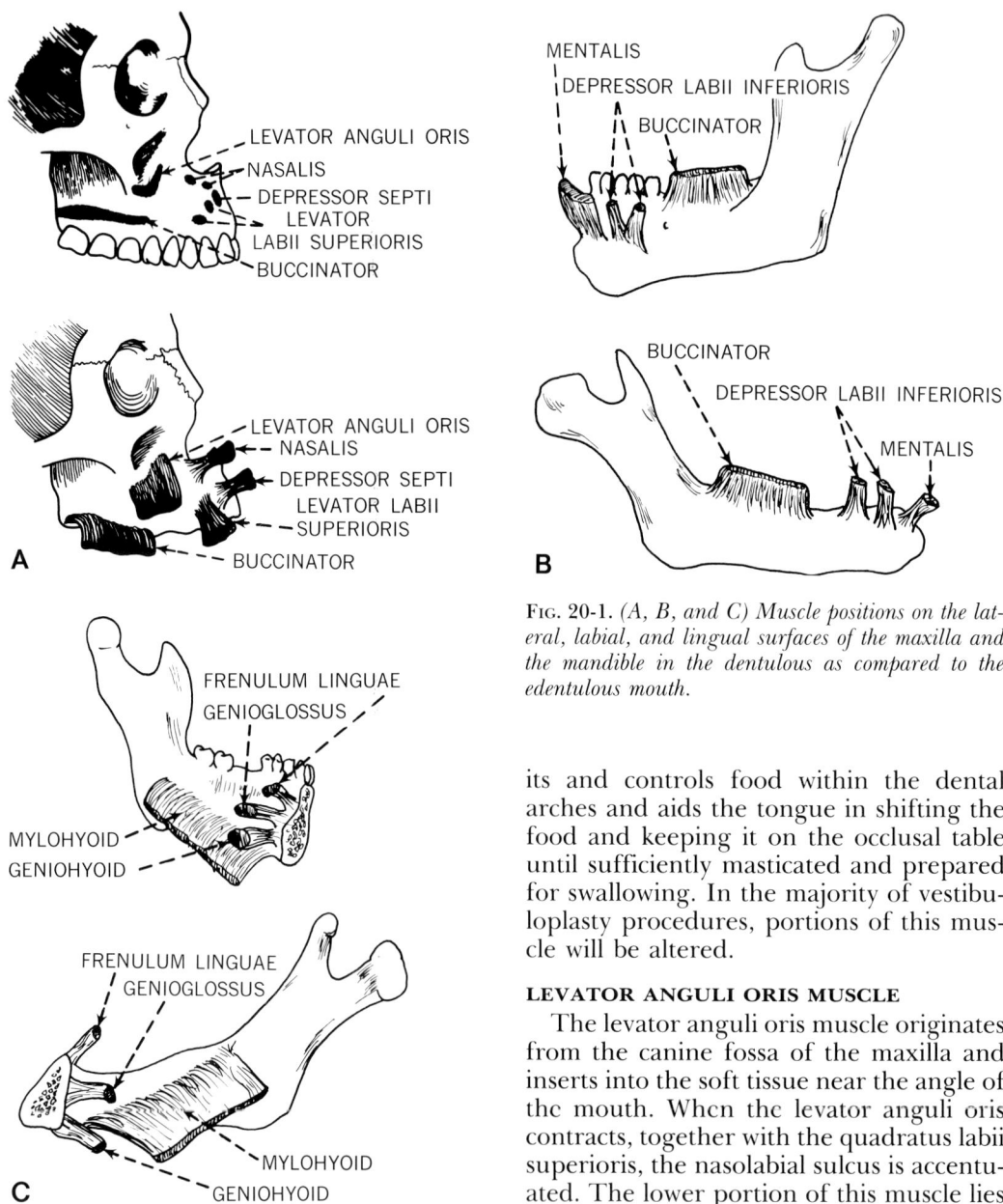

FIG. 20-1. *(A, B, and C) Muscle positions on the lateral, labial, and lingual surfaces of the maxilla and the mandible in the dentulous as compared to the edentulous mouth.*

its and controls food within the dental arches and aids the tongue in shifting the food and keeping it on the occlusal table until sufficiently masticated and prepared for swallowing. In the majority of vestibuloplasty procedures, portions of this muscle will be altered.

LEVATOR ANGULI ORIS MUSCLE

The levator anguli oris muscle originates from the canine fossa of the maxilla and inserts into the soft tissue near the angle of the mouth. When the levator anguli oris contracts, together with the quadratus labii superioris, the nasolabial sulcus is accentuated. The lower portion of this muscle lies beneath the facial artery; therefore, surgical procedures affecting the two muscular origins may result in brisk arterial hemorrhage. However, blunt rather than sharp dissection of the tissues often avoids severing of the vessel.

LEVATOR LABII SUPERIORIS MUSCLE

The levator labii superioris muscle is a small muscle band that arises from the outer alveolar process of the maxilla. It has two points of origin just above the lateral and cuspid teeth, and inserts into the fibers

BUCCINATOR MUSCLE

The buccinator muscle of the cheeks derives its name from Latin, in which it means "trumpeter." It originates from the outer alveolar process of the maxilla, the external oblique line of the mandible, and the pterygomandibular raphe. The terminal fibers blend into the orbicularis oris muscle anteriorly and the pterygomandibular raphe posteriorly. The buccinator lim-

of the orbicularis oris muscle. Its function is of little concern and probably serves only to tense the lip.

NASALIS AND DEPRESSOR SEPTI MUSCLES

The nasalis and depressor septi muscles have a fairly low point of origin on the maxilla and frequently are severed in alveoloplasty procedures. However, their function is restricted almost completely to the action of the alae of the nose (Fig. 20-1).

MENTALIS MUSCLE

The mentalis is an elevator of the chin and arises from the incisive area on the outer surface of the mandible. Its function is valuable in tensing and raising the lower lip in facial expression. During surgical procedures in this area, particularly vestibuloplasty, which is a supraperiosteal procedure, the entire muscle origin should not be sacrificed. Complete supraperiosteal dissection of this muscle results in a drooping of the soft tissues of the chin. This is referred to as chin ptosis and is extremely unesthetic. In the surgical approach to this portion of the mandible for osseous surgery, the degloving technique is subperiosteal and therefore permits reattachment without interfering with muscle function.

DEPRESSOR LABII INFERIORIS MUSCLE

The depressor labii inferioris muscle originates from the incisive fossa and inserts into the deep fibers of the lower lip. This muscle is located closer to the inner mucosae than the skin surface and often is involved in flaps designed to deepen the sulcus.

MYLOHYOID MUSCLE

The origin of the mylohyoid muscular basket for support of the tongue is from the mylohyoid ridge, which is the same as the internal oblique ridge. A median fibrous raphe between this paired muscle serves as the insertion for the muscle fibers that pass medially and posteriorly from their bony origin. Mylohyoid action raises the hyoid bone and also the floor of the mouth, thus enabling the tongue to exert pressure against the palate aiding in deglutition. This muscle plays a minor role in depressing the mandible. It appears that most of this muscle can be sacrificed in sur-

gical procedures without complication, as long as the genioglossus muscle remains attached to the genial tubercle. During the procedure of lowering the floor of the mouth, the mylohyoid is carefully approached and sectioned close to its point of origin. This is a supraperiosteal technique, and after careful repositioning of the overlying mucosa, portions of the muscle probably reattach. Special care must be exercised when transecting the posterior portion of the muscle, since the lingual nerve is in close relation in this area.

GENIOGLOSSUS MUSCLE

The genioglossus is a powerful extrinsic muscle of the tongue. This paired muscle arises from the superior genial tubercles, with its upper anterior fibers radiating toward the tip of the tongue and its remaining fibers passing back to the dorsum of the tongue and down to the upper border of the hyoid bone. When the upper fibers contract, the tip of the tongue is lowered and brought forward. The inferior fibers exert a pull on the hyoid bone, raising it and drawing it forward. Because this is an important muscle for proper manipulation of the tongue, the entire attachment should not be sacrificed in surgical procedures, although the superior portions of it may be sectioned without causing apparent limitation of the tongue.

GENIOHYOID MUSCLE

Originating from the lower genial tubercle and inserting into the anterior surface of the body of the hyoid bone, the geniohyoid muscle functions when the hyoid bone is fixed. It then acts as a depressor of the mandible. Its motor innervation is supplied by the loop of the cervical plexus between the first two cervical nerves by way of the sheath of the hypoglossal nerve.

TRIGEMINAL NERVE

The dentist performing preprosthetic surgery must be aware of the anatomic relationships of the branches of the trigeminal nerve to the area of surgical dissection. Few postoperative sequelae are as problematic as are nerve dysesthesias. Patients frequently pursue legal recourse as a result of lip or tongue anesthesia or paresthesia following oral surgery.

The close proximity of the lingual nerve

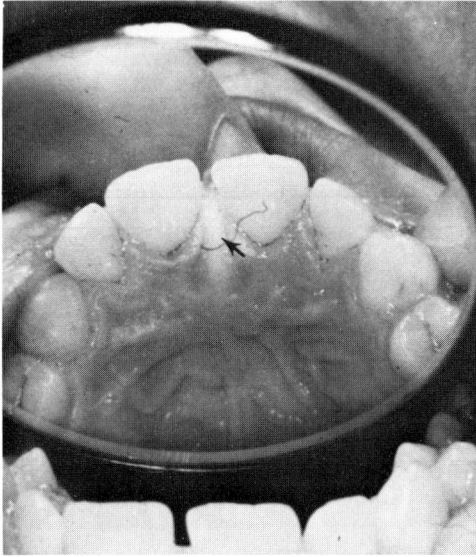

FIG. 20-2. *Technique to determine lingual attachment of the frenulum. Note tissue blanching on the lingual.*

to the medial aspect of the mandible in the molar region and the relationship of the mental foramen and nerve to anticipated incisions should be reviewed with the patient prior to surgery.

A common complaint of patients following maxillary labial vestibular extension procedures is parasthesia involving the upper lip. If the surgical dissection extends into the soft tissues of the upper lip, the terminal fibers of the infraorbital nerve may be cut, resulting in dysesthesia of the lip. Less commonly, fibers of the greater palatine and nasopalatine nerves may be

injured, resulting in altered sensation on the palate. When the dentist anticipates that a branch of the trigeminal nerve may be surgically manipulated during preprosthetic surgical procedures, the patient must be informed of the possibility of altered sensation in the area of surgery. These dysesthesias may be temporary or permanent.

FRENULA

Frenula are bands of connective tissue rarely muscular in nature. They usually consist of mucosal folds in the labial, buccal, and occasionally the lingual surface of the alveolar ridge (Fig. 20-2). They act as flexible checkreins, limiting the movement of the lips, cheeks, and sometimes the tongue. A diastema between the maxillary incisors may appear due to the frenulum; however, when the lateral and canine teeth erupt this space almost always closes. If not, frenectomy is indicated. As the alveolar bone resorbs, the frenum attachments become more limiting and may need to be lengthened or excised (Fig. 20-3).

Surgical Correction of Soft Tissue Abnormalities

FRENECTOMY

The maxillary labial frenum may interfere with the peripheral seal of dentures and they may become frequently traumatized; however, the routine resection of labial frenula is rarely indicated in preprosthetic surgery. It is occasionally necessary to reduce the broad frenum at-

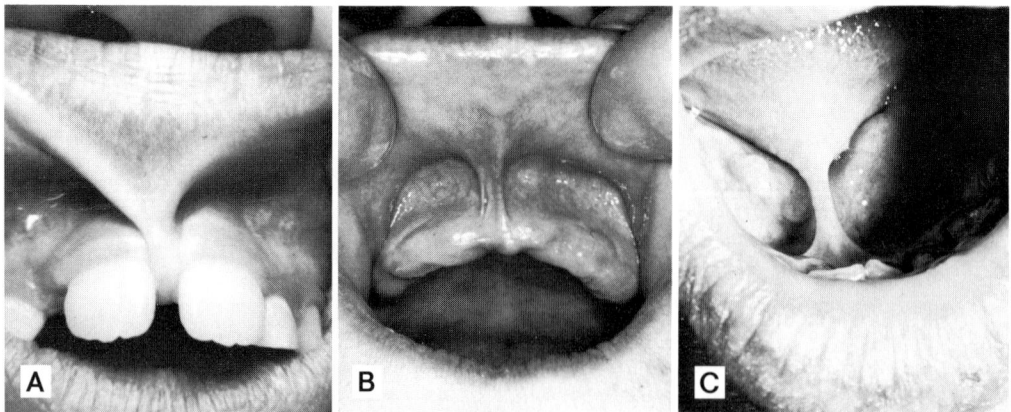

FIG. 20-3. *(A and B) Maxillary frenulum attachments. (C) Lingual frenulum attachment to tongue.*

tachment that extends between the maxillary central incisors and becomes confluent with the nasopalatine papillae. The frenum occupying the space between the central incisors may have to be excised, frequently in combination with orthodontic closure of the diastema.

The indications and timing of the excision of a lingual frenum that has resulted in ankyloglossia have been controversial. No clear evidence shows that ankyloglossia is invariably responsible for abnormal speech. However, because the high lingual frenum attachment can cause periodontal problems between the mandible central incisors, and because psychologists believe children should have tongue freedom, most surgeons recommend that a lingual frenectomy be performed prior to the time a child enters school. Speech pathologists may request earlier excision of the lingual frenum if significant speech abnormalities exist.

Speech considerations in ankyloglossia are important; however, the parent must be informed that other factors play a role in abnormal speech development and that the release of the lingual frenum may not in itself resolve the child's speech abnormality.

Several techniques are available for labial frenectomy. Vertical or elliptical excision from the base of the frenulum attachment is a good method; the lip portion is closed by undermining the lateral borders and suturing together. It is important to excise the frenum to periosteum to the depth of the labial fold. The first suture placed is inserted at the height of the fold through mucosa, periosteum and out through mucosa on the opposite side. When this suture is tied, it adapts the mucosa to the periosteum and to the depth of the labial sulcus. The sutures from the first to those at the crest of the ridge should also include periosteum. The remaining sutures should be confined to the labial mucosa. The electrocautery unit may also be used to sever the attachment, and has the advantage of minimizing bleeding (Fig. 20-4).

Z-plasty is used to correct wide fibrous bands and muscle. A vertical incision is made along the length of the frenulum and the muscosa is then undermined bilat-

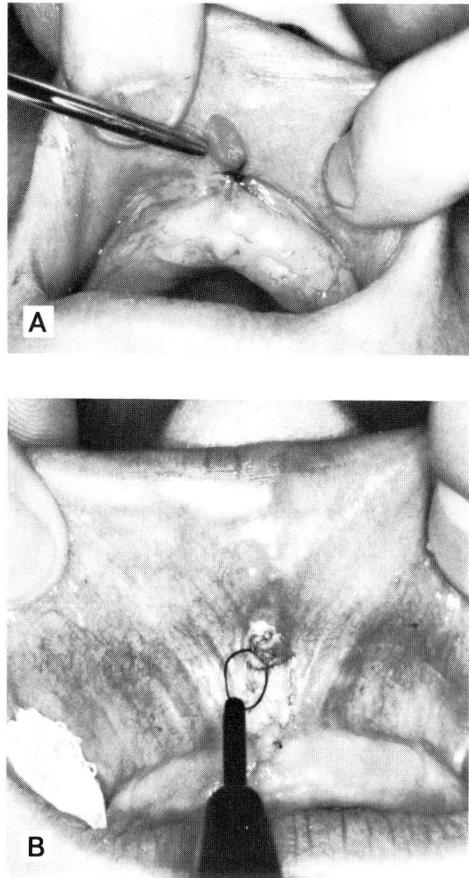

FIG. 20-4. (A) Elliptical excision technique for removal of frenulum; horizontal suture in place following the excision. (B) Frenectomy by electrocautery.

erally. Two lateral incisions are made at approximately 60°; one on each side at opposite ends of the vertical incision—the three incisions resembling the letter "Z." The flaps are then transposed and sutured, thus obliterating the fibrous band and creating a deeper labial fold (Fig. 20-5).

The hemostat technique is another method for removing the labial frenulum. One clamp is applied to the lip portion of the frenulum and one to the ridge portion, with the tips of the clamps meeting in the depth of the fold. A scalpel is then passed beneath the clamps, removing the frenulum. The lip portion is sutured and the ridge portion is not. A surgical pack dressing or oral bandage may be placed in the alveolar void for a few days (Fig. 20-6).

To determine the need for excision of the lingual attachments of a labial frenu-

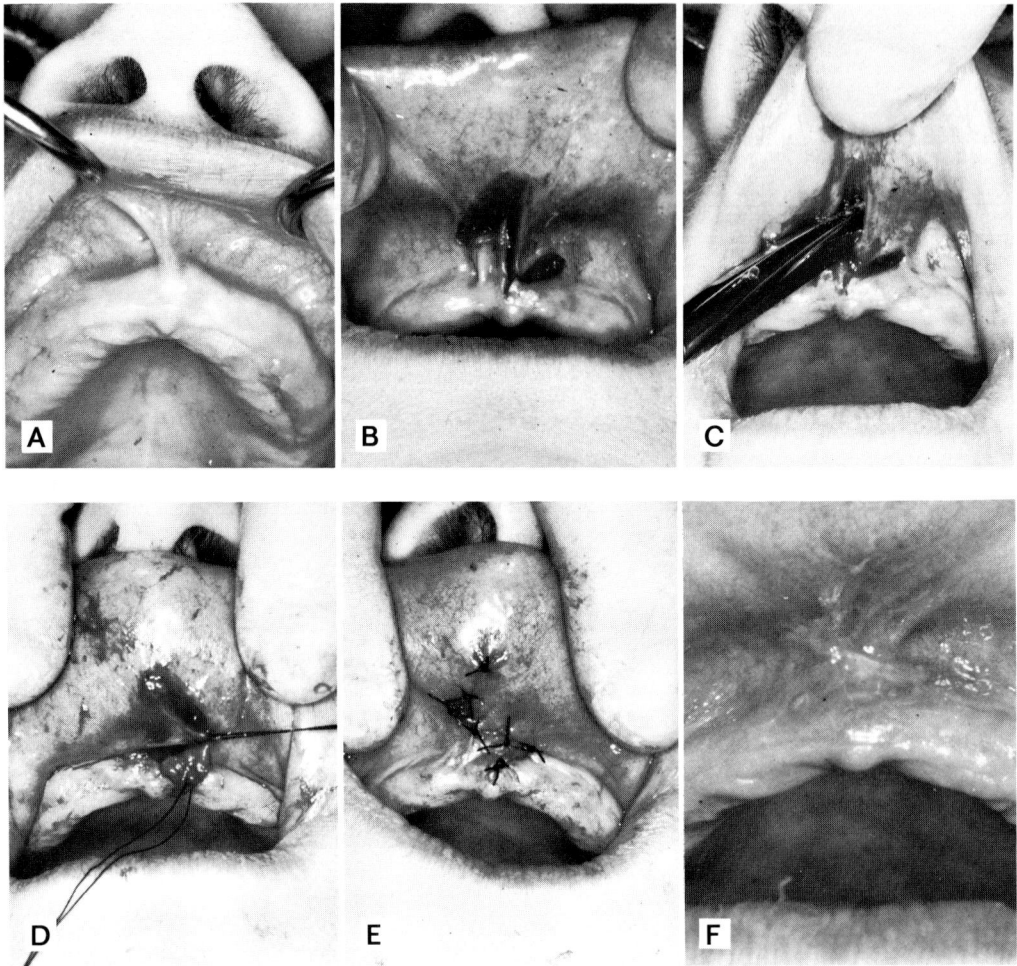

FIG. 20-5. *(A) Frenulum to be corrected by* **Z**-*plasty. (B) Incision outlined in the form of a "Z." (C) Undermining of flaps. (D) Transposition of flaps. (E) Flaps sutured into new position. Note lengthening. (F) After suture removal.*

lum when a diastema continues after lateral and cuspid tooth eruption, place traction on the lip and observe whether blanching occurs on the lingual aspect of the teeth in the nasopalatine region (Fig. 20-2). If so, excision of the lingual attachment is also indicated. In some instances the bony septa between the maxillary incisors may also have to be removed; this can be accomplished by carefully passing a tapered fissure or ½ round bur a short distance between the teeth. A periodontal pack can then be placed to control bleeding and to relieve pain. In cases of small muscle attachments on the buccal, an inverted semilunar incision can be made at

the base of the muscle attachment (Fig. 20-7). This supraperiosteal incision should be made with minimal undermining and, once accomplished, the incised attachment is raised and sutured to the periosteum (Fig. 20-8).

Lingual frenulum attachments on the tongue cause various degrees of ankyloglossia, which may interfere with speech and certainly limit the tongue in its cleansing ability. Although most surgeons prefer the elliptical excision technique, the **Z**-plasty, or the **V-Y** advancement may be acceptable procedures. It is important to limit the depth of the incision at the junction of the floor of the mouth and the

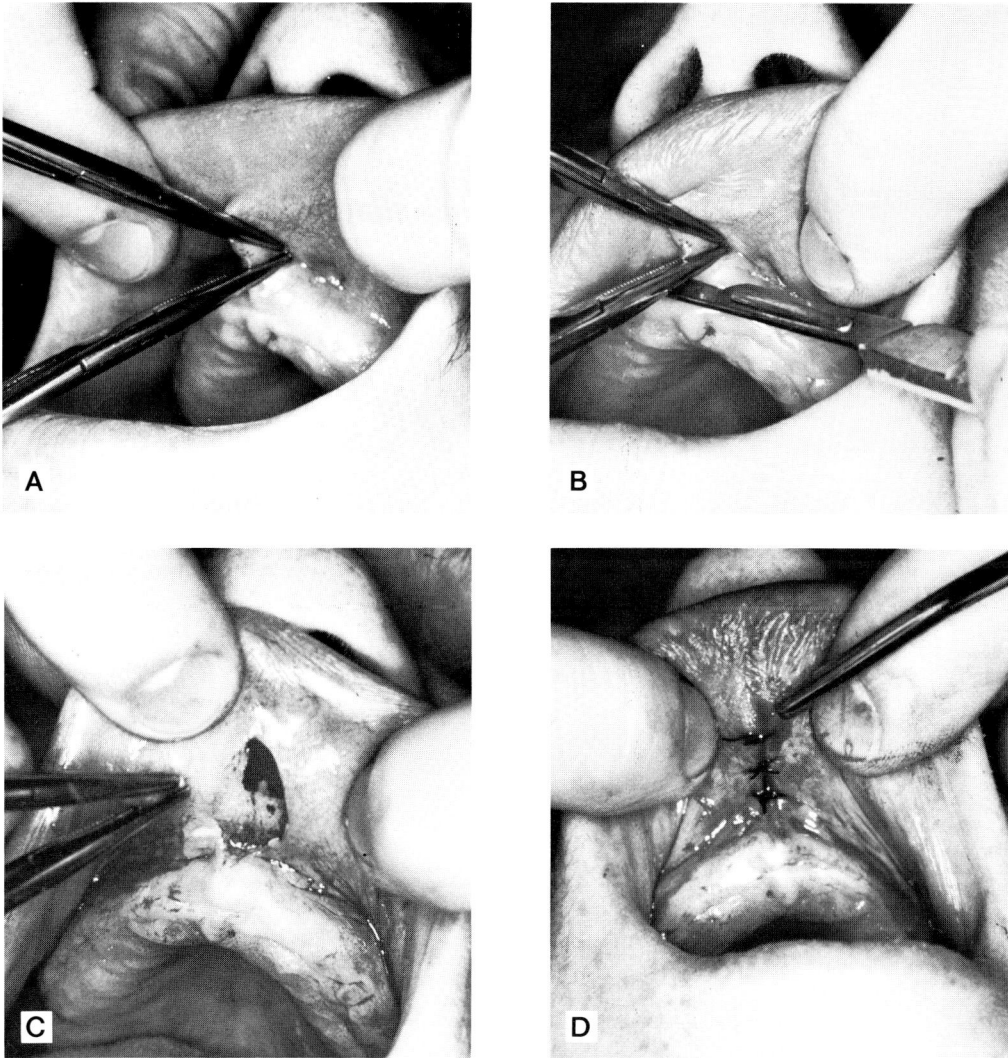

Fig. 20-6. *(A) Hemostats in place for frenectomy. (B) Ridge incision of frenulum is made first. (C) Frenulum excised. Note elliptical shape of wound. (D) Sutures in place (lip portion only).*

tongue to avoid the orifices of the subman-dibular ducts and the terminal branches of the sublingual arteries. It is also wise to in-form the parents that immediate speech improvement should not be anticipated. Only after speech therapy will marked improvement be noted (Fig. 20-9). Lingual frenectomies are easily performed at the time of mandibular extractions (Fig. 20-10). Elimination of the lingual frenum prior to denture construction minimizes the frequency of mandibular denture dis-lodgement during tongue function.

TUBEROSITY REDUCTION

Surgical correction of the bulbous tuber-osity is performed primarily to provide sta-bility of the prosthesis and to increase pos-terior interarch vertical-dimension (Fig. 20-11A). The tuberosity can best be re-duced by an elliptical incision with minimal undermining and the removal of two in-verted triangles of tissue. The wedge-shaped incision is made first through the center of the tuberosity to a depth where contact is made with the crest of the alveo-lar ridge. After this wedge is removed, the

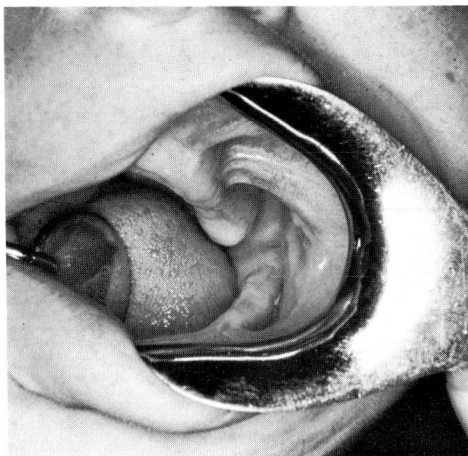

FIG. 20-7. *Low muscle attachments on the left maxilla.*

surgeon estimates the inverted V or triangle of undermined tissue necessary to be removed on both the buccal and lingual aspects of the tuberosity (Fig. 20-11B). This undermining is necessary for the tuberosity to be narrowed buccalpalatally and for primary closure to be accomplished. This technique provides both a lateral and a vertical reduction of the tuberosity. Bone removal, if necessary, is accomplished at the same time (Fig. 20-11C, D, and E). Prior to bone reduction, x-rays must be evaluated to determine the relationship of the maxillary sinus to the area of surgery. It is occasionally necessary to reduce the bone in the tuberosity to the level of the antral membrane; however, great care must be exercised so that the lining is not perforated, potentially resulting in an oroantral fistula. Once adequate soft

and hard tissue reductions have been accomplished, the flaps are sutured primarily. Another technique for tuberosity reduction is merely to "decapitate" that portion of the soft tissue tuberosity that is pendulous or hanging down (Fig. 20-12A). If the tuberosity is composed entirely of soft tissue, this horizontal excision can be accomplished with slight contouring and minimal hemorrhage. In such instances the primary goal is to increase vertical dimension while maintaining a good solid base for the prosthesis (Fig. 20-12B).

The greatest error made in tuberosity reduction surgery is the inadequate reduction of the soft and hard tissues. Prior to closure it is wise to assess the amount of interarch space that has been gained. The dentist should be able to pass a dental mirror horizontally between the tuberosity and retromolar pad of the mandible when the patient closes to the desired vertical dimension.

HYPERPLASTIC TISSUE

Flabby hyperplastic tissue beneath a poorly fitting prosthesis may create a difficult surgical problem (Fig. 20-13). If the denture can be removed for 7 to 10 days prior to surgery, the edema and inflammation may subside sufficiently to make the procedure considerably less difficult and may result in less of a surgical correction. A variety of corrective procedures are available, such as excision (Fig. 20-13 B, C, and D), removal by electrocautery, or special flap designs plus undermining and repositioning with the excision of the excess tissue. The latter is referred to as the draping procedure. Because the hypertrophied or

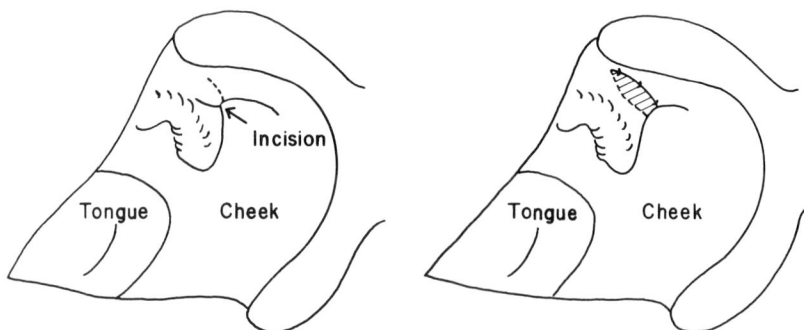

FIG. 20-8. *Incision for raising the muscle attachment.*

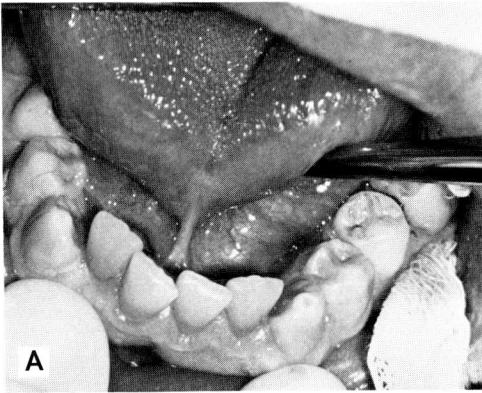

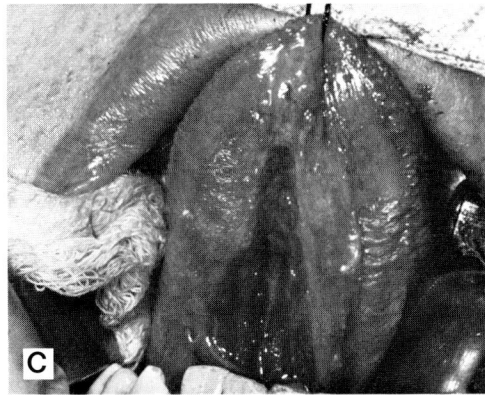

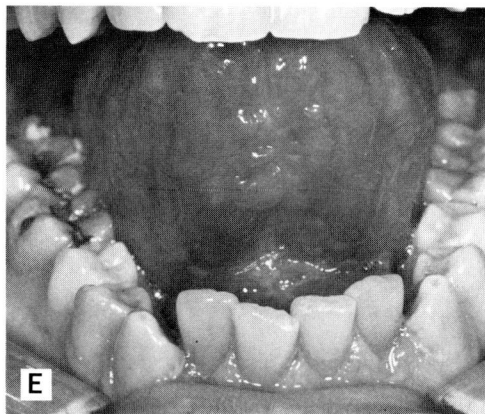

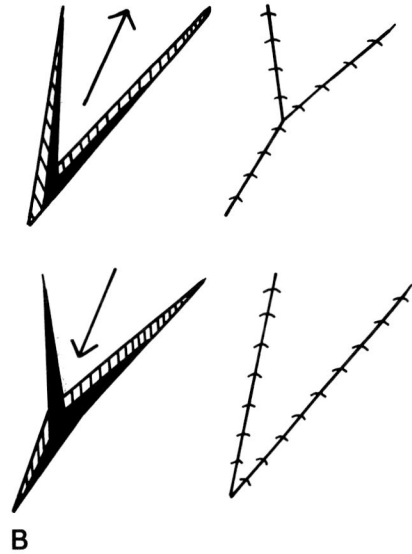

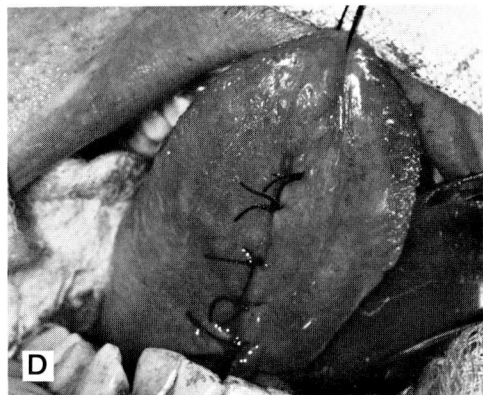

FIG. 20-9. *Ankyloglossia. (A) Clinical appearance in a 21-year-old man. (B) The* **V-Y** *advancement flap. (C) Surgical correction by* **V-Y** *incision. (D) Sutures in place. (E) Three-month postoperative result. Note freedom of tongue movement.*

hyperplastic folds of tissue have a continuous epithelial covering, an incision can be made on the crest of the ridge and the soft tissue flap reflected. Undermining is continuous until all folds and wrinkles are free. The entire flap is then pulled out as a drape (Fig. 20-14A) and the excess tissue excised. The new flap margin is then su-

tured (Fig. 20-14B), and the denture reinserted as a splint.

Although small rolls of hyperplastic tissue can also be simply excised and allowed to heal by granulation, most surgeons prefer to reconstruct extensive areas of excision immediately with a split thickness skin graft. The graft is usually harvested from

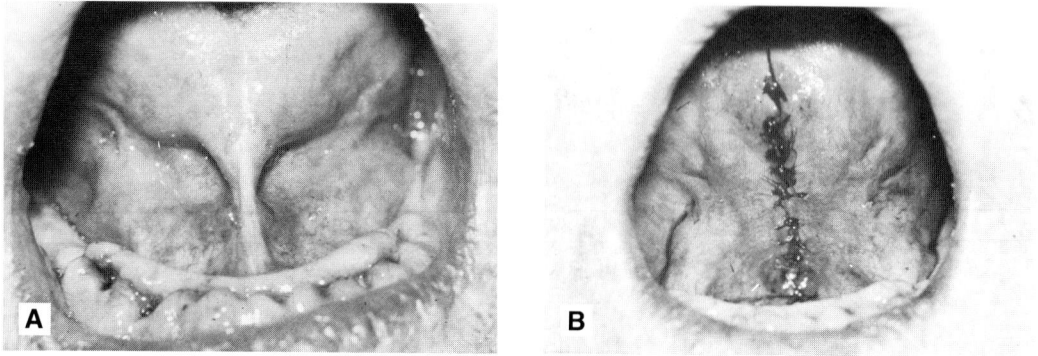

FIG. 20-10. (A and B) Lingual frenectomy performed at time of extraction.

the thigh and held in position for 10 to 14 days with the patient's denture or a surgical splint. The placement of the skin graft increases the vestibular depth and limits the recurrence of the hyperplastic tissue. Although malignant transformation is uncommon, the hyperplastic tissue that has been excised should be submitted for histopathologic examination.

INFLAMMATORY PAPILLARY HYPERPLASIA

Inflammatory papillary hyperplasia has specific characteristics. It appears on the palate and apparently is due to denture injury. In most instances there is an associated anterior-posterior shift to the denture. Its cause may relate to the relief provided in the vault during denture con-

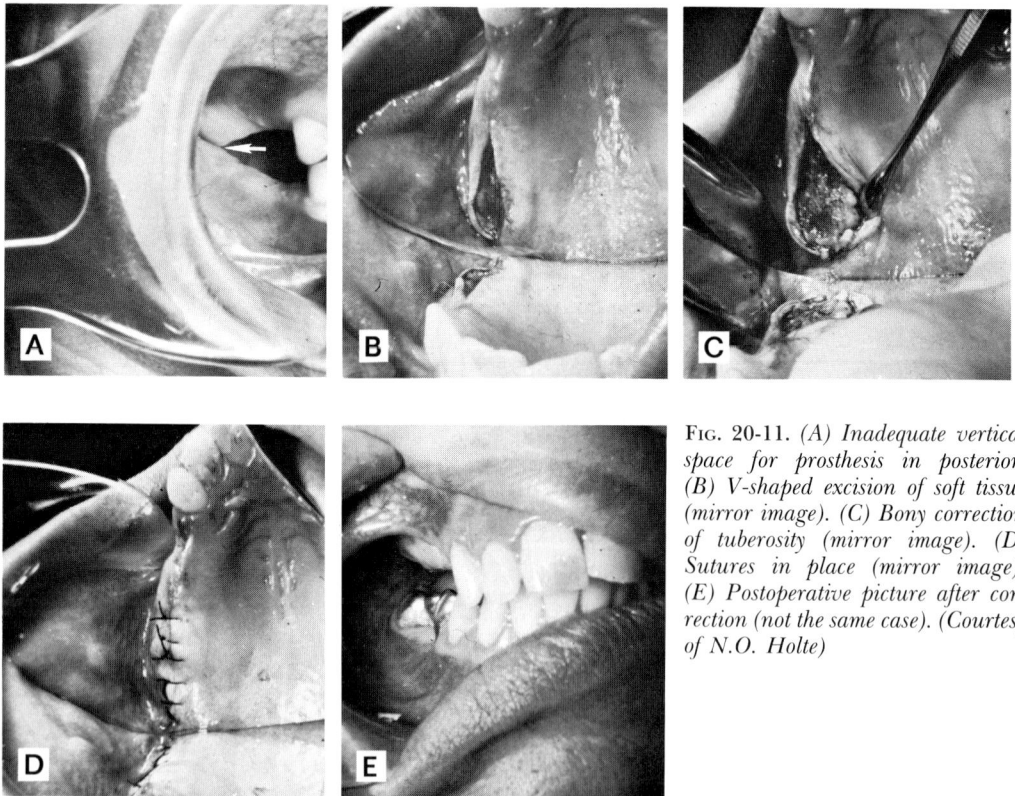

FIG. 20-11. (A) Inadequate vertical space for prosthesis in posterior. (B) V-shaped excision of soft tissue (mirror image). (C) Bony correction of tuberosity (mirror image). (D) Sutures in place (mirror image). (E) Postoperative picture after correction (not the same case). (Courtesy of N.O. Holte)

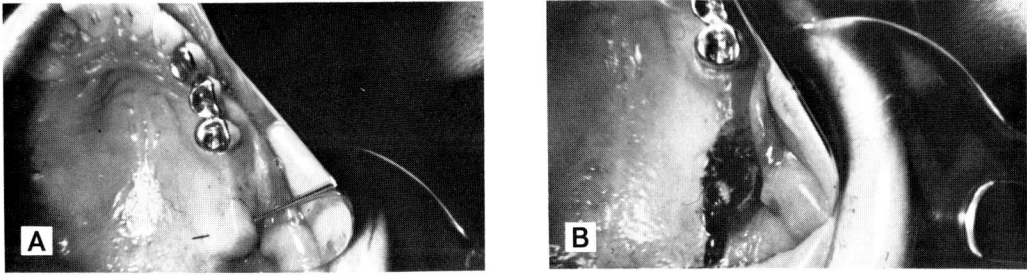

FIG. 20-12. (A) Probe in place shows that the tuberosity is composed entirely of soft tissue. (B) Complete excision of the tuberosity by decapitation. Note raw bleeding surface.

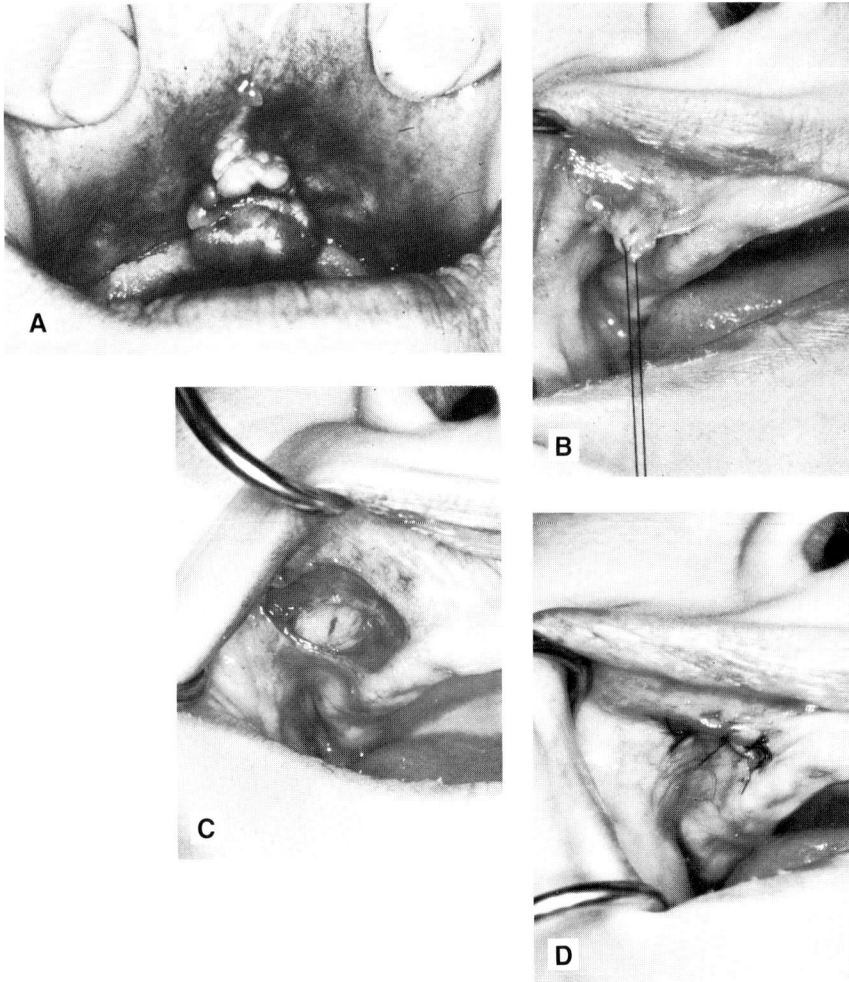

FIG. 20-13. (A) Maxillary fibrous hyperplasia with associated inflammation. (B) Preoperative view of soft tissue mass. (C) Lesion excised. (D) Postoperative view.

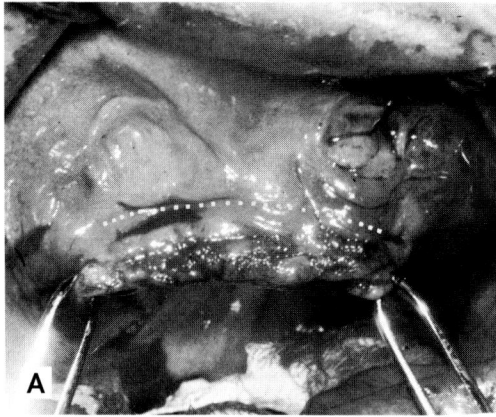

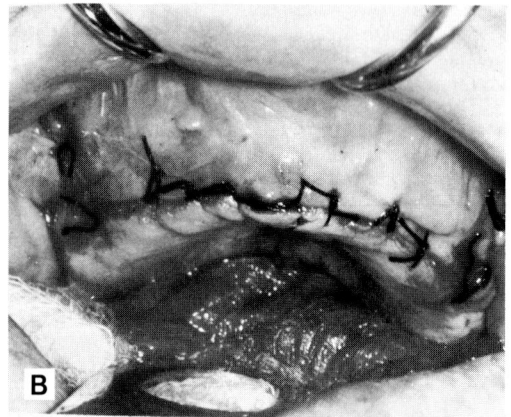

FIG. 20-14. *(A) Many tissue folds resulting from ill-fitting denture; draping procedure following undermining. (B) Excision of excess tissues sutured in new position.*

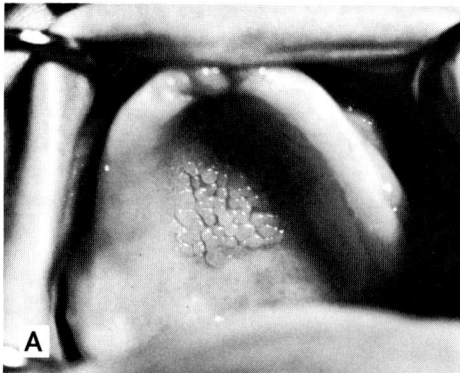

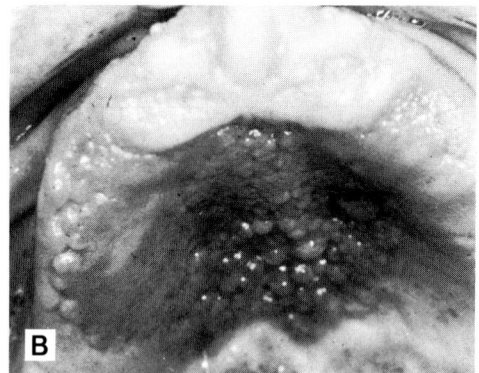

FIG. 20-15. *(A and B) Inflammatory papillary hyperplasia. Note numerous small papillary-like structures.*

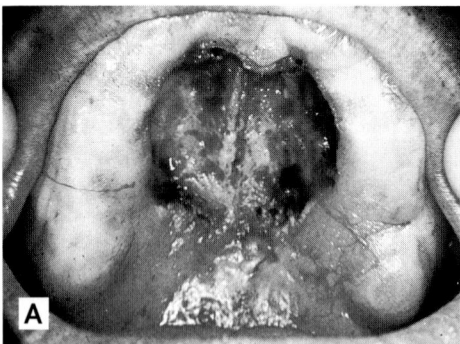

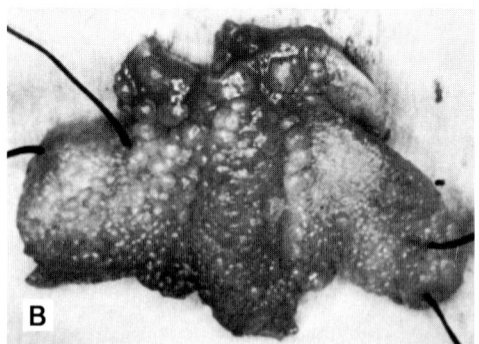

FIG. 20-16. *(A) Excision of the palatal lesion including the periosteum. (B) Surgical specimen.*

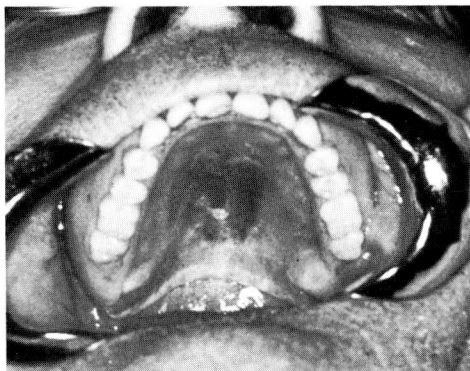

FIG. 20-17. *Denture is reinserted and used as a protective covering; clear acrylic vault permits good visualization.*

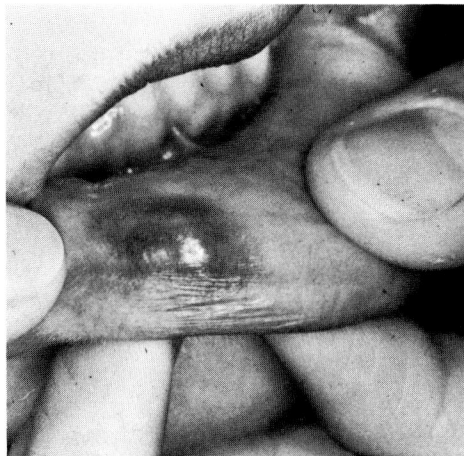

FIG. 20-19. *Small hemangioma of the lip.*

struction, which affects the amount of suction and pressure on the palate. The lesion worsens with time and appears reddened, sore, and raspberry-like (Fig. 20-15A). One can play a stream of air on the lesions and note the small pedunculated stalks of tissue (Fig. 20-15B). Food and tissue fluid become embedded in the base and crevices of the lesion, adding to the injury and irritation. It is desirable to have the patient leave the denture out or to reline it with a soft tissue treatment material prior to surgery, thus decreasing the size of the lesions and limiting the amount of associated inflammation. The lesion may be stripped supraperiosteally with the broad end of a periosteal elevator, abraded with the high-speed drill using a large vulcanite surgical bur, or excised (Fig. 20-16). The electrocautery unit might also be used. The denture

should be relined with a soft reline material and immediately inserted as a protective splint (Fig. 20-17).

SOFT TISSUE TUMORS

A variety of soft tissue tumors occur within the oral cavity. Surgical management follows the same principles for the handling of all soft tissue.

Papillomas may be found on the tongue, cheek, or palate and are usually small pedunculated growths treated by excision (Fig. 20-18).

Hemangiomas appear as dark red or purplish compressible tumor masses located on lips, cheeks, or tongue (Fig. 20-19). Treatment is by excision and/or the injection of a sclerosing solution. Incisional biopsy should not be performed because of profuse bleeding that is difficult to control; aspiration of a suspected hemangiomatous lesion is a safer diagnostic method.

Lipomas may occur in the oral cavity but are uncommon. A lipoma occurs so slowly and painlessly that it can attain a fairly large size before the patient may be aware of it. Usually found in the cheek or the floor of the mouth, they are composed of yellow fatty tissue with a soft, doughy consistency (Fig. 20-20).

Occasionally, *pigmented lesions* may be found in the oral cavity. If a change in pigmentation has occurred, these lesions should be removed only by wide excision and considered potentially malignant until proved otherwise (Fig. 20-21).

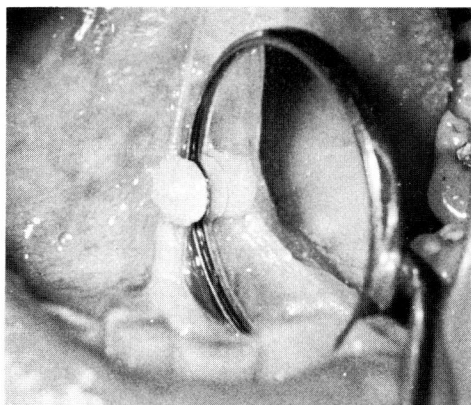

FIG. 20-18. *Papilloma. (Courtesy of R. Gorlin)*

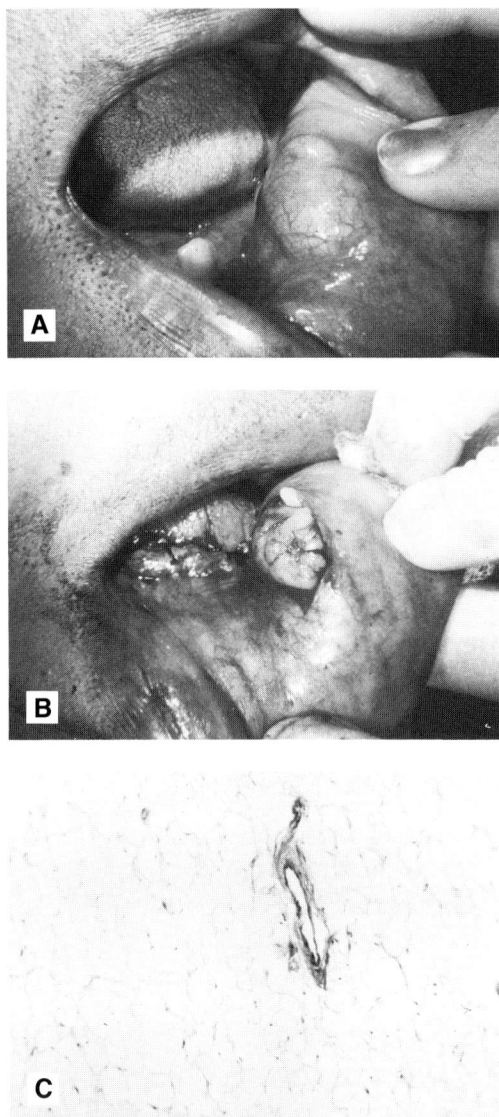

FIG. 20-20. (A and B) Lipoma of buccal soft tissue. (C) Histology of the lipoma.

The *mucocele* usually results from salivary secretion retention, and appears most commonly on the lower lip. It is best removed by elliptical excision, which is less likely to rupture the lesion and makes its dissection less complicated. This is followed by slight undermining and closure with interrupted sutures (Fig. 20-22). Care should be taken to remove adjacent glands that have been violated in the surgery to limit the potential for recurrences.

The *ranula* is a soft tissue swelling of the floor of the mouth related to obstruction of one or more minor salivary glands (Fig. 20-23). The term "ranula" comes from the resemblance of this swelling to the color and consistency of the undersurface of a frog (Fig. 20-24). Treatment consists of establishing adequate drainage of the obstruction by creation of an epithelialized tract, marsupialization, or extirpation of the sublingual salivary gland.

Large *lesions of the tongue* can be removed by excision, and with extensive undermining, primary closure can be accomplished (Fig. 20-25). Diagnosis and treatment of white lesions continue to be controversial, and the terms describing these lesions vary among medical and dental clinicians. However, most agree that red and white keratotic lesions should be evaluated by biopsy and histopathologic examination. The great majority are benign but a significant number can be precancerous or frankly cancerous, making such vigilance worthwhile.

Vestibuloplasty

Preprosthetic surgery includes the minor surgical corrections previously discussed, such as frenectomies and tuberosity reductions, and the surgical correction of bony abnormalities of the jaws to pro-

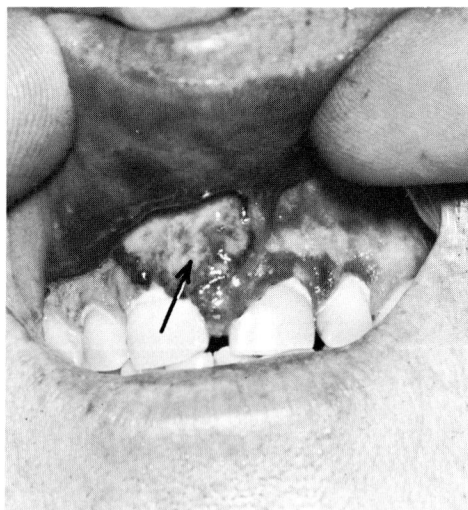

FIG. 20-21. *Malignant melanoma. (From: Catlin, D.: Mucosal melanomas of the head and neck. Am. J. Roentgen., 99, 1967.)*

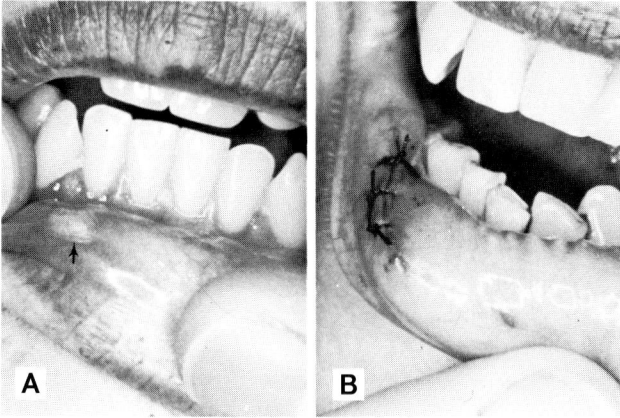

FIG. 20-22. *(A) Mucocele of the lip. (B) Undermined enclosure with sutures in place following excision.*

vide an improved denture base. In addition, a denture-wearing patient may need increased sulcus depth accomplished by vestibuloplasty. The number of people age 65 and over in the United States is expected to increase from 25 million to 30 million between 1980 and 1990. Recent estimates indicated that over 33 million people were edentulous. These figures indicate the number of persons probably wearing a partial or full prosthesis that is likely to be inadequate (Fig. 20-26).

The life span has been extended as a direct result of medical knowledge and the control of many diseases. Likewise, comparable advancement in the knowledge of surgical procedures and the safety under which they can be performed has occurred.

Vestibuloplasty is necessary when no sulcus depth is available for prosthetic retention and support, as when alveolar resorption has been extensive, or when muscle,

frenula, and mucosal attachments occur on or near the crest of the ridge (Fig. 20-27). A number of techniques can be utilized to improve the alveolar ridges for denture bearing and to increase the sulcus depth in relation to the alveolar process and muscle attachments. These techniques include repositioning of the mucosa, as in Kazanjian and Clark's technique, and the procedures relying on immediate epithelial transfer of either mucosa or skin. Finally, ridge rebuilding by bone in extreme cases of alveolar bone atrophy may also be required.

Prior to selecting the surgical procedure, the dentist must classify the degree of the patient's osseous deformity. The reconstructive procedure of choice depends frequently upon the degree of bone loss as exemplified in the following classification.

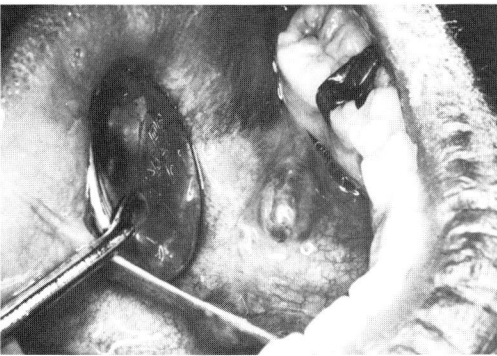

FIG. 20-23. *Superficial ranula of the floor of the mouth.*

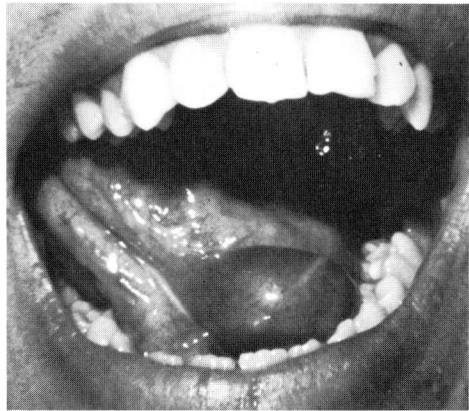

FIG. 20-24. *Ranula. Note the dark color and nature of fluctuance.*

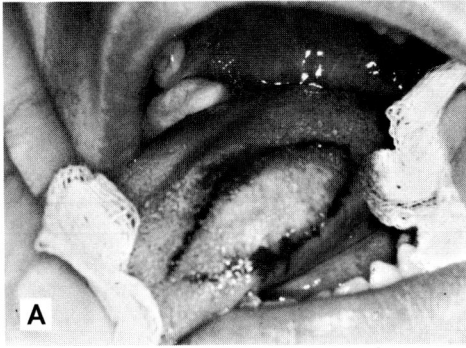

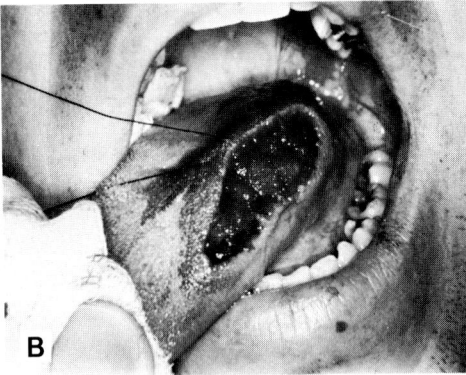

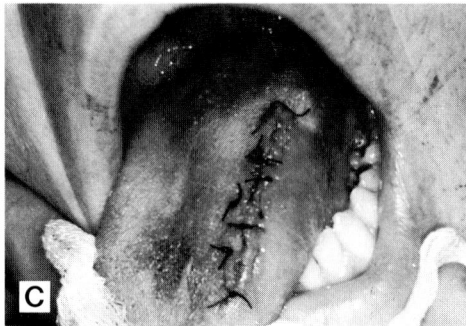

FIG. 20-25. (A) White lesion of tongue with incision lines marked. (B) Lesion excised. (C) Adequate closure by undermining and use of mattress sutures.

Rehabilitation of a patient with a Class I or II deformity can usually be accomplished by one of the soft tissue vestibuloplasty procedures; however, those with Class III or IV deformities generally require mandibular augmentation with bone and/or alloplasts such as hydroxylapatite (HA).

The submucous procedure for vestibuloplasty as advocated by Obwegeser is best

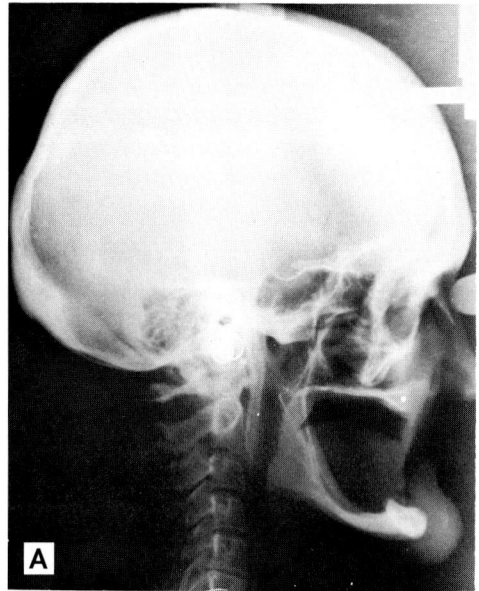

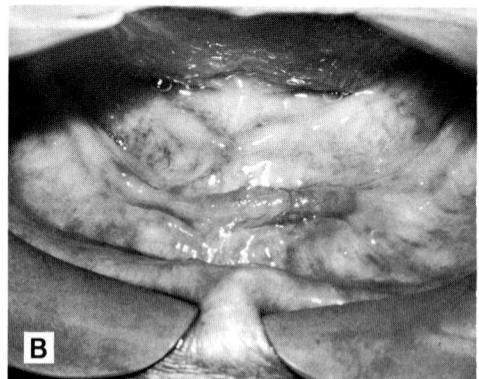

Class	Definition
I	The alveolar ridge is adequate in height but shows significant undercut areas and insufficient width.
II	The alveolar ridge is deficient in both height and width and presents a knife-edge appearance.
III	The alveolar ridge has been resorbed to the level of the basal bone of the mandible of maxilla.
IV	The mandible or maxilla presents with severe resorption; there is impending pathologic fracture.

FIG. 20-26. (A) Lateral cephalogram showing severe alveolar bone loss. Note prominent genial tubercles remaining. (B) Photograph of inadequate ridge.

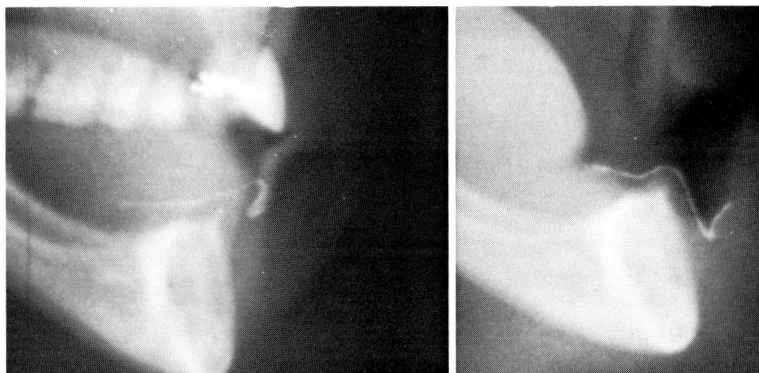

FIG. 20-27. *Barium tracing of anterior sulcus depth before and after vestibuloplasty.*

for increasing sulcus depth of the anterior maxilla.[3] A vertical incision is made in the midline just through the mucosa, permitting a blind supraperiosteal dissection with

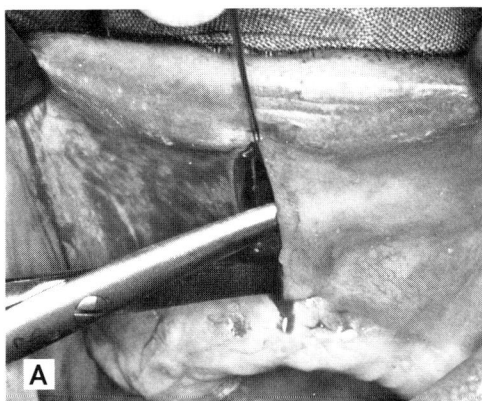

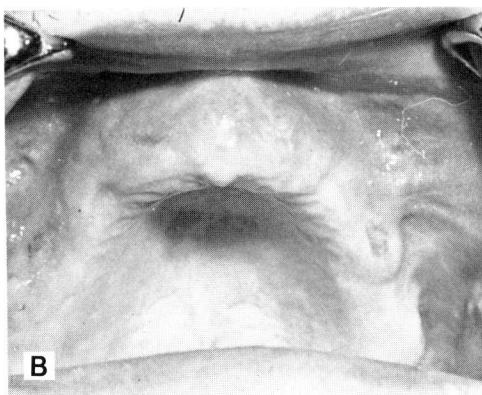

FIG. 20-28. *(A and B) Submucous procedure for vestibuloplasty of anterior maxilla. See text for description. (Courtesy of E. Steinhauser)*

scissors. After all attachments have been released, the tissue is tacked high in the vestibular depth and a denture or surgical template is pressed against the new ridge and held in place by a perialveolar wire or palatal screw (Fig. 20-28).

The secondary epithelialization method involves the reflection of a supraperiosteal flap from the labial aspect of the ridge or the preparation of a mucosal flap on the inner surface to heal by secondary intention. A rubber catheter is then inserted in the depth of the newly created sulcus and held in place by through-and-through sutures to the skin held in place by buttons. After 7 to 10 days, the sutures and catheter are removed, and within 4 to 6 weeks a new prosthesis can be made (Fig. 20-29). Experience has shown, however, that at least 50 percent of the gained surgical depth is slowly lost. A similar procedure is accomplished by carefully dissecting the mucosal flap free from the periosteum and suturing at the new level, creating as much sulcus as possible (Fig. 20-30).

A more accurate method involves the utilization of a previously constructed splint. This is accomplished by taking a compound impression of the existing ridge and carving on the model the degree of extension that is potentially possible surgically, and then constructing a splint to fit the model. The surgery is accomplished as planned and the splint inserted and retained by bone screws or circumzygomatic or mandibular wiring (Fig. 20-31).

The immediate extension technique has many advantages similar to those of the

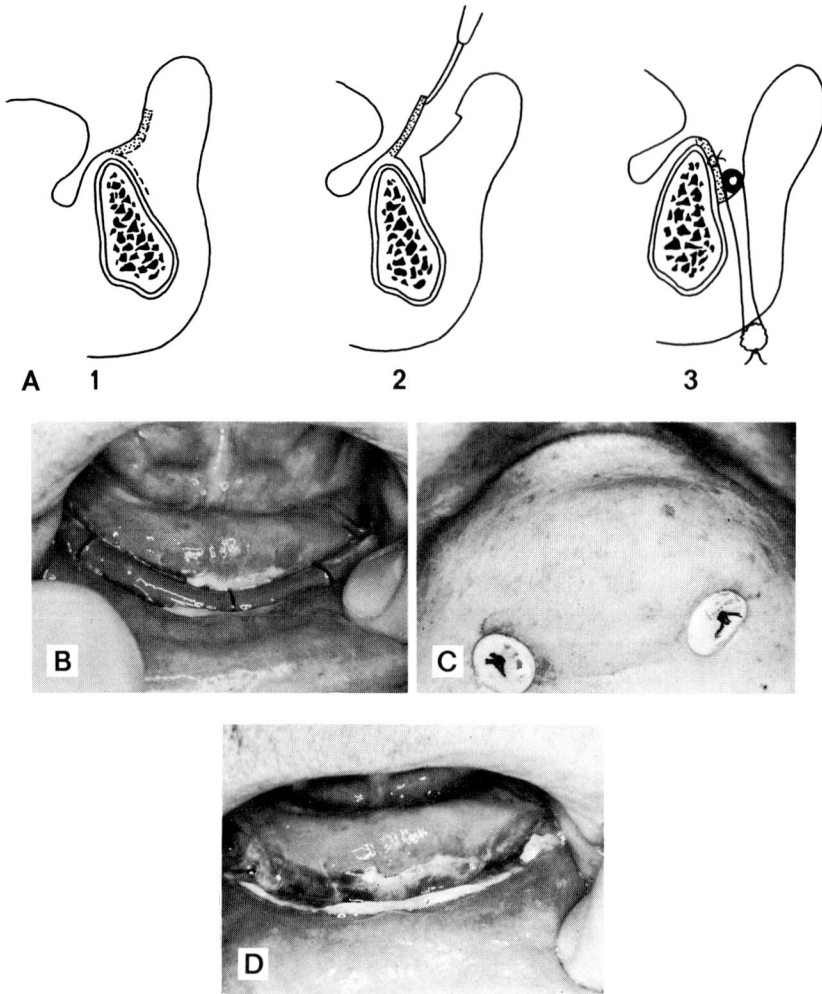

FIG. 20-29. *(A) Secondary epithelialization technique. (B) Mucosa from lip attached to rubber tubing. (C) Tied to buttons on skin surface. (D) Seven days postoperative, tubing is removed. Note increased vestibule.*

immediate denture. The incision is made directly over the crest of the ridge through periosteum and gently curves into the mucobuccal fold distal to the areas where the extension is desired. The mucoperiosteal flap and muscle attachments are carried superiorly and buccally to the desired, or limit of, extension. This leaves a raw bony surface to be covered by the splint. This area becomes filled with a blood clot that forms granulation tissue and finally epithelializes over the exposed bone. It is important that the periphery of the over-extended denture be thick and well rounded to prevent fissuring and undue irritation. In the maxilla, a single retention screw in the midline of the palate is often

sufficient to stabilize the splint (Fig. 20-32). In the lower arch, at least two screws are necessary; however, three are advantageous, one in each of the retromolar pad areas and the other in the midline.

The swinging of buccal mucosal flaps with a pedicle base has also been a successful method of vestibuloplasty (Fig. 20-33). In such instances, the flap design is marked out on the cheek surface, keeping a broad base near the crest of the ridge in the retromolar area (Fig. 20-34). The flap (designated by a solid black dot in Fig. 20-35) is incised and freed to its base and then transferred into the new surgical site (designated by an open white dot), extending the sulcus. The donor site is then under-

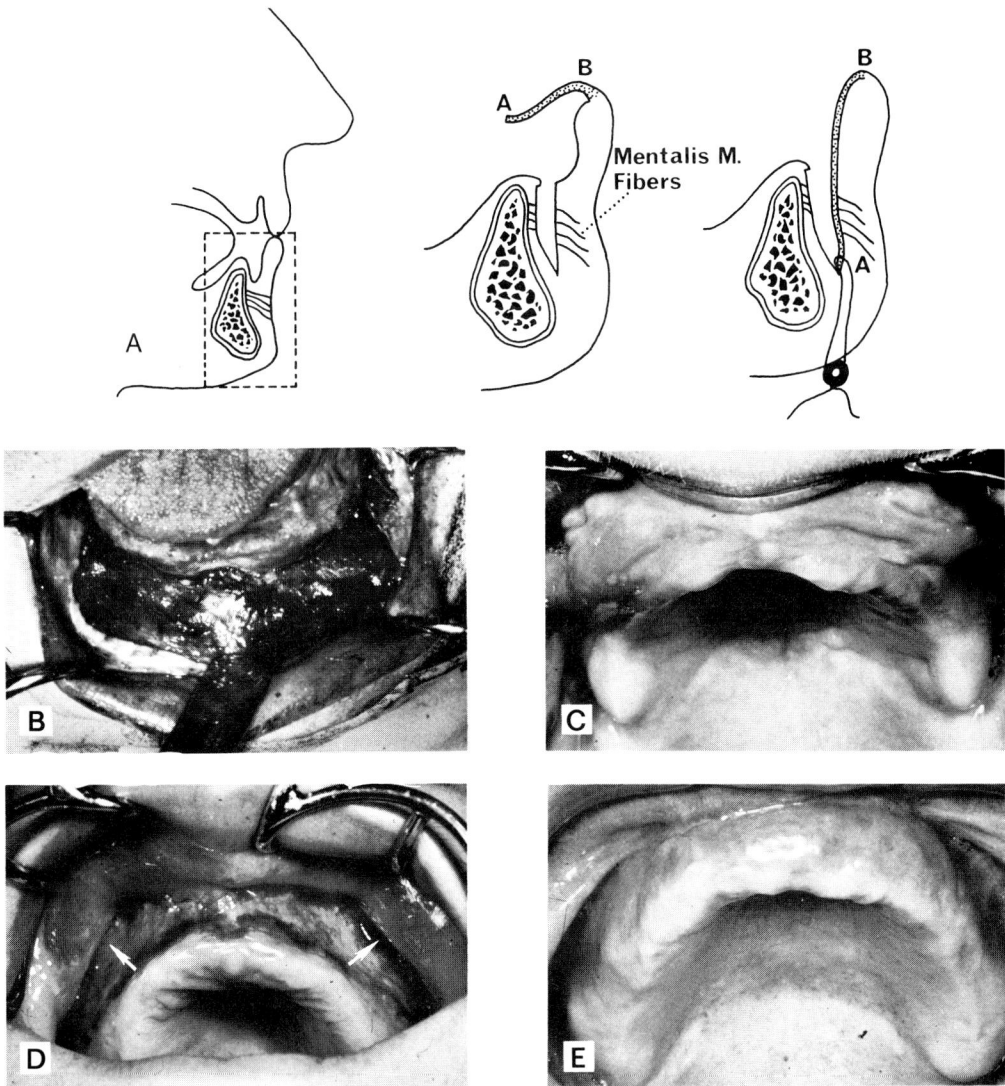

FIG. 20-30. *(A) Secondary epithelialization technique, taking supraperiosteal flap from alveolar ridge of mandible. (B) Secondary epithelialization technique for mandibular ridge. (C) For maxillary ridge. (D and E) Pre- and postoperative views. (Courtesy of E. Steinhauser)*

mined and closed by sutures (Fig. 20-36). Again, an overlying splint is inserted and held in place by circummandibular sutures or screws (Fig. 20-37).

Surgical Correction of Bony Anomalies

Surgical procedures for the management of bony lesions or other hard tissues of the oral cavity are not particularly different from any other surgical procedure: the same careful and meticulous technique is indicated for all surgery. However, the removal of such conditions as the odontoma (Fig. 20-38), ossifying fibroma (Fig. 20-39), and tori (Fig. 20-40) or generalized exostoses is among the more difficult bony surgical procedures to execute and can produce prolonged postoperative problems.

The removal of palatal and bilateral lingual mandibular exostoses (tori) is usually indicated prior to denture construction. The mucosa overlying these exostoses is extremely thin and cannot withstand chronic irritation from an overlying pros-

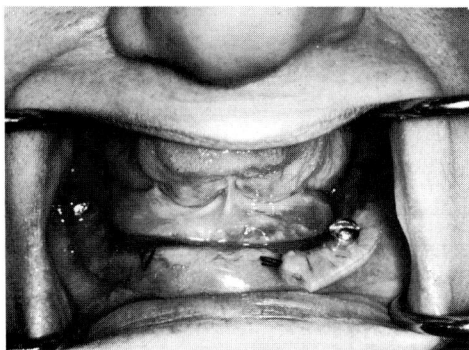

FIG. 20-31. *Preconstructed acrylic splint with overextension.*

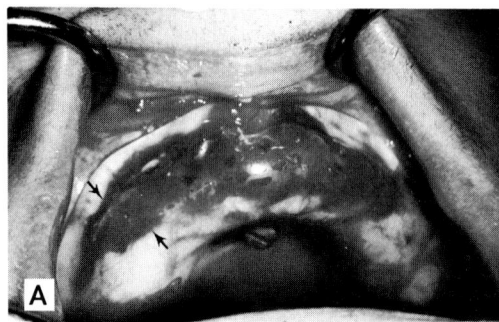

FIG. 20-33. *Pedicled mucosal grafts from the parietes.*

thesis. Ulcers develop as a result of denture-induced trauma. These lesions heal slowly because of the thinness of the mucosa and the poor blood supply to the area secondary to the cortical nature of the underlying bone. Occasionally, tori must be removed in patients with a full complement of teeth, merely because of chronic trauma to the mucosa overlying the exostoses.

The operative approach to these calcified structures is by means of the reflection of a mucoperiosteal flap, exposing them for excision by either the chisel or the bur. Some mandibular tori can be removed in toto, while palatal tori generally require a sectioning technique. In the case of an exostosis or torus, the intent may not always be complete removal, but simply trimming or smoothing the bulky mass to accommodate a prosthesis.

The most common enlargement of the palate is that of the torus palatinus. This condition has never been reported as a malignant growth; it is removed primarily

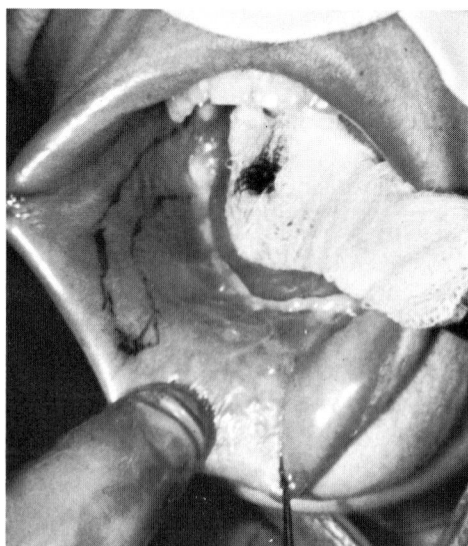

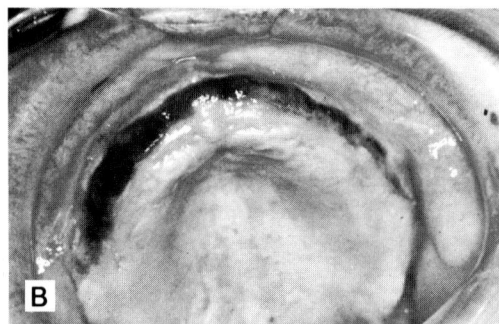

FIG. 20-32. *(A) Immediate extension technique using retention screws. (B) Splint removed. Granulating tissue marks degree of vestibular extension.*

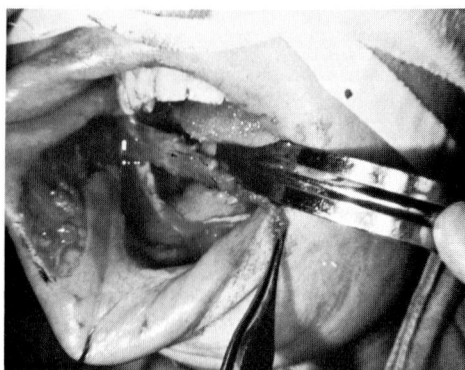

FIG. 20-34. *Unilateral vestibular inadequacy due to trauma. Depth of vestibule was increased by pedicle graft.*

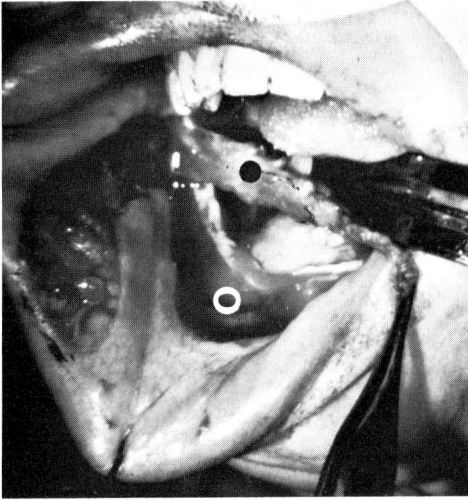

FIG. 20-35. *Pedicle graft taken from right cheek; host site also prepared.*

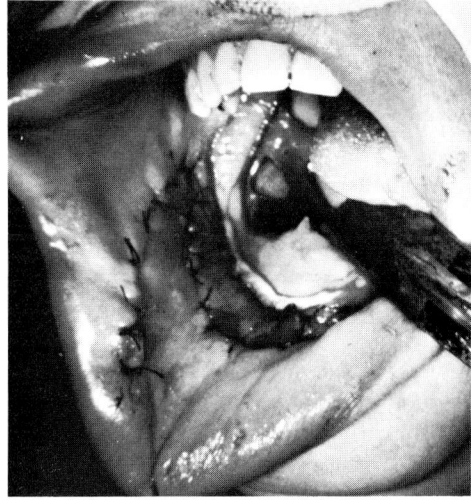

FIG. 20-36. *Pedicle sutured into new position and donor site closed.*

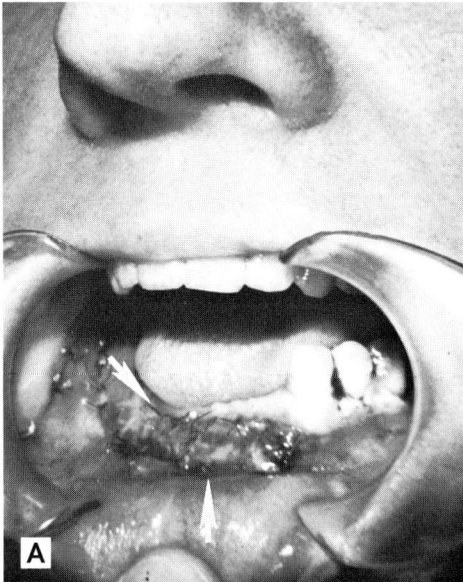

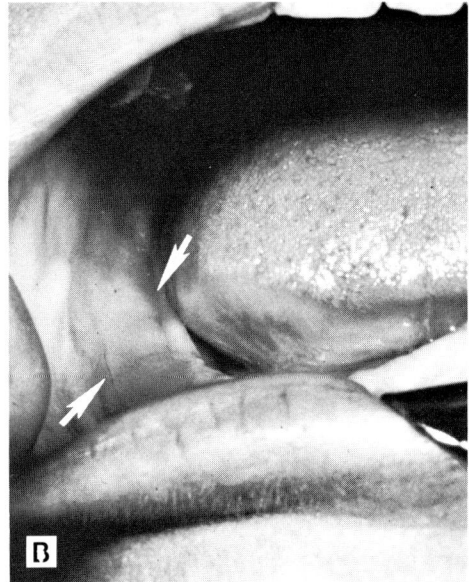

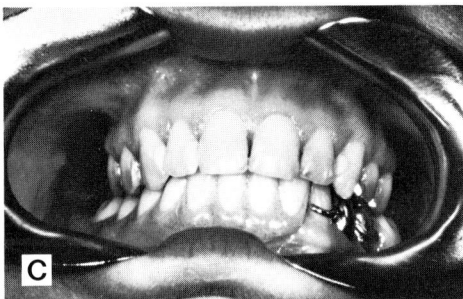

FIG. 20-37. *(A) Seven-day postoperative view of pedicle graft. (B) Two-month postoperative view of pedicle graft. (C) Prosthesis in place.*

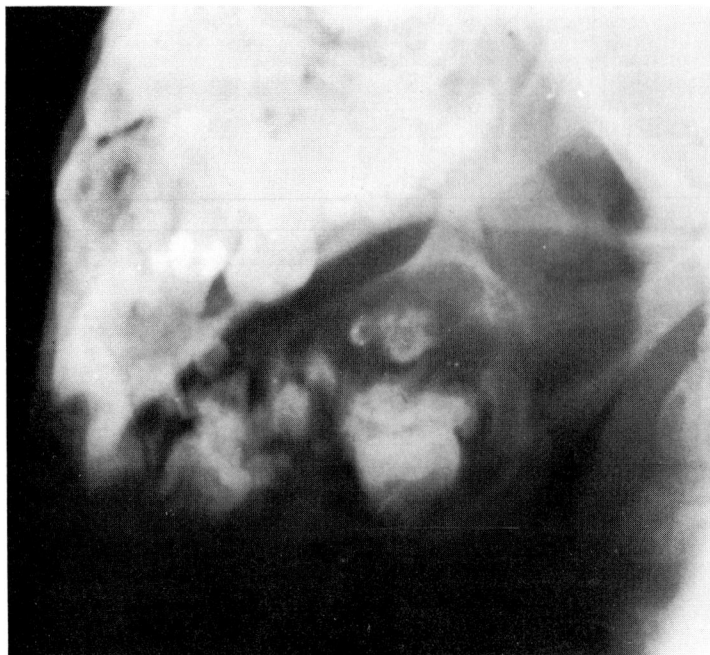

FIG. 20-38. *Odontoma involving the body and ramus of the mandible in a 10-year-old boy.*

to prevent irritation to the overlying mucosae and to permit the reception of a prosthesis. Its presence has been reported as
high as 20 and 25 percent.[4] Palatal tori are
more prevalent than the mandibular tori,
with no sex or race difference.[5] These
bony masses have been known to increase

in size during the first three decades of life
but stabilize after that with no considerable
change.

When discovered for the first time, this
growth of the palate often creates great
anxiety in the patient. A cancer phobia
may exist, and considerable reassurance
and sometimes surgical removal may be
necessary to satisfy such a patient. A frequent complaint may be that of trauma
(Fig. 20-41). The bony growth, which occurs in the midline, takes considerable
abuse from the mastication of food against

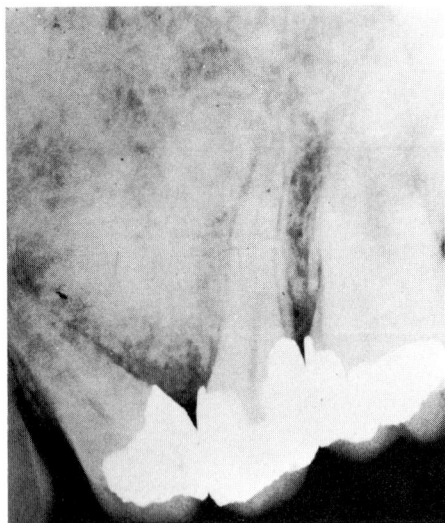

FIG. 20-39. *Ossifying fibroma in a 48-year-old
woman. Note divergence of roots in teeth.*

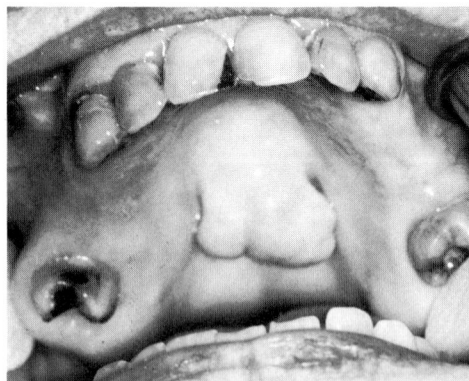

FIG. 20-40. *Torus palatinus.*

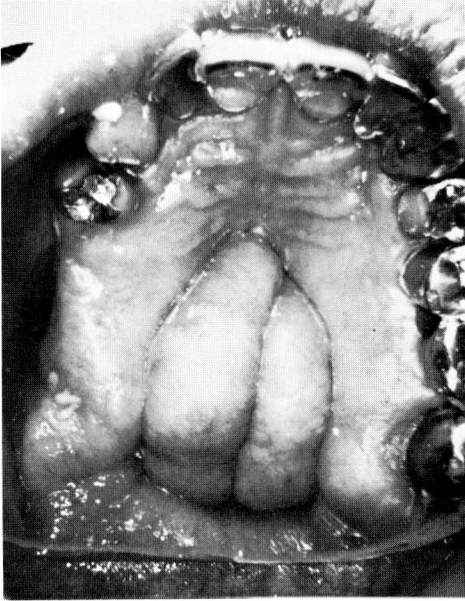

FIG. 20-41. *Burn on midline of palate.*

the roof of the mouth by the tongue as well as from food passing through the oral cavity. Since the torus may extend posteriorly as far as the postdam area and occur lobulated and in a variety of shapes, it may also interfere with a prosthesis, preventing peripheral seal of the denture (Fig. 20-42). The surgical management for the reduction of the torus can be done under local or general anesthesia.

The double Y midline incision probably provides the best surgical access. This flap design preserves the nerve and blood supply to the flap entering from the nasopalatine and the bilateral greater palatine foramina. The mucoperiosteal flap is extremely thin and tears easily, so it must be handled gently. A traction suture may be helpful (Fig. 20-43).

Injection of a local anesthetic near the base of the bony protuberance controls hemorrhage into the area, while injection of the anesthetic fluid beneath the periosteum makes the dissection easier. The growth mass is then sectioned into segments by means of the high-speed drill with each segment removed separately (Fig. 20-44).

A unibevel chisel may also be used to remove the individual segments. The torus is not removed in one large piece because

of the possibility of fracturing the nasal floor. The injudicious use of a chisel in removing the posterior portions of the torus may result in a bony separation at the junction of the maxilla and the palatine bones. The high-speed drill may also be used to reduce the entire mass, utilizing copious irrigation. Smoothing of the raw bony surface is accomplished by rongeurs and files or rotary bone burs, and debridement is done by irrigation (Fig. 20-45A and B). The tissues are closed with mattress sutures (Fig. 20-45C).

A surgical splint is used to protect the flap during the first few postoperative days (Fig. 20-46). The splint not only physically protects the tissues from injury and food debris, but prevents dependent hematoma formation beneath the flap, which would retard the healing process.

In preparing the splint, the surgeon should trim the cast himself to note the appropriate bony reduction necessary during the surgical procedure. If inadequate relief is provided, pressure will be exerted against the wound. One can also insert a ball of gauze soaked in tincture of benzoin and held in place with a number of sutures criss-crossed from one side of the arch to the other like a basket. If teeth are present, they are used to anchor the criss-crossing sutures.

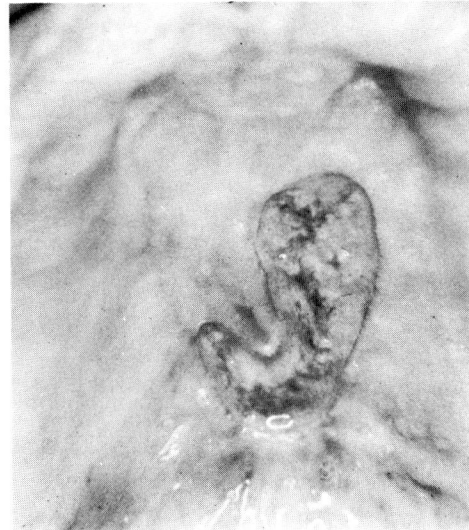

FIG. 20-42. *Maxillary torus showing lobulations, undercuts, and posterior extension.*

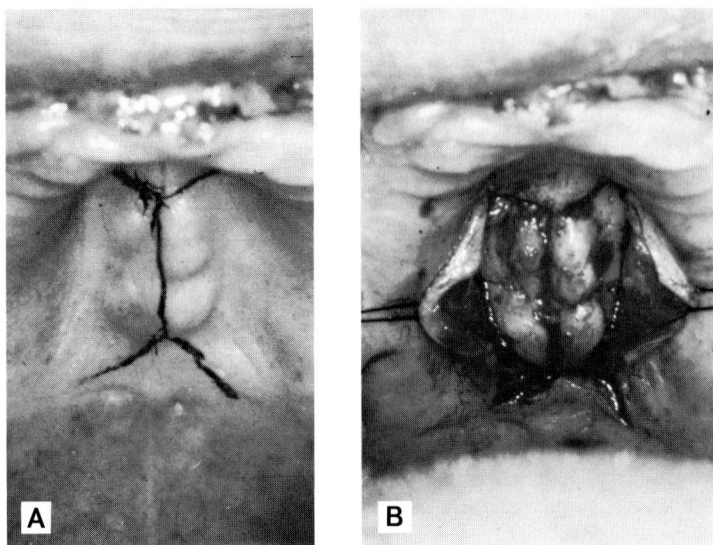

FIG. 20-43. *(A) Torus showing outline of incision for the surgical approach. (B) Flap reflected and traction sutures used to hold the flap.*

Mandibular tori are similar to the palatal tori except for location. They occur less frequently, develop above the mylohyoid muscle attachment, and occur bilaterally in most instances (Fig. 20-47). Their removal is similar to that for palatal tori, except when they occur with a narrow base, as on a pedicle. In this case, the chisel is best utilized.

Rarely can mandibular tori be tolerated by the denture-wearing patient. It is most appropriate to reduce these exostoses with a rotary reduction bur or a unibevel chisel at the time of the extraction of the posterior teeth. Great care must be exercised in the reflection of the overlying soft tissues. A seemingly minor tear or "button hole" of the mucosa results in increased postoperative pain and delayed healing.

Once the tori have been exposed, they can be removed with a chisel if a narrow base is present. A natural cleavage point exists at the junction of the torus and the mandible. If the osteotome is placed at the junction of the exostosis and the mandible with the bevel facing away from the lingual cortex, and if the chisel is tapped carefully but firmly with a mallet, the torus separates cleanly from the body of the mandible (Fig. 20-48).

The major complicating aspect of this procedure is that of access: a sufficiently long incision must be made to provide good vision and surgical access. This may include an incision from the molar area to the midline (Fig. 20-49). In bilateral tori removal it is desirable, if possible, to leave the mucoperiosteum attached to the midline. There is also less space for hematoma formation if the mylohyoid muscle is not stripped away and the excess flap is re-

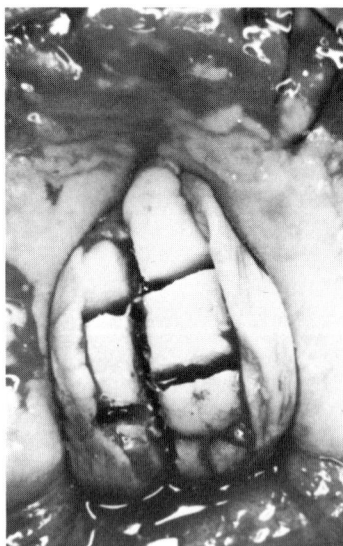

FIG. 20-44. *Torus showing the bony mass sectioned by the high-speed drill.*

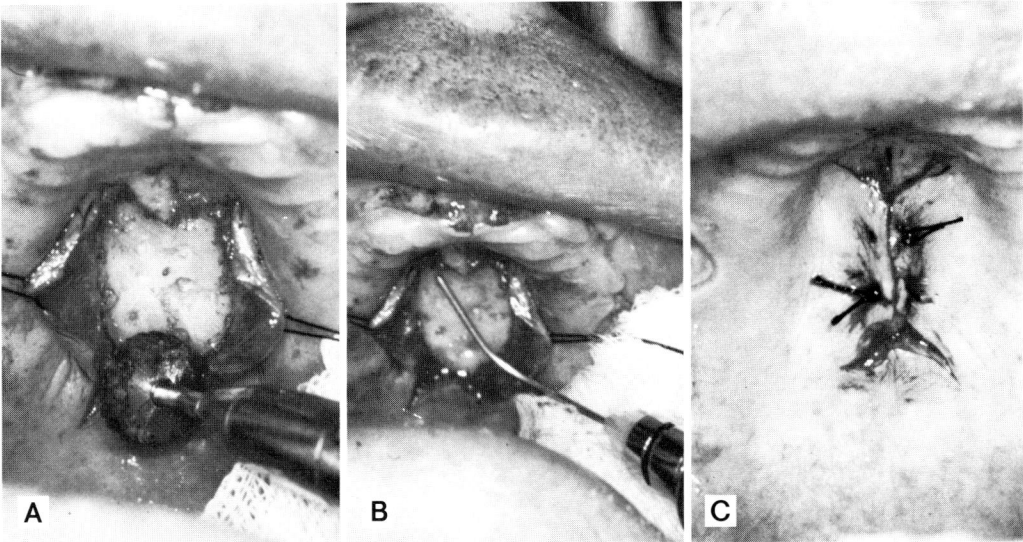

FIG. 20-45. (A) Smoothing of the bony surgical site with rotary high-speed instrument. (B) Final toilet of the wound with saline solution. (C) Flap returned and mattress suture used to evert the flap.

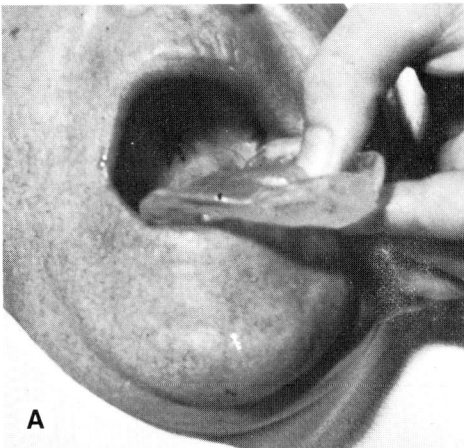

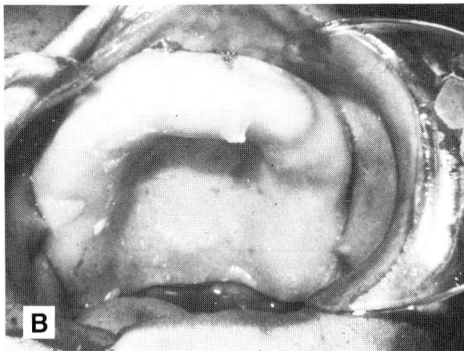

FIG. 20-46. (A) Full arch acrylic splint inserted for postoperative comfort and protection to the wound. (B) Palatal splint protects soft tissues during healing phase.

moved from the incised margin and sutured firmly.

A previously constructed acrylic splint is the best way to ensure tissue adaptation and to limit edema and hematoma formation (Fig. 20-50). The presence of the salivary ducts and the lingual nerve, and the ease with which postoperative edema and infection occur in the floor of the mouth, add to the concern regarding any surgery in this area.

The surgical removal of multiple exostoses is basically no different than that for tori, except that exostoses occur with no uniformity as to location. They also may appear singularly around the arch or in multiple formation (Fig. 20-51). The relationship of osteomas as a part of Gardner's

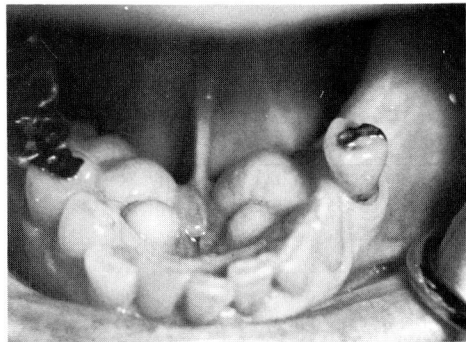

FIG. 20-47. Multiple mandibular tori.

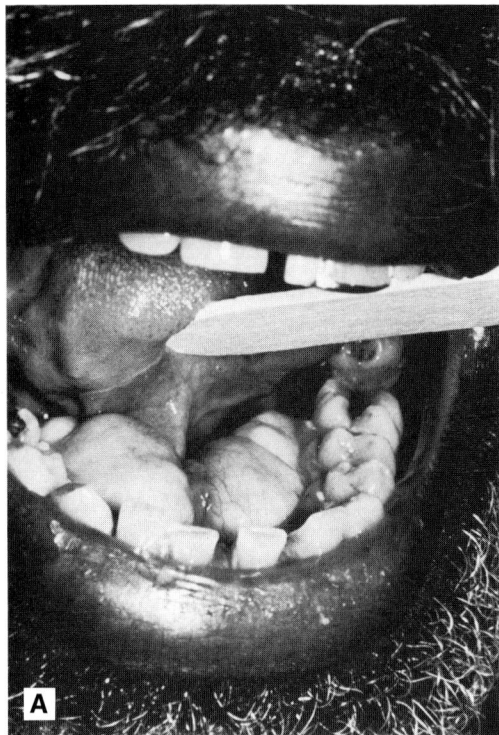

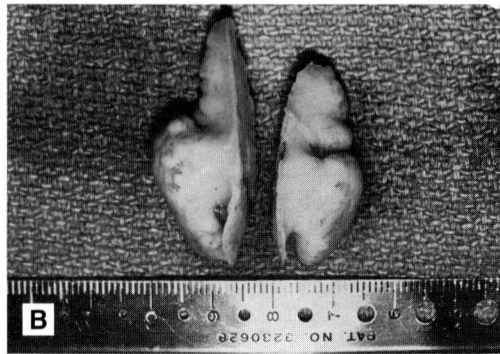

FIG. 20-48. *(A and B) Large mandibular tori removed en bloc with osteotome. (C) Lingual splint used to eliminate dead space between tissue and bone.*

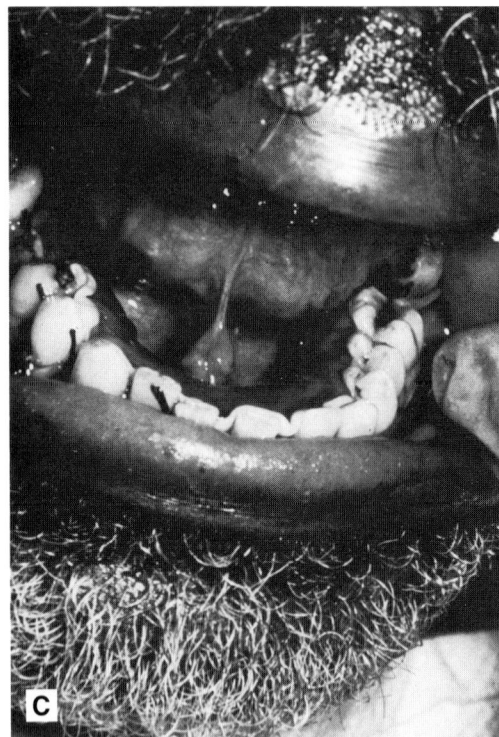

syndrome should be considered, particularly if supernumerary teeth are present.[4] The term "enostosis" appears in the literature. In contrast to exostosis, it is a similarly dense radiopaque ossification except that it is confined within the cortical walls and is not palpable (Fig. 20-52).

The bony maxillary tuberosity is reduced to increase the vertical space between the arches and to remove undercut in preprosthetic surgery (Fig. 20-53). The bone of this area is usually cancellous and can be reduced easily with rongeurs or files. An excess amount of mucoperiosteal flap may

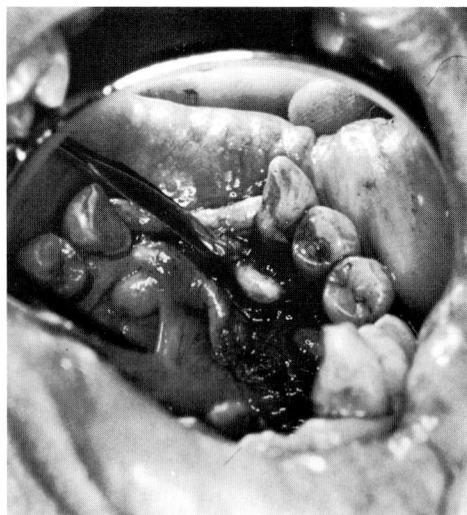

FIG. 20-49. *Surgical removal of mandibular tori (mirror image). Note incision length.*

The genial tubercle is a normal anatomic protuberance on the lingual symphysis of the mandible that corresponds to the attachment of the genioglossus and the geniohyoid muscles. During the process of

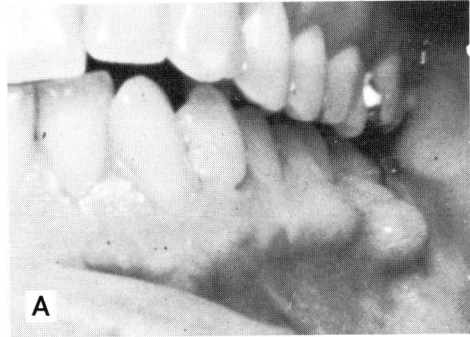

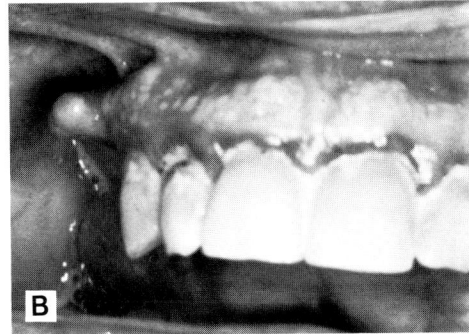

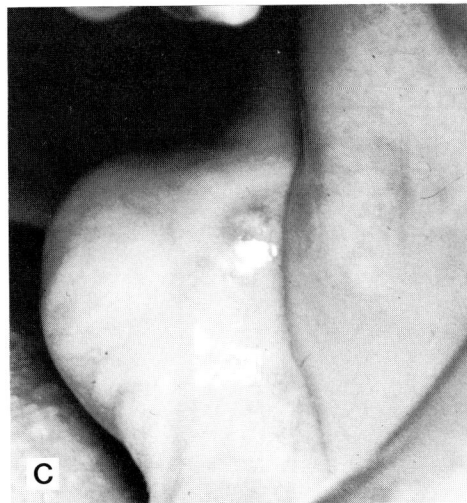

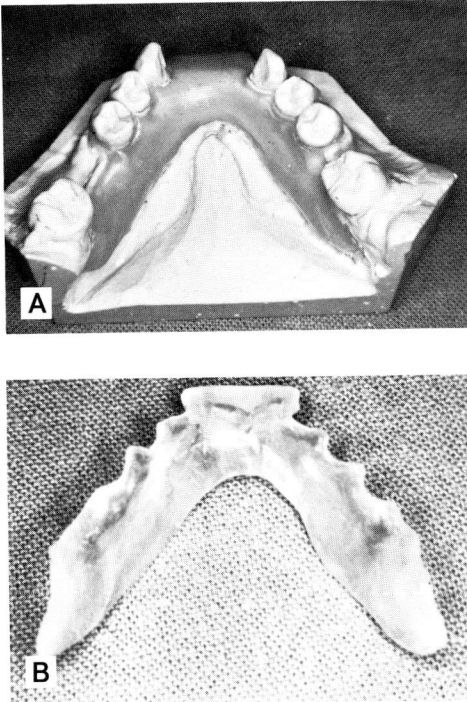

FIG. 20-50. *(A) Model showing reduction of tori and wax-up for splint construction. (B) The acrylic splint.*

be present, necessitating a wedge excision for appropriate closure.

The mylohyoid ridge, or the internal oblique line, is a bony prominence that frequently interferes with the prosthesis (Fig. 20-54). Its removal is somewhat more difficult and the tissues must be handled delicately. The mucoperiosteal flap is reflected following a horizontal incision on the crest of the ridge. When the muscle fibers come into view, they can be sectioned with the scissors or stripped with a periosteal elevator. The bony prominence is then reduced using the chisel or file until the sharpness and/or undercut is removed.

The term "endoalveolar crest" is not often used, but refers to the bony prominence lingual to the mandibular third molar (Fig. 20-54). This bony balcony is not the same as the mylohyoid ridge. There is no muscle attachment to it, and it should be reduced at the time of the third molar removal. When this is not done, the bony projection may become sharp, irritate the tongue, and interfere with the prosthesis (Fig. 20-55).

FIG. 20-51. *(A) Multiple mandibular exostoses. (B) Maxillary buccal exostoses. (C) Large lingual exostosis in edentulous patient opposite the third molar area.*

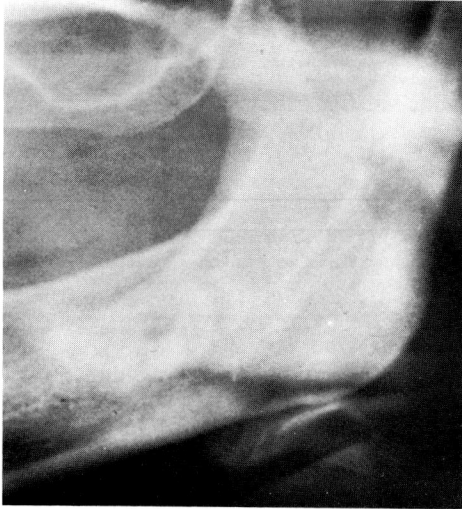

FIG. 20-52. *Enostosis in body of the mandible.*

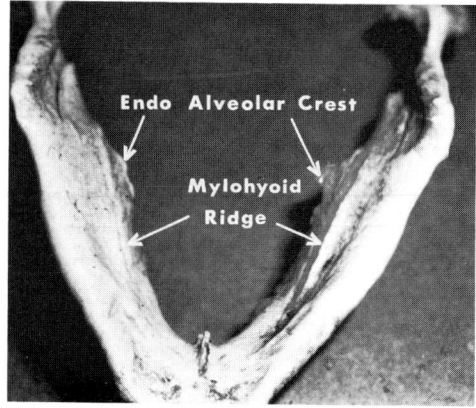

FIG. 20-54. *Mylohyoid ridge and endoalveolar crest.*

ridge atrophy or alveolar bone resorption, these bony prominences and their muscle attachments may appear entirely on the crest of the ridge (Fig. 20-56). They may interfere with the prosthesis, necessitating their removal and lowering of the muscle attachment (Figs. 20-57 and 20-58).

A sharp, spiny, knife-like ridge may be painful for a patient (Fig. 20-59), but surgery on it should be avoided. Any surgery may result in total loss of the ridge, making prosthodontic construction more difficult. Denture adjustment or special prosthetic

construction may be indicated to provide patient comfort.

SKIN GRAFTING

Although all techniques have varying degrees of success, the vestibular extension methods described previously in the chapter frequently result in the eventual loss of much of the extension gained. This is caused by a gradually increasing fibrosis of

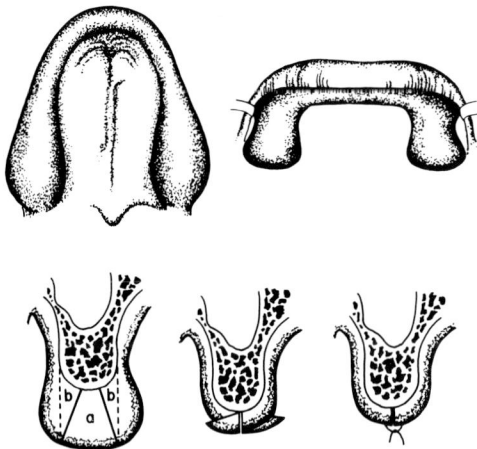

FIG. 20-53. *Tuberosity—buccal undercut—demonstrating the wedge resection method for surgical correction.*

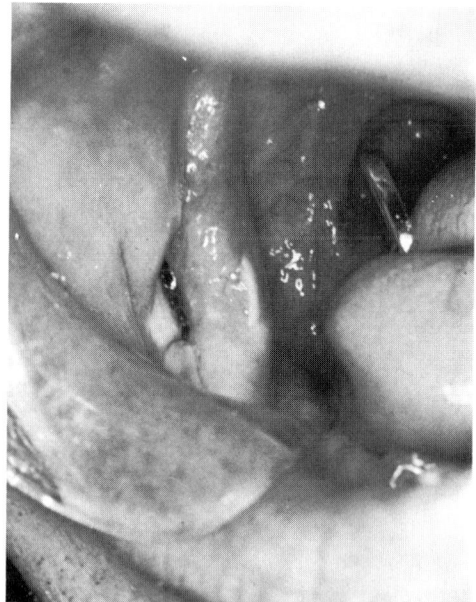

FIG. 20-55. *Ulceration of the lingual mucosa due to sharp endoalveolar crest not reduced at time of surgery.*

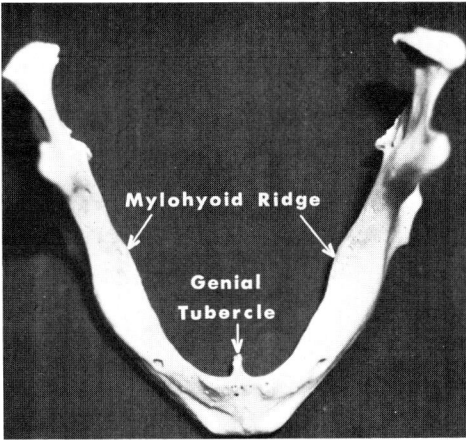

FIG. 20-56. *Mandible showing mylohyoid ridge and genial tubercle.*

exposed granulation tissue and resultant progressive contraction. However, this loss seems to be minimized when a split-thickness skin graft is used in conjunction with the vestibuloplasty. In such instances, the successful skin graft depends on rapid revascularization, which in turn depends on the vascularity of the host bed and adequate fixation of the grafted skin to the periosteum.

The actual procedure of using skin in the oral cavity to prevent infection or scar formation, or to cover defects from tumor surgery or trauma, dates back to the late nineteenth century. The Thiersch graft for defects of the buccal mucosa were among

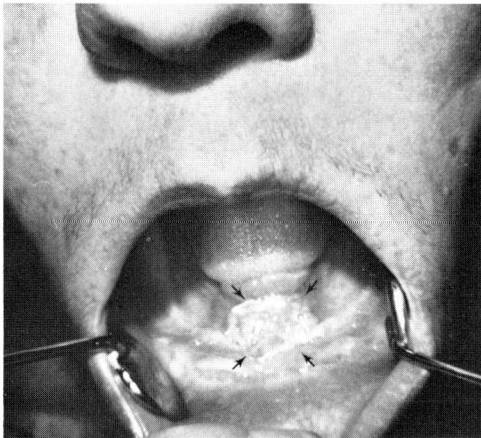

FIG. 20-58. *Technique for lowering the genioglossus muscle. (A and B) Genioglossus muscle is isolated. (C) Muscle is cut free. (D) A circumferential nonabsorbable suture is passed with a stop knot (■). The suture around the muscle is tied beneath the stop knot. (E) Muscle is repositioned. (F) Ten days later, the circumferential suture is removed in a reverse manner.*

the first used.[6] Skin grafting was later described by Moskowicz and Esser in the early twentieth century.[7,8] Pichler, in 1931, presented probably the best series of covering intraoral defects with skin to prevent

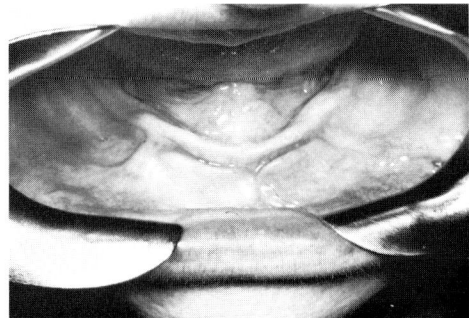

FIG. 20-57. *Need for genial tubercle reduction and muscle lowering.*

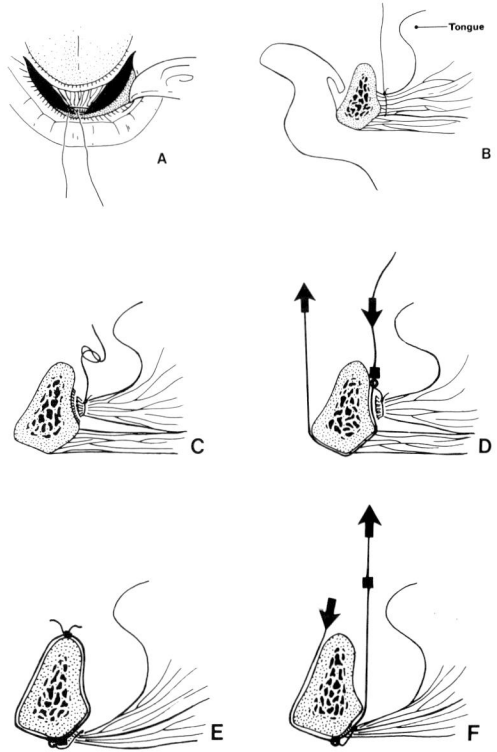

FIG. 20-59. *Knife-like mandibular ridge.*

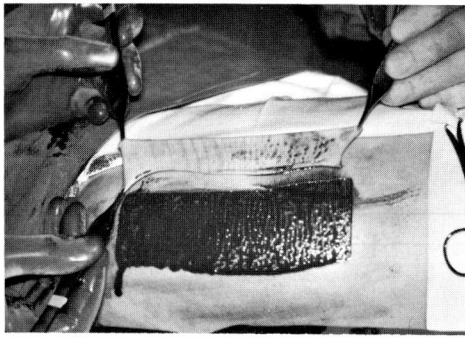

FIG. 20-60. *Split-thickness skin graft taken from the thigh.*

scarring and shrinkage of the soft tissue.[9]

Obwegeser improved the "buccal inlay technique" originally described by Gillies.[10] This was the beginning of extensive skin grafting in the oral cavity for ridge extension procedures. In recent years, vestibuloplasty utilizing the split-thickness skin graft has gained considerable success.

Technique. Prior to surgery, the clinician takes impressions of the alveolar ridge and constructs a duplicate plaster or stone model. A lateral cephalogram is also taken to provide accurate information on bony contours and outline. The duplicated cast is contoured to permit construction of the tray, allowing adequate relief in the area of the mental nerves. The buccal and labial aspects are extended along the entire length of the periphery. If the patient has a

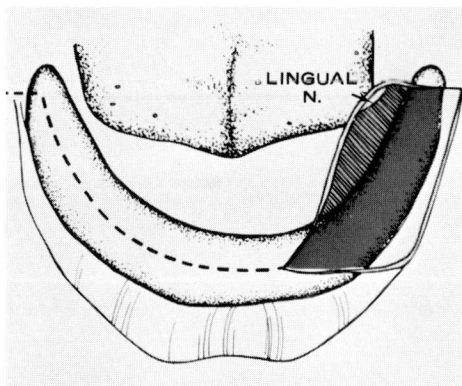

FIG. 20-61. *Schematic drawing showing incision for vestibuloplasty with skin graft. Note extension of incision at 90° angle into vestibule; also note location of lingual nerve.*

denture, this can be modified at the time of surgery and used as the surgical splint.

The dermatome is used to take skin from the outer aspect of the thigh or buttocks. Care is taken to select an area devoid of hair. Transplanted hair follicles will survive thus creating a nuisance for the patient. A split-thickness graft best measures approximately 0.015 to 0.018 inch in thickness (Fig. 20-60). Although a full-thickness graft undergoes less contracture, the split-thickness has a higher degree of "take" and, when placed directly against periosteum, undergoes minimal shrinkage. The graft is wrapped in a saline-solution-soaked gauze and the donor site covered with an appropriate dressing.

The recipient site is prepared in the following manner. The buccal, labial, and lingual tissues are injected with a local anesthetic solution containing a vasoconstrictor, and an incision is made on the crest of the ridge throughout the arch (Fig. 20-61). It is carried through the mucosae only, without cutting into the periosteum, and the labiobuccal supraperiosteal flap is reflected by careful dissection (Fig. 20-62A and B). If the periosteum is perforated, small bur holes can be placed in the cortical plate. This provides a means by which medullary endothelium can revascularize the graft.

The incision for lowering the floor of the mouth is made in a sweeping manner at the junction of the lingual attached and unattached gingivae, extending from the retromolar area to the midline. The lingual nerve is near the posterior limit of this incision (Fig. 20-62C). The mylohyoid muscle is cut free from its attachment, and the remaining lingual depth can be established by using the finger to strip away attachments of the submandibular gland and other visceral tissues in this area (Fig. 20-62D). The superior and lateral parts of the genioglossus muscle are also incised, but the entire muscle is not detached. Sutures are then placed, using awls to draw the mucosal margins of both the lingual and labial buccal surfaces together near the lower, or inferior, portion of the body of the mandible, upon which the skin graft will be applied (Fig. 20-62E, F, and G). The previously constructed splint or denture is lined with dental compound and carried to

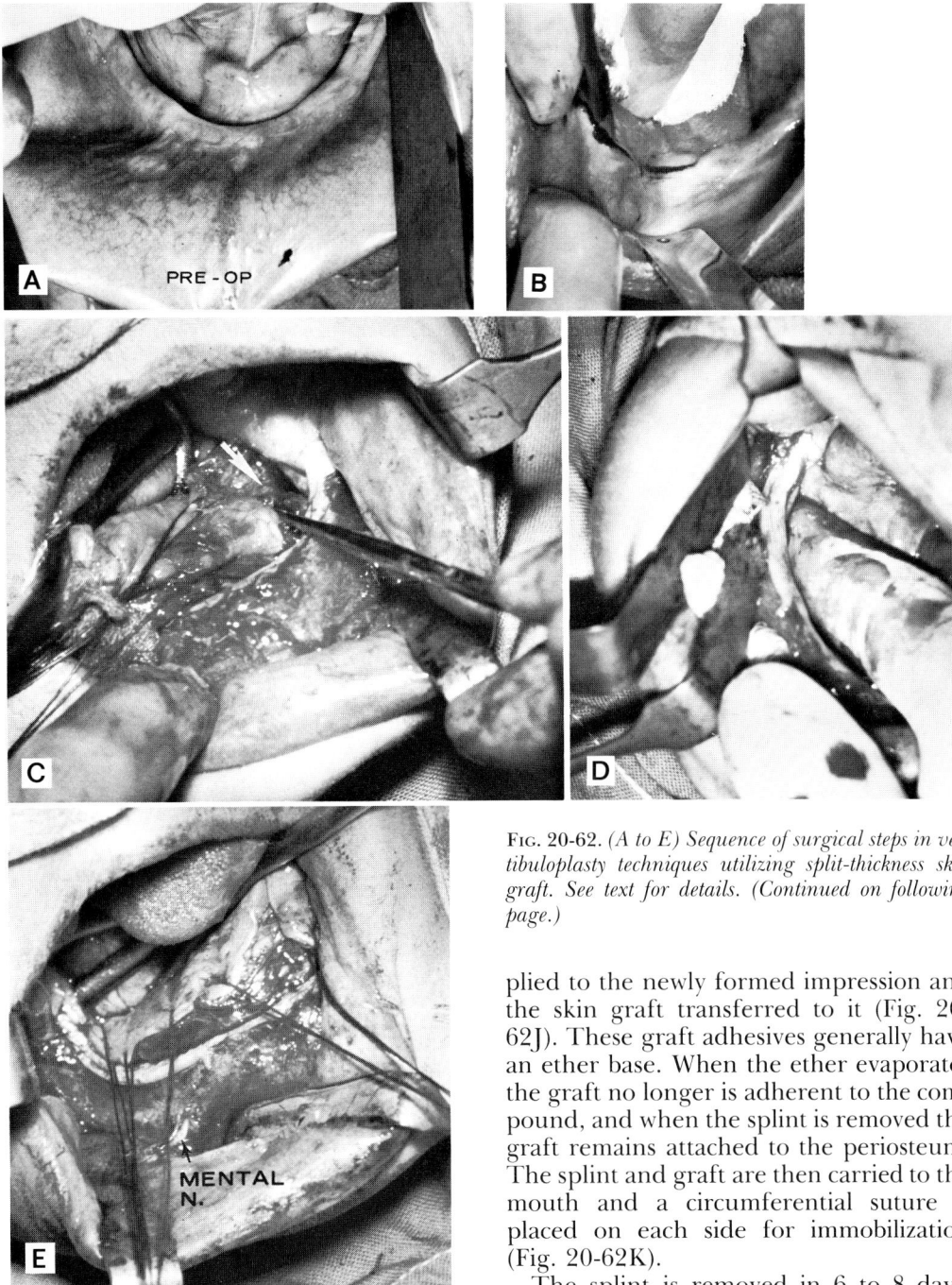

Fig. 20-62. *(A to E) Sequence of surgical steps in vestibuloplasty techniques utilizing split-thickness skin graft. See text for details. (Continued on following page.)*

plied to the newly formed impression and the skin graft transferred to it (Fig. 20-62J). These graft adhesives generally have an ether base. When the ether evaporates the graft no longer is adherent to the compound, and when the splint is removed the graft remains attached to the periosteum. The splint and graft are then carried to the mouth and a circumferential suture is placed on each side for immobilization (Fig. 20-62K).

The splint is removed in 6 to 8 days, when a "take" should be evident. A new prosthesis can be constructed in 6 to 8 weeks (Fig. 20-62L, M, and N). It is desirable for the patient to wear the splint until the new denture is constructed to limit any change in vestibular depth. Skin grafts can also be utilized to increase the vestibular depth in the maxilla (Fig. 20-63).

the mouth and an impression taken (Fig. 20-62H). This is immediately cooled and examined for reasonable accuracy. It can be further improved by the use of gutta-form (Obwegeser) for the final impression (Fig. 20-62I). A skin graft adhesive is ap-

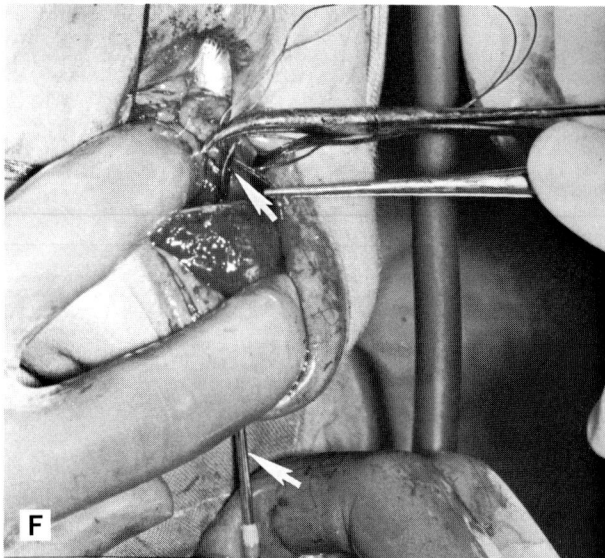

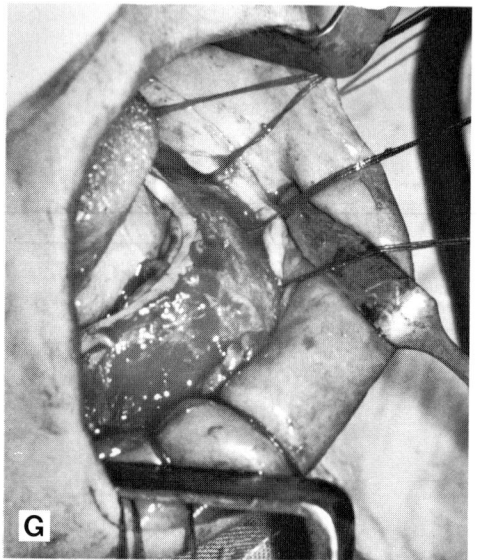

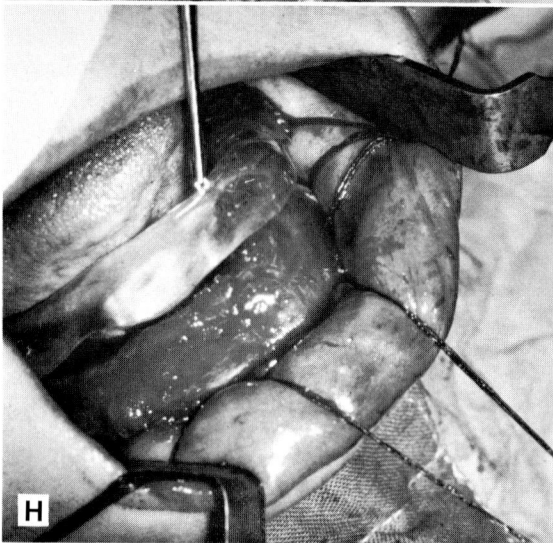

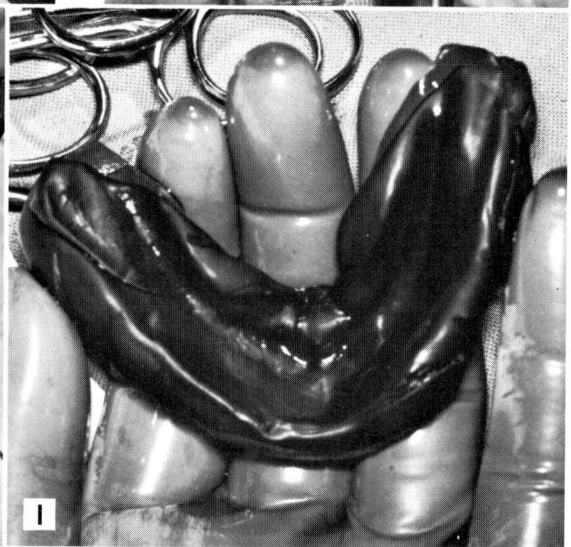

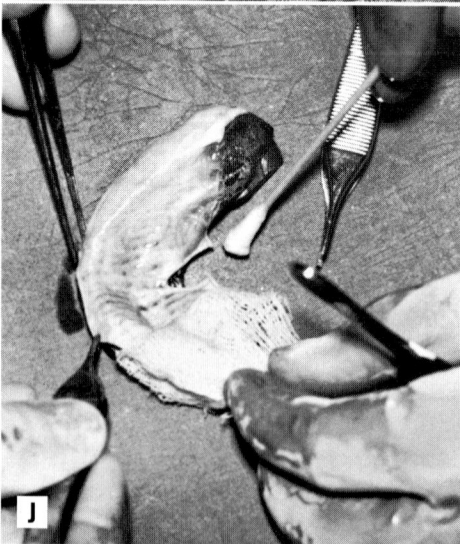

FIG. 20-62 (continued). (F to J) Vestibuloplasty technique utilizing split-thickness skin graft. See text for details. (Continued on facing page.)

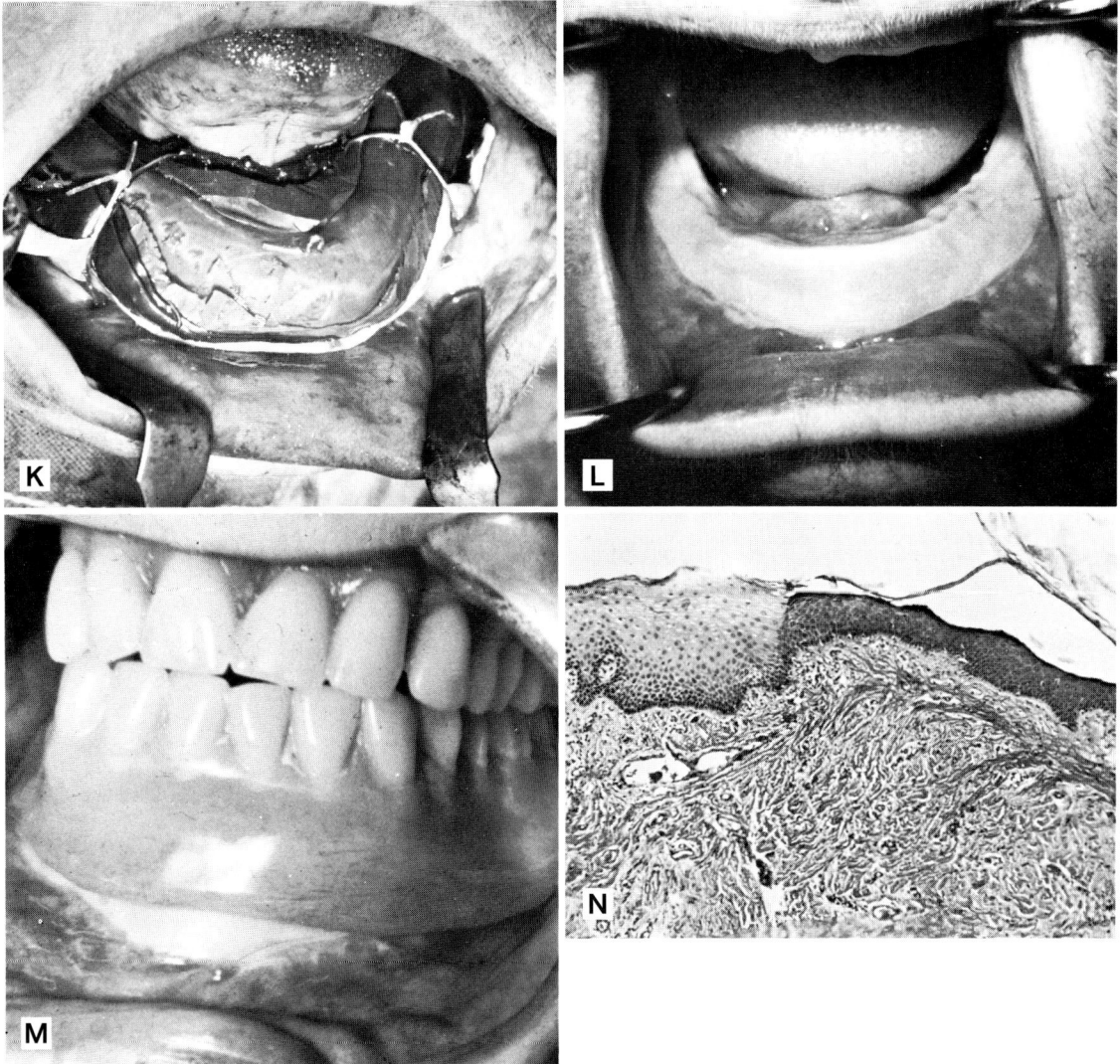

FIG. 20-62 (continued). *(K to M) Vestibuloplasty technique utilizing split-thickness skin graft. See text for details. (N) Histologic section of mucosa and skin. Note thickness of skin (on right) compared to mucosa (on left) for denture-bearing surface.*

Mucosal grafts are successful and more nearly reproduce the normal ridge tissue (Fig. 20-64). If the required vestibuloplasty is extensive, however, adequate mucosa may not be available. The mucosal strip graft is acquired from cheek, lips, and palate. The palatal donor site, however, can be a source of chronic irritation and inflammation while a large buccal donor site may scar and limit the patient's maximum opening. Steinhauser recommends mucosal grafting mainly in the atrophic maxilla, because adhesion and retention of the den-ture are more favorable with mucosa than with the skin grafting.[11] However, it should be remembered that the vertical height of the ridge is more important in maxillary denture retention than is the depth of the labial sulcus. An extensive labial skin or mucosa graft in a patient who has lost the majority of his maxillary alveolar ridge height does little to improve the maxillary denture retention and function.

BONE REBUILDING

In more severe cases of mandibular

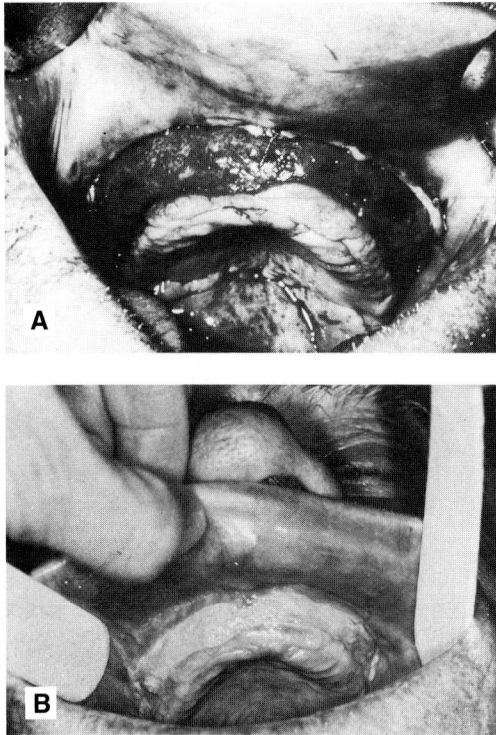

Fig. 20-63. *(A) Maxillary labial vestibuloplasty. (B) With skin graft.*

ridge atrophy—when it is not possible to increase the vestibular space by any of the aforementioned procedures—bone rebuilding may be necessary. This may be accomplished by the use of rib, cartilage, or iliac crestal bone with varying degrees of success.

Blocks of iliac crestal bone may be used to reconstruct the mandible (Fig. 20-65). Occasionally, a second procedure consisting of a vestibuloplasty with skin graft may be necessary once the bone graft has healed. (Fig. 20-66).

Significant bone resorption has occurred (89 percent in some cases) within 4 years after surgery.[12] However, most patients have indicated acceptable results. Although some of the ridge height has been lost, a broad bony base seems to replace the previous knife-like, painful ridge, thus permitting the wearer of the prosthesis more comfort (Fig. 20-67). The greatest problem with iliac crest grafts relates to donor site morbidity. The most common forms are pain, paresthesia, and gait abnormalities.

Autogenous rib has also been used, particularly in the maxilla. The rib donor site usually causes less postoperative morbidity than the iliac crest site unless pneumothorax occurs. However, rib resorption is usually more extensive than that of iliac crest and is probably a result of less bone marrow. (Fig. 20-68).

It has been observed that when mandibular bone graft augmentation is followed by an implant that stabilizes the prosthesis, bone loss can be minimized. The bone graft is allowed to heal and mature for 6 months prior to implant insertion. Theoretically, the stabilized implant denture produces more evenly distributed stress on the grafted bone, thus limiting the amount of pressure resorption (Fig. 20-69).

Alloplastic Implants in Reconstructive Preprosthetic Surgery

Prior to 1975 the concept of "implants" in preprosthetic surgery was viewed with skepticism if not with blatant professional animosity. The results of implant procedures were extremely poor (less than 50 percent, 5-year survival), and dentists who advocated implant use were severely criticized for their lack of professionalism. However, during the past 15 years interest in implant surgery has increased and, because of improved materials and techniques, implants have achieved credibility within the dental profession.

The patient (usually female) with severe mandibular resorption can now be totally reconstructed without bone or skin grafts. These potentially morbid surgical procedures are being replaced by procedures that augment the mandible with bone substitute materials (hydroxylapatite), followed by the insertion of transosseous implants. This combined approach provides the patient with improved alveolar ridge height and a mechanism for the stabilization of the prosthesis without the morbidity associated with bone and skin grafting.

HA is an inert material and chemically similar to bone. The current technique for its use in maxillary and mandibular augmentation involves the application of anterior vertical incisions followed by the development of bilateral subperiosteal tunnels.

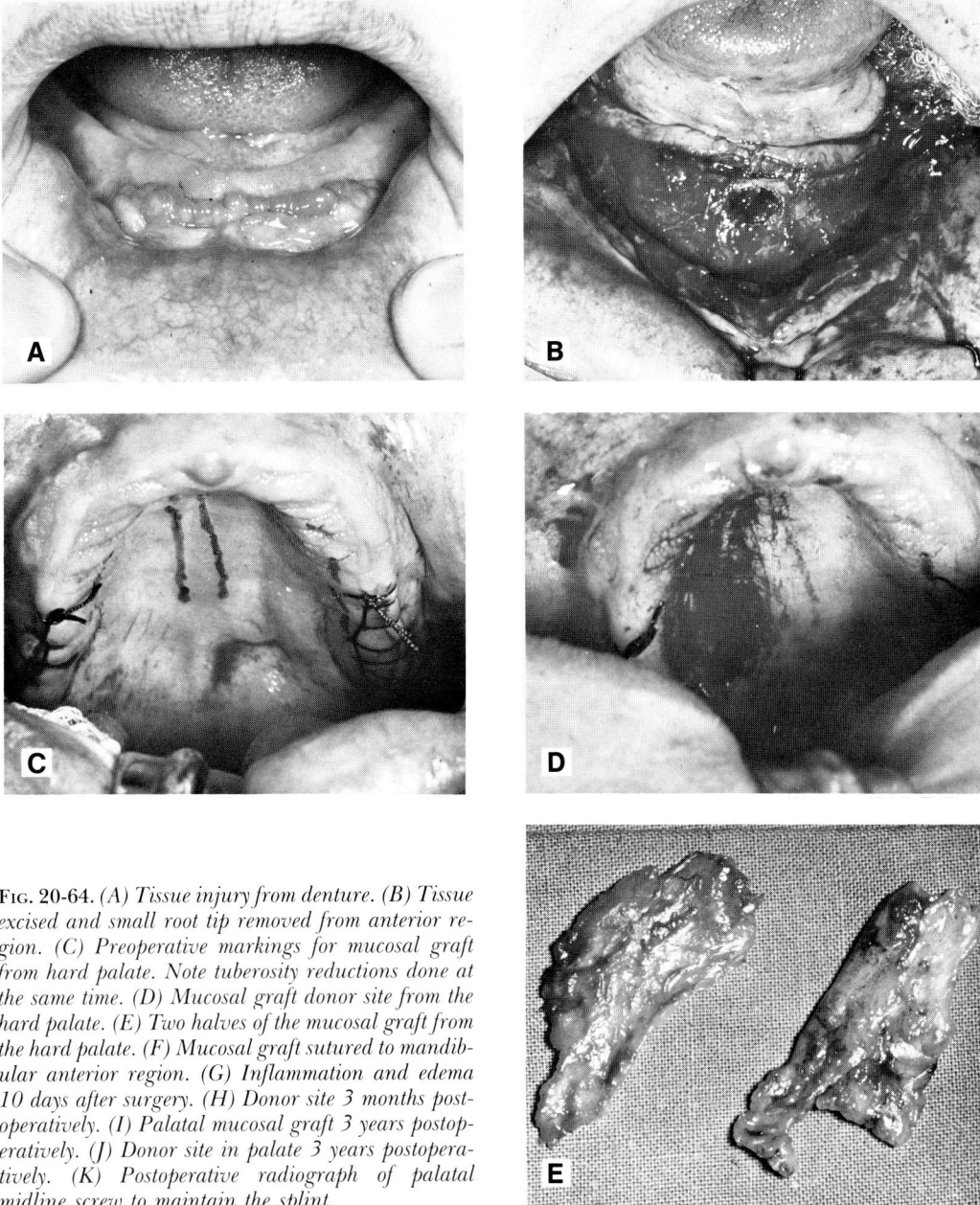

FIG. 20-64. *(A) Tissue injury from denture. (B) Tissue excised and small root tip removed from anterior region. (C) Preoperative markings for mucosal graft from hard palate. Note tuberosity reductions done at the same time. (D) Mucosal graft donor site from the hard palate. (E) Two halves of the mucosal graft from the hard palate. (F) Mucosal graft sutured to mandibular anterior region. (G) Inflammation and edema 10 days after surgery. (H) Donor site 3 months postoperatively. (I) Palatal mucosal graft 3 years postoperatively. (J) Donor site in palate 3 years postoperatively. (K) Postoperative radiograph of palatal midline screw to maintain the splint.*

The HA is then inserted by an injection technique, and the newly formed ridge is covered for 14 to 21 days with a surgical splint. During this time the HA particles are engulfed principally by dense connective tissue providing for an increased vestibular depth and improved denture-bearing area (Fig. 20-70). HA can also be mixed with particulate corticocancellous bone chips which have been harvested through a small opening made in the patient's iliac crest (Fig. 20-71). This technique increases the volume of material available for ridge augmentation and increases the probability that the HA will be surrounded by bone rather than by fibrous connective tissue.

A problem with the use of HA has been the lack of control of the particles at the time of surgery. It is not uncommon to see patients with HA augmentation in which

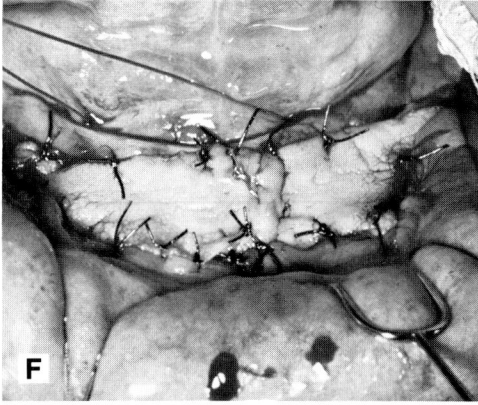

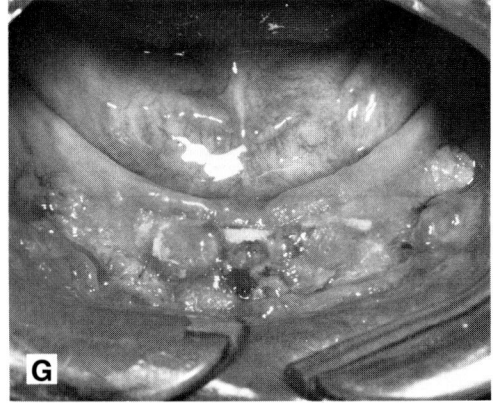

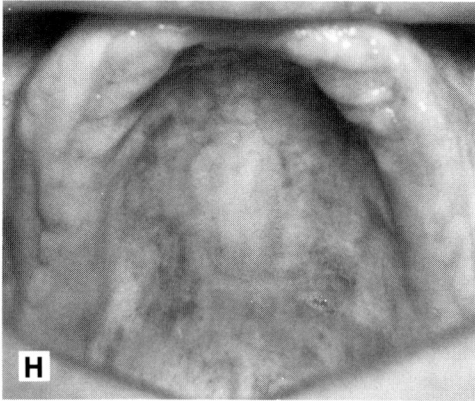

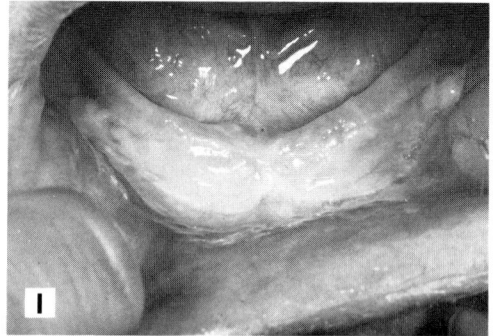

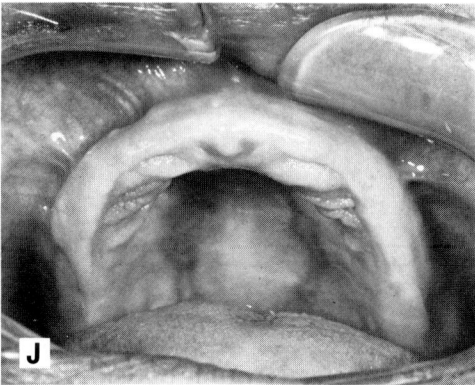

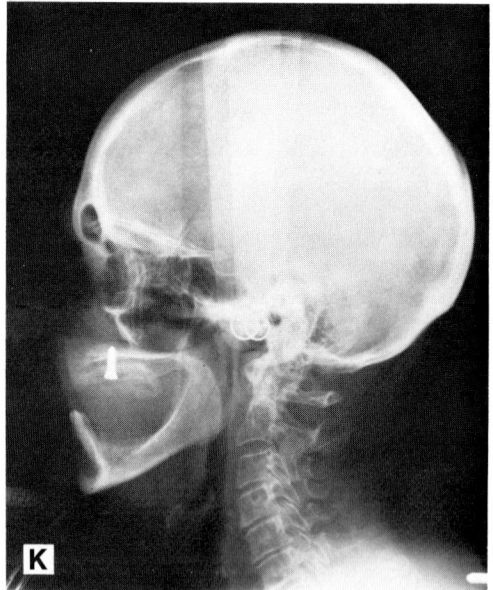

FIG. 20-64 (continued). *See legend on page 397.*

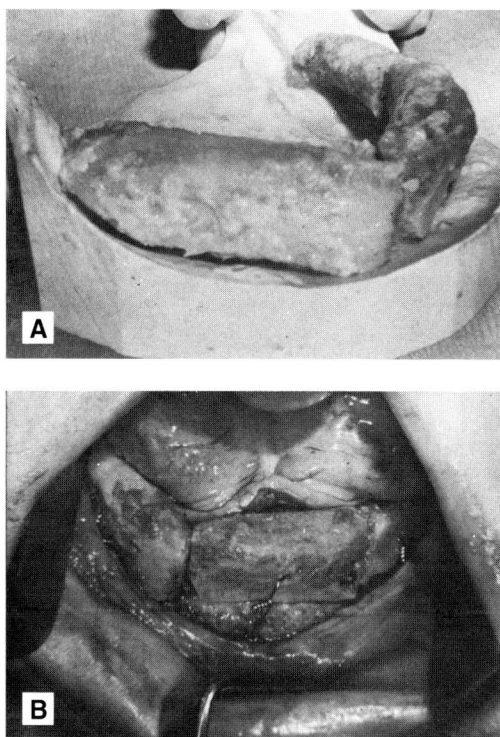

FIG. 20-65. *(A) Blocks of iliac crestal bone formed on sterilized model in the operating room. (B) Blocks stabilized with circummandibular wires.*

the material has flowed into unintended anatomic areas, e.g., floor of mouth and buccal soft tissues. It now appears that, as a result of improved technology, the reconstructive surgeon can insert this material in a more stable "block" form.

In the patient with a mandibular vertical height of 9 mm or more, reconstruction can be best achieved with the use of endosseous or transosseous implants. With the development of biologically acceptable materials (titanium) and improved surgical and prosthetic techniques, implants inserted in a medically acceptable patient now have a 95 percent 10-year survival rate. Patients with systemic medical problems such as diabetes mellitus or severe metabolic bone disorders must be evaluated carefully prior to their acceptance as implant patients.

The ideal reconstructive implant material should be biologically acceptable, strong, and should lend itself to osseous

integration. This direct and intimate contact between bone and implant is critical to implant survival. Various types of titanium endosseous implants are placed transorally and have been shown to exhibit integration between the bone and implant material.

A transosseous implant that meets the criteria of biologic acceptability and osseous integration is the mandibular staple bone plate (Fig. 20-72). This implant has a 20-year history of clinical acceptability. The staple is inserted by means of a extraoral approach. After a submental incision has been made, five or seven parallel holes are placed in the mandible with a low-speed, high-torque drill. The staple bone plate is then inserted, tapped to place, and fasteners are inserted on the threaded transosteal pins (Fig. 20-73). The patient's current denture is then modified to accept the transosseous pins and relined with a soft reline material. The patient

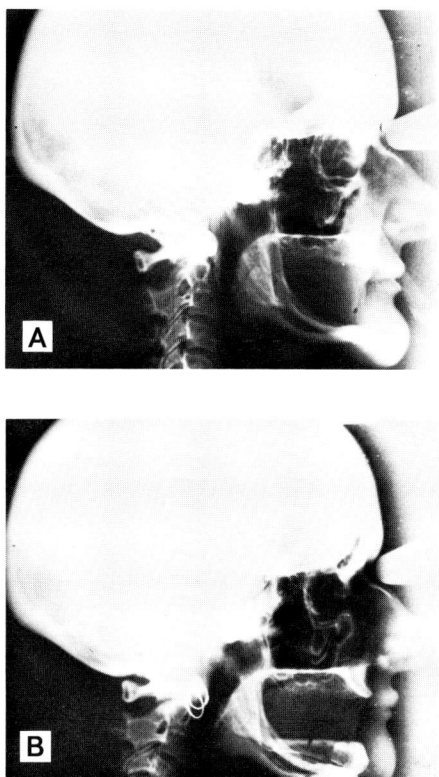

FIG. 20-66. *(A) Preoperative cephalogram of 38-year-old patient. (B) Cephalogram following ridge augmentation with iliac bone crest.*

FOLLOW-UP STUDY ON RIDGE AUGMENTATION PROCEDURE

MALE PATIENTS

	1	2	3	4	5	6	7	8	9	10	11	12	17	29	30	38	41
CASE #1			*23%								69%		77%	77%			
CASE #2		14%					*67%				89%				100%		
CASE #3		32%		*				32%									
CASE #4					22%		25%			*		67%					
CASE #5	0%	*7%			13%				35%								

% OF RESORPTION – (IN MONTHS) ILIAC CREST

A

* INDICATES THE DATE THE SKIN GRAFT PROCEDURE WAS DONE

ILIAC CREST GRAFT
5 PATIENTS–AVERAGE AUGMENTATION

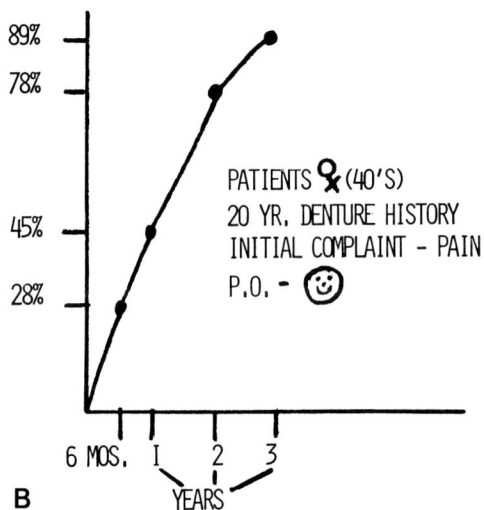

89%
78%
45%
28%

PATIENTS ♀ (40'S)
20 YR. DENTURE HISTORY
INITIAL COMPLAINT – PAIN
P.O. – ☺

6 MOS. 1 2 3
YEARS

B

FIG. 20-67. *Documented studies of bone resorption of patients receiving a bone graft for ridge augmentation. (Courtesy of Wang and Waite)*

functions with a soft diet for 8 weeks, and at that time a precision appliance is constructed (Fig. 20-74). When the new prosthesis is constructed, it is imperative that the denture is tissue borne and does not apply vertical force to the implant during function. The 10-year survival rate of staple bone plates exceeds 95 percent.

Because the intermediate pins of the staple are 9 mm in length, the minimum height of a patient's mandible must be 9 mm prior to staple insertion. If the mandibular height, as measured on a cephalometric x-ray, is less than 9 mm, a ridge augmentation procedure with HA can be performed. It is usually advisable to wait 6 to 8 weeks following HA augmentation before inserting the staple bone plate (Fig. 20-75).

Postoperative Problems

Postoperative problems in preprosthetic surgery are extremely variable. Preoperative assessment of the patient's systemic health can help predict the potential for postoperative problems. Systemic problems such as diabetic mellitus, severe osteoporosis, and other metabolic diseases can adversely alter the patient's response to surgery.

In regard to surgical procedures in the maxilla, the anatomic location of the tissues involved and their venous drainage are significant. The extension of infection by this route can result in encephalitis, brain abscess, meningitis, and cavernous sinus thrombosis.

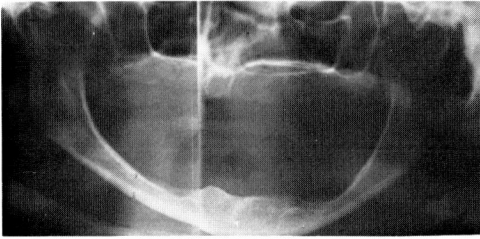

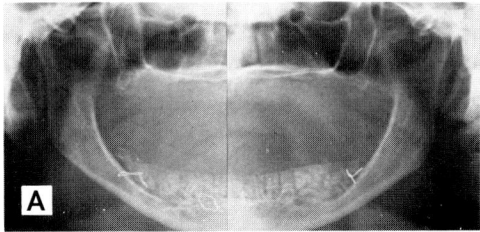

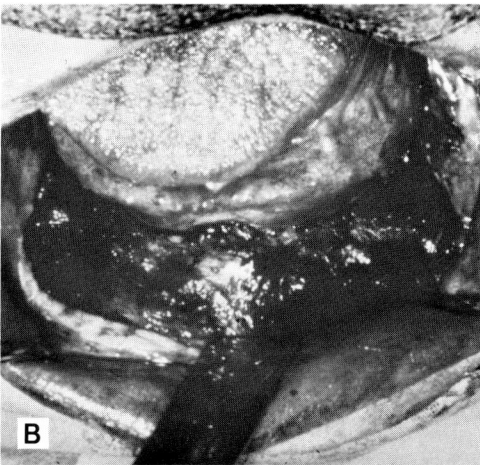

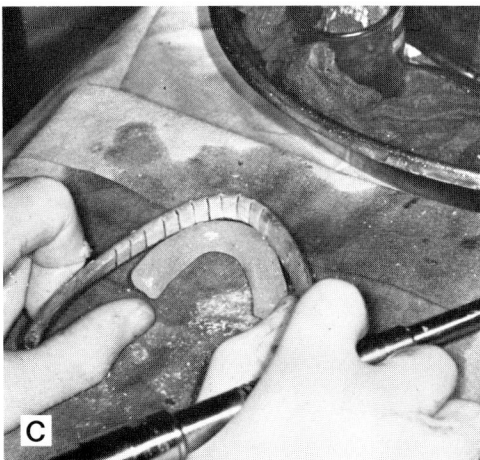

FIG. 20-68. (A) Preoperative and one-year postoperative radiographs of a 40-year-old patient who had rib graft to mandible for pain of lower jaw and inadequate sulcus and ridge. (B) Surgical preparation of mandibular ridge to receive rib graft. (C) Patient's rib (autogenous graft) is contoured to fit a prepared model for placement to the atrophied mandibular bone.

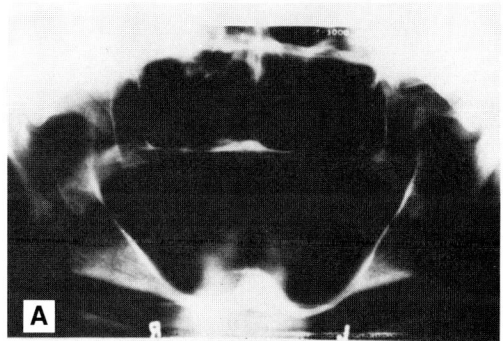

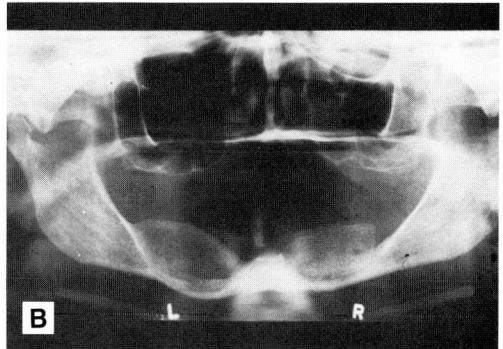

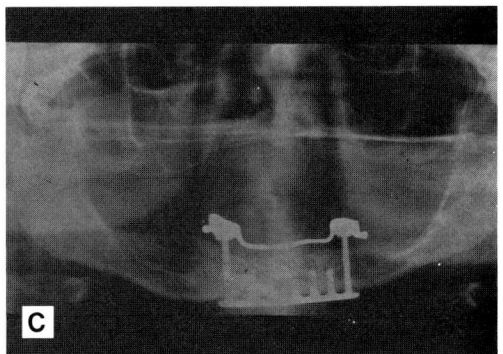

FIG. 20-69. (A) Severely resorbed mandible. (B) Reconstruction with iliac crest bone graft. (C) Minimal bone loss at 10 years because of denture stability provided by implant.

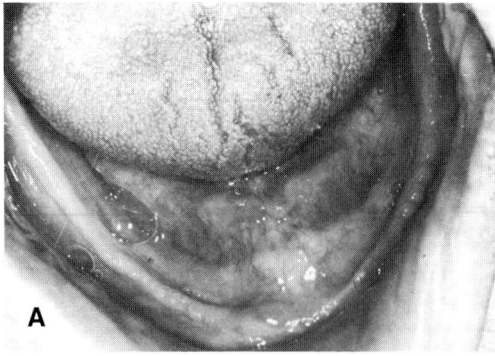

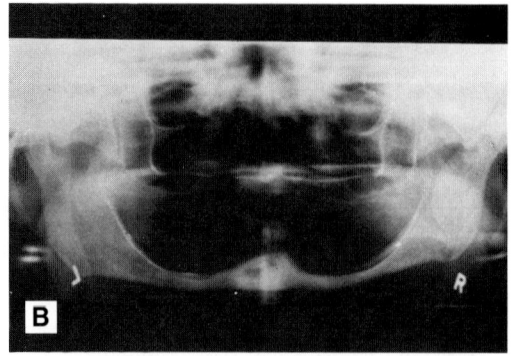

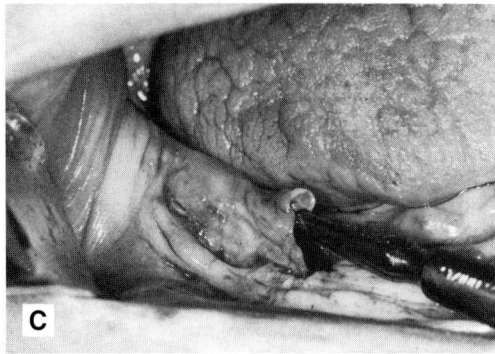

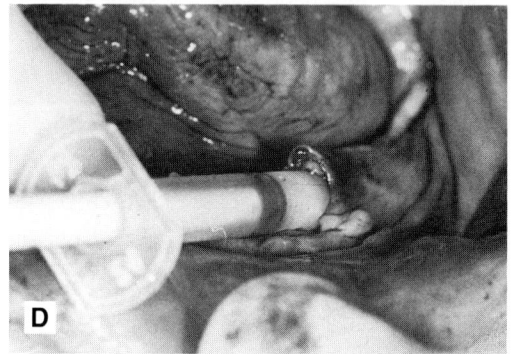

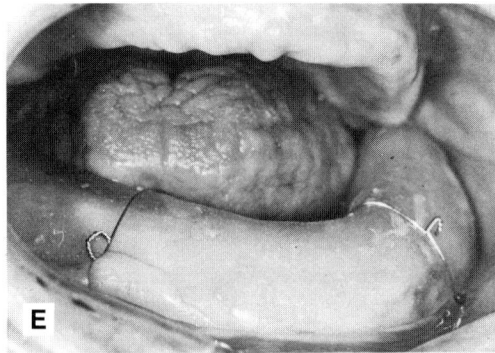

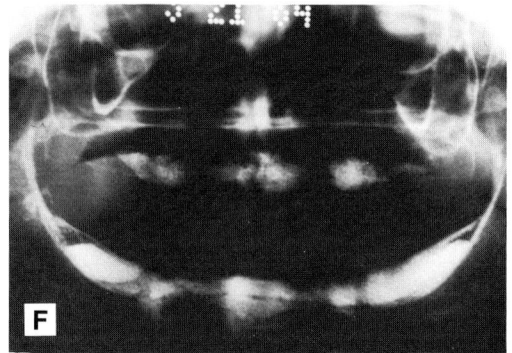

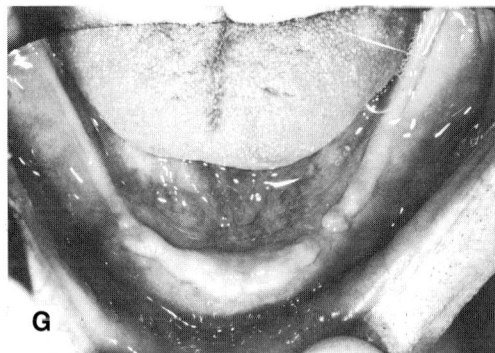

FIG. 20-70. (A) Fibrous alveolar process. (B) Secondary to marked mandibular atrophy. (C) Tunnel created. (D) Hydroxylapatite injected. (E and F) Acrylic splint is used to maintain HA on superior aspect of mandible. (G) Marked improvement in vestibular depth following HA augmentation.

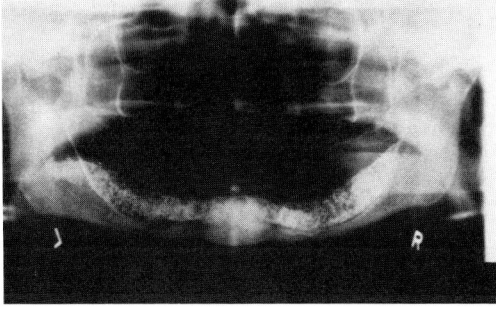

FIG. 20-71. *Panorex of HA-particulate bone graft combination. Notice multiple radiolucent areas occupied by the bone.*

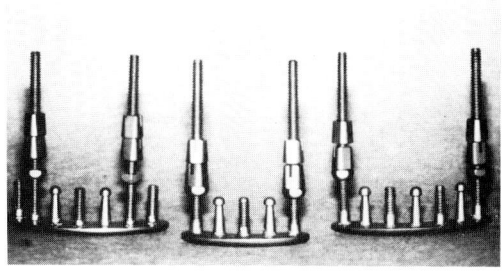

FIG. 20-72. *The three types of staple bone: 5 pin, 7 pin, and modified 7 pin.*

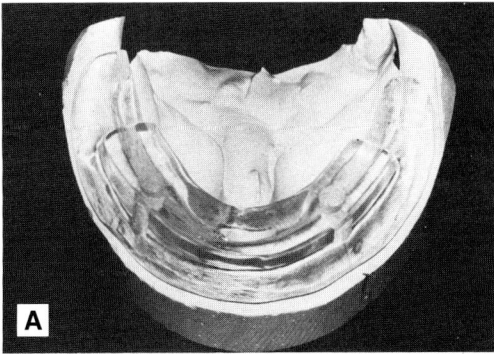

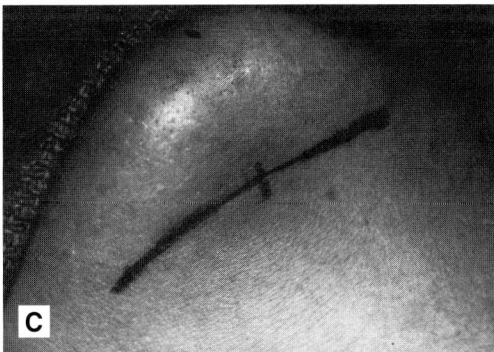

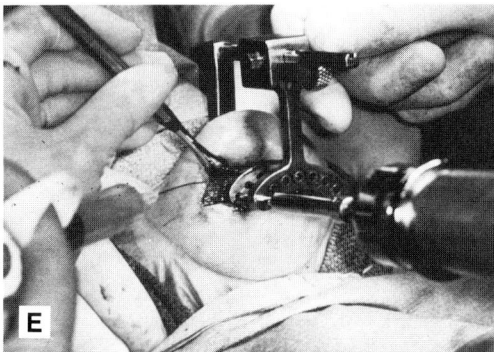

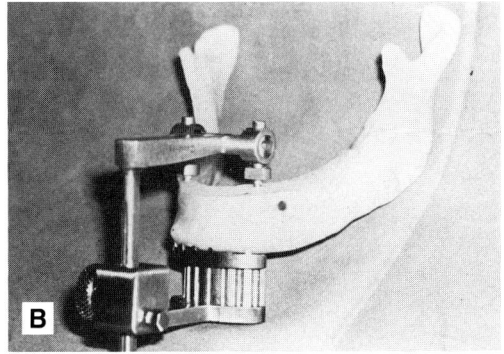

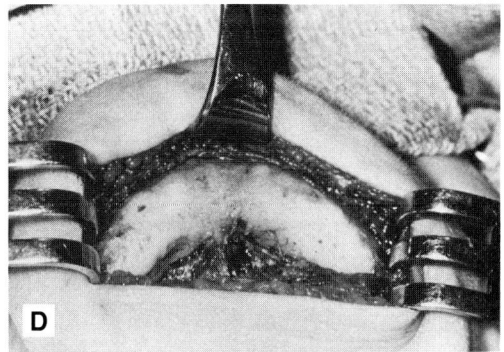

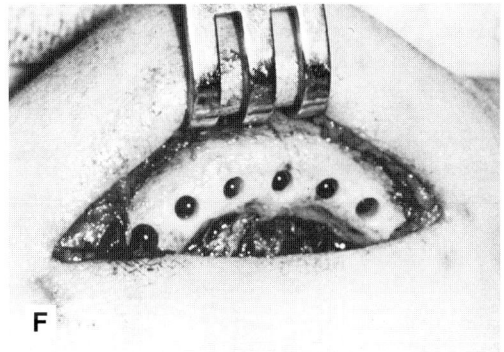

FIG. 20-73. *(A and B) Acrylic splint is used as a template for the staple drill guide at time of surgery. (C and D) A submental approach is used to expose the mandibular symphysis. (E and F) With the drill guide seven parallel holes are placed.*

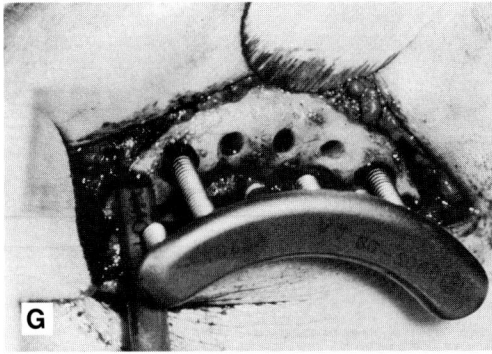

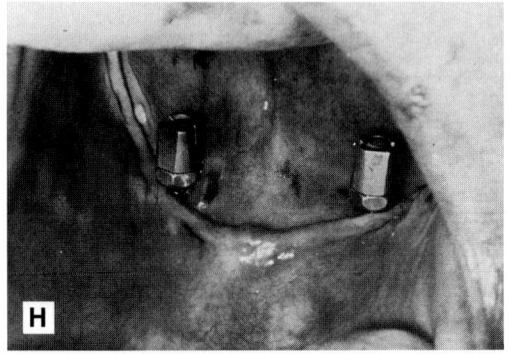

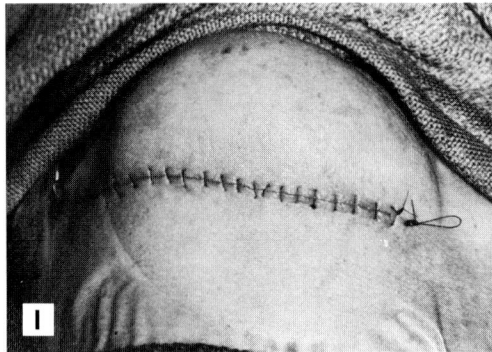

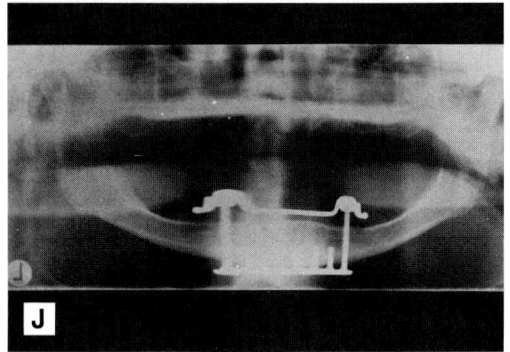

FIG. 20-73 (continued). (G) Staple is inserted. (H) Fasteners are applied to the transosteal pins. (I) Incision is closed. (J) Postoperative x-ray shows staple in proper position.

Antibiotic coverage is most important in these cases, as well as the appropriate use of heat and cold. Antibiotic therapy is appropriate whenever skin and bone grafting procedures are performed. Careful attention to oral hygiene, general hydration, and nutrition is most important. Cortisone administered intravenously during the procedure and for 2 days postoperatively aids in the control of edema. Carefully planning the procedure, using sharp incisions, and giving meticulous attention to proper suturing materially aid in the success of these procedures.

The biologic acceptability of hydroxylapatite and dental implants has considerably reduced the morbidity previously associated with preprosthetic surgery. The exposure and loss of HA crystals does not necessarily mean the loss of the total implant. The exfoliation of several crystals in the first 7 to 10 days is not uncommon following HA insertion. Exposure of a bone graft, however, may ultimately result in loss of the entire graft.

Although the 10-year survival rates of the currently used osseous integrated implants exceed 90 percent, cases occur in which the implants must be removed. The most common indications for removal are infection and mobility. It is possible to obtain resolution of an infection associated with an implant with antibiotics if the implant is stable; if it is not, the infection will not resolve until the implant has been removed.

References

1. MacIntosh, Robert B., and Obwegeser, Hugo L.: Preprosthetic surgery: A scheme for its effective employment. J. Oral Surgery, 25:397, 1967.
2. Shapiro, H. H.: Maxillofacial Anatomy, Philadelphia, J. B. Lippincott Co., 1954.
3. Obwegeser, H.: Surgical preparation of the

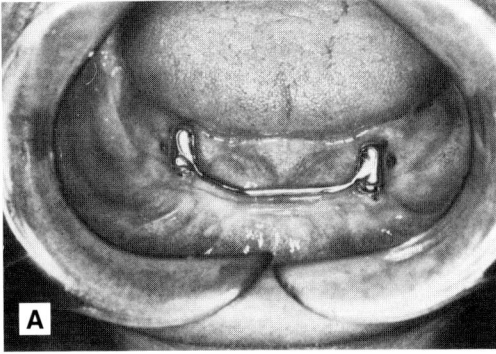

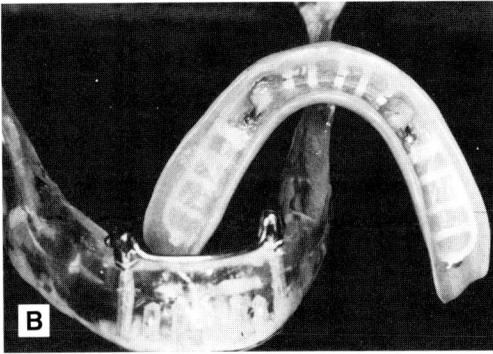

FIG. 20-74. *(A) The superstructive using a precision attachment is constructed eight weeks following staple insertion. (B) Plastic mandible and denture disclosing the prosthetic reconstructive concepts.*

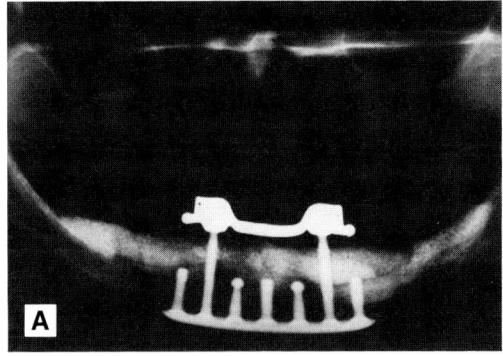

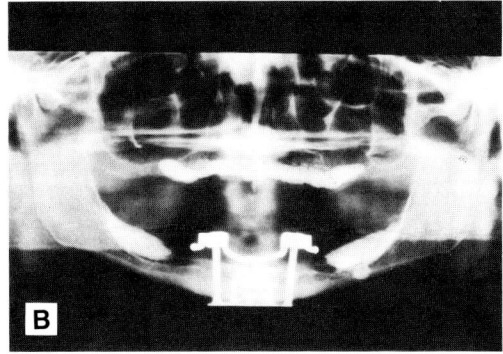

FIG. 20-75. *(A) Staple can be placed through HA, or (B) HA can be used with the staple to augment deficient areas of the maxilla or mandible.*

maxilla for prosthesis. J. Oral Surgery, *22:*127, 1964.

4. Shafer, W. G., Hine, M.K., and Levy, B. M.: Oral Pathology. 1st Ed. Philadelphia, W. B. Saunders Co., 1983.

5. Kolas, S., et al.: The occurrence of torus palatinus and torus mandibularis in 2478 dental patients. Oral Surgery, *6:*1134, 1953.

6. Thiersch, K.: Uber die feineren Anatomischen vcranderungen bei aufheilung von haut auf granulationen. Arch. Klin. Chir., *17:*318, 1874.

7. Moszkowicz, L.: Uber Verpflanzung Thiersch' scher Epidermislappchen in die Mundhohle. Arch. Klin. Chir., *108:*216, 1916.

8. Esser, J. F. S.: Studies in plastic surgery of the face. Ann. Surgery, *65:*297, 1917.

9. Pichler, H., and Trauner, R.: Die Alveolarkammplastik. F. Stomat., *28:*675, 1930.

10. Gillies, H. D.: Plastic Surgery of the Face. London, Oxford University Press, 1920.

11. Steinhauser, E. W.: Free transplantation of oral mucosa for improvement of denture retention. J. Oral Surgery, *27:*955, 1969.

12. Wang, J. H., and Waite, D. E.: Evaluation of the surgical procedure of sagittal split osteotomy of the mandibular ramus. J. Oral Surg. Oral Med. Oral Pathol. *38:*167, 1974.

Selected Reading

Boyne, P. J.: New concepts in facial bone healing and grafting procedures. J. Oral Surgery, *27:*557, 1969.

Suzuki, M., and Sakai, T.: A familial study of torus palatinus and torus mandibularis. Am. J. Phys. Anthrop., *18:*263, 1960.

CHAPTER 21

The Temporomandibular Joint

JOHN J. DELFINO

Anatomy and Function

The temporomandibular joint (TMJ) has many unique and functional features that separate it from the other joints of the body. As a result, its anatomy is highly specific for the complex functional demands of mandibular movement required in mastication, speech, and deglutition.

The TMJ forms the bilateral movable attachments of the mandible with the skull. Because it has the dual properties of a hinged (ginglymoid) and gliding (arthrodial) attachment, it is termed a ginglymoarthrodial joint. It is a freely mobile joint with superior and inferior joint compartments separated by an interposed meniscus. The articulating surfaces of the inferiorly positioned mandibular condyle and the superiorly positioned glenoid fossa of the temporal bone are lined with dense fibrocartilage, not hyaline cartilage as found in most other joints. The joint cavities are also lined with synovial membrane, producing a constant flow of lubricating fluid from the villi that protrude from the anterior and posterior meniscus to the attachments to the mandibular condyle and temporal bone.

The meniscus serves as a cartilagenous structure between the mandibular condyle and the glenoid fossa and articular eminence of the temporal bone. As a result of this relationship, it acquires both a convex and concave configuration that produces varying densities and thicknesses of menis-

cal tissue. The central region of the meniscus, the *pars gracilis*, is composed of thin (1 to 2 mm thickness) and avascular collagen. The anterior projection of the meniscus, the *pes meniscus*, is substantially thicker and highly vascular. This is due to its attachment superiorly to the articular eminence and superior head of the lateral pterygoid muscle and inferiorly to the condyle by way of synovial membrane at the superior margin of the inferior head of the lateral pterygoid muscle.

The posterior extension and attachment of the meniscus is quite thick and broad and has become known as the *bilaminar zone*. It is composed of two strata of fibers with an interposed zone of neurovascular and loose, areolar connective tissue. The superior stratum, containing dense, thick elastic fibers oriented in an anteroposterior direction, is attached to the posterior wall of the glenoid fossa and squamotympanic suture. The inferior stratum has a markedly different composition with dense fibrous tissue with few elastic fibers connecting it to the posterior head and neck of the condyle (Fig. 21-1). The meniscus is tightly attached to the condyle through attachments at the medial and lateral poles.

These internal joint structures are surrounded by a *capsule* of dense collagen tissue on the medial, lateral, and posterior walls of the joint. Superiorly, the capsule attaches to the tympanic plate medially and the inferior border of the zygomatic pro-

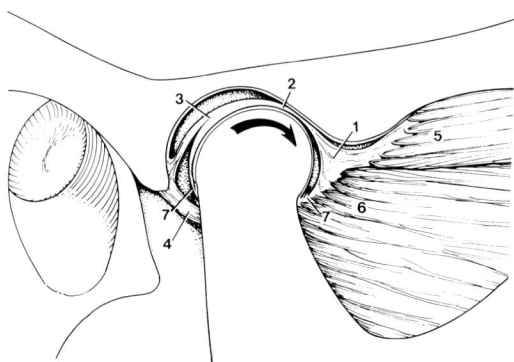

FIG. 21-1. *Sagittal view of the temporomandibular joint. (1) pes meniscus. (2) pars gracilis. (3) bilaminar zone. (4) posterior capsule. (5) superior head of lateral pterygoid muscle. (6) interior head of lateral pterygoid muscle. (7) synovial villi.*

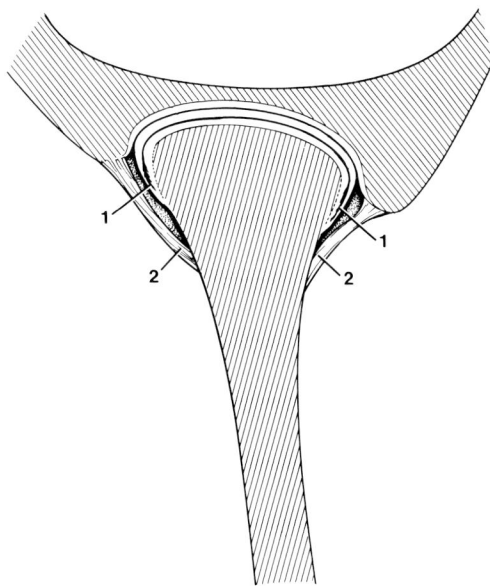

FIG. 21-2. *Frontal view of the temporomandibular joint. (1) Meniscal attachments to condyle. (2) Capsular attachments to condyle.*

cess laterally. Inferiorly, capsular fibers attach to the condylar neck, independent of the meniscus, in both medial and lateral positions (Fig. 21-2). Posterior capsule extends from the typanic plate to the posterior surface of the condyle. Note the abscence of an anterior capsular wall which may predispose the TMJ to hypertranslation and meniscal stretch injuries in traumatic episodes. Laterally and medially the capsule is reinforced by the temporomandibular ligament (collateral ligament). This strong ligament originates at the lateral and inferior aspect of the zygomatic process and inserts into the lateral neck of the condylar process. Both the capsule and the temporomandibular ligament have a certain degree of laxity so that the condyle retains translatory capabilities but that excessive lateral condylar displacement is resisted. The sphenomandibular and stylomandibular ligaments are accessory structures with no functional significance to the TMJ.

Sensory innervation of joint structures is by the mandibular division of the fifth cranial nerve, principally the auriculotemporal branch, which supplies the medial, lateral, and posterior capsule and meniscus. Anterior joint innervation is through the masseteric and deep temporal branches. Vascular supply is obtained through the external carotid system by way of terminal branches of the superficial temporal and the mandibular portion of the internal maxillary arteries.

Internal joint function is a complex interplay of movement between the condyle and meniscus, which at certain points is completely diametric. Initial opening is primarily a hinge movement with an anterior clockwise rotation of the condyle and a static positioning of the meniscus (Fig. 21-3A). As opening or protrusive movements increase, the condyle accompanied by the meniscus, because of its attachments to the medial and lateral poles of the condyle and adduction of the superior head of the lateral pterygoid muscle, moves inferior and anterior along the posterior slope of the articular eminence. This movement of the meniscus creates a degree of tension in the bilaminar zone, primarily in the superior stratum, which is permitted by its high elastin content (Fig. 21-3B). In addition, a potential space is created between the stratum of the bilaminar zone in the vascular areolar tissue that rapidly fills with blood due to the negative pressure of the vacated glenoid fossa.

As the forward phase of translation continues, the tensile limit of the bilaminar zone and its temporal attachment is reached and further anterior positioning of the meniscus is not permitted despite continued condylar movement. As a result,

A

B

C

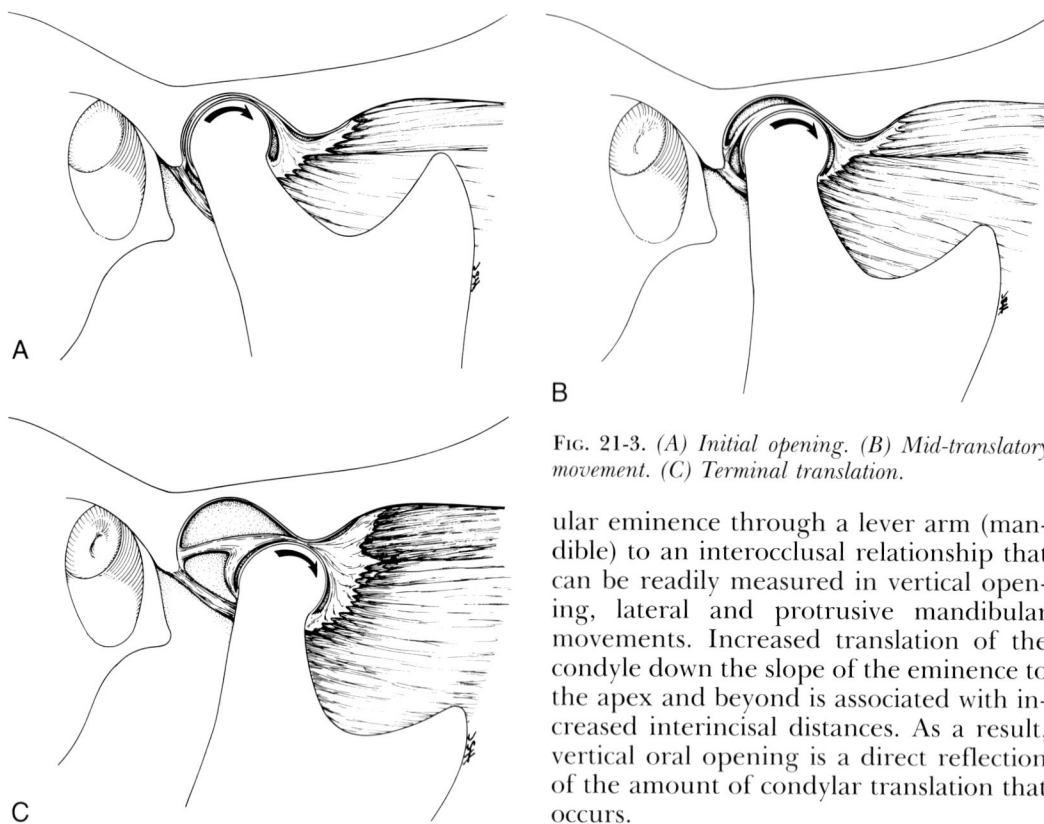

FIG. 21-3. *(A) Initial opening. (B) Mid-translatory movement. (C) Terminal translation.*

the meniscus rotates posterior to the advancing condylar head (Fig. 21-3C). This anteroposterior meniscal movement during translation allows intimate contact to be maintained between the superior margin of the meniscus and articular eminence as well as to avoid serving as an obstruction at the latter phases of translation. Thus, it can be appreciated that the meniscus is a truly dynamic component of the joint and an important consideration in normal function. In pathologic changes of the meniscocondylar complex, meniscal position and movement are amplified concerns.

Closing movements are essentially a reversal of the aforementioned sequence. As the condyle resumes a centric position within the glenoid fossa, vascular decompression occurs between the stratum of the bilaminar zone. Meniscal return occurs through its lateral and medial condylar attachments but also is aided by the elastic recoil of the stretched superior stratum.

This joint system permits a clinical assessment of function by transmitting the degree of condylar translation on the artic-

ular eminence through a lever arm (mandible) to an interocclusal relationship that can be readily measured in vertical opening, lateral and protrusive mandibular movements. Increased translation of the condyle down the slope of the eminence to the apex and beyond is associated with increased interincisal distances. As a result, vertical oral opening is a direct reflection of the amount of condylar translation that occurs.

Growth and Development

The mandible develops as an intramembranous bone lateral to the cartilage of the first branchial arch (Meckel's cartilage). Its appearance, along with muscle and teeth buds, can be seen as early as the third week in the embryonic facial region. Development of the temporomandibular joint follows, which eventually becomes a mobile suture between the developing membranous temporal and mandibular bones. Such positioning necessitates that the temporomandibular joint have tremendous adaptive capabilities to respond to the stresses of various local developmental and functional influences.

The condyle has been investigated extensively as a facial growth center. For many years it was believed that the condyle acted as the major growth center of the mandible, causing it to grow inferiorly and anteriorly. Evidence accumulated by experimental and clinical studies, however, does not fully support this contention. Rather, the condyle appears to be similar to the epiphyses of the long bones, which act as regional centers of growth that continually adapt and remodel during their development. The functional demands placed on the temporomandibular joint are greater and more sustained, however, as it must cope with an ever-changing occlusion in addition to progressive skeletal facial development. Injury, therefore, to the developing temporomandibular joint structures does not predictably result in aberrant mandibular growth disturbances or long-term joint dysfunction. In the adult, however, the joint structures are far less adaptive than in children, and excessive functional loads frequently produce pathologic changes and resultant dysfunction.

Temporomandibular Joint Dysfunction

Pain and dysfunction of the TMJ affect a significant number of individuals. Because of the high affliction incidence, a voluminous amount of written material has been generated in the past half century. The literature is so abundant and diversified that its review is not only uninviting, but has led many to propose that no further explanations of dysfunction and treatment be forthcoming without scientific evidence. Therefore, discussion of TMJ dysfunction is presented with current and accepted concepts.

Classification

Trauma to joint structures is clearly the major contributing factor in most cases of joint dysfunction and, as such, serves as a convenient classification system. Although variations in the magnitude and duration of traumatic insult result in variable expressivity of dysfunction, its extracapsular origin is overwhelmingly preponderant. Thus, one must bear in mind that most TMJ dysfunction problems (excluding true intracapsular origins of dysfunction, i.e., rheumatoid arthritis, developmental condylar dysplasias, neoplasias, etc.) represent a range of progressive pathology in which internal structural damage of the joint and clinical dysfunction are the end sequelae.

MACROTRAUMA

Macrotrauma results from rapid and/or excessive application of force to the mandible or adjoining craniofacial areas. A marked increase in intracapsular pressure occurs which, in conjunction with condylar displacement, exceeds the limits of the soft tissue attachments of the joint. These actions result in an acute stretch or tear injury to the meniscus and capsule with resultant internal joint hemorrhage. Common causes include trauma from motor vehicle accidents, sports activities, social altercations, falls, difficult exodontia, prolonged oral procedures, excessive opening for mastication, yawning, or laughter, endotracheal intubation, and propped oral opening for intraoral or pharyngeal surgery.

Macrotrauma produces immediate acute symptoms in a previously normal patient, or macrotrauma of a lesser degree results in an acute exacerbation of a preexisting chronically damaged joint. Conditions produced include:

1. Joint effusion, secondary adhesions
2. Capsulitis, meniscitis, myositis, synovitis
3. Fracture of the condylar head or neck
4. Internal meniscal derangement
5. Osteoarthritis
6. Ankylosis (fibrous, osseous)

MICROTRAUMA

Microtrauma, by far, accounts for the majority of patients who develop internal injuries and damage. It has an insidious onset, chronic symptomatology, usually a protracted course, and often recruits adjacent facial and cervical areas producing symptoms that make an accurate diagnosis difficult. Because proper joint function depends upon a delicate balance and interplay of many craniofacial factors, disruption of any element in this system may result in aberrant muscular coordination of joint function and ultimate internal derangement. Microtraumatized joints are characterized by chronic inflammation of the capsule and meniscus, osteoarthritic hard tissue changes, and deranged meniscocondylar function.

The etiology of microtrauma has been widely debated and many factors have been implicated. These factors may be categorized as morphologic (occlusion, muscular activity, facial skeletal relationship) and psychologic (emotion, stress, central neurophysiologic transmitters). Current evidence implicates masticatory muscle hyperactivity in producing persistent chronic trauma to the soft tissue of the joint. This muscular hyperactivity may be secondary to either local morphologic causes (malocclusion, perioral habits) or more centrally mediated (stress). Prolonged activity of the superior head of the lateral pterygoid causes persistent anterior traction on the meniscus, particularly enhanced during translation. This may result in stretch injuries of the posterior attachment, loss of its elastic properties, and eventual disruption of meniscocondylar coordination in translation, with internal derangements as the end result. The exact etiologic pathway for masticatory muscle hyperactivity, however, remains unclear, and the best understanding at present is a multifactorial view of a number of interlocking morphologic and psychologic factors.

Microtrauma results in a progressive range of pathology and symptoms which eventually involves both extra- and intracapsular joint structures. Resulting conditions include:

1. Myofascial pain dysfunction syndrome (muscle spasm)
2. Muscle splinting
3. Myositis, mcniscitis, synovitis
4. Internal meniscal derangements
5. Osteoarthritis

NONTRAUMA

Nontraumatic etiologic factors comprise a small number of infrequently encountered intracapsular pathologic states. These may be summarized as follows:

1. Developmental anomalies
   a) condyle
      1) agenesis
      2) hypoplasia
      3) hyperplasia
   b) temporal bone
      1) pneumatization
2. Arthritides
   a) rheumatoid
   b) psoriatic
   c) infectious
   d) gouty
3. Neoplasia
   a) benign
      1) chondroma
      2) osteochondroma
      3) osteoma
      4) synovial chondromatosis
      5) fibrous dysplasia
      6) myoma
   b) malignant
      1) osteosarcoma
      2) rhabdomyosarcoma
      3) multiple myeloma
      4) metastatic disease
      5) synovial sarcoma

In addition to true joint pathology, a variety of extracapsular conditions may resemble joint pathosis in terms of pain and aberrant mandibular function. These conditions include:

1. Similar pain
   a) odontitis
   b) pericoronitis
   c) otitis media
   d) tinnitus
   e) parotiditis
   f) maxillary/frontal sinusitis
   g) facial neuralgias (i.e., trigeminal neuralgia, etc.)
   h) temporal arteritis
   i) Eagle's Syndrome (elongated styloid process)
2. Decreased oral opening
   a) facial/odontogenic infections
   b) contiguous tumors (hemangioma, lymphangioma, neurofibroma)
   c) osteochondroma of coronoid process
   d) depressed zygomatic arch fracture
   e) myositis ossificans
   f) scleroderma
   g) tetanus
   h) extrapyramidal reaction
   i) hysteria
3. Inability to close
   a) myasthenia gravis
   b) Bell's palsy
   c) extrapyramidal reaction

Symptoms and Clinical Findings

Temporomandibular joint symptoms are variable and are, of course, dependent upon their etiologic basis. However, they may be grouped into three general categories: pain, altered mandibular function, and the elicitation of joint noise. One or all three of these symptomatic categories may be simultaneously involved.

The majority of patients have some degree of pain, and this symptom usually encourages them to present for treatment.

The pain most commonly is localized to the preauricular area and may be bilateral in distribution. It can be produced by digital palpation of the condyles or by mandibular movement. Headaches, localized to the temporofrontal area or extending to involve the entire unilateral face, parietal, and occipital areas, are a common complaint. Otalgia and tinnitus are also variable findings and may occasionally be the only symptom that the patient experiences. The presentation of the triad of preauricular pain, headaches, and ear symptoms is not uncommon and most patients have at least two of these pain symptoms in varying combinations.[1]

Alterations of normal mandibular movement occur in most, but not all, cases.[2] Decreased oral opening with deviation of the mandible to the affected side is a characteristic finding. Muscle spasm or splinting, meniscal derangements, joint adhesions, and inflammatory changes of the capsule affect joint mobility in various ways. As a result, clinical range of motion is variably expressed in joint pathosis and must be carefully assessed. The amount of opening (interincisal distance minus the vertical overlap of the teeth), amount of lateral movement (based on the midlines of the central incisors), and the presence of deviation (as noted within the first 20 to 25 mm of movement) in opening and closing should be measured.

Joint noise may be evident either audibly or through auscultation. Two main types of noise are usually generated—clicking or popping, and crepitation. Clicking noises, associated with meniscocondylar incoordination, commonly occur with anterior meniscal displacement with reduction. Crepitation can be related to degenerative arthritic changes, fractures, and meniscal perforations differs clearly from the opening and closing clicks of meniscal derangement patients. Both types of joint noise indicate pathologic changes, but crepitation is far more ominous and suggests significant internal damage.[3]

Occlusal disharmony is often implicated in joint pathology and may be a significant clinical finding.[4] It can be an obvious observation such as in loss of posterior vertical support or in open bite relationships found in joint effusions resulting from macrotrauma. Usually it requires more careful assessment for potential interceptive occlusal contacts. All patients should be evaluated for prematurity in centric relation, existence of nonfunctioning contacts, degree of posterior guidance in protrusion, and evidence of occlusal wear.

Radiographic Diagnosis

Treatment of temporomandibular joint dysfunction has historically been controversial because of an inability to assess intracapsular pathology accurately and reliably. Radiography, the only currently accepted method of nonsurgical intracapsular investigation, serves as the primary diagnostic adjunct in the evaluation of symptomatic temporomandibular joints. Radiographic diagnostic modalities may be divided into several basic types: conventional, tomographic, and contrast studies. However, all have limitations because of the small size of the joint, its location within dense craniofacial structures, and its complex anatomic structure and function. It is imperative that the capabilities of each radiographic method be understood in an effort to maximize obtainable diagnostic information while reducing patient radiation exposure and expense.

CONVENTIONAL RADIOGRAPHY

Prior to present times, the use of transcranial radiographic techniques (Lind-

FIG. 21-4. *Transcranial temporomandibular joint films in closed and opening positions.*

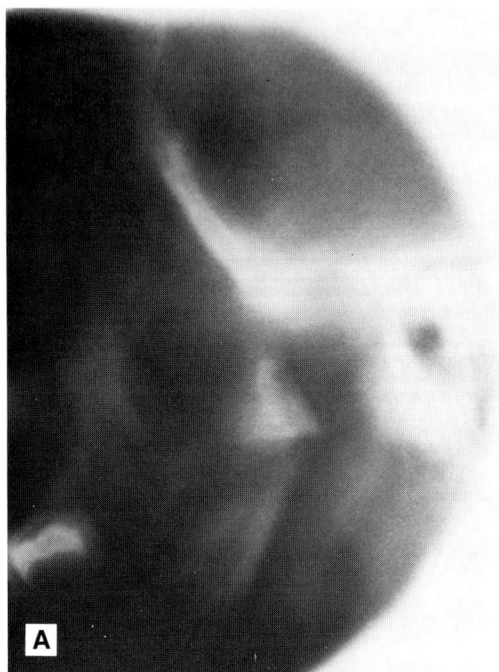

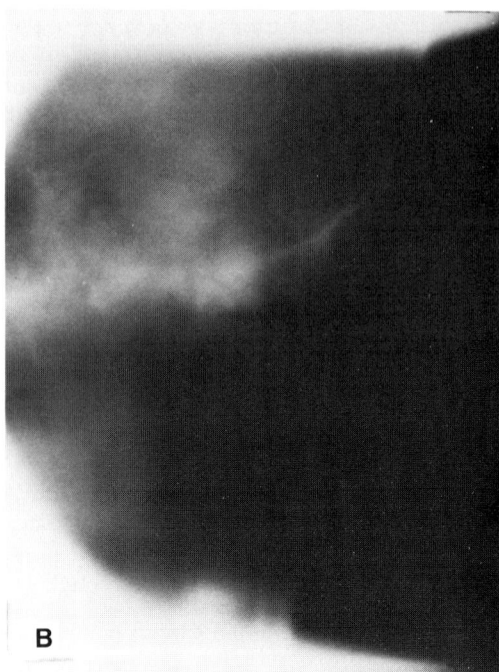

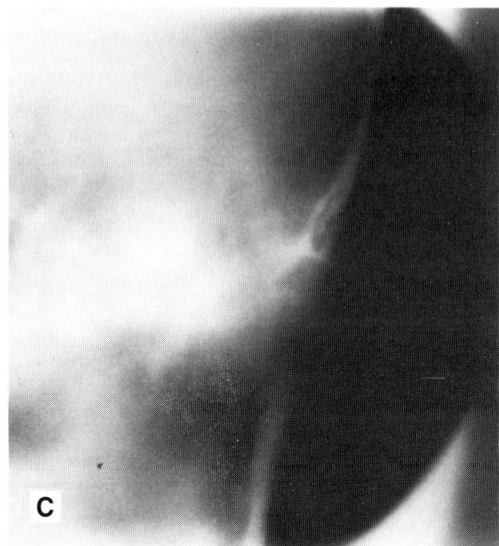

FIG. 21-5. *Tomograms of patient with subcondylar fracture with displacement. (A) Inferior displacement of condylar segment evident in lateral view. (B) Medial displacement also evident in frontal view. (C) Frontal view of contralateral normal joint.*

tion about hard tissue structures. However, the entire joint is not visualized nor is there any information concerning soft tissue pathology. Thus, transcranial films are most appropriately utilized as a screening examination when hard tissue pathology is suspect.

Another conventional film of value is the cephalometric view. This film is a true lateral radiograph of the temporomandibular joint in relation to the skull, midface, mandible, and occlusion. It is best used as an adjunctive aid to evaluate the contribution of facial skeletal relationships to existing joint dysfunction.[7]

TOMOGRAPHY

Tomography is a method of evaluating anatomic structures through a series of cuts or slices taken at different levels in the sagittal and frontal planes. The technique blurs all surrounding structures that do not lie in the desired plane. As a result of the complex skull anatomy surrounding the joint, tomography is a good method of evaluation. The central two thirds of the

blom, Greecock, Gillis, McQueen techniques) was the standard in TMJ radiography.[5,6] To circumvent the superimposition of surrounding joint structures, these techniques directed the radiation source posterior and superior from the contralateral ear. The resultant films produced images of the lateral half of the condyle and fossa (Fig. 21-4). Because most pathology occurs in the lateral half of the joint,[1] transcranial radiography does provide useful informa-

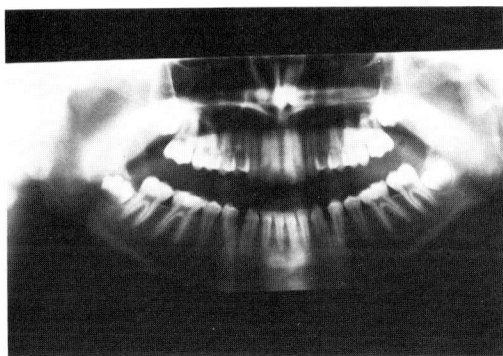

Fig. 21-6. *Pantographic view of left subcondylar fracture. One can easily compare both joints simultaneously.*

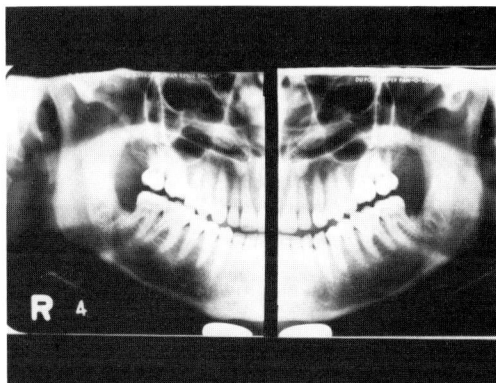

Fig. 21-7. *Pantographic view. Note smaller deformed left condyle as compared to the right.*

joint are well defined with sharp contours, whereas the lateral or peripheral structures are blurred (Fig. 21-5). These properties give tomography superiority over transcranial techniques in pathologic detection and support its use in the diagnosis of suspected arthritic changes.[8-10] However, like transcranial radiography, it fails to evaluate the soft tissue or the dynamics of the joint.

Pantographic radiography is a form of tomography with an arc movement of the radiation source around the patient, and the view is used for better evaluation of the mandible. It can evaluate both joints simultaneously and permits measurements of the relative size of each side of the mandible. However, condylar anatomy is distorted and only the medial aspect of the joint is viewed. As a result, pantographic views are of most value in the evaluation of macrotraumatized joints (Fig. 21-6) to rule out fractures and in cases of mandibular developmental growth disturbances (Fig. 21-7).

CONTRAST STUDIES

All of the previous radiographic techniques fail to evaluate the soft tissue elements of the joint. The introduction of contrast material into the inferior joint space (arthrography) followed by the evaluation of the contrasted images produced through the dynamics of videofluoroscopy or in conjunction with tomography (arthrotomography) has resulted in new insights into meniscal form and function. Arthrography has significantly advanced

concepts of internal joint pathology by clearly demonstrating that the pathophysiologic mechanism is a form of intra-articular derangement characterized by anterior displacement of the meniscus as a result of abnormality of its posterior ligamentous attachment.[11,12,13] This has resulted in an understanding of a range of progressive pathology as evidenced by arthrography; meniscal dislocation with reduction [Fig. 21-8(1)], meniscal dislocation without reduction (Fig. 21-9), and meniscal dislocation without reduction and loss of integrity (perforation) (Fig. 21-10). This concept is now widely accepted, and recent evidence substantiates a high statistical correlation between arthrographic diagnosis and actual joint pathology.[1,14,15]

Arthrography should be used whenever clinical signs and symptoms suggest aberrant clinical function or prior conventional films reveal anticipated pathology. Evidence of localized pain and a restriction or deviation of mandibular movement justify arthrographic evaluation.

Presently, the modality of computed tomography has been applied to the temporomandibular joint. As with arthrography, significant accuracy rates have been reported in the detection of internal derangements[16,17] (Fig. 21-11). Computed tomography offers the advantages of negating superimposition of surrounding structures, simultaneous evaluation of all joint structures, and ability to scan small, well-defined areas. Its major drawback is the difficulty in evaluating three-dimensional structures and relationships on a

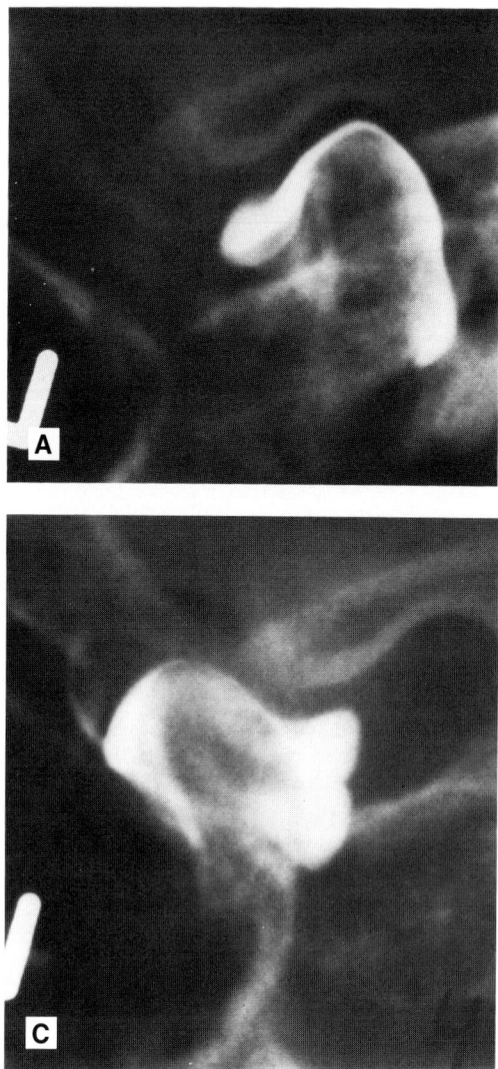

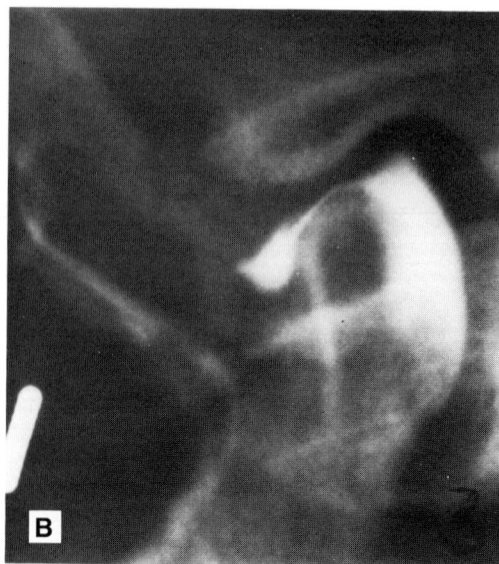

FIG. 21-8(1). *Arthrogram demonstrating meniscal dislocation which reduces. (A) Closed position. (B) Mid-opening position. Note bulge (anterior recess) of contrast material anterior to condylar head providing transient obstruction to further translation. (C) Terminal translation. A click or pop noise, which can be visualized by video fluoroscopy, occurs as a result of aberrant coordination between anterior condylar and posterior meniscal movement. The meniscus then reduces allowing normal or hypernormal condylar range of motion at terminal translation.*

two-dimensional display screen. Computed tomography provides an alternative diagnostic modality for the patient who refuses or has technical difficulties with an arthrographic examination. More research is needed, however, to fully assess the capabilities of computed tomography prior to its use as a primary imaging modality in suspect internal derangements.

Early results of the use of magnetic resonance imaging (MRI) have shown remarkable detail of the meniscus and bilaminar zone tissues [Fig. 21-8(2)]. Additional advantages of this modality include its noninvasiveness and lack of radiation hazard. Further studies are necessary, however, to explore fully its diagnostic potential and role in the evaluation of temporomandibular joint disease.

Treatment

It is doubtful that any other disease has been so variably treated as temporomandibular joint problems. Much has been learned from what we now recognize as inappropriate treatment utilized in the past. These lessons, in conjunction with improved diagnostic modalities and skills, have resulted in therapeutic regimens with a more sound physiologic basis.

CONSERVATIVE TREATMENT

Conservative treatment is best thought of as any treatment that is reversible. It is generally reserved for joint injuries that are transient (joint effusions) or reversible (myofascial pain dysfunction), or incipient pathology (anterior mensical dislocation with reduction). The following conditions

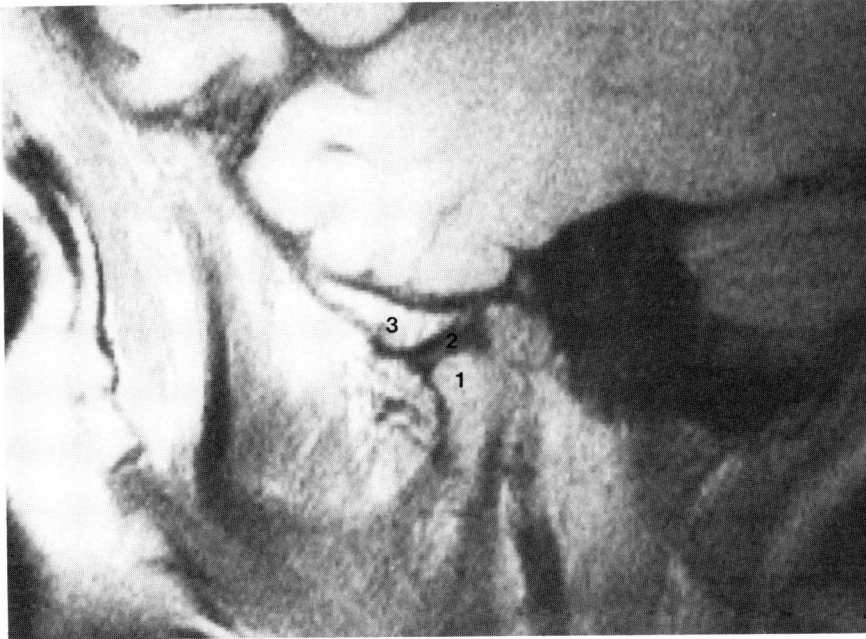

FIG. 21-8(2). *Example of magnetic resonance imaging of the TMJ. (1) Condyle; (2) articulare disc; (3) eminence.*

are believed to be amenable initially to conservative and/or supportive therapy:

1. Joint effusion
2. Condylar fractures (depending upon age of patient and degree of displacement)
3. Capsulitis, meniscitis, myositis, synovitis
4. Myofascial pain dysfunction syndrome
5. Muscle splinting
6. Internal derangements (anterior meniscal dislocation with reduction only)
7. All arthritides except infectious and severe osseous degeneration in rheumatoid arthritis

Conservative treatments are described in the following paragraphs.

Rest. Rest is accomplished by placing the patient on a liquid or soft diet and voluntarily restricting his range of motion. This may be aided by intermaxillary fixation with interarch elastics. Decreased joint mobility allows the resolution of inflammatory changes and edema as well as hemorrhagic exudate.

Thermal Applications. The application of cold is reserved for acute injuries to minimize inflammation, hemorrhage, and edema. It may be applied continuously for the first 24 hours. After the first 24 hours in an acute injury or chronic inflammation and muscle pain, intermittent moist heat is recommended to increase circulation to the affected structures and promote muscle relaxation.

Pharmaceutical Agents. Pharmaceutical agents provide a conservative modality that offers many benefits in the production of analgesia, muscle relaxation, and in reducing inflammation. Many of the current agents are significant improvements over those of the past and their utilization is better understood.

Most complaints of pain may be adequately controlled by non-narcotic peripherally acting analgesics such as acetylsalicyclic acid (buffered 0.6 g q.i.d.) or acetaminophen (500 mg q.i.d.) as well as narcotic centrally acting analgesics such as acetaminophen with codeine (300 mg/ 30 mg/q 4h). Patients who require increased doses or demand more potent narcotics must be viewed suspiciously.

Relaxation of masticatory muscles, particularly in myofascial pain dysfunction, is an effective adjunctive aid. All relaxant agents used exhibit a centrally acting sedative effect, which combined with a peripheral skeletal muscle inhibition accounts for the effectiveness of these agents. Primary

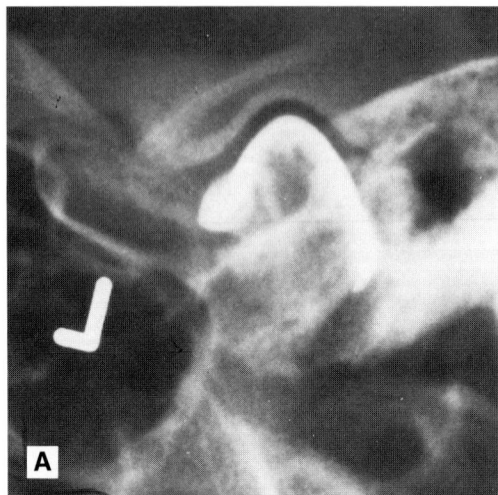

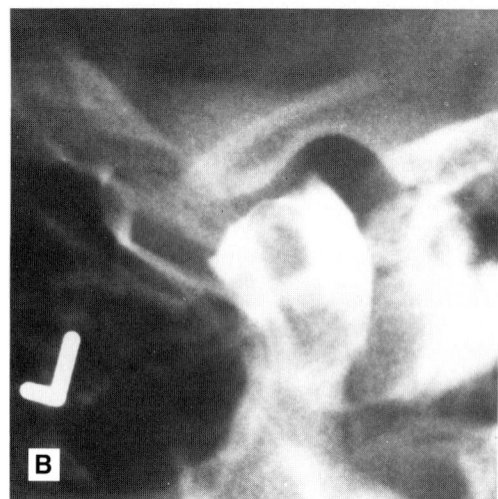

FIG. 21-9. *Arthrogram of meniscal dislocation without reduction. (A) Closed position. (B) Condyle unable to continue translation to anterior position of meniscus which will not reduce or move posteriorly.*

domethacin (25 mg q.i.d.) are effective compounds but should be limited to short term use (7 to 10 days) secondary to their potential toxic effects, primarily including gastrointestinal symptoms (pain, nausea, diarrhea, peptic ulcer, bleeding, and perforation). Ibuprofen (400 mg q.i.d.), an over-the-counter medication, appears to be equally effective but with fewer complaints of gastrointestinal distress. Glucocorticoids, also, have demonstrated dramatic abilities to reduce inflammatory changes of

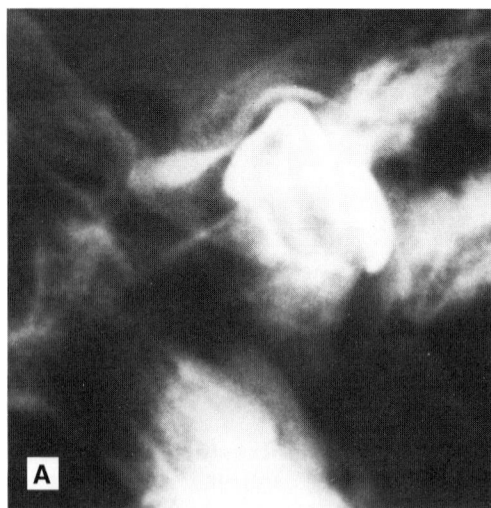

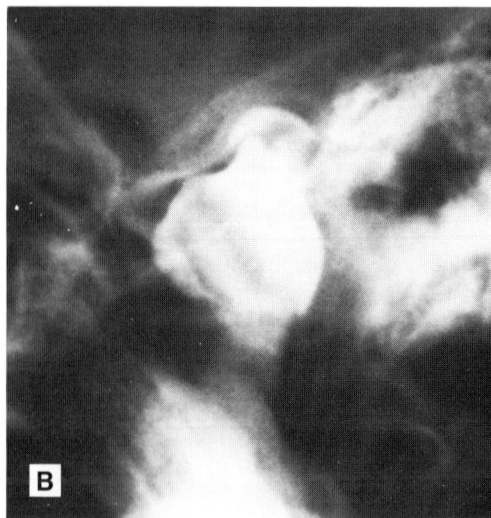

FIG. 21-10. *Arthrogram demonstrating dislocation with meniscal perforation. (A) In closed position, note fill of superior joint space with contrast material outlining the meniscus. (B) Anterior meniscal dislocation without reduction.*

centrally acting muscle relaxants such as methacarbamol (750 mg t.i.d.) and chlorzoxazone (250 mg t.i.d.) or benzodiazepine derivatives such as diazepam (2 mg q.i.d.) and chlordiazepoxide (5 mg q.i.d.) appear to be equally effective.

The ability to reduce soft tissue inflammation (muscle, ligament, synovium) in a reliable and efficacious fashion is a more recent pharmaceutical development. Acute and chronic injuries alike may benefit from these effects. Salicylates, as previously mentioned, and salicylate-like agents such as phenylbutazone (100 mg q.i.d.) and in-

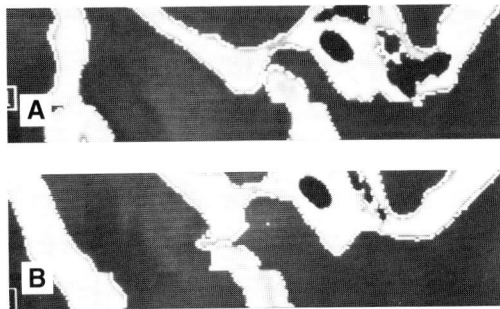

FIG. 21-11. *Computed tomographic reconstruction of the TMJ. (A) Mid-opening. (B) Terminal translation. Note outline of different density material anterior to condylar head representing a dislocation without reduction.*

soft tissue. Agents such as cortisone (25 mg t.i.d.), prednisone (5 mg t.i.d.), and dexamethasone (.75 mg t.i.d.) have been extensively used in the past decade. Due to their significant and potentially lethal effects when used in chronic high dosages, however, their use should be limited to those patients that fail to respond to other agents, and then only for short periods until other modalities may be instituted.

Injection Therapy. In the past, injection therapy utilizing local anesthetics, steroids, and sclerosing agents has been used intracapsularly. It is now clear that these injections have created more damage than long-term benefits. The deleterious effects of steroids (osteoporosis, retarded healing) and sclerosing agents (scarring, fibrosis, chronic inflammatory changes) are well recognized, and their use can no longer be recommended. Local anesthetics may be used to effect a conduction block of the auriculotemporal nerve as a diagnostic aid or to treat an acute painful episode. If discomfort persists, intracapsular injection may be done to differentiate whether the joint is the actual source of pain. In general, however, intra-articular injections of any agent should be avoided to prevent the likelihood of increasing joint damage.

Physical Therapy. After acute inflammation and edema have subsided, gentle stretching exercises are recommended to gradually increase the range of mandibular motion and elongate previously shortened muscle fibers. The patient may do this manually in vertical, lateral, and protrusive movements, augmented by heat and mus-

cle relaxants. With some patients, a physical therapy facility or therapist helps to ensure compliance and proper execution of the stretch maneuvers.

Ultrasonic treatments, particularly when scarring, fibrosis, and hypomobility of joint structures exist, may be helpful. Its benefits are probably due to the deep penetration of heat, which produces an increase in local circulation and the mechanical breakdown of adhesed tissue.

Occlusal Therapy. Occlusal stents function primarily as diagnostic aids. They are designed to allow the patient to function without interference from interceptive occlusal contacts. As the stent is worn, it is adjusted periodically as the occlusion and neuromuscular factors change. If the stent gives complete relief, it can be expected that occlusal adjustment will do the same. If the stent fails to resolve the painful symptoms after 4 to 6 weeks' use, it can be discarded as another etiologic factor is involved.[18,19]

Occlusal coverage (Niteguard) may also be used to promote muscle relaxation, eliminate premature contacts that may initiate bruxism, and protect the occlusion from further iatrogenic wear.[20] In addition to providing a structural interface between occlusal surfaces, it elongates the musculature through the creation of an interarch occlusal gap. They are usually worn at night and may be used for months to years.

Occlusal equilibration may be conducted with some confidence if the patient has responded to occlusal coverage. It must be remembered that equilibration is, in fact, an irreversible therapy and should be considered carefully prior to initiation. Appropriate equilibration will effect mandibular repositioning into a more physiologic state.

In addition to these conservative modalties, biofeedback, hypnosis, acupuncture, and psychotherapy are being applied to temporomandibular joint problems. However, there is insufficient scientific evidence at this time to purport them as effective techniques.

SURGERY

Surgery of the temporomandibular joint is indicated in the following conditions:
1. Internal derangements

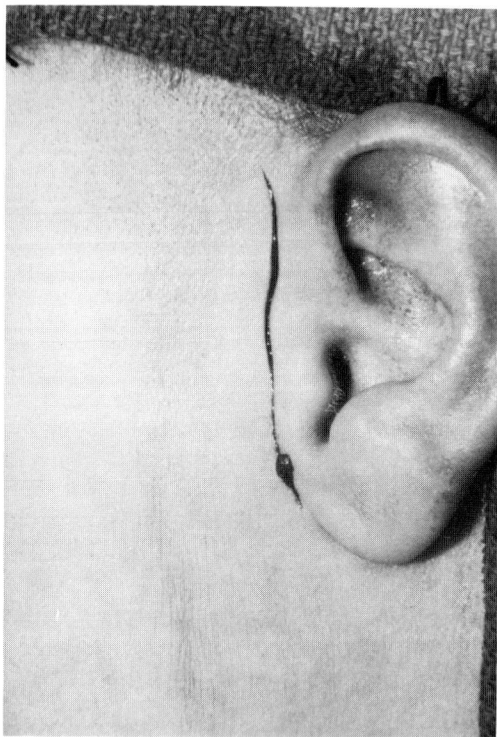

FIG. 21-12. *Preauricular incision.*

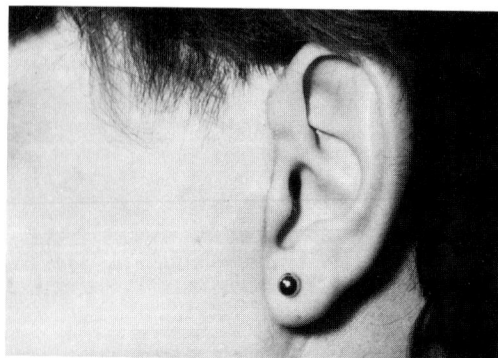

FIG. 21-13. *Preauricular incisional scar 6 weeks post-operatively.*

a) meniscal dislocation with reduction that does not respond to conservative measures

b) meniscal dislocations without reduction, loss of meniscal integrity

2. Condylar dislocations (hypermobility)
3. Ankylosis
4. Condylar fractures
5. Developmental and degenerative deformities

Although the TMJ is a superficial structure that lies anterior to the ear, unhindered access is hampered by branches of the facial nerve and the parotid gland. As a result, multiple incisional approaches have been devised from the lateral, posterior, and inferior directions. The preauricular incision (Fig. 21-12) has been the most commonly used. It provides maximum exposure both laterally and anteriorly. A visible scar remains but it is usually quite cosmetic (Fig. 21-13). In an effort to enhance cosmesis, an endaural modification of the preauricular incision has been devised. The inferior part of the incision follows the superior and anterior meatal wall, thus masking incisional scar.

In view of the excellent cosmetic results with the standard preauricular incision, endaural modifications are rarely used. The postauricular incision is made posterior to the ear, followed by anterior dissection with division of the cartilagenous canal. A flap, containing the entire external ear, is reflected anteriorly providing excellent exposure of posterior joint structures. Although it has the advantage of a hidden scar, problems can be encountered with adequate anterior joint exposure, stenosis of the auditory canal, and prolonged auricle anesthesia. The submandibular incision, made 2 to 3 cm below the angle of the mandible is the approach of choice for procedures involving manipulation of the condylar neck, coronoid notch, or lateral ramus.

Internal Derangements. Internal derangements are characterized by pathologic changes of meniscocondylar function, resulting in loss of compliance and integrity of the meniscus and osteoarthritic changes of the condyle and articular eminence. These have been most successfully repaired by the reconstructive arthroplastic techniques of *articular eminectomy*[21,22] and *high condylectomy.*[23-25] Both employ the concept of intracapsular decompression through reduction of either the superior or inferior bony component. The meniscus is then reduced in size and repositioned.

Technique. Following the induction of general anesthesia, the preauricular area is shaved, prepped, and draped in a sterile fashion. An epinephrine solution (1:100,000) is injected subcutaneously to maximize hemostasis. After an appropriate

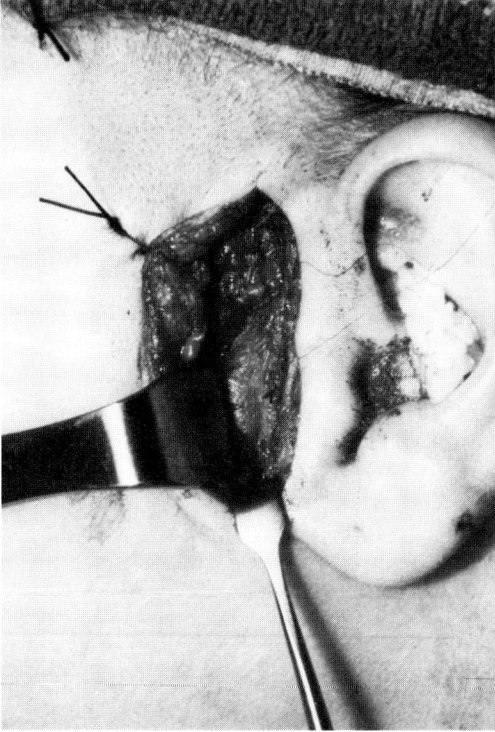

FIG. 21-14. *Anterior skin flap developed and sutured. Temporalis fascia overlying lateral joint capsule exposed.*

time interval to allow optimal effect of the epinephrine, a preauricular incision is made with a gentle S-shaped vertical incision immediately anterior to the ear, extending from its superior to inferior attachment along the medial surface of the tragus. An anterior skin flap is developed subcutaneously and sutured back, providing exposure to the deeper subcutaneous tissues (Fig. 21-14). These deeper tissues are then dissected to expose the temporal fascia. Anatomic structures encountered include the superficial temporal artery and vein, the transverse facial artery, and the auriculotemporal nerve. This dissection is accompanied by nerve stimulation to safely locate any facial nerve branches, which may then be retracted anteriorly. The condyle and zygomatic arch are localized by palpation, and sharp dissection is used to incise the fascia and expose the periosteum of the lateral fossa and eminence. The periosteum is then sharply incised, and subperiosteal elevation is used to reflect the capsular tissues and enter the superior joint compartment. The meniscus is sepa-

rated from all aspects of the superior osseous structures, and its superior surface may be inspected (Fig. 21-15).

Superior joint decompression may be achieved through reduction of the articular eminence. A prominent and steeply angulated eminence is often found in meniscal displacements with or without reduction, and its reduction improves meniscocondylar coordination. With the use of an osteotome and mallet or an air-driven handpiece, the eminence is vertically reduced and the posterior slope lessened, markedly increasing the functional joint space (Fig. 21-16). Infrequently, pneumatization of the temporal bone exists and air cells are exposed with eminence reduction, producing a vacuolated and irregular superior surface. The voids can be filled and smoothed with acrylic material to restore a uniform surface.[26]

Often in internal derangements of long duration, there are significant degenerative changes of the condyle. Such pathology may be managed by inferior joint decompression and recontouring through a

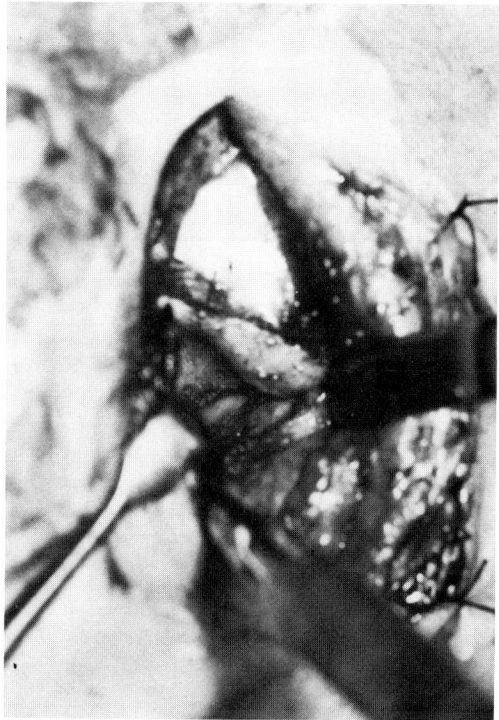

FIG. 21-15. *Superior compartment and articular eminence exposed.*

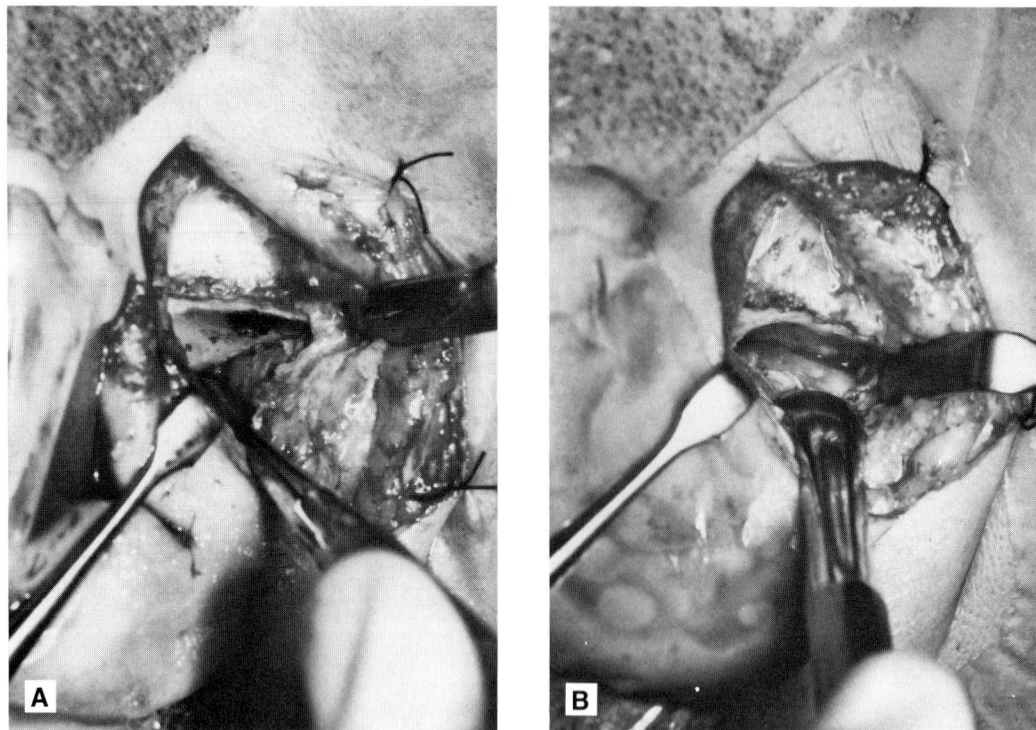

FIG. 21-16. *(A) Articular eminence reduced and angulation of posterior slope decreased producing gradual change between depth of glenoid fossa and apex of eminence. (B) Note increased anterior (functional) joint space and improved view and accessibility to the superior aspect of the meniscus.*

high condylectomy procedure. Upon capsular exposure, it may be incised through an L- or H-shaped design that later facilitates closure. The inferior joint compartment is entered and the condyle exposed, aided by specialized retractors (Fig. 21-17). The condylar head is then reduced 4 to

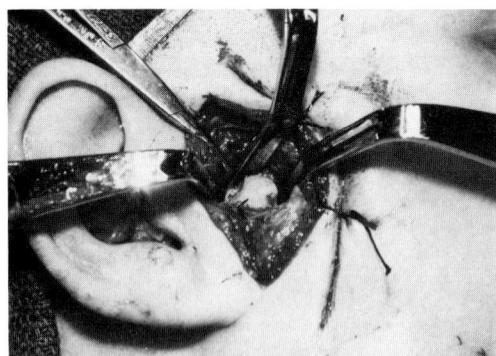

FIG. 21-17. *Condyle exposed and retracted in preparation for high condylectomy.*

5 mm, preserving some medial bone to limit the amount of stripping of the lateral pterygoid muscle—thus enhancing postoperative function. The remaining condylar head is smoothed with bone files or a rotary instrument.

The meniscus frequently suffers stretching and thinning of the posterior attachment tissues with inflammatory hyperplasia of tissue or an actual loss of integrity resulting in a perforation or complete detachment. If possible, perforations are best managed by primary closure with a nonresorbable suture material (Fig. 21-18). Complete detachments are usually not amenable to reapproximation and primary closure, and are best handled by meniscectomy and alloplastic replacement. In addition, redundant meniscal tissue may be reduced and the entire meniscus posteriorly repositioned by wedge resection of either the superior lamina or full thickness of the bilaminar zone.[27]

The capsule is then closed and the fascia

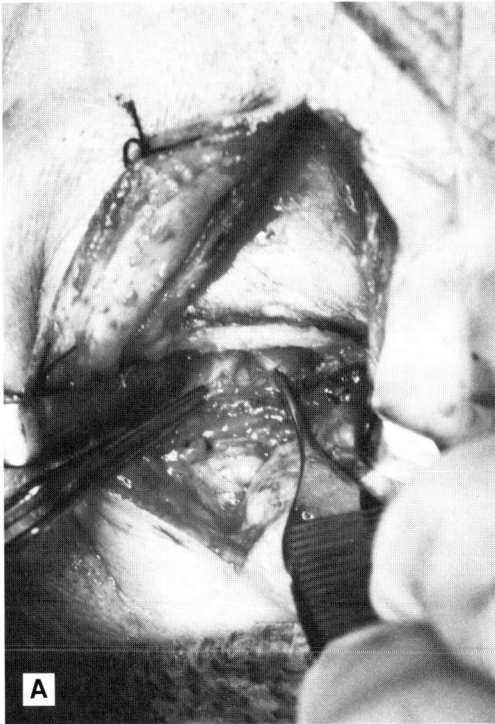

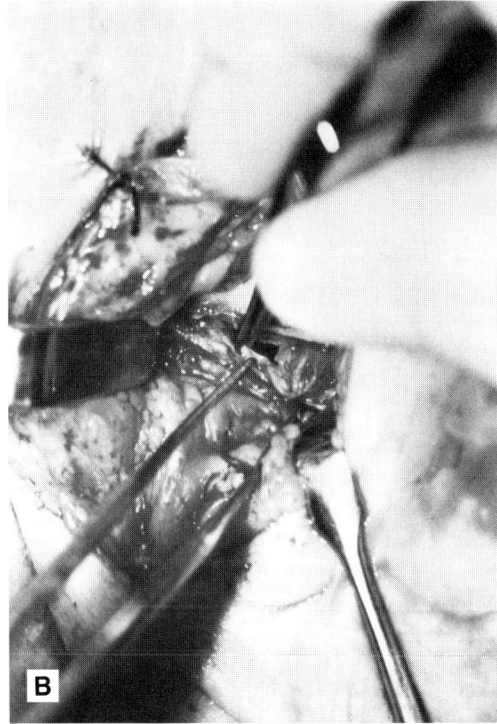

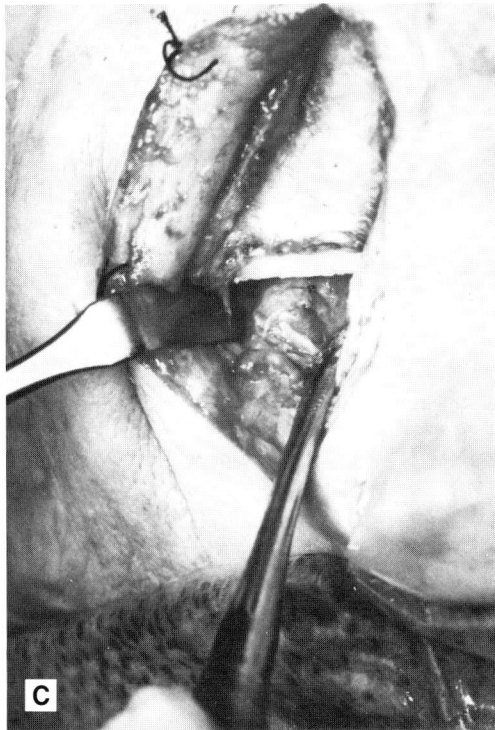

FIG. 21-18. *(A) Partial tear of lateral aspect of the meniscus. (B) Perforation of central aspect of the meniscus. (C) Primary suture repair of meniscal perforation.*

and subcutaneous tissues reapproximated in multiple layers with resorbable suture. The skin is sutured either with interrupted or a subcuticular technique (Fig. 21-19). A pressure dressing is applied and left on for 24 hours. Restricting full range of motion through a soft diet is effected for the first 48 hours. Gentle and gradually increasing physical therapy is begun thereafter. The use of pre-, intra-, and postoperative antibiosis is not necessary with these procedures.[28]

Condylar Dislocations (Hypermobility). Dislocation of the mandible occurs whenever the condyle translates beyond the articular eminence. This is usually not a problem unless the condyle cannot be retracted back over the eminence, which can result from muscle contraction and locking of the condyle in that position. These conditions can usually be treated locally with manual maneuvers, infiltration of local anesthetics into the surrounding musculature, or intravenous muscle relaxants to induce reduction. Rarely, the administration of a general anesthetic may be necessary for long-standing dislocations. Surgical open reductions have been reported in

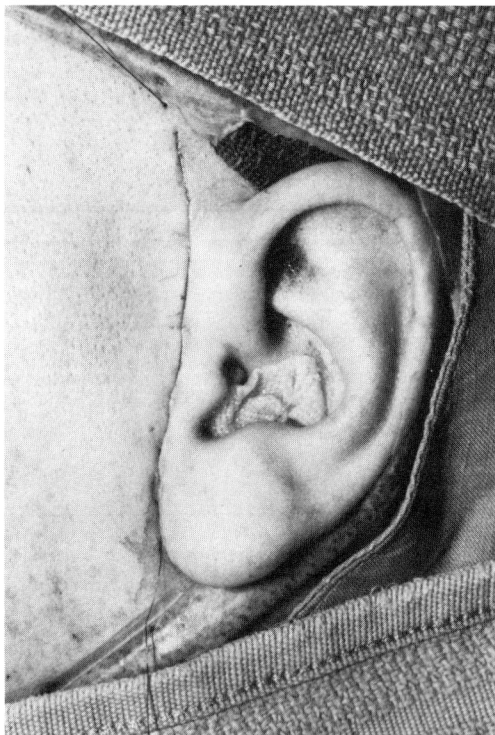

FIG. 21-19. *Subcuticular closure of preauricular incision.*

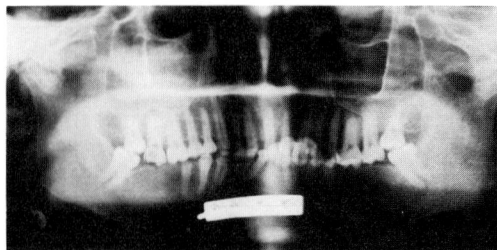

FIG. 21-20. *Bilateral joint ankylosis secondary to macrotrauma. The patient had a history of bilateral subcondylar and symphysis fractures initially repaired with a compression bone plate and intermaxillary fixation. The patient never regained the ability to open after release of fixation.*

a few select cases, either through a preauricular approach to distract the condyle directly or a submandibular approach to apply inferior traction at the angle.

Condylar dislocations pose two significant long-term considerations. Even in a single occurrence that reduces, meniscal stretch or tear may occur ultimately resulting in internal derangement that may require future repair. Chronic, persistent dislocations pose a similar risk, but even if meniscocondylar function is not damaged, increased laxity of the supporting structures occurs, creating a cycle of repetitive dislocations. If the patient cannot easily reduce his dislocations, significant disability ensues.

Several surgical procedures have been used successfully in the treatment of chronic dislocations. Both zygomectomy,[33] in which an osteotomy is used to lower the anterior slope of the eminence, and bone grafting to the eminence, enlarge the articular eminence, which then serves as an obstacle to anterior dislocation of the condyle. An opposite approach is the eminectomy,[34] which removes the anatomic obstruction to posterior condylar movement after terminal translation. Despite the obvious contradiction in approach of these procedures, both have high degrees of success that may be due principally to capsular scarring and fibrosis from entrance into the intracapsular space.

Ankylosis. Fortunately, ankylosis of the temporomandibular joint is relatively uncommon. Unfortunately, any degree (partial or complete) or type (fibrous, osseous) of ankylosis results in a nonfunctional joint that can be managed only through surgery and intensive postoperative rehabilitation. By far, ankylosis is induced through macrotrauma. The accumulation of blood, both above and below the periosteum of the joint, promotes scar tissue or bony union. Other causes include infection, advanced arthritis, and radiation exposure.

Diagnosis of ankylosis is relatively easy. Condylar translation is clinically missing and vertical opening is severely restricted. Radiographs reveal complete obliteration or opacification of the joint space and, in severe cases, ossification of the entire capsule (Fig. 21-20).

Technique. Two basic types of surgical procedures are employed in the treatment of ankylosis. Gap arthroplasty refers to those operations in which a joint space is recreated at either the site of the preexisting space or at a level below the previous space in which no substance is interposed between the recreated bony surfaces. Interpositional arthroplasty also recreates a joint space but has, in addition, the introduction of an autogenous or alloplastic material in the gap.

A gap arthroplasty involves exposure of

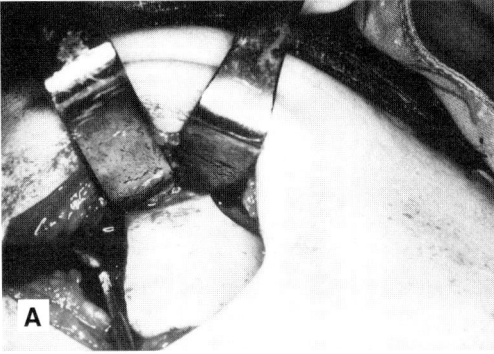

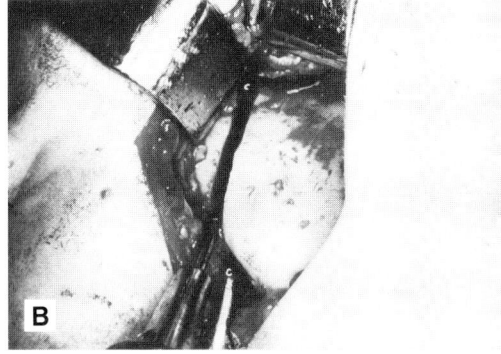

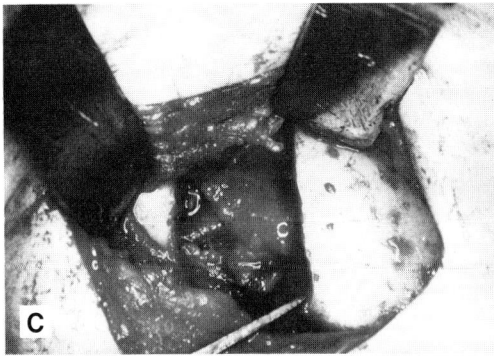

FIG. 21-21. *Submandibular joint approach. (A) Complete osseous ankylosis. (B and C) Osteotomy with ostectomy in creation of a new joint space at a lower level in preparation for placement of interpositional material.*

have been claimed with fascia, fat, muscle, skin, cartilage, acrylic, vitallium, titanium, tantalum, silastic, and teflon. Furthermore, these have been attached successfully to the fossa or superior ramus utilizing screws, wires, plates, and pins (Fig. 21-22). Recently metallic condylar prostheses have been used alone[31] (Fig. 21-23) or in conjunction with fossa implants for total joint

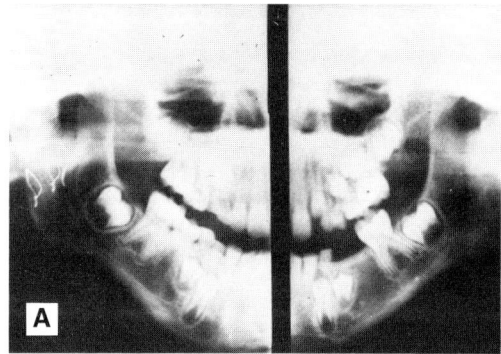

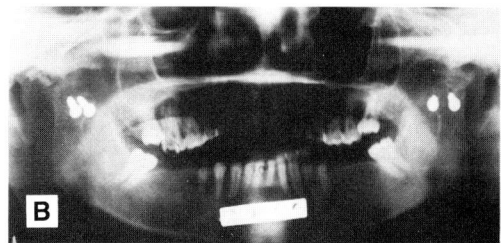

the joint through the previously described preauricular incision and a submandibular incision if lower access is desired. An osteotomy and/or fibrous tissue removal through the preexisting joint space is carried out or a lower level of osteotomy with removal of the condylar head will result in a space of 1 to 3 cm between the zygomatic arch and the superior margin of the ramus (Fig. 21-21). In addition, there must be consideration of the coronoid process and its temporal muscle attachment for it is usually fibrosed, providing an extracapsular source of limitation of mobility. Gaps through the preexisting joint space require the addition of a coronoidectomy procedure to increase movement effectively. Recreation of a lower joint space automatically includes transection of the coronoid process.

Most clinicians agree, however, that the recurrence of ankylosis is markedly decreased when the gap is interposed with material.[29] In addition, the risk of loss of vertical height of the ramus is decreased. As such, interpositional arthroplasties are preferred. However, opinion is divided as to whether autogenous or alloplastic materials should be used[30] and good results

FIG. 21-22. *(A) Postoperative radiograph of silastic interpositional arthroplasty held into position by wire ligatures. (B) Postoperative radiograph of silastic interpositional arthroplasty by screw fixation.*

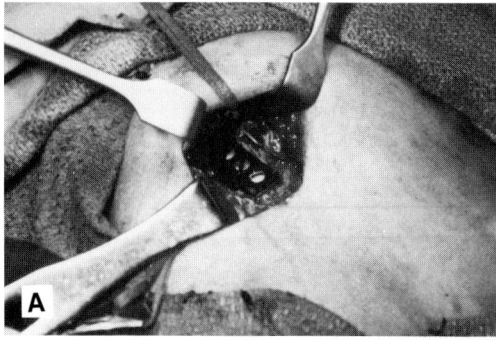

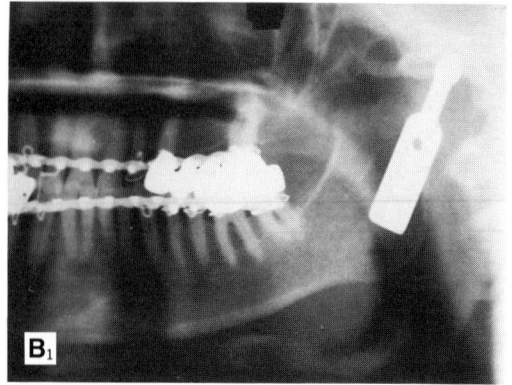

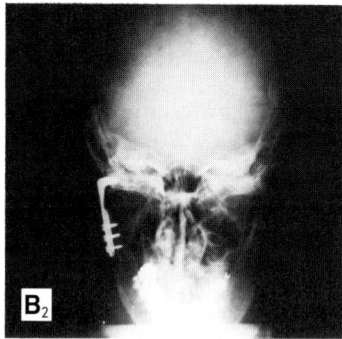

FIG. 21-23. (A) Condylar prosthesis placed through submandibular approach. (B) Postoperative radiographic views of condylar prosthesis: (1) Frontal. (2) Pantographic.

reconstruction[32] (Fig. 21-24). In our experience, new bone may continue to be deposited from the fossa area when condylar prostheses are used alone, and we prefer complete joint replacement including the fossa prosthesis to prevent this recurrence possibility.

A most important factor in successful reestablishment of postoperative function is physiotherapy. It is begun as soon as pain and edema subside and the patient is capable of mandibular mobilization. This is best done in cooperation with a therapist

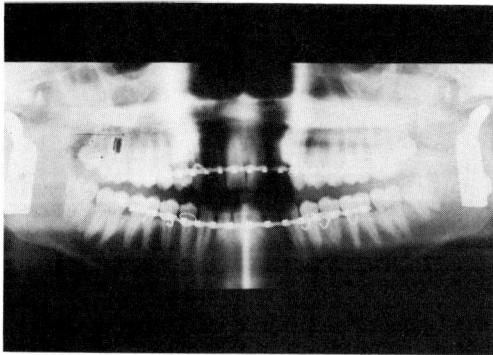

FIG. 21-24. Bilateral total joint replacements (fossa and condyle) secondary to severe osseous degeneration from rheumatoid arthritis.

and may have to be done for several months postoperatively.

Fractures. The majority of condylar fractures can be satisfactorily treated by closed reduction, utilizing intermaxillary fixation with early mobilization. This is possible when the condyle is nondisplaced or favorably displaced within the fossa anteromedially. When the fractured condyle becomes displaced from the fossa, such as into the middle cranial fossa or external auditory canal, or when there is lateral extracapsular displacement or foreign bodies intruding into the joint space, open reduction may be necessary for adequate osseous repositioning and the reestablishment of a functional alignment.[36] These indications apply to both children and adults, although pediatric patients have a far greater adaptive response to poor condylar positioning than adults.

Surgical repositioning of a displaced condyle is a difficult and frequently troublesome procedure. Direct access to the fracture is precluded by the position of the facial nerve and parotid gland. As a result, surgical approaches vary depending upon the level of the fracture site. In low subcondylar fractures, a submandibular approach may be satisfactory. A fracture at a higher level may require a combined submandibular and preauricular approach to locate and position the segments effectively. Either method, however, never really produces easy access.

Once located and repositioned, the condylar segments require internal stabilization if ones desires nonfixation or early mobilization. This may be done with wires, pins, or plates,[37-40] but is, again, technically difficult due to the indirect access required. If acceptable segment position is obtained, one may circumvent the application of internal fixation provided 4 to 6 weeks of intermaxillary fixation are allowed.

Developmental and Degenerative Deformities. Joint deformities characterized by absence, hypoplasia, or loss of the condylar component occur either through developmental aberration (trauma to growth center, hemifacial microsomia, Treacher Collins syndrome) or arthritic disease (rheumatoid, seronegatives). They are usually associated with decreased condylar and ramus height, which produces a concomitant facial skeletal deformity and apertognathia.

Historically, surgical rehabilitation has produced variable results, secondary to a lack of a completely satisfactory reconstructive method that is biocompatible, anatomic in form, and functionally based. However, the recent advent of total joint reconstruction with condyle and fossa prostheses[32] has produced reliable results in condylar reconstruction with simultaneous correction of apertognathia and mandibular retrognathia. It not only recreates a potentially functional joint but reliably restores vertical ramus height.[31] Its use, however, should be reserved for adult patients over the age of 18, in whom facial growth is essentially complete. In a child or young adult, a more biologic material such as costochondral grafts[35] offers the capability of responding to the dynamics of ongoing growth. In addition, this joint reconstructive system cannot presently be adapted to the decreased size of pediatric anatomy.

References

1. Delfino, J. J. and Eppley, B. L.: Radiographic and surgical evaluation of internal derangements of the temporomandibular joint. J. Oral Maxillofac. Surg., *44:*260, 1986.
2. Roberts, C.A., et al.: Mandibular range of motion versus arthrographic diagnosis of the temporomandibular joint. Oral Surg., *60:*244, 1985.
3. Oster, C., et al.: Characterization of temporomandibular joint sounds. Oral Surg., *58:*10, 1984.
4. Mongini, F.: Anatomic and clinical evaluation of the relationship between the temporomandibular joint and occlusion. J. Prosth. Dent., *38:*539, 1977.
5. Updegrave, W. J.: Improved roentgenographic technic for the temporomandibular articulation, JADA, *40:*391, 1950.
6. Grewcock, R. J. G.: A simple technique for temporomandibular joint radiography. Br. Dent. J., *94:*152, 1953.
7. O'Ryan, F., and Epker, B. N.: Temporomandibular joint function and morphology: Observations on the spectra of normalcy. Oral Surg., *58:*272, 1984.
8. Bean, L. R., Omnell, K. A., and Oberg, T.: Comparison between radiologic observations and macroscopic tissue changes in temporomandibular joints. Dentomaxillofac. Rad., *6:*90, 1977.
9. Stanson, A. W., and Baker, H. L.: Routine tomography of the temporomandibular joint, Rad. Clin. N. Am., *14:*105, 1976.
10. Rosenberg, H. M., and Silha, R. E.: TMJ radiography with emphasis on tomography. Dent. Photo. and Rad., *55:*1, 1982.
11. Farrar, W. B., and McCarty, W. L.: Inferior joint space arthrography and characteristics of condylar paths in internal derangements of the TMJ. J. Prosth. Dent., *41:*548, 1979.
12. Katzberg, R. W., et al.: Arthrography of the temporomandibular joint. AJR, *134:*995, 1980.
13. Murphy, W. A.: Arthrography of the temporomandibular joint. Rad. Clin. N. Am., *19:*365, 1981.
14. Bronstein, S. L., Tomasetti, B. I., and Ryan, D. E.: Internal derangement of the temporomandibular joint: Correlation of arthrography and surgical findings. J. Oral Surg., *39:*572, 1981.
15. Graham, G. S., Ferraro, N. E., and Simms, D. A.: Perforations of the temporomandibular joint meniscus: arthrographic, surgical and clinical findings. J. Oral Maxillofac. Surg., *42:*35, 1984.
16. Helms, C. A., Katzberg, R. W., Morrish, R., and Dolwick, M. F.: Computed tomography of the temporomandibular joint meniscus. J. Oral Maxillofac. Surg., *41:*512, 1983.
17. Sartoris, D. J., Neumann, C. H., and Riley, R. W.: The temporomandibular joint: True sagittal computed tomography with meniscus visualization. Radiology, *150:*250, 1984.
18. Beard, C. C., and Clayton, J. A.: Effects of occlusal splint therapy on TMJ dysfunction. J. Prosth. Dent., *44:*324, 1980.
19. Goharian, R. K., and Neff, C. A.: Effect of

occlusal retainers on temporomandibular joint and facial pain. J. Prosth. Dent., *44:*206, 1980.

20. Mejiias, J. E., and Mehta, N. R.: Subjective and objective evaluation of bruxing patients undergoing short-term splint therapy. J. Oral Rehabil., *9:*279, 1982.

21. Mercuri, L. G., Campbell, R. L., and Shamaskin, R. G.: Intra-articular meniscus dysfunction surgery. A preliminary report. Oral Surg., *54:*613, 1982.

22. Weinberg, S: Eminectomy and meniscorhaphy for internal derangements of the temporomandibular joint. Oral Surg., *57:*241, 1984.

23. Henny, F. A.: Surgical treatment for the painful temporomandibular joint, JADA, *79:*171, 1969.

24. Cherry, C. O., and Frew, A.: High condylectomy for treatment of arthritis of the temporomandibular joint. J. Oral Surg., *35:*235, 1977.

25. Dunn, M. J., Benza, R., Moan, D., and Sanders, J.: Temporomandibular joint condylectomy: a technique and postoperative follow-up. Oral Surg., *51:*363, 1981.

26. Tyndall, D. A., and Matteson, S. R.: Radiographic appearance and population distribution of the pneumatized articular eminence of the temporal bone. J Oral Maxillofac. Surg., *43:*493, 1985.

27. Hall, M. B.: Meniscoplasty of the displaced temporomandibular joint meniscus without violating the inferior joint space. J. Oral Maxillofac. Surg., *42:*788, 1984.

28. Eppley, B. L., and Delfino, J. J.: Prophylactic antibiotics in temporomandibular joint surgery. J. Oral Maxillofac. Surg., *43:*675, 1985.

29. Topazian, R. G.: Comparison of gap and interposition arthroplasty in the treatment of temporomandibular joint ankylosis. J. Oral Surg., *24:*405, 1966.

30. Moorthy, A. P., and Finch, L. D.: Interpositional arthroplasty for ankylosis of the temporomandibular joint. Oral Surg., *55:*545, 1983.

31. Kent, J. N., et al.: Temporomandibular joint prosthesis: a ten-year report. J. Oral Maxillofac. Surg., *41:*245, 1983.

32. Kent, J. N., and Zide, M. F.: Wound healing: bone and biomaterials. Otolaryngol. Clin. North Am., *17:*309, 1984.

33. Boudreau, R. G., and Tideman, H.: Treatment of chronic mandibular dislocation. Oral Surg., *41:*169, 1976.

34. Irby, W. B.: Surgery of the temporomandibular joint. *In* Current Advances in Oral Surgery. St. Louis, C. V. Mosby Co., 1974.

35. Kennett, S.: Temporomandibular joint ankylosis: the rationale for grafting in the young patient. J. Oral Surg., *31:*744, 1973.

36. Zide, M.F., and Kent, J.N.: Indications for open reduction of mandibular condyle fractures. J. Oral Maxillofac. Surg., *41:*89–98, 1983.

37. Tasanen, A., and Lamberg, M.A.: Transosseous wiring in the treatment of condylar fractures of the mandible. J. Maxillofac. Surg., *2:*200–203, 1976.

38. Koberg, W., and Momma, W-G: Treatment of fractures of the articular process by functional stable osteosynthesis using miniaturized dynamic compression plates. Int. J. Oral Surg., *7:*256–262, 1978.

39. Cadanet, H., et al.: Osteosynthesis of subcondylar fractures in the adult. J. Maxillofac. Surg., *11:*20–25, 1983.

40. Wennogle, C.F., and Delo, R.I: A pin-in-groove technique for reduction of displaced subcondylar fractures of the mandible. J. Oral Maxillofac. Surg., *43:*659–665, 1985.

CHAPTER 22

Correction of Dentofacial Deformities

Larry M. Wolford and Frank W. Hilliard

To study the phenomena of disease without books is to sail an uncharted sea, while to study books without patients is not to go to sea at all. Sir William Osler

Orthognathic surgery (or surgical orthodontics) is the science and art of correcting dentofacial deformities with a combination of tooth movement (orthodontics) and repositioning of the jaw structures (surgery). Orthodontic treatment alone is primarily a movement of the teeth within their bone base. Orthodontics can correct some discrepancies in the skeletal relationship of the upper and lower jaws, but the correction may be limited. Orthodontic treatment of a skeletal problem is naturally more successful when the patient is growing, but case selection should be made very carefully. Three basic dimensions should be considered when evaluating the relationship of the upper and lower jaws to each other, and most importantly to the face:

1. Vertical—The heights of the upper and lower jaw and facial proportions
2. Horizontal—The profile positions of the upper and lower jaws and soft tissue form
3. Transverse—The widths and symmetries of the upper and lower jaws and associated soft tissues

If disharmony between the upper and lower jaws (and the face) is moderate to severe, a more ideal result may be acheived by combining orthodontic treatment with jaw surgery. The orthodontist must align the teeth with braces, and then the surgeon repositions the upper and/or lower jaw to a more ideal predetermined position. Orthodontic treatment is completed after the surgical procedure has healed. The specialties of orthodontics and oral and maxillofacial surgery have blended their efforts to achieve optimal functional and aesthetic results for patients with dentofacial deformities. The support of the general dentist, prosthodontist, periodontist, endodontist, pedodontist, and our medical colleagues has afforded patients the opportunity to receive "state of the art" care in correcting these deformities. The specialists involved must be able to diagnose correctly, establish a treatment plan, and execute the recommended treatment.

The three areas that require expertise in order to achieve optimum results for patients include:

1. *Diagnosis.* A complete diagnosis of all existing related problems identified in the patient evaluation, radiographic evaluation, dental model analysis, and other indicated evaluations. Without a correct diagnosis, treatment may be incomplete and successful results cannot be assured.
2. *Treatment planning.* The treatment plan takes into consideration all the factors identified in the diagnosis, as well as patient concerns and reasons for con-

sidering orthognathic surgery. It outlines the sequence of treatment to be performed by all health care professionals involved. In defining the treatment plan, a thorough knowledge of the many types of dentofacial deformities and the treatment modalities available to correct them is essential.

3. *Treatment.* Therapeutic management must be carried out as planned, without omitting steps or unnecessarily changing the timing sequence. Total correction of dentofacial deformities usually involves several members of the health care team.

Research studies and innovative ideas in oral and maxillofacial surgery and orthodontics have permitted significant advances to occur within a very short time. This chapter includes a brief history of the field, which provides insight into some of the many contributions to this special area of patient care. Also included is an expansion of the three basic areas outlined above and presentation of some of the more common disorders and their management.

History

It is not known when the first surgical procedures were performed. Few articles were published in the early 20th century. One of the first persons to publish an intraoral setback of the mandible was Hullihen in 1848.[1] He utilized intraoral body osteotomies. One of the next known recorded surgeries was referred to by Edward H. Angle in his orthodontic book published in 1907.[2] He discussed two cases in which the lower jaw was repositioned posteriorly by bilateral body ostectomies. One operation, performed around 1898, involved bilateral mandibular body ostectomies, in which the lower jaw was resectioned in the first bicuspid area bilaterally and the anterior part of the mandible moved posteriorly. This case was reported successful, but a case subsequent to it was a total failure, with the patient near death and finally having almost total loss of the mandible through necrosis. The early pioneers in this surgery were extremely brave, but lacked the sterility, instrumentation, and antibiotics necessary to achieve predictable results. For many years, the emphasis for correcting facial deformities focused primarily on mandibular body surgery.

Anterior maxillary surgery was introduced in 1921 by Cohn-Stock,[3] and total maxillary surgery was first described by Wassmund in 1927.[4] These procedures were not used extensively, and not much appeared in the literature until the late 1960s. In the late 1960s and early 1970s, significant advances were made in orthognathic surgery as orthodontists and oral surgeons began working together more closely to achieve optimal functional and aesthetic results. Three classic textbooks, directed entirely to orthognathic surgery, were written by Hinds and Kent, 1974;[5] Epker and Wolford, 1980;[6] and Bell, Profitt, and White, 1980.[7] Hundreds of articles and book chapters have been published about correcting dentofacial deformities.

Considerations for Orthognathic Surgery

The four fundamental reasons for considering orthognathic surgery are function, aesthetics, stability, and treatment time.[8]

Functional problems often coexist with aesthetic deformities. Functional concerns may include occlusion, mastication, speech, muscle function, the temporomandibular joint (TMJ), etc. Functional deformities that benefit from treatment are depicted later in this chapter. When functional problems are corrected, aesthetics can be either enhanced or worsened, depending on the surgical procedures chosen. The design for correction of the functional problems obviously should be directed toward optimal aesthetics.

Aesthetics may be the primary concern for many patients. When a moderate to severe musculoskeletal deformity occurs, usually the facial balance is not ideal and it is almost impossible to achieve acceptable aesthetics with orthodontics alone. It is important to assess carefully existing musculoskeletal and dental deformities so that the orthodontic mechanics and surgical techniques permit optimal aesthetic and functional results. These are depicted later in this chapter.

Stability is a definite consideration for surgical orthodontic treatment because the stability of results achieved by combined treatment in certain deformities is far superior to orthodontic or surgical management alone. The use of stable orthodontic mechanics, together with the proper selection and execution of the surgical techniques, should provide stable and predictable results. Identifying the potential for stability in patients is important in order to provide optimal treatment and long-term stability. The combination of surgery and orthodontics seems to provide improved predictability of results when the techniques are properly applied.

Treatment time may be reduced with combined surgery and orthodontics when correcting certain dentofacial deformities as compared to attempting to correct the malocclusions strictly orthodontically. With the combined approach, the orthodontics are designed to align teeth over the basal bone and then surgically to reposition the jaw structures into proper functional and aesthetic balance. In some cases, treatment time may be lengthened because of extensive orthodontics necessary and the interruption of the orthodontic management for the surgical procedures. Also, if unstable orthodontic mechanisms or surgical techniques have been introduced, long-term retention may be necessary.

Diagnosis

Patient Evaluation

Four primary areas for patient evaluation that provide the most diagnostic information include patient concerns, clinical evaluation, radiographic evaluation, and dental model analysis.

Additionally, some patients may require speech, audiometric, psychologic, medical, and other evaluations. The oral and maxillofacial surgeon and/or orthodontist must be able to recognize the need for these additional evaluations.

PATIENT CONCERNS

It is of utmost importance to determine the patient's feelings about the existing problems and his expectations for treatment results. In treatment planning we must address the patient's concerns so that the treatment results satisfy the patient. It is hoped that the preliminary patient as-

sessment will alert the orthodontist and oral and maxillofacial surgeon to that patient with pathologic psychosis or unrealistic expectations.

CLINICAL EVALUATION

Clinical evaluation of the patient should be done with the patient either standing or sitting in a straight-backed chair directly opposite the examiner. The patient's head should be oriented so that clinical Frankfort horizontal, i.e., a line from the tragus of the ear and the bony infraorbital rim, is aligned relatively parallel to the floor. The patient's mandible should be placed in a centric relation, with the condyles properly seated in the fossa and the teeth lightly touching together. The lips should be relaxed and not forced together (Fig. 22-1). The relaxed lip position is very important, particularly in patients with vertical facial excesses. If the lips are forced together, it is difficult to evaluate the degree of vertical deformity and the soft tissue morphology. On the other hand, if the lips are overclosed, as seen in vertical maxillary deficiencies, the patient should be evaluated with the condyles in centric relation, with

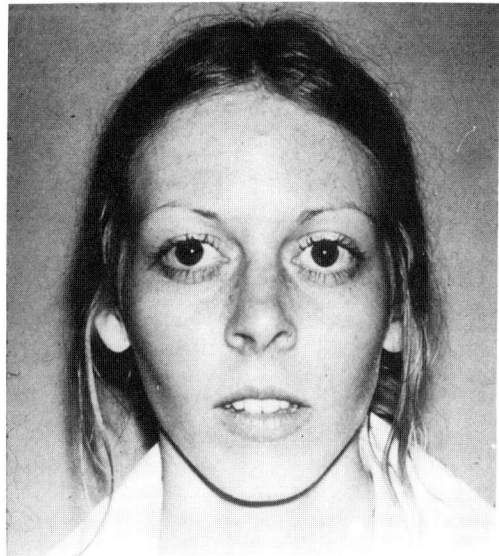

FIG. 22-1. *It is important in assessing patients to be sure that the lips are completely relaxed and the occlusion is in centric relation. Head posture should be oriented so that clinical Frankfort horizontal (tragus of the ear to infraorbital bone rim) is parallel to the floor.*

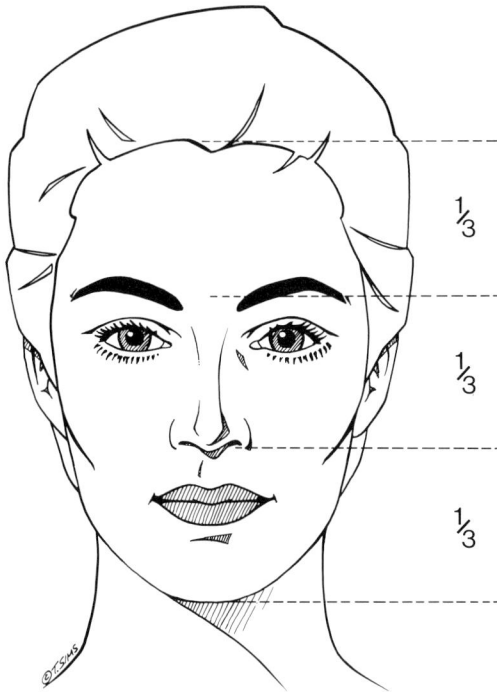

FIG. 22-2. *The face is divided into thirds. The upper third is from the bridge of the nose superiorly. The middle third is from the bridge to the base of the nose. The lower third is from the base of the nose to the bottom of the chin.*

the jaws open until the lips begin to separate so that tooth-to-lip and soft tissue morphology can be assessed.

The face is divided into thirds (Fig. 22-2). The upper third is from the forehead superiorly, the middle third is from the area between the eyebrows to the base of the nose, and the lower third is from the base of the nose to the under surface of the chin. Because surgical orthodontic management basically alters the lower third of the face, this chapter focuses on the evaluation of these aspects. The middle and upper thirds of the face can be surgically altered, but this requires additional special training for the surgeon.

Frontal View. The frontal view is important to assess because it is usually how the patient sees himself. The forehead, eyes, orbits, and nose are evaluated for harmony. The upper lip is measured from the base of the nose (subnasale) to the inferior part of the upper lip (upper lip stomion). The normal length is 22 mm ± 2

mm for males and 20 mm ± 2 mm for females (Fig. 22-3). With the lips relaxed, the normal amount of tooth exposed below the upper lip is 1 to 4 mm. (Fig. 22-4).[9] These measurements are significant if the upper jaw position is to be surgically altered. The facial midline, nasal midline, upper lip, dental midlines, and chin midline should be concurrent, and the face should have reasonable symmetry from the left to the right side (Fig. 22-5). When the midlines are not properly aligned or the face is asymmetrical, the diagnosis and treatment plan should include surgical-orthodontic correction of these aspects.

The alar base width (width of the nose) is altered when upper jaw surgery is performed. Ideally, when a line is dropped from the medial canthal tendon area of the eye perpendicular to a pupillary line, the alar base should fall on that line ± 2 mm (Fig. 22-6). If the patient has vertical deficiencies, the lips may be overclosed and distorted and should also be evaluated with

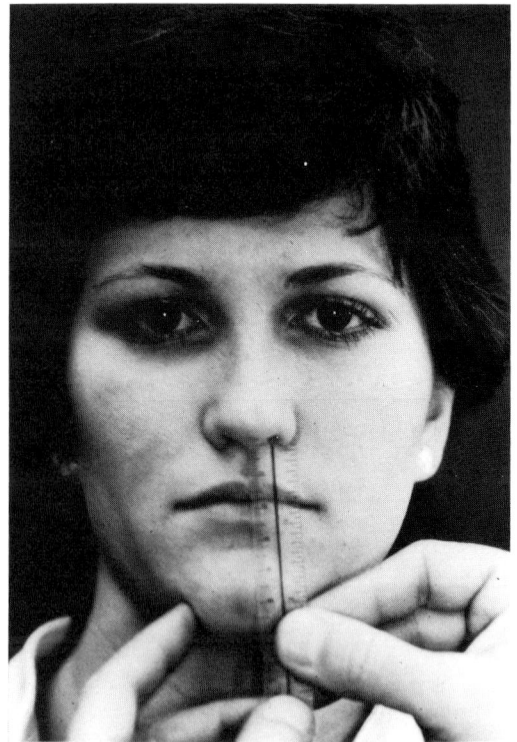

FIG. 22-3. *Upper lip length is measured from the base of the nose to the inferior aspect of the upper lip (upper lip stomion).*

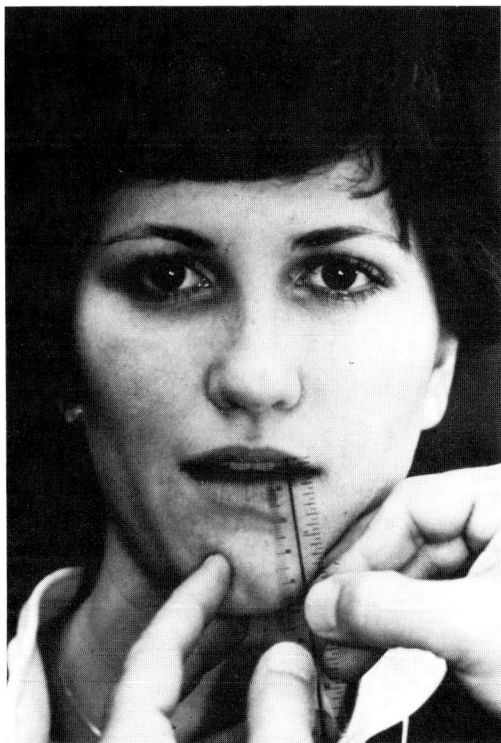

FIG. 22-4. *Upper tooth-to-lip relationship is measured from the incisor edge to the inferior aspect of the upper lip.*

the jaws opened slightly until the lips start to separate with the condyles in centric relation. This allows evaluation of the soft tissues and dental osseous relationship.

Although the smile is important to examine and evaluate because it may be one of the patient's primary concerns, it is important not to make vertical maxillary position determinations from the smile (Fig. 22-7). The anteroposterior position of the maxilla, the inclination of the anterior dentoalveolus, and muscle function affect the amount of upper lip elevation and could give false information relative to vertical types of deformities.

Lateral View. The lateral view is probably of most value in determining vertical and anteroposterior problems of the jaw structures (Fig. 22-8). The distance from glabella (medial aspect of the eyebrows) to the base of the nose and base of the nose to the soft tissue chin should be equal,[9] providing the upper lip is of normal length. If a line is dropped from subnasale perpen-

dicular to the clinical Frankfort horizontal line, the chin should be 3 mm ± 3 mm posterior to that line.[10] The interrelationships of the bony and soft tissue structures surrounding the orbit and globe are evaluated for excesses or deficiencies. Morphology of the nose, upper lip, and cheeks is evaluated relative to their interrelationships with one another. The position of the lower lip and chin should be assessed relative to established anteroposterior and vertical standards. Generally, the distance from the top of the lower lip to the bottom of the chin should be slightly more than twice the length of the upper lip. The chin-neckline and angle are important for evaluation of the position of the chin and head posture.

Oral Examination. The interrelationships of the teeth are evaluated in centric occlusion and, more importantly, in centric relation. Gentle pressure is used to ensure that the condyles are properly seated. This is the jaw position that the surgeon must plan and work from at the time of surgery.

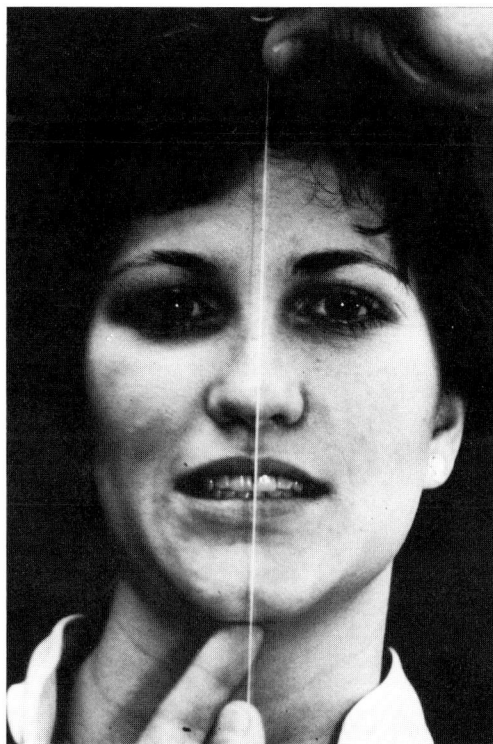

FIG. 22-5. *Midlines of the face, nose, upper lip, maxillary and mandibular dental midlines, and chin midline are evaluated in relation to one another.*

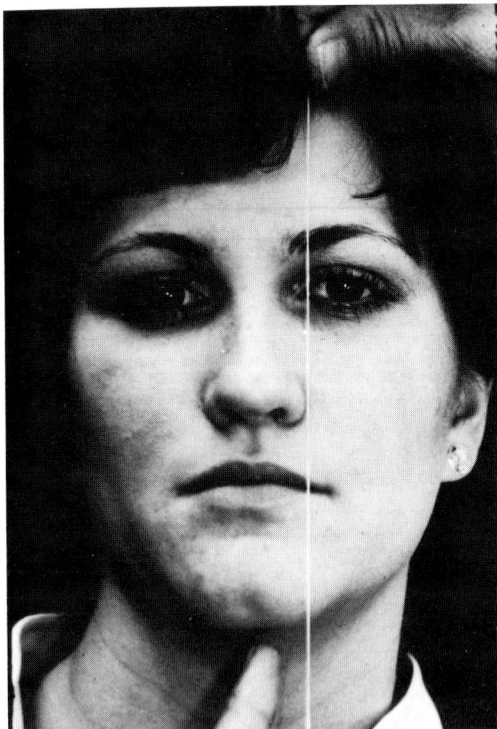

FIG. 22-6. *A line dropped from the medial canthal area to perpendicular to the pupillary plane should fall within 1 to 2 mm of the base of the nose.*

Transverse problems, including crossbites, crowding of the arches, the curves of the occlusion (curve of Spee), arch symmetry, health of the gingiva, the type of occlusion (i.e., Class I, II, or III and their appropriate subdivisions), and the overall health of the teeth (i.e., missing teeth, decay, etc.) are aspects to examine (Fig. 22-9). The buccal tipping of posterior teeth (curve of Wilson) is also important to assess, particularly in the upper arch. Periodontal considerations should be assessed because with some orthodontic mechanics and particularly surgery in the anterior part of the mandible, significant worsening of preexisting periodontal problems can occur.

Temporomandibular Joint. The temporomandibular joint should be assessed thoroughly to determine any preexisting problems that may be present. This establishes a base line to follow the progress of joint function throughout treatment or establish the necessity for TMJ treatment. The basic concerns relative to the joint in-

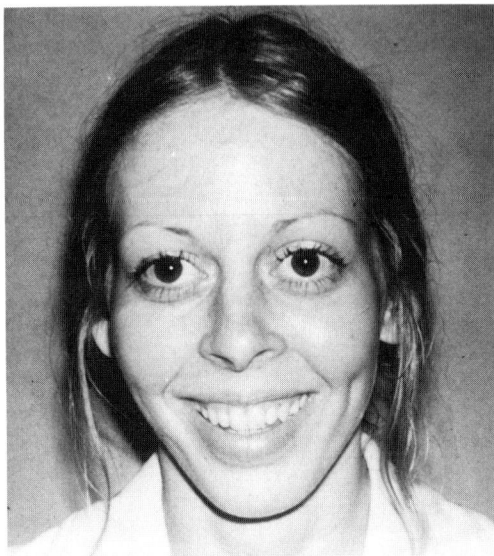

FIG. 22-7. *Although the smile may be a major concern for the patient, it is important not to treatment plan vertical changes from the smile pattern.*

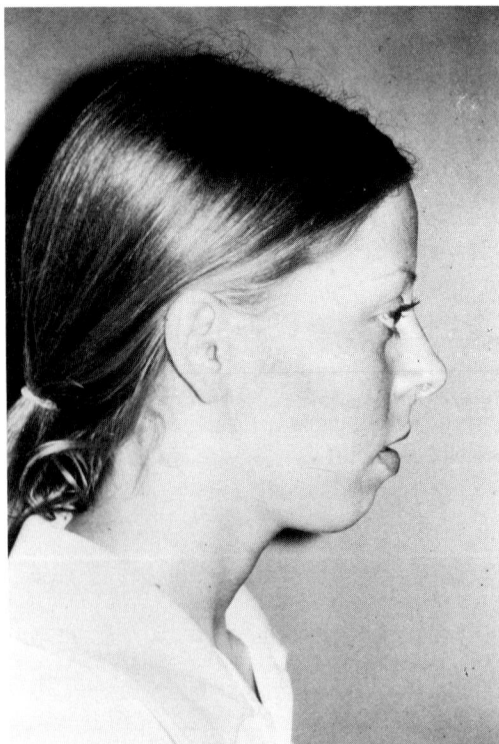

FIG. 22-8. *The profile view is helpful for determining A-P and vertical skeletal deformities.*

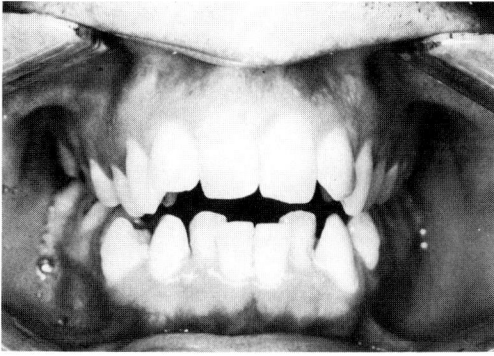

FIG. 22-9. *The occlusion must be evaluated in centric relation because this is where the surgeon and orthodontist must plan from. In this case, an anterior open-bite and bilateral posterior cross-bites exist. The lower anterior arch is crowded.*

clude its functional abilities, any limitations of function created by the joint, and noises such as clicking and popping that may denote articular disc displacement. Crepitation may indicate osteoarthritis or perforations through the disc or bilaminar zone or other pathologic conditions. Also, it should be determined whether or not the patient has a history of headaches or other pain associated with the head and neck area. In cases with preexisting TMJ problems, a complete assessment for an accurate diagnosis and appropriate treatment recommendations should be done.

RADIOGRAPHIC EVALUATION

The three most routine radiographs used in the diagnosis of dentofacial de-

formities are cephalometric, panographic, and periapical.

A cephalometric radiograph is a lateral x-ray taken at a fixed distance from the patient (Fig. 22-10). The patient is placed within a machine with the lips in repose, in centric relation, with the teeth lightly touching and taken so that the soft tissue profile as well as the teeth and bone can be seen on the subsequent x-ray. This permits analysis of the patient's profile, soft tissue, bone, and teeth (Fig. 22-11).

If the patient has an "over-closed" bite, the lips will also be "over-closed" when the teeth are together. For better radiographic evaluation of the soft tissue in these patients, an additional cephalometric radiograph should be taken with the jaws opened until the lips begin to separate, keeping the condyles in a centric relation. A cephalometric x-ray in this position gives accurate soft tissue morphology and a measurable tooth-to-lip relationship that are very important in treatment planning. Numerous detailed cephalometric analyses have been developed from studies of average or "normal" subjects in which standard angular and lineal measurements have been established. Some common cephalometric landmarks are demonstrated in Figure 22-12 and defined in Table 22-1. Whatever analysis is utilized, it is impor-

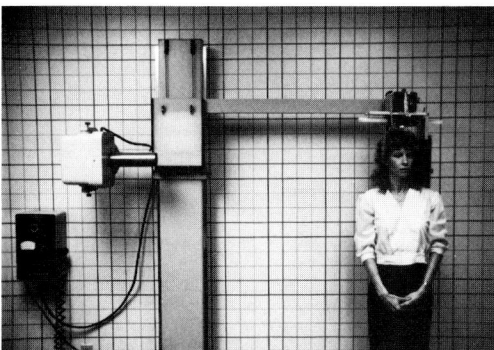

FIG. 22-10. *A cephalometric film is being taken on a patient. A fixed focal distance of 6 feet is used, which yields approximately 8 percent magnification of the X-ray film as compared to the patient's actual size.*

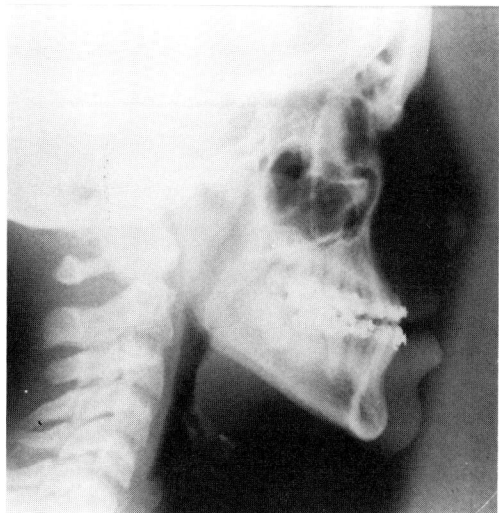

FIG. 22-11. *The cephalometric radiograph should be taken with a technique that shows the soft tissue profile image as well as the dento-osseous structures.*

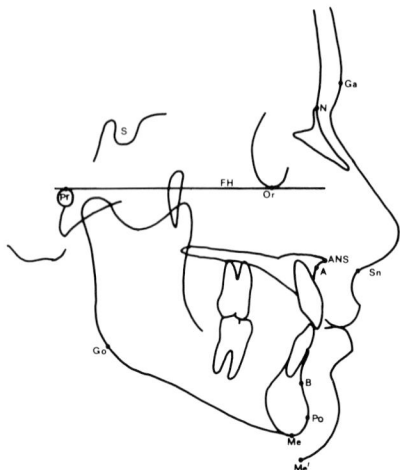

FIG. 22-12. *The basic landmarks necessary for a ceph-alometric analysis of an orthognathic surgery case.*

tant to know that occasionally a significant difference can occur between the clinical evaluation and the numerical values obtained from the cephalometric analyses. When a significant difference occurs, the clinical evaluation is more important relative to treatment planning. In these cases, the cephalometric numbers that are uncorresponding should be disregarded. Ceph-

alometrics tempered with good clinical judgment can be valuable in completing the diagnosis and establishing a treatment plan.

Eleven cephalometric interrelationships are routinely used to permit a very rapid diagnostic assessment and provide the basic information necessary to correct most dentofacial deformities. This concise analysis provides guidelines for establishing treatment goals orthodontically and surgically.

1. *Upper tooth to upper lip relationship*[9] is normally 1 to 4 mm (Fig. 22-13A, #1). It must be correlated with upper lip length to achieve the best facial harmony. The longer the upper lip, then the treatment goal would be for less tooth exposed (1 to 2 mm) after treatment; the shorter the upper lip, then more tooth should be exposed (3 to 5 mm) in order to maintain optimal vertical facial balance and aesthetics.

2. *Upper lip length* is measured from the base of the nose (subnasale) to the inferior part of the upper lip, upper lip stomion (Fig. 22-13A, #2). The normal length of an adult male lip is 22 mm ± 2 mm, and for a female it is 20

TABLE 22-1. Cephalometric landmarks

Ga (glabella): The most prominent point of the forehead

Sn (subnasale): The most posterior superior point on the nasolabial curvature

Me (soft tissue menton): The most inferior point on the soft tissue of the chin

N (nasion): The point formed by the frontonasal suture

ANS (anterior nasal spine): The most anterior point of the nasal floor

A (subspinale): The point of greatest concavity of the maxilla between anterior nasal spine and maxillary dental alveolus

B (supramentale): The point of greatest concavity of the mandible between mandibular dental alveolus and pogonion

Me (menton): The most inferior point on the mandibular symphysis

Or (orbitale): The most inferior point of the orbital rim

Go (gonion): The point located by bisecting the angle formed by tangents to the posterior border of the ramus and inferior border of the mandible

Pr (porion): The most superior point on the curvature of the bony ear canal (internal auditory meatus)

S (sella): The midpoint of sella turcica

Po (pogonion): The most anterior point on the mandibular symphysis

FH (Frankfort): Anatomic porion—orbitale plane

(From: Wolford, L.M., et al.: Surgical Treatment Objective: A Systematic Approach to the Prediction Tracing. St. Louis, C.V. Mosby Co., 1984.)

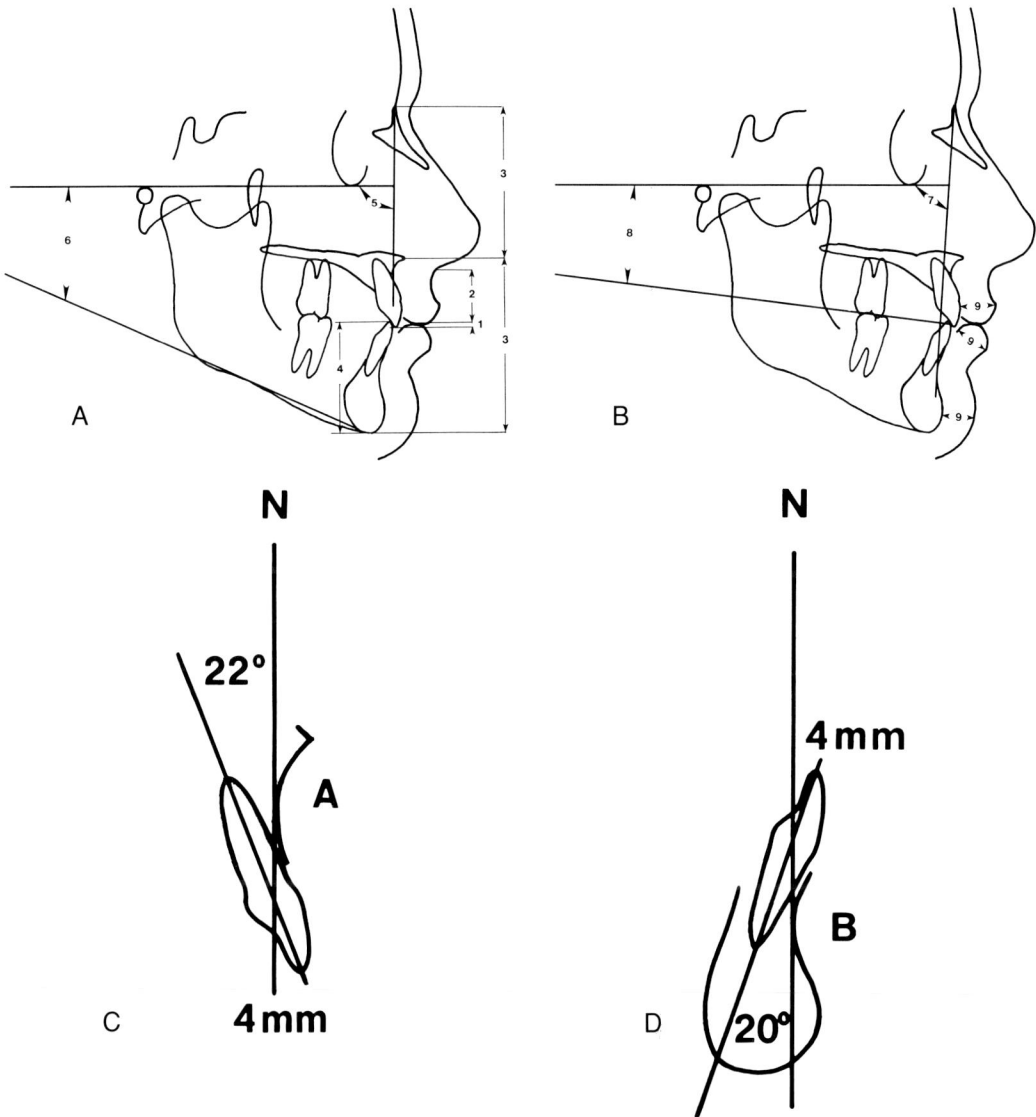

FIG. 22-13. *(A and B) Osseous and soft tissue cephalometric interrelationships. (C and D) Ideal incisor position.*

mm ± 2 mm. Upper lip length is the basis for establishing vertical facial dimensions since it cannot be easily altered.

3. *Vertical bony height of the face*[11] is measured from nasion to anterior nasal spine and from anterior nasal spine to menton (Fig. 22-13A, #3). The normal values are 53 mm from nasion to anterior nasal spine and 65 mm from anterior nasal spine to menton. However, the important interrelationship is a 5:6 ratio, provided that the upper lip

is totally normal in length. If the upper lip is excessively long or short, the vertical height ratio will be less meaningful.

4. *Lower anterior dental height*[11] is measured from the lower incisor tip to the inferior border of the mandible (Fig. 22-13A, #4). The average lower anterior dental height for males is 44 mm ± 2 mm; for females, 40 mm ± 2 mm. Usually, for optimal facial balance, this length is approximately twice the upper lip length. If the upper lip is

longer than average, the lower anterior dental height should be longer than average so that the facial dimensions correlate.

5. *Maxillary depth*[12] is a measurement of a line from nasion to point A (NA line) and the angle it forms with Frankfort horizontal (Fig. 22-13A, #5). Normally, it is 90° ± 3°. This gives information on the anteroposterior (AP) position of the maxilla relative to the cranial base structures.

6. *Frankfort mandibular angle*[13] is the angle created by a line from menton through gonion relative to Frankfort horizontal (Fig. 22-13A, #6). Normally it is 25° ± 5°. This angle influences the diagnosis of the existing facial type and is also of value in determining treatment procedures.

7. *Mandibular depth*[12] is the angle formed by a line from nasion through point B of the mandible and the Frankfort horizontal plane (Fig. 22-13B, #7). Normally it is 88° ± 3°. This gives information relative to the A-P position of the mandible in regard to the cranial base structures.

8. *Occlusal plane angle*[14] is a line drawn tangent to the molar and bicuspid occlusal surfaces and the angle it creates with Frankfort horizontal (Fig. 22-13B, #8). The normal angle is 8° ± 4°. The occlusal plane angle has significant influence on aesthetic and functional results, particularly when double jaw surgery is performed.

9. *Soft tissue thickness*[9] of the upper lip, lower lip, and chin area is normally 11 to 14 mm, but more importantly there should be a 1:1:1 ratio (Fig. 22-13B, #9). The upper lip is measured from the labial surface of the incisor to the most protruding part of the upper lip. The lower lip is measured from the mucocutaneous junction across the lip curvature toward the lower incisor tip. Soft tissue thickness of the chin is measured from bony pogonion to soft tissue pogonion. Differences in soft tissue thickness may affect the subsequent treatment performed. The vertical soft tissue thickness between hard and soft tissue menton is 7 mm ± 3 mm.

10. *Upper incisor angulation*[15] relates to the long axis of the incisor to the NA line and is normally 22° ± 2° (Fig. 22-13C). The labial surface of the incisor tip should be 4 mm ± 2 mm anterior to the NA line.

11. *Lower incisor angulation*[15] relates the long axis of the incisor to the NB line and is normally 20° ± 2° (Fig. 22-13D). The labial surface of the incisal tip should be 4 mm ± 2 mm anterior to the NB line.

Panographic radiographs can help to assess tooth alignment, root angulation, and existing pathology. Periapical films aid in assessing caries, periodontal concerns, and root alignment. Tomographic x-rays, CT scans, magnetic resonance imaging (MRI), or other imaging techniques may also be indicated if TMJ pathology is suspected.

DENTAL MODEL ANALYSIS

Dental model analysis is very important in determining orthodontic treatment goals as well as in defining surgical treatment. Ten basic aspects should be analyzed.[16]

1. *Arch length* determines the amount of mesiodistal tooth structure present in regard to the amount of arch length available. This assessment is to determine if teeth need to be extracted or space created.

2. *Tooth size analysis* relates the mesiodistal widths of the upper teeth to the lower teeth. This analysis is used primarily to determine discrepancies in the anterior six teeth. In dentofacial deformities a significant number of patients have an anterior tooth size discrepancy. This usually means that the lower teeth are large relative to the upper teeth. In other words, if the teeth are properly aligned and positioned within the arch, it would be impossible to obtain a Class I cuspid relationship with surgery, but instead a slight Class II cuspid relationship would be the result.

There are various ways to assess whether this discrepancy exists. The Bolton's analysis is a method to correlate the widths of the upper and lower anterior six teeth. If the upper six teeth are summated into the mesial distal width at the contact level and divided into the lower anterior six teeth width, a numerical value would be derived called the intermaxillary (Bolton's) index with a median of 77.5 ± 3.5.[17] Simple mathematics allows the determinations for the amount of adjustment necessary in order to get the teeth into a Class I position. If alterations of tooth size are to be done in the lower arch (i.e., recontouring mesial and distal contacts, decreasing axial inclination, etc.), the length of the upper arch is multiplied by 77.5 percent to give the ideal lower arch length for the anterior six teeth. If alterations for the tooth size problem are to be done in the upper arch, the lower arch is multiplied by 1.3 to give the dimensions of the ideal upper arch. The actual upper arch length is subtracted from the ideal upper arch length to give the numerical value for the amount of alteration to be done in the upper arch (i.e., creating spacing around lateral incisors, distally angulating incisor root tips, etc.). If spaces are created, they can later be eliminated with dental restorations.

A dental arch set-up can be performed, cutting out each tooth independently and setting it up onto the dental arch appropriately. This procedure must be done carefully, however, as it is easy to tilt the crowns to get them to fit together better even though tooth size problems may exist. Occlusal mapping is a method using acetate paper to trace out each arch separately in an ideal set-up if the teeth were properly aligned in the arch. Overlaying the sheets of acetate paper will permit evaluation of tooth size problems.

3. *Tooth position* is best evaluated by correlating the dental models with the cephalometric radiograph. For stable results in orthognathic surgery, it must be decided if the teeth are in an ideal axial inclination and properly positioned over the basal bone or what treatment would be required to properly position them.

4. *Arch width analysis* means to place the models in the position that is to be achieved at the time of surgical correction and assess the transverse problems that may or may not exist. For example, if the patient is a true skeletal Class III, position the models in a Class I position and evaluate for any transverse problems. This analysis will help in determining preoperative orthodontic mechanics and appropriate surgical procedures.

5. *Curve of occlusion* (curve of Spee) significantly influences whether the curve of occlusion in the arches will be corrected orthodontically, if surgical intervention will be helpful, or if extractions will be necessary (Fig. 22-14). With no spacing and no extractions, routine orthodontic leveling of the occlusion may cause the incisors to become more angulated, and the incisor tips to move forward. This new position may or may not be desirable. Surgical leveling of the arches is faster without increasing the angulation of the teeth and may be considered more stable.

6. *Cuspid-molar position* evaluation is essential to determine the way the occlusion presently functions, but important to determine how the teeth will be aligned at surgery. It is usually preferred to have a Class I cuspid and molar relationship; however, a Class II molar relationship is very acceptable. A Class III molar relationship is less desirable but even in some cases this may be indicated. Determination of final cuspid-molar interrelationships between the arches will be influential in treatment planning.

7. *Overbite/overjet relationship* may dictate the orthodontic mechanics and surgical techniques. Open-bite problems may significantly influence the preoperative orthodontic design. The amount of overjet influences the orthodontic mechanics and the surgical AP repositioning of the jaw structures. Therefore, it is necessary to determine the amount of correction to be accomplished by the preoperative orthodontics and the amount to be corrected by surgery.

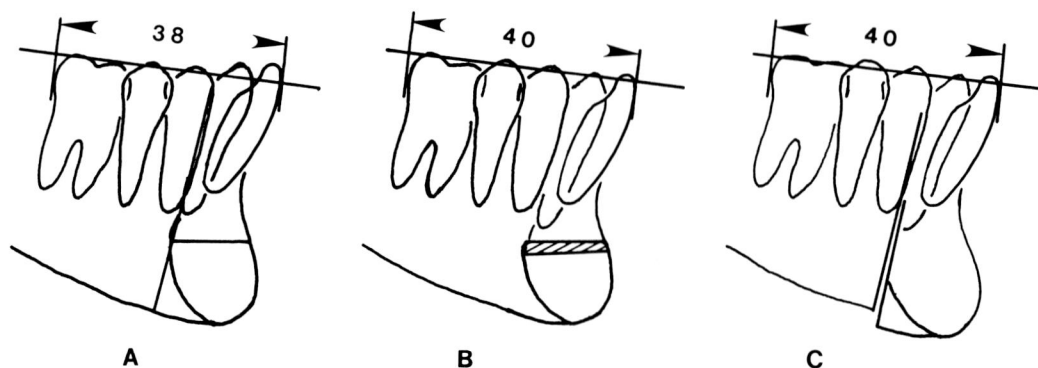

FIG. 22-14. *(A) An accentuated curve of Spee is often present in various dentofacial deformities. It can be leveled orthodontically or surgically. (B) It can be leveled with a subapical ostectomy to reposition the anterior six teeth inferiorly. (C) Bilateral body osteotomies can be performed to lower the anterior six teeth and chin as a unit.*

8. *Tooth arch symmetry* establishes the left-right symmetry within each arch. Significant asymmetries may exist, such as the cuspid on one side being more anterior than on the opposite side. This problem often occurs when a tooth is missing unilaterally in the arch, but can occur for other reasons. Correction of this type of problem may require special orthodontic mechanics, unilateral extraction or additional surgery (i.e., cutting the arch into segments) to establish arch symmetry.

9. *Buccal tooth tip* (curve of Wilson) must be assessed relative to the position of the occlusal surfaces of the maxillary posterior teeth, particularly in a medial-lateral direction. When maxillary posterior teeth are tipped buccally, it is difficult for the orthodontist to expand the arch and also correct the buccal tipping. These combined movements may be easier to correct surgically with better stability. This problem influences the design of the orthodontics and surgical procedures.

10. *Missing, broken down, or crowned teeth.* Identification of these teeth influences treatment design. If a tooth is unrestorable and requires extraction, its area may be a potential osteotomy location, extraction space closed orthodontically, or it may be helpful to maintain it to improve stability during surgical fixation with removal post-surgery.

Treatment Planning

Problem List

Before a treatment plan can be developed, a list of all existing problems is established on the basis of the clinical, radiographic, dental model, and other indicated evaluations. The definitive treatment plan, based on the existing problems, can be formulated. The problem list should include all functional, aesthetic, and dental problems present.

Initial Surgical Treatment Objective

An initial surgical treatment objective (STO)[18] is constructed from the cephalometric tracing to illustrate the desired orthodontic tooth movements, indicated surgical procedures, and resulting profile prediction. The initial STO is created prior to treatment to help establish a detailed treatment plan. A final STO is constructed after the presurgical orthodontics are complete and prior to surgery to define the exact movements of the jaws or segments thereof.

In constructing the initial STO, the desired orthodontic movements of the teeth are drawn on the cephalometric tracing in a different color pencil, thus establishing the preliminary orthodontic goals (Fig. 22-15). Surgical reference lines (lines depicting the actual surgical cuts) are also drawn on the original cephalometric tracing (Fig. 22-16A). A second sheet of acetate tracing paper is then used to demonstrate the ac-

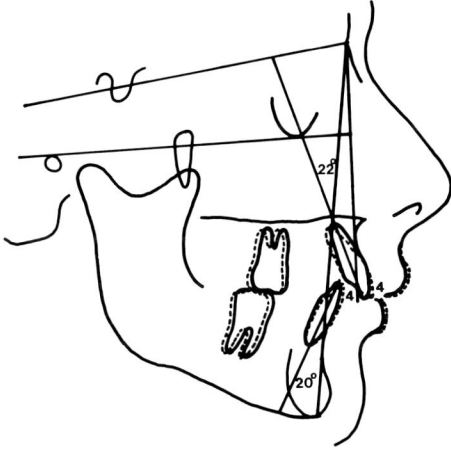

FIG. 22-15. *Orthodontic movements can be predicted and inserted on the original cephalometric tracing as a preliminary predetermination of preoperative tooth position.*

tual surgical procedures that are indicated to achieve the desired functional and aesthetic results (Fig. 22-16B). The teeth, bony structures, and soft tissues are repositioned in the new relationships relative to the stable, unaltered cranial structures. This helps solidify the orthodontic goals and surgical treatment objectives and provides a visual aid to the patient for his appreciation.

Definitive Treatment Plan

The definitive treatment plan is formulated from the patient's concerns, clinical evaluation, radiographic evaluation, and dental model analysis.

Once the treatment plan is established, the oral and maxillofacial surgeon or orthodontist should send a letter to all health professionals involved in the treatment, explaining in detail the problem list and recommended treatment.

The general sequence of the various health care professionals involved follows.

DENTAL AND PERIODONTAL TREATMENT

Any indicated periodontal and general dental care related to maintaining teeth or improving dental health should be performed prior to orthodontic and surgical intervention. The objective is to maintain as many of the teeth as possible and stabilize the periodontium. Periodontal treatment that may be required prior to the or-

thodontic and surgical treatment would be confined to deep scaling and curettage, and gingival grafting to provide attached gingiva, particularly in the anterior mandibular area. Major periodontal flap sur-

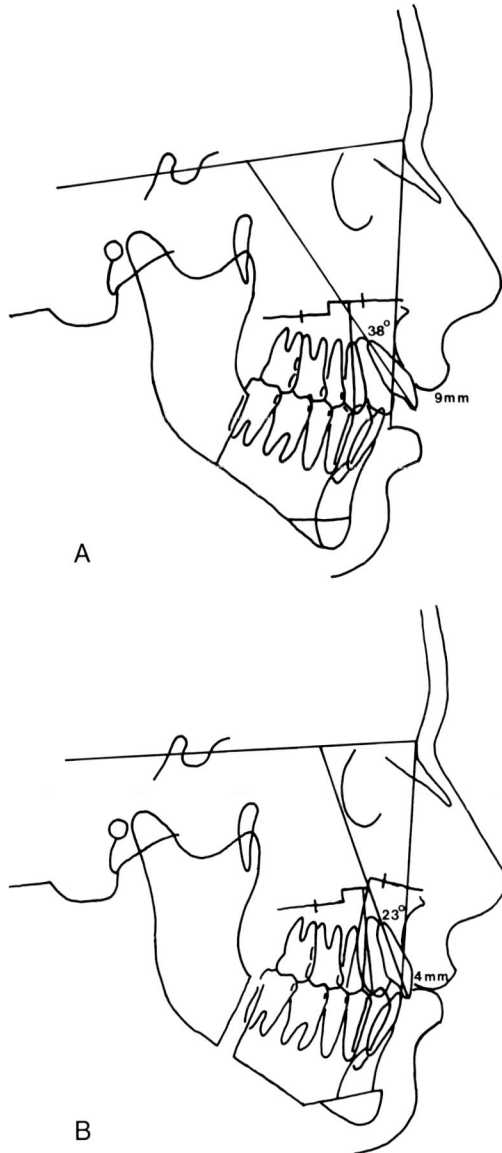

A

B

FIG. 22-16. *An STO can also be performed to determine profile changes with various surgical procedures. (A) Cephalometric tracing of this patient demonstrates a mandibular A-P deficiency and a vertical maxillary excess. (B) Mandibular deficiency is corrected with a mandibular advancement and a chin augmentation. The maxillary vertical excess is corrected by moving the maxilla superiorly and removing the first bicuspid teeth.*

gery is often deferred until after surgical orthodontic treatment is completed, but can be done earlier if necessary. No permanent crowns, bridges, or inlays should be done prior to the orthodontics and surgery. Rather, temporary crowns should be placed until the orthodontics and surgery are completed. The reason for this is that the occlusal interrelationships may be significantly altered with the orthodontics and surgery, and any crowns or bridges made prior to that treatment may have to be redone following the completion of the orthognathic procedures.

EXTRACTIONS

Extractions required for the orthodontics (i.e., bicuspids) should be done at this time. Impacted third molars, particularly the lower third molars, should be removed at least 9 to 12 months prior to mandibular ramus surgical procedures, especially when mandibular sagittal ramus osteotomies are being considered. The lingual cortical plate is often thin or may be weakened during removal of the third molars, and could cause a fracture through the third molar area at the time of surgery, creating a significant complication, if sufficient healing time is not allowed.

PREOPERATIVE ORTHODONTICS

The orthodontist is responsible for moving the teeth to more desirable positions in preparation for the surgical repositioning. Because teeth should fit reasonably well at the time of surgery, the amount of preoperative orthodontic treatment varies depending on the individual case requirements. Preoperative orthodontic treatment may be completed in 3 to 4 months or, in the more difficult malocclusion, 16 to 20 months. Dental compensations are nature's response to skeletal jaw growth discrepancies. As an example, in Class III malocclusion the lower incisors are generally tipped lingually and the upper incisors tipped labially (Fig. 22-17A). The dental compensation must be removed prior to surgery by moving the lower incisors labially and the upper incisors lingually, making the skeletal deformity and dental malocclusion even more apparent (Fig. 22-17B). Orthodontic repositioning of the teeth properly over the basal bone prior to

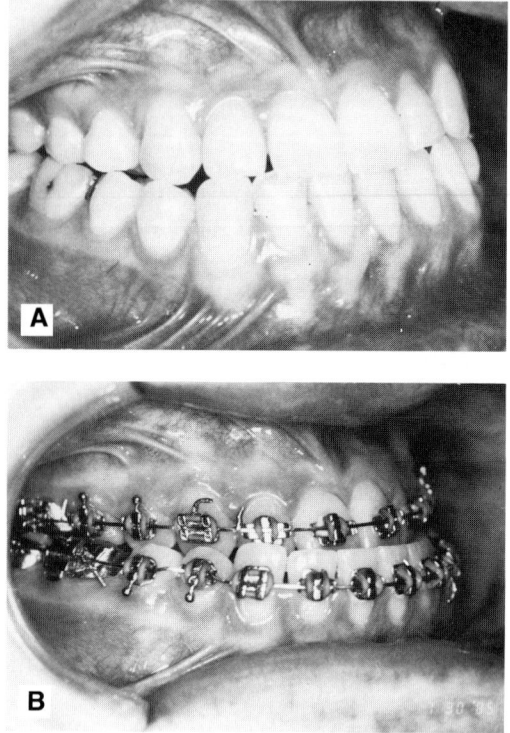

FIG. 22-17. (A) This patient has a mandibular prognathism but has significant dental compensations with the lower incisors tipped excessively lingually and the maxillary incisors overangulated labially. The dental compensations partially mask the true skeletal deformity. (B) The preoperative orthodontics were designed to position the teeth properly over their basal bone structures. This has made the occlusion much worse and the obvious skeletal deformity more apparent.

surgery also permits the lower jaw to be surgically set back a greater distance providing better skeletal balance.

Preoperative Orthodontic Appliances. Because intermaxillary fixation is necessary at the time of surgery, it is helpful for the orthodontic appliance to provide a means for easy fixation. Auxiliary wires or hooks may be soldered to the arch wire. Specialized appliances (brackets) are also available that provide a gingival extension for the intermaxillary fixation (Fig. 22-18A). Special ligature tie wires with extensions may be used to secure the arch wire to the bracket while also providing a means of fixation (Fig. 22-18B). All of the above methods are advantageous for attachment of elastics after the fixation is removed.

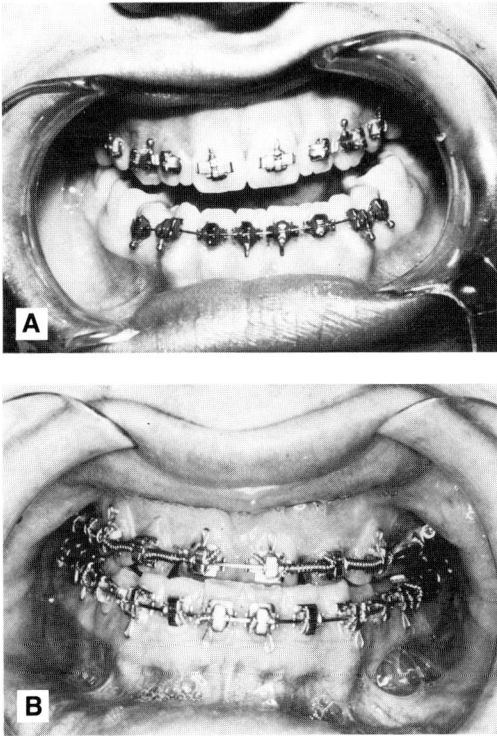

FIG. 22-18. *(A) Some orthodontic appliances are manufactured with gingival extensions for use in orthognathic surgery. (B) Special ligature tie wires with extensions can also be used.*

Preoperative Orthodontic Goal. The goal position of the teeth is established by completion of an initial STO as previously discussed. The orthodontic mechanics are then designed to achieve this cephalometric goal position. The primary responsibilities of the preoperative orthodontic treatment are:

1. *Position the teeth over their respective basal bone* (alveolus) or segments of bone if sectional surgery is indicated. The desired dental positions are established primarily by the initial STO and secondarily by dental model analysis. If extractions are necessary, the resulting space will generally be closed with the preoperative orthodontic treatment when nonsegmental surgery is planned. If segmental procedures are indicated, the spaces may be eliminated orthodontically or surgically, depending on the design.

2. *Align and level the teeth* within their respective arches or segments of arches as determined by dental model analysis. In cases with extreme curves of occlusion, the leveling can be accomplished with a segmental surgical procedure, usually with better stability than leveling orthodontically. In Figure 22-19A and B, the maxillary incisors were leveled and aligned in one segment and the cuspids and posterior teeth aligned with the segmented arch wire. The extreme maxillary curve can then be leveled with the surgical procedure (Fig. 22-19C), usually improving long-term stability.

3. *Adjust for tooth size discrepancies.* If the Bolton analysis indicates a significant tooth size discrepancy, the surgeon may not be able to achieve a Class I cuspid relationship at the time of surgery unless appropriate orthodontic adjustments are made beforehand. In some cases it may be indicated to reduce the width of the lower anterior teeth by recontouring (Fig. 22-20A). At other times it may be indicated to open spaces between the upper anterior teeth, usually adjacent to the lateral incisors (Fig. 22-20B). These spaces can be eliminated with restorative dentistry postoperatively.

4. *Correct rotated teeth.* The determination of dental rotations is made from the dental models. When a rotation does not interfere with the establishment of the desired skeletal relationship as determined by feasibility model surgery, the rotation may be corrected with the postsurgical orthodontics.

5. *Create divergence of roots adjacent to surgical sites.* If interdental osteotomies are planned, it is necessary for the orthodontist to tip the adjacent tooth roots away from the planned bone cut to prevent damage at the time of surgery (Fig. 22-21A and B). Panographic and periapical x-ray films are necessary to make this determination.

6. *Coordinate upper and lower arch widths.* In some cases transverse arch width discrepancies can be corrected with stable and predictable orthodontic movements. The width requirements are determined from the dental models and the preoperative orthodontic mechanics

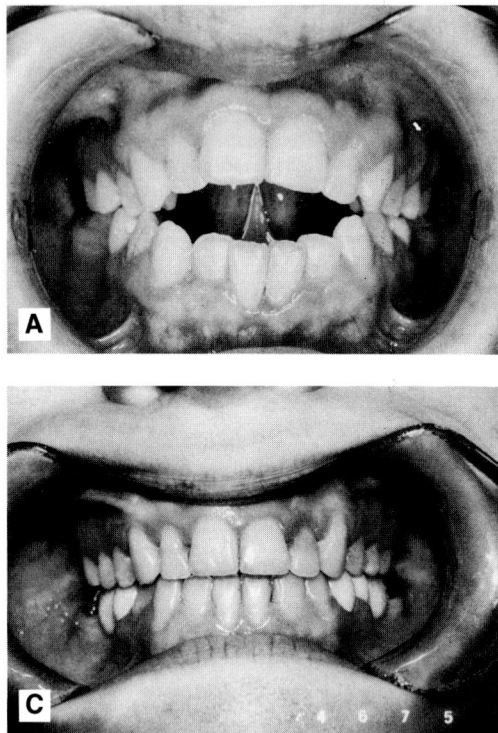

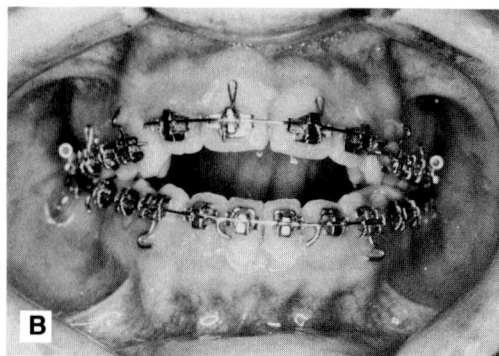

FIG. 22-19. (A) This patient has an extreme accentuated curve of Spee in the upper arch that would be unstable if leveled orthodontically. (B) Segmental arch wire is used to align the four incisors at an elevated occlusal plane and the posterior teeth, including the cuspid, at a lower occlusal plane level. This is utilizing stable orthodontic mechanics so that the arch can be leveled surgically. (C) After treatment, following a 3-piece maxilla to level the bite plane, the photo shows a stable result.

designed to avoid unstable movements and undesirable tipping of teeth. If the orthodontic movements would be unstable or in moderate to severe width incompatibility, the transverse correction would probably be more stable with a surgical correction.

As the preoperative orthodontic treatment progresses, new diagnostic records are taken to determine the feasibility and timing of surgery. It may be necessary to perform model surgery and complete an STO to determine the necessity and extent of continued presurgical orthodontic treatment. When the surgical evaluation records indicate the desired surgical result can be achieved, the patient is scheduled for surgery.

SURGERY

Surgical procedures to correct the existing musculoskeletal deformities must be selected carefully to provide the best functional and aesthetic results and stability of the achieved results. Following the preoperative orthodontics and prior to surgery, new records are taken including patient reevaluation, cephalometric and panographic radiographs, dental models, and other evaluations as indicated. A final STO is constructed to define the final position of the jaw structures and profile prediction (Fig. 22-16). Surgery is performed on the dental models to determine how the jaw structures will be repositioned to achieve the desired results. If the model surgery is done with a facebow mounting on an anatomic articulator and the actual movements are recorded accurately, this information, along with that gained from the STO, can be taken and duplicated at the time of surgery, yielding a predictable result (Fig. 22-22). Surgery is designed to reposition the basal bone and/or dentoalveolar segments into more normal interrelationships.

POSTOPERATIVE ORTHODONTICS

The orthodontics can be resumed in 2 to 6 weeks after surgery if rigid skeletal fixation is used or in 6 to 10 weeks if nonrigid skeletal fixation is used. The teeth and osseous segments can move very rapidly during the first few months following surgery. Therefore, the orthodontist should see the patient every week or two for adjustments during the first 2 months of postoperative orthodontic treatment so that these

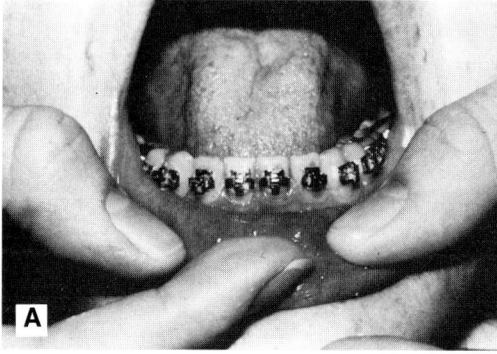

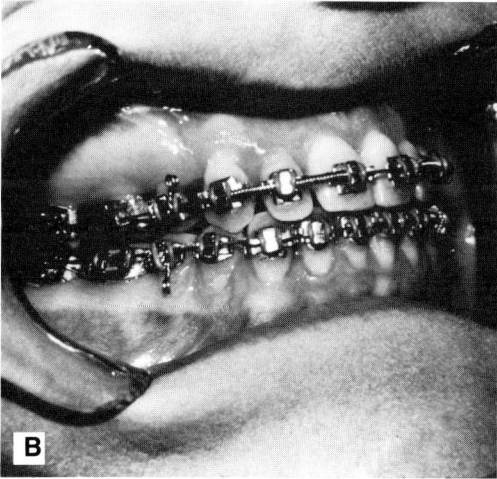

FIG. 22-20. *Tooth size discrepancies are found commonly in dentofacial deformities. (A) Mesial distal width of the lower anterior teeth has been reduced by recontouring. (B) Space has been created around the upper lateral incisor to compensate for tooth size discrepancy.*

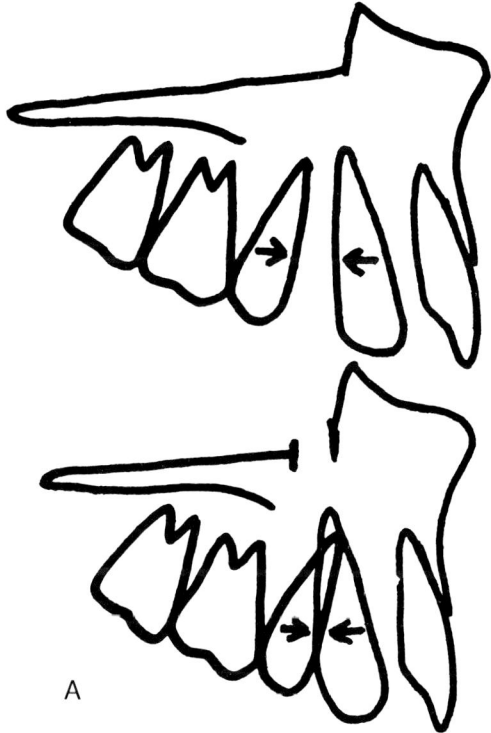

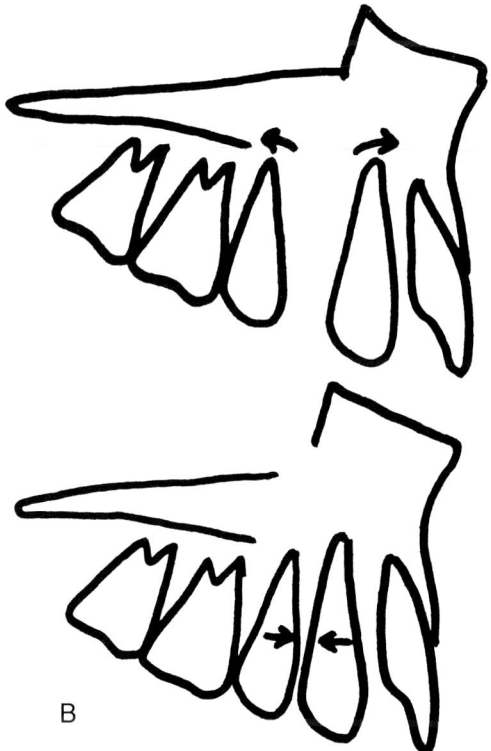

FIG. 22-21. *(A) Roots are slightly convergent, and space between the apices is inadequate to close the extraction space without damaging the roots. (B) The cuspid root is tipped forward, and the bicuspid root is tipped posteriorly to provide space between the roots to perform an ostectomy.*

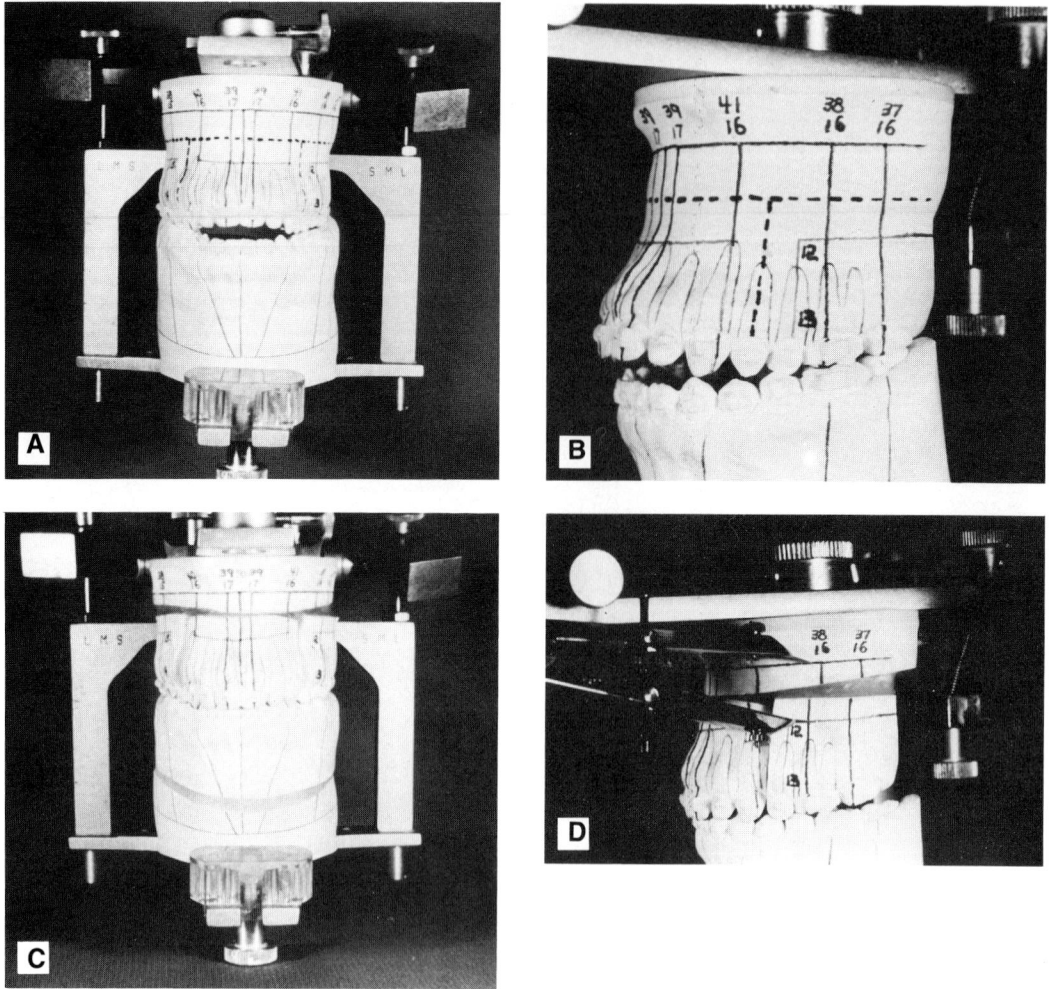

FIG. 22-22. *Models are mounted by means of a facebow on an anatomic articulator. (A) Frontal view. (B) Lateral view. Appropriate reference lines are placed. (C) Frontal view. Model surgery is completed accurately to depict actual movements of the maxillary segments and the mandible. (D) Lateral view.*

changes can be closely monitored. Once the initial healing phase is over and the occlusion remains stable, the appointment intervals can be extended to 3 to 5 weeks. As the teeth are moved to their final positions, the bones and muscles continue to heal and adapt to the repositioning. This final healing and positioning of the teeth generally takes from 4 to 10 months of postoperative orthodontic treatment. Routine orthodontic mechanics are used to fin-

ish and detail the occlusion. Retainer design should consider the surgical procedures and orthodontic mechanics used in each case.

DEFINITIVE PERIODONTAL AND GENERAL DENTAL MANAGEMENT

Any definitive periodontal treatment such as major flaps can now be performed. Lastly, crowns and bridges and prosthetic replacements are done at this stage to com-

FIG. 22-23. *This 38-year-old woman was diagnosed as having mandibular A-P deficiency and a right TMJ articular disc dislocation. (A) Frontal view demonstrates good vertical facial proportions. (B) A-P deficiency of the mandible is noted. (C) Patient demonstrates a deep overbite anteriorly caused by hypereruption of the lower anterior teeth. (D and E) Class II cuspid-molar relationship is noted. (F) The cephalometric analysis shows a mandibular A-P deficiency and slight vertical anterior mandibular excess.*

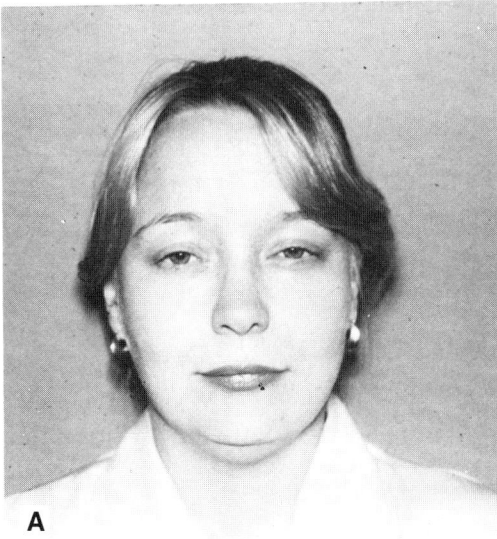

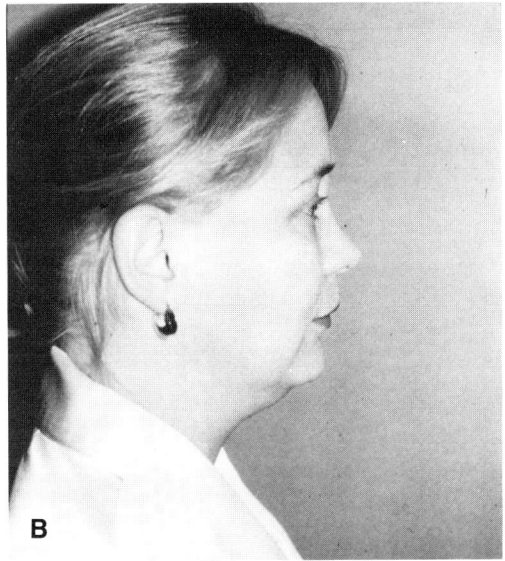

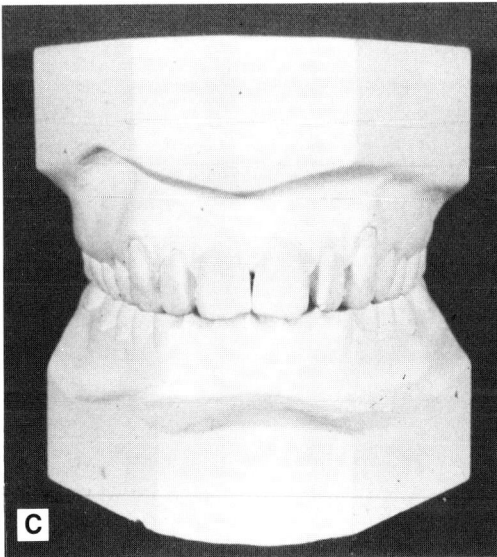

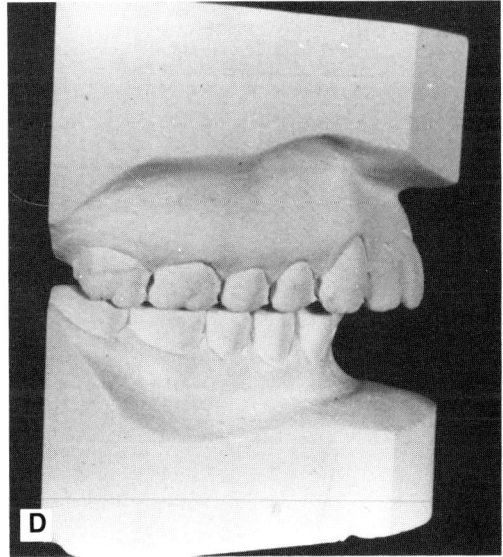

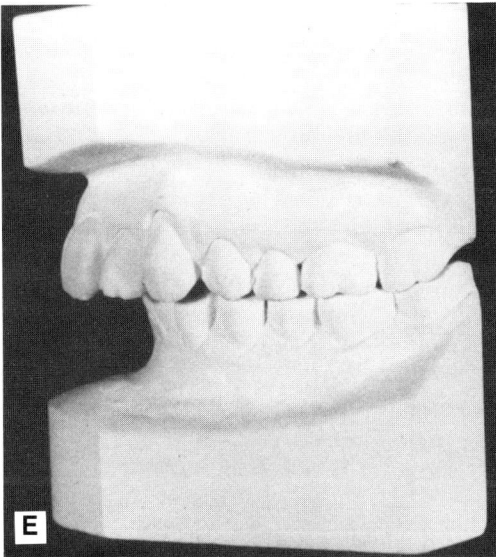

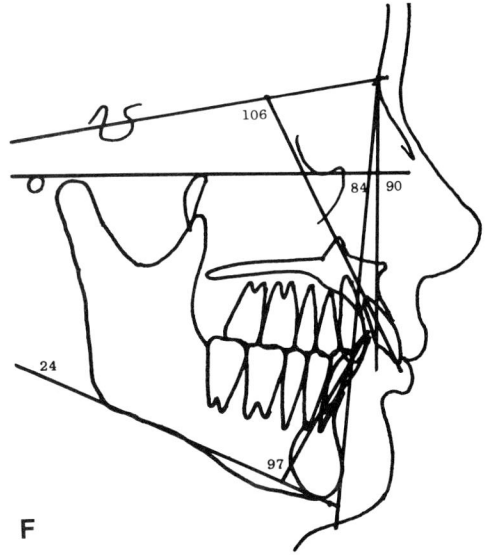

plete the treatment. Other treatment (i.e., rhinoplasty, speech therapy, etc.), as indicated, would follow.

Surgical Treatment

Numerous kinds of dentofacial deformities, involving the bone and soft tissue of the maxilla, mandible, and midfacial structures in all three planes of space, can occur. These deformities can usually be identified in the young child and should be monitored through the early years. The orthodontic concerns are varied for each of these deformities. This section presents some basic deformities, their combinations, and the orthodontic and surgical management.

Some terminology used includes:

Deficiency: underdevelopment (hypoplasia), retrognathism

Excess: overdevelopment (hyperplasia), prognathism

Osteotomy: bone cut with no bone removed

Ostectomy: bone cut with bone removed

Genioplasty: surgical alteration of the chin

Mandibular subapical: a bone cut below the apices of the teeth, but above the inferior border of the mandible, combined with 2 vertical cuts between teeth to mobilize and reposition a dentoalveolar section

Segmental osteotomy (ostectomy): separating the dento-osseous arch into segments

Rigid fixation: using bone screws and/or bone plates to hold the jaw segments in their new position

Intermaxillary fixation: wiring the jaws together

Mandibular Deficiency

Anteroposterior deficiency is a common mandibular deformity. It is usually diagnosed clinically by the chin and lower jaw being retruded (Fig. 22-23A and B). Patients frequently demonstrate crowding in the lower anterior arch and an accentuated lower curve of occlusion (Fig. 22-23C, D, and E). Cephalometrically, mandibular depth is less than average, the chin is usually recessive to cephalometric criteria, and the lower anterior teeth may be over angulated (Fig. 22-23F).

The basic orthodontic principle is to align and level the arches, and this may or may not require extractions. Lower incisors should be uprighted over basal bone, and any tooth size discrepancy appropriately managed with the preoperative orthodontic treatment. Correction of the skeletal deformity is achieved usually by surgery in the ramus area to lengthen the mandible. A bilateral mandibular ramus sagittal osteotomy is one of the common procedures used to lengthen the lower jaw. The surgery is performed inside the mouth. The ramus is sagittally sectioned and the jaw lengthened by telescoping the anterior part of the mandible forward, with an overlapping bony interface being maintained (Fig. 22-24A and B). The teeth are placed into occlusion and wired together. The bone segments are stabilized to each other in the new position with bone screws or stainless steel wire. The bone screws provide a rigid fixation to the ramus, and with this technique the jaws are usually wired together for only a couple of days. If stainless steel wires are used to stabilize the segments, the jaws are wired together for 6 to 8 weeks. Stable and predictable results can be achieved with mandibular advancement (Fig. 22-23G through L).

Mandibular deficiency can also occur in the vertical direction. The primary cephalometric criterion for diagnosing this deformity is when the anterior mandibular height (the tip of the lower incisor to the inferior border of the mandible) is less than normal. Average height in females is 40 mm and in males 44 mm, but this must be correlated to the upper lip length and other vertical facial measurements. This

FIG. 22-23. *Continued. (G through K) The establishment of good facial harmony and a functional Class I cuspid-molar relationship after treatment. Treatment involved: 1. Preoperative orthodontics to align and level the upper arch. Lower teeth aligned at two occlusal plane levels, with lower incisors kept at an elevated level. 2. Surgery: Right TMJ articular disc plication; anterior mandibular subapical ostectomy to lower the four incisors; bilateral mandibular ramus osteotomies to advance it. 3. Postoperative orthodontics to finish and retain the occlusion. (L) Superimposition of pre- and postoperative cephalometric radiographs demonstrates overall functional and aesthetic changes achieved.*

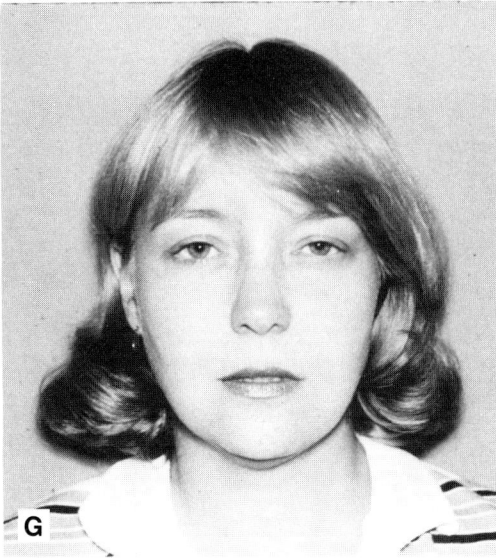

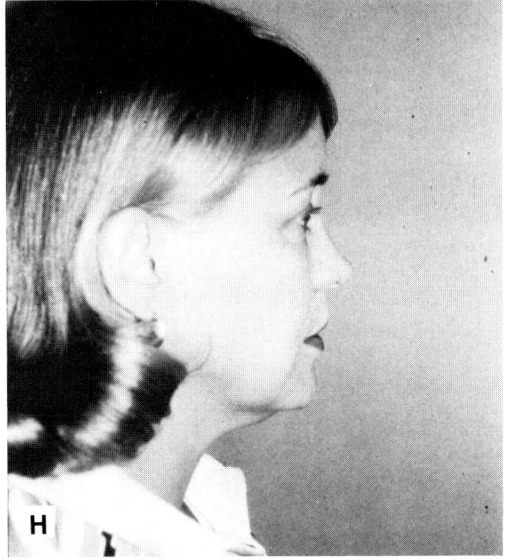

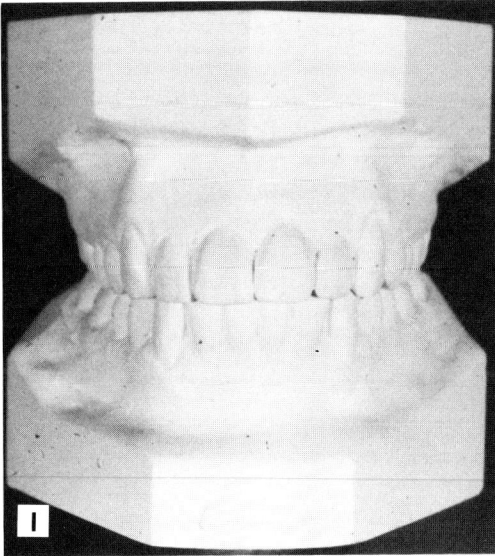

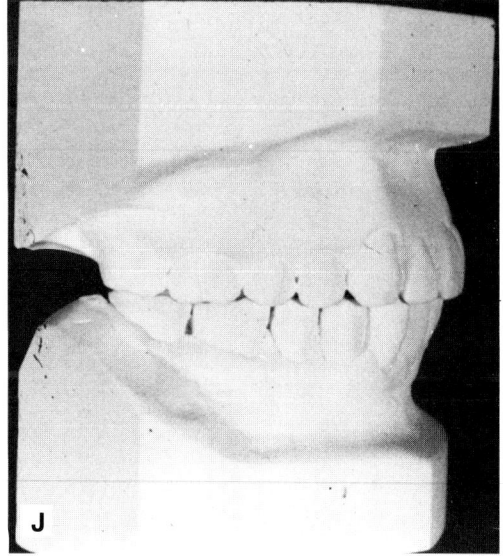

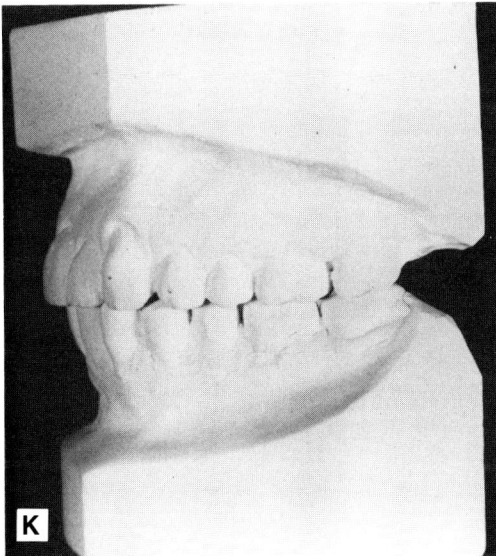

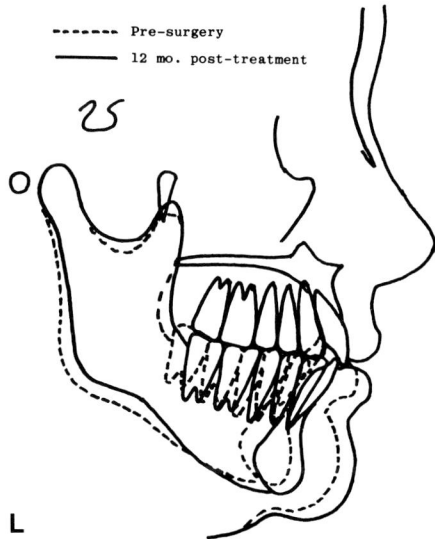

------- Pre-surgery
———— 12 mo. post-treatment

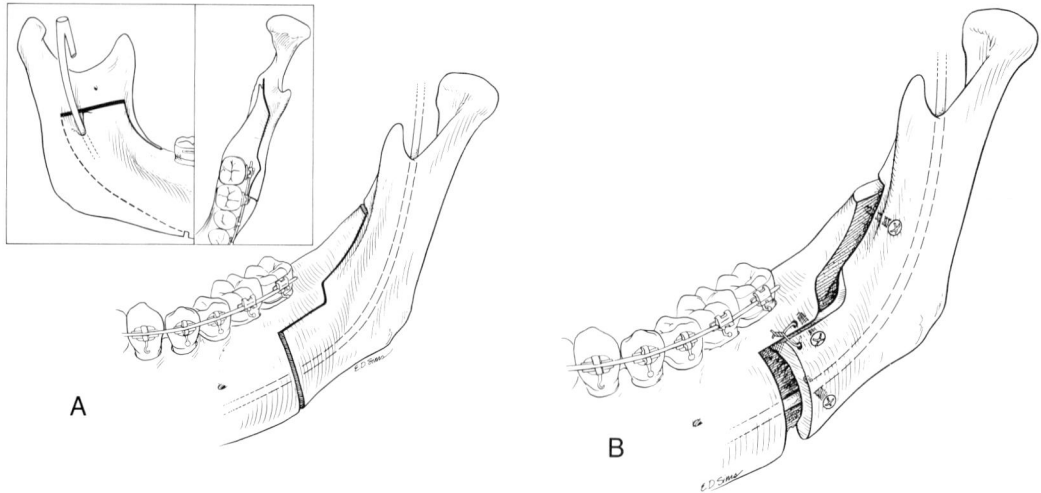

FIG. 22-24. *A common method to reposition the mandible forward or backward. (A) The bony cuts are illustrated for the sagittal split osteotomy of the ramus. (B) The segments are usually stabilized with bone screws that remain permanently.*

deformity is usually corrected by vertically lengthening the chin area either by alloplastic or synthetic bone augmentation to the inferior border or by doing a horizontal osteotomy to the anterior part of the chin and rotating it downward. The gap is then filled either with bone or with hydroxyapatite (synthetic bone). Chin surgery is usually done intraorally.

If transverse mandibular deficiency also occurs, it can be corrected by doing additional vertical osteotomies through the symphysis and body area or doing total mandibular subapical segmental osteotomies to allow expansion of the dental arch.

Mandibular Excess

Mandibular excess in the anteroposterior dimension is also referred to as mandibular prognathism and is manifested usually by a prominent lower jaw and chin (Fig. 22-25A and B). This basically means that the lower jaw has overgrown in an anterior direction relative to the rest of the facial structures. Although a myriad of dental and aesthetic variations can occur with this deformity, those most common are the lower teeth angled lingually and a Class III malocclusion (Fig. 22-25C and D). There frequently are anterior and bilateral posterior crossbites. Cephalometrically, the mandibular depth is greater than normal (larger than 88° angle) (Fig. 22-25E).

Preoperative orthodontics for this type of deformity is usually directed towards uprighting the lower teeth over the basal bone. Quite often the patient's appearance and bite may worsen prior to surgery because of aligning teeth appropriately over basal bone, which may cause the lower lip to be more protrusive and increase the negative overjet. The upper incisors are often overangulated and extractions may be required to properly position them orthodontically over basal bone. As the teeth are brought back over the basal bone, the anteroposterior discrepancy between the maxillary and mandibular incisors becomes much worse (Fig. 22-17A and B), and the upper lip may move posteriorly.

The lower jaw can be set posteriorly by ramus or body ostectomies. The two most common ramus procedures are the vertical oblique ostectomy (Fig. 22-26A and B) and the mandibular ramus sagittal ostectomy. The procedure is done similar to a mandibular advancement (Fig. 22-24A and B), except the anterior part of the mandible is set backwards. The ramus sagittal ostectomy permits the use of rigid fixation (bone screws) so that the patient's jaws are wired together for a couple of days or less. The vertical oblique ostectomy usually requires the jaws to be wired together for about 6 to 8 weeks. The mandible can also be set posteriorly by doing bilateral body

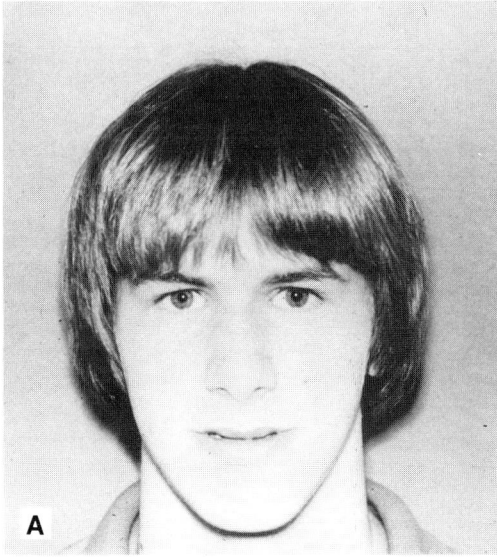

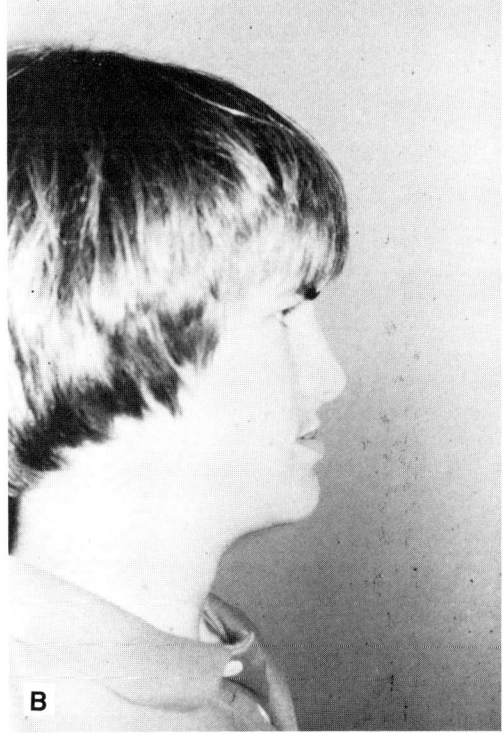

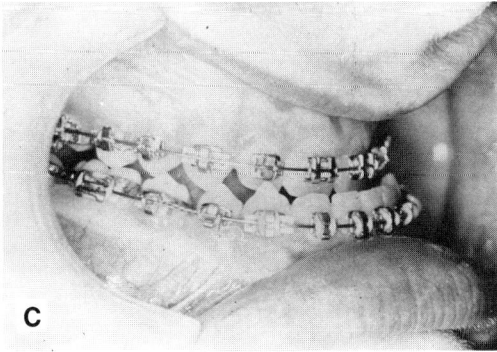

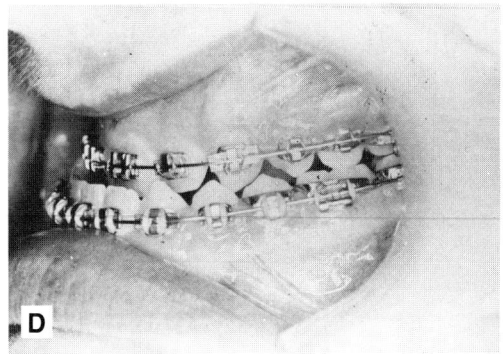

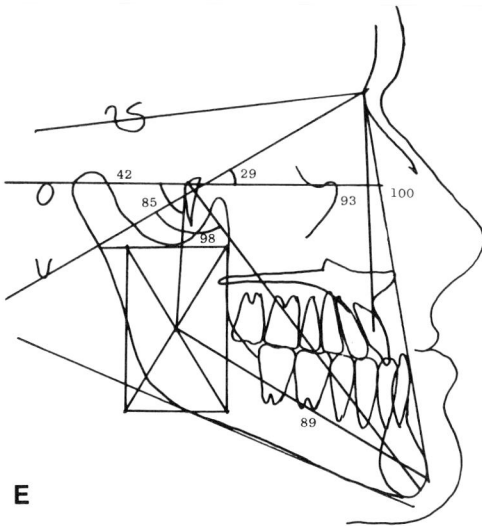

FIG. 22-25. This 16-year-old patient was concerned about his functional and aesthetic appearance. (A) Frontal view shows prominence of chin. (B) Mandibular prognathism is readily seen with the prominence of the lower jaw. (C and D) Class III occlusal relationship is noted. (E) Cephalometric evaluation demonstrates mandibular prognathism.

---- Pre Surgery (age 15.5 yrs.)
—— 2.7 yrs. Post Surgery (18.0 yrs.)

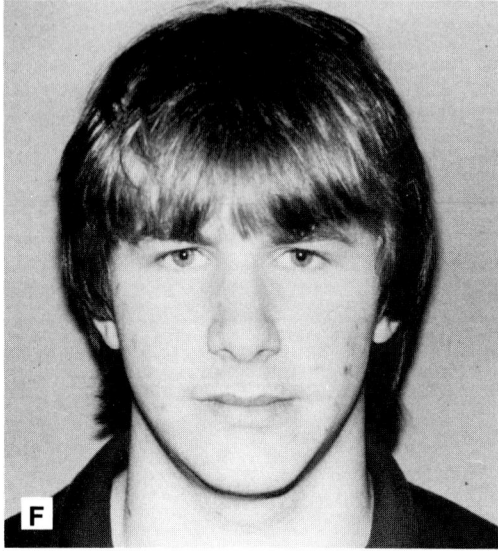

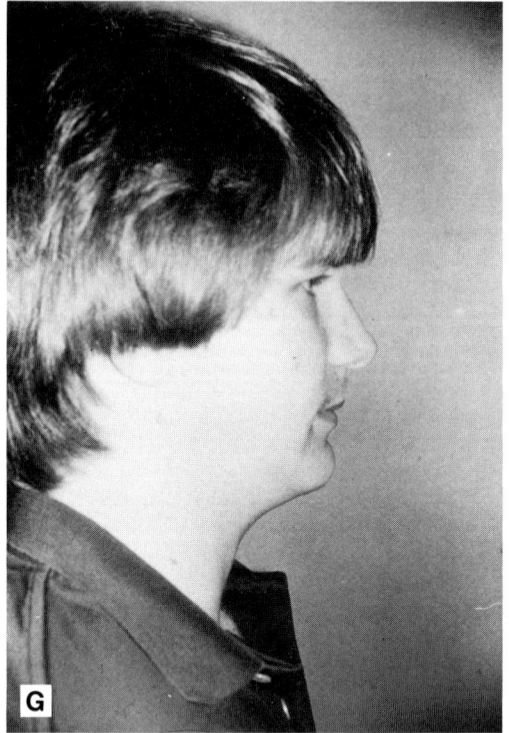

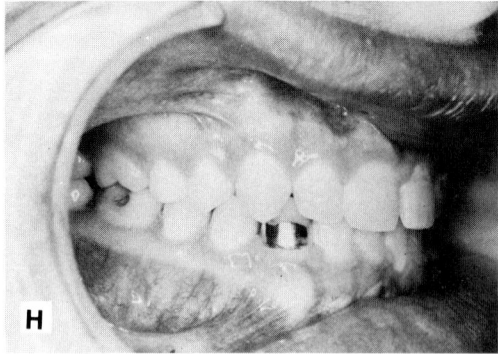

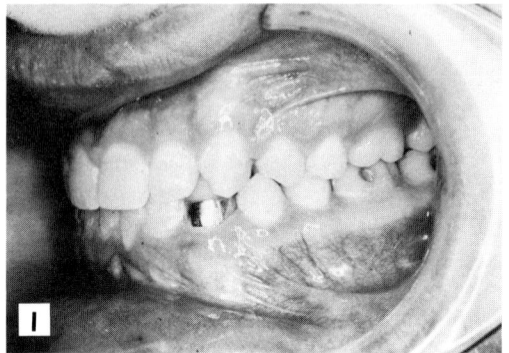

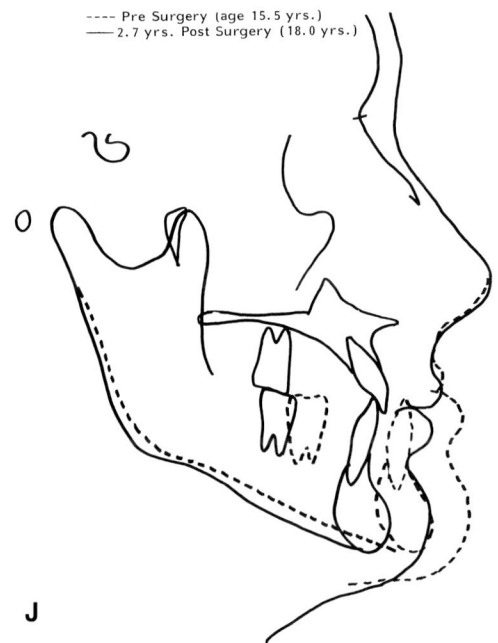

FIG. 22-25. *Continued. (F through I) Post-treatment results. Treatment plan included: 1. Preoperative orthodontics to align and level arches. 2. Surgery—bilateral mandibular ramus ostectomies to set it backward. 3. Postoperative orthodontics to refine and retain occlusion. (J) Superimposition of pre- and postoperative cephalometric radiographs demonstrates the aesthetic and functional results achieved. (Orthodontics by Dr. Clay Ellis.)*

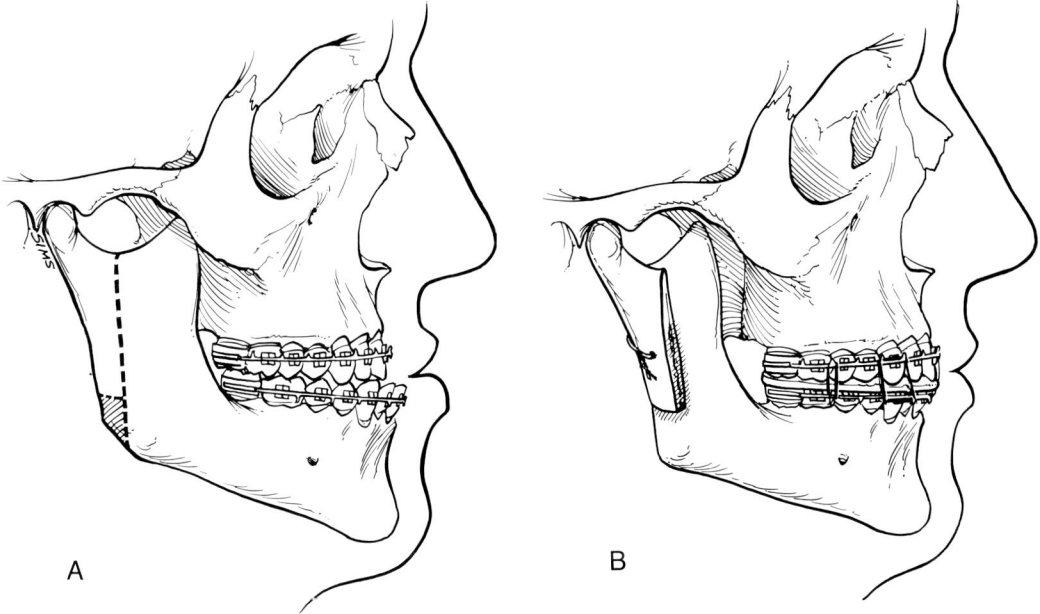

FIG. 22-26. (A) The vertical oblique osteotomy can be done intraorally or extraorally. It consists of making a vertical osteotomy from the sigmoid notch down toward the angle of the mandible. (B) This allows the lower jaw to be set posteriorly, overlapping the condyle segments on the anterior part of the lower jaw.

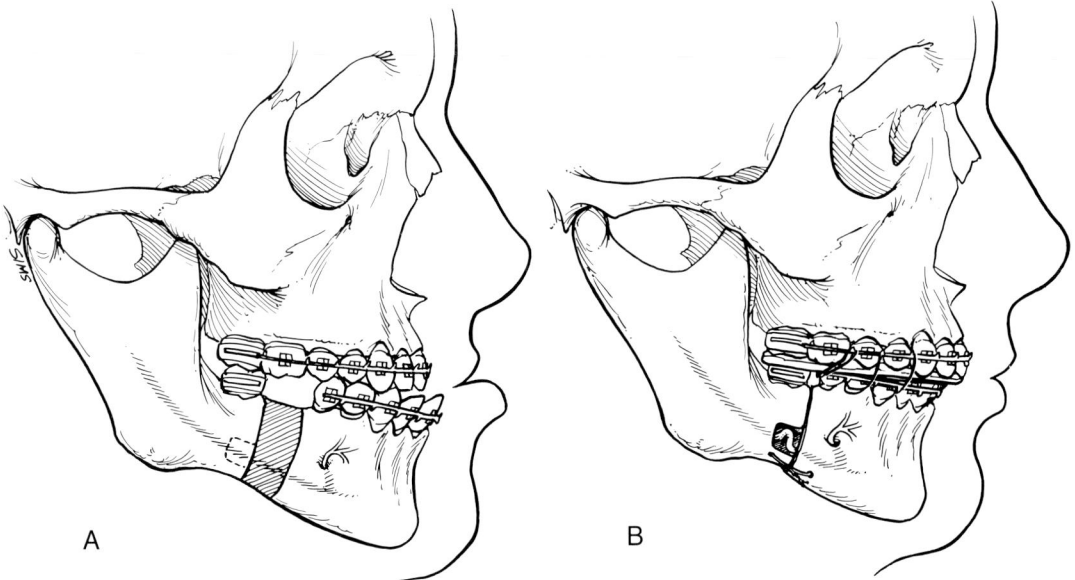

FIG. 22-27. (A) Mandibular body ostectomies can be performed to set the mandible backward by removing a full thickness section of the mandible, usually in the bicuspid or molar area. (B) The mandible is set back and can be stabilized with interosseous wires or bone plates.

ostectomies, removing dental alveolar bone vertically from the alveolar ridge completely through the inferior border of the mandible, and moving the anterior part of the mandible posteriorly (Fig. 22-27A and B). Usually the occlusion dictates which technique would provide the best functional and aesthetic result. With proper planning and treatment, optimal functional and aesthetic results can be achieved (Fig. 22-25F through J).

The mandible can be excessive in a vertical direction also and is usually diagnosed by an increased lower anterior dental height. This condition can be corrected by performing an anterior mandibular horizontal ostectomy, removing a wedge of bone above the chin area, and then rotating the chin superiorly.

Transverse excess in the mandible can occur in Class I, II, or III skeletal relationship and is diagnosed when the mandibular dental arch is too wide in comparison to a normal maxillary arch width. The mandibular width can be reduced by symphysis or body osteotomies in conjunction with the ramus ostectomies.

Maxillary Deficiency

Maxillary deficiency can occur vertically, anteroposteriorly, and transversely. In vertical maxillary deficiency, the upper jaw, either at the palatal level or at the dental alveolar level (which is most common), has exhibited less than normal vertical growth. Usually a lack of tooth exposure is evident when the upper lip is relaxed. Normal upper tooth to upper lip is 1 to 4 mm. These patients may look edentulous, the lower jaw may appear relatively strong, and the lips look over-closed (Fig. 22-28A and B). Vertical maxillary deficiency is often coupled with A-P maxillary deficiency, making the upper lip look retruded. In the patient with maxillary deficiency, the upper lateral incisor may be small, or occasionally partial anodontia could occur (Fig. 22-28C, D, and E). The occlusion may have a reverse deep-bite or posterior open-bite. Cephalometrically, maxillary depth may be less than normal, mandibular depth may be greater than normal, and the lower third facial height will be less than normal (Fig. 22-28F).

The orthodontics indicated for these patients is to align the teeth over the respective basal bone as a unit or in segments. Surgery is designed to bring the maxilla downward to establish normal tooth-to-lip relationship and forward to establish a Class I cuspid relationship (Fig. 22-29A and B).

Transverse problems can also be corrected at the same time by sectioning the upper jaw into two or more pieces. In this manner, the maxilla or sections thereof can be repositioned into an ideal functional relationship. The upper jaw can be stabilized in its new position by a number of methods. The use of small bone plates and screws to attach the mobilized segments to the stable maxilla is a very effective method. Gaps created between the bone segments and the stable part of the facial structures must be grafted either with bone or hydroxyapatite (synthetic bone) to give a stable result. Following orthognathic surgery, patients with deformed teeth or partial anadontia may require extensive reconstructive dentistry (Fig. 22-28G through L).

Maxillary Excess

Maxillary excess can occur in all three planes of space. Vertical maxillary excess, a common dentofacial deformity, is characterized by an increased lower third facial length and usually an excessive exposure of upper tooth and gingiva, particularly when the individual smiles (Fig. 22-30A and B). There may be an associated anterior open-bite. These patients may have posterior cross-bites and an accentuated curve of occlusion in the maxilla, with the anterior teeth of the maxilla being much higher than the posterior teeth. Crowding may occur in both arches (Fig. 22-30C, D, and E). Cephalometrically, the lower third of the face is elongated and the mandible is rotated down and backward, making it appear retruded (Fig. 22-30F).

Orthodontically, the design of mechanics is to align the teeth over basal bone. This may require a segmental alignment of the maxillary arch; for example, aligning the bicuspids and molars in one segment on each side and aligning the cuspids and incisors in another segment. It is not uncommon to align the maxilla in three or four separate segments so that surgically

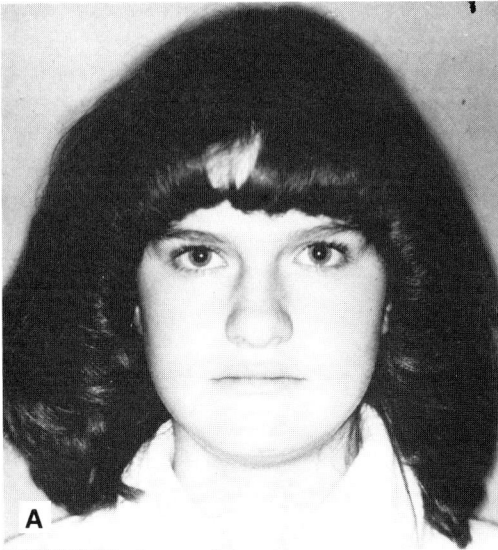

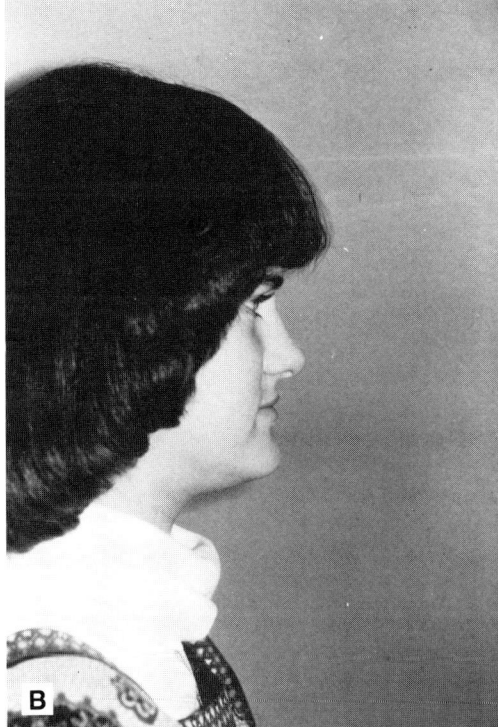

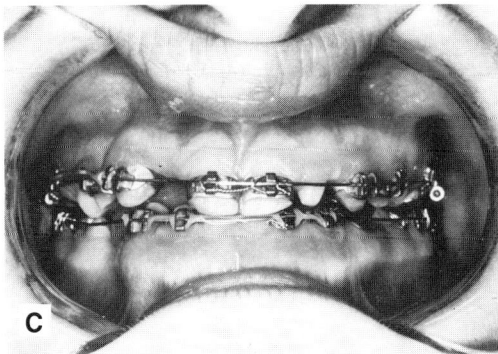

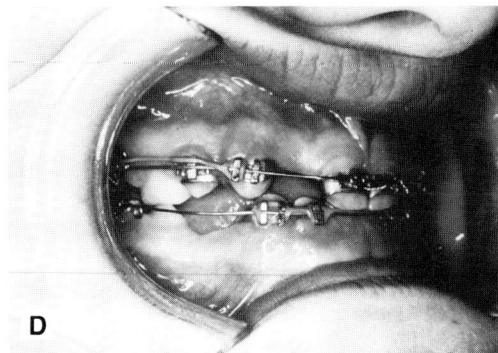

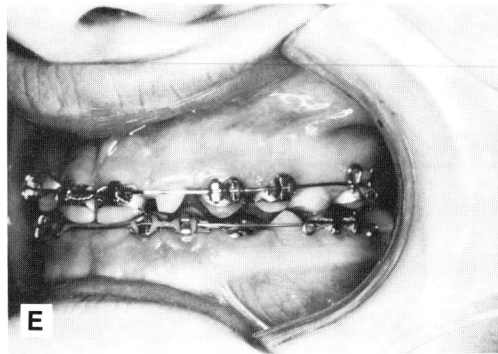

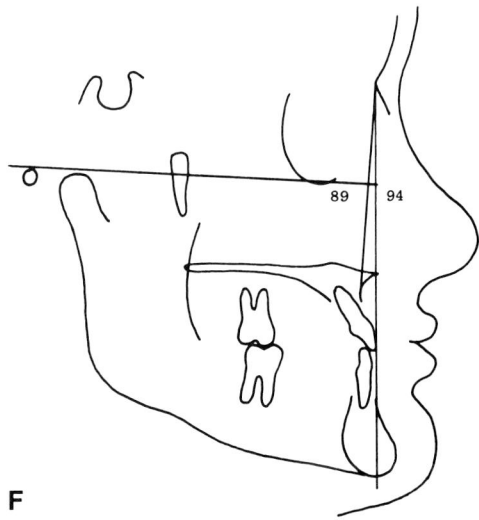

FIG. 22-28. (A and B) This 15-year-old patient was diagnosed as having vertical maxillary deficiency and vertical mandibular deficiency. (C, D, and E) She demonstrates a Class III occlusion and has partial anodontia in the upper arch. (F) Cephalometric evaluation demonstrates vertical maxillary and mandibular deficiency.

--- Presurg. (Age 13.2 yrs.)
— 1.4 Yrs. Postsurg. (Age 14.6)

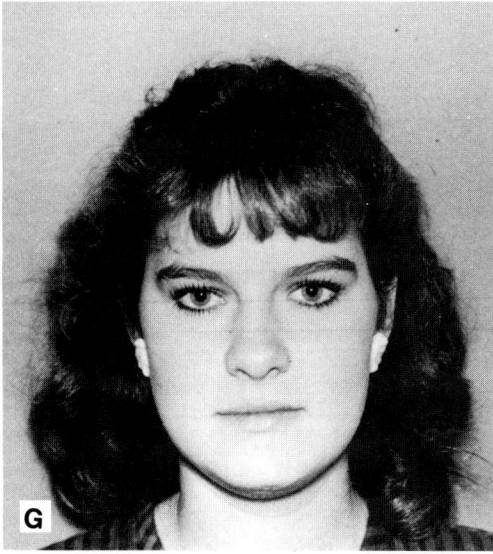

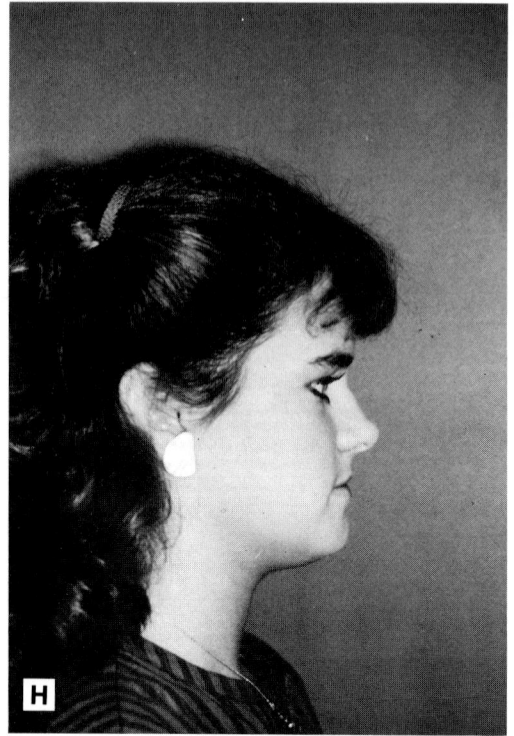

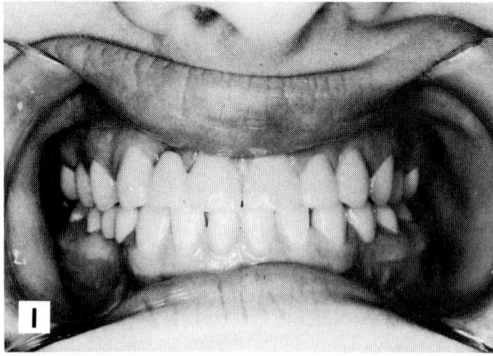

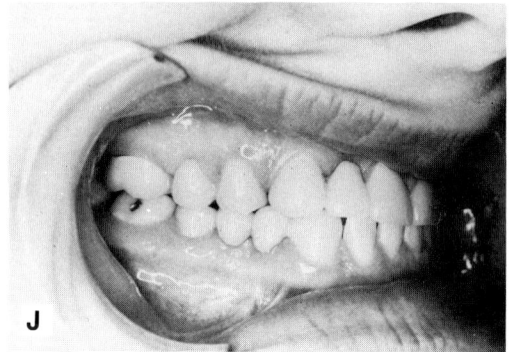

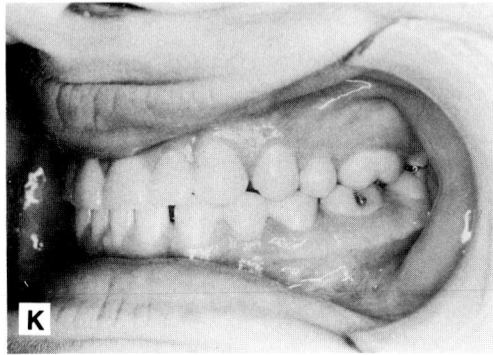

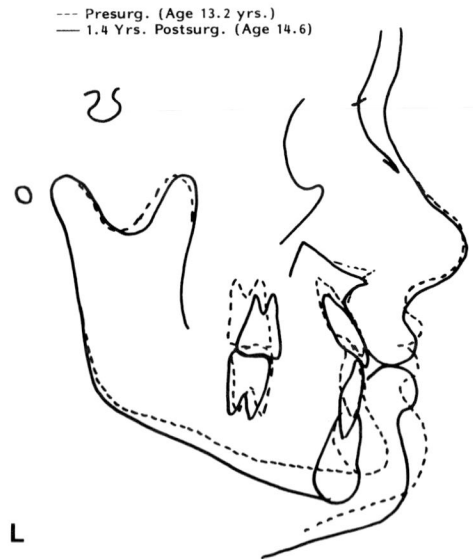

FIG. 22-28. *Continued. (G through K) This patient was treated in the following manner: 1. Preoperative orthodontics to align and level the maxillary and mandibular arch. 2. Surgery—downgraft of maxilla to increase vertical dimension; downgraft of chin with slight posterior repositioning to increase vertical prominence and decrease A-P prominence. 3. Postoperative orthodontics to refine occlusion. 4. Reconstructive prosthetics to replace missing teeth in maxillary arch. (L) Superimposition of pre- and postoperative radiographic tracings demonstrates the overall change achieved.*

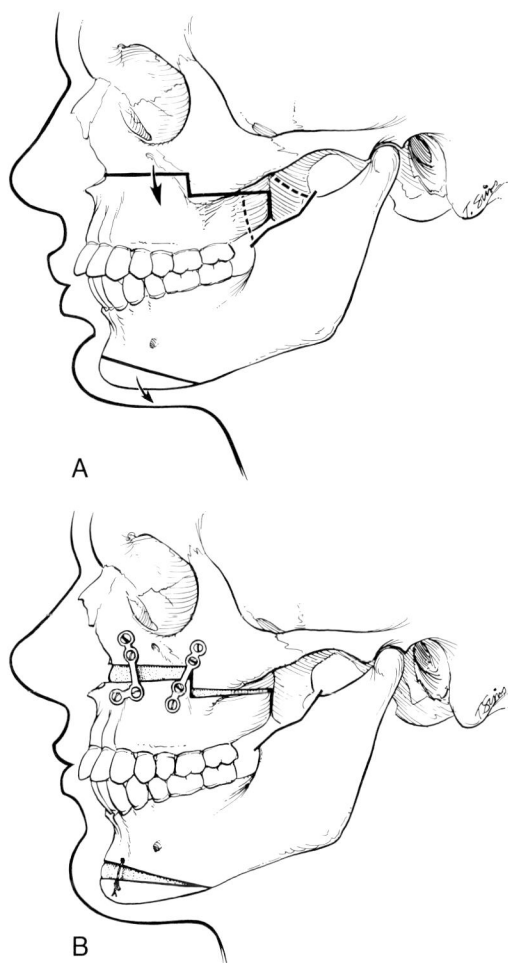

A

B

FIG. 22-29. *(A) Anteroposterior and vertical maxillary deficiency as well as vertical mandibular deficiency. (B) Downgrafting and advancing the maxilla with rigid skeletal stabilization is illustrated. A horizontal osteotomy through the chin area will permit the chin to be rotated downward to increase the anterior mandibular height. Bone grafts or synthetic bone is used to fill in the gaps created by the movements.*

these individual segments can be repositioned to provide good arch form, good function, and long-term stability.

Surgery is usually performed at the LeFort I level, approximately 5 mm above the apices of the teeth. The surgical design may incorporate a maxillary step osteotomy to provide a more predictable result (Fig. 22-31A). The maxilla can be moved upward by moving the entire dental alveolus and palate, or the palate can be maintained in its original position and only the

dental alveolus moved upward so that the functional nasal airway is not decreased. A predetermined amount of bone is removed from the lateral maxillary wall (Fig. 22-31A and B), the pterygoid plates are separated from the tuberosity of the maxilla, the nasal septum is released from the maxilla, and the lateral nasal walls are cut to facilitate mobilization of the maxilla. The maxilla can be segmentalized with palatal and interdental bone cuts. The segmentalization of the maxilla allows expansion or narrowing of the maxilla and leveling of the maxillary occlusal plane. The maxilla can be narrowed or widened by doing a cut through the palatal bone and either expanding with bone or hydroxyapatite grafting (Fig. 22-32) or removing bone from the palate and narrowing it. The maxillary mobilized segments are repositioned as planned by placing them into an acrylic occlusal splint (fabricated from the surgery previously done on the dental models) and wiring the upper and lower teeth together. The segments are secured to the stable maxillary bone with bone plates, or with other stabilizing techniques using wires and/or pins. With careful planning and surgery, predictable results with optimal function and aesthetics can be achieved, as illustrated in Figure 22-30G through L.

Double Jaw Surgery

The deformities that have been described and others can occur in any combination (i.e., maxillary A-P deficiency and mandibular A-P excess, anterior maxillary vertical excess, posterior maxillary vertical deficiency, maxillary transverse deficiency, mandibular A-P deficiency, etc.). Probably the majority of patients have a combination of deformities affecting both jaw structures that may require surgery on both jaws to correct the existing functional and aesthetic deformities (Fig. 22-33A through L). Double jaw surgery is much more complex than single jaw surgery.

Both jaws are surgically separated from the cranial base and must be repositioned appropriately in all three planes of space. Usually one jaw is mobilized and stabilized using the other jaw as a stable positional reference. Then the second jaw is mobilized and stabilized in its final position,

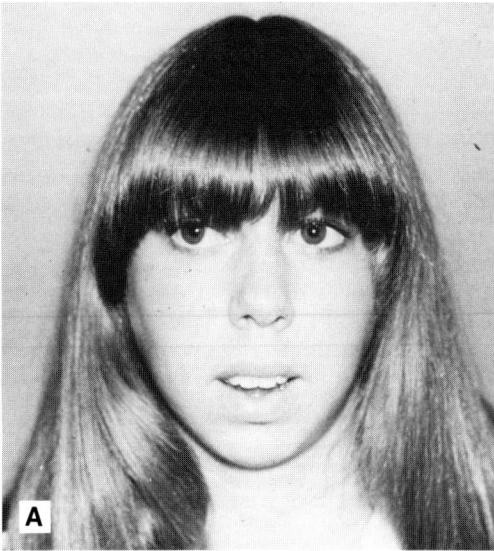

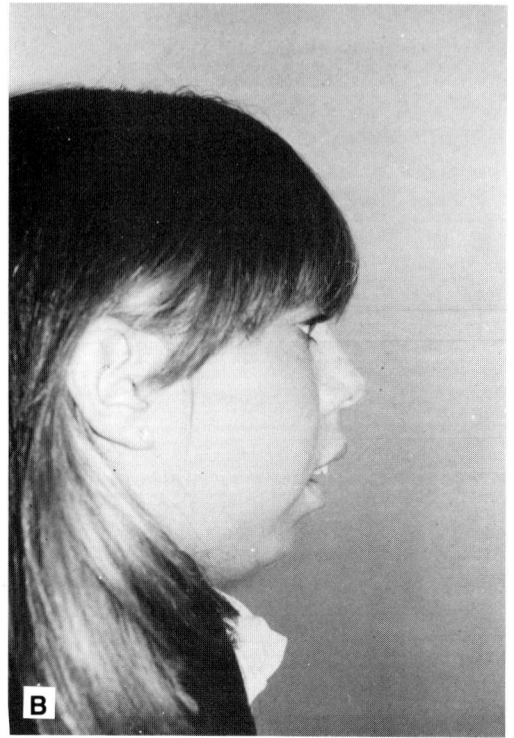

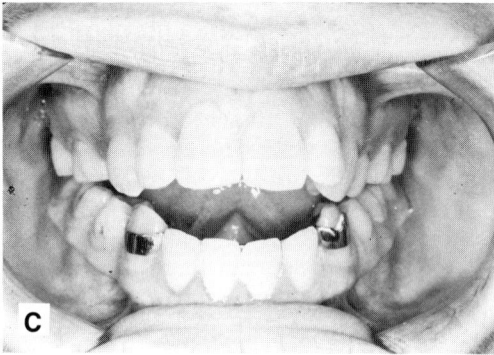

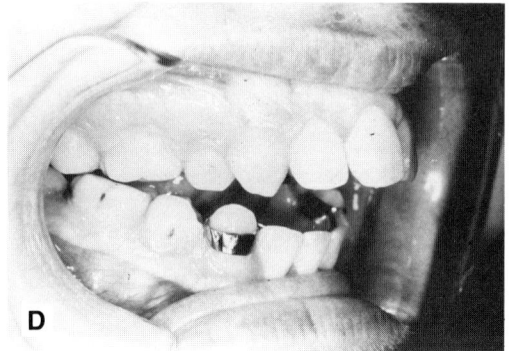

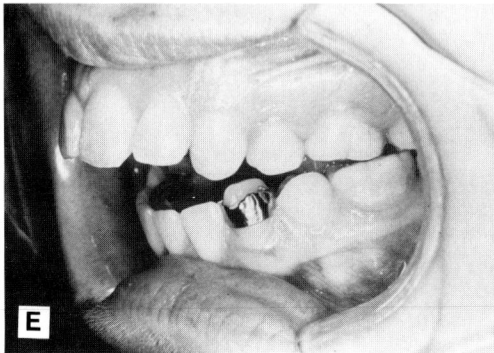

FIG. 22-30. *(A and B) This patient demonstrates excessive vertical growth of the maxilla as evidenced by the tooth-to-lip relationship. (C, D, and E) Class II occlusal relationship and an anterior open bite are often seen in this patient type. (F) Vertical excess in the maxilla is obvious. This causes the mandible to rotate downward and backward, decreasing the prominence of the lower jaw.*

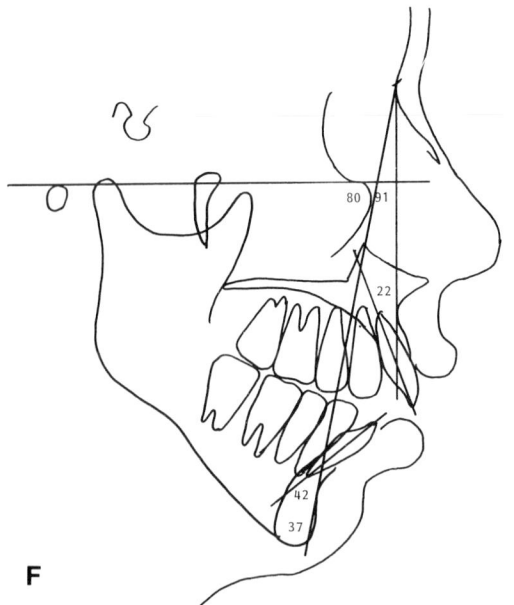

F

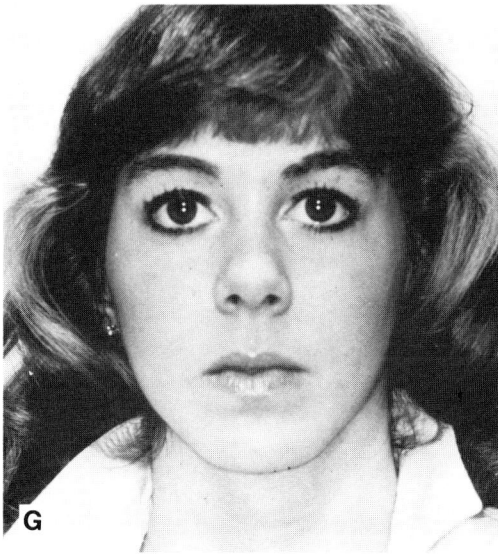

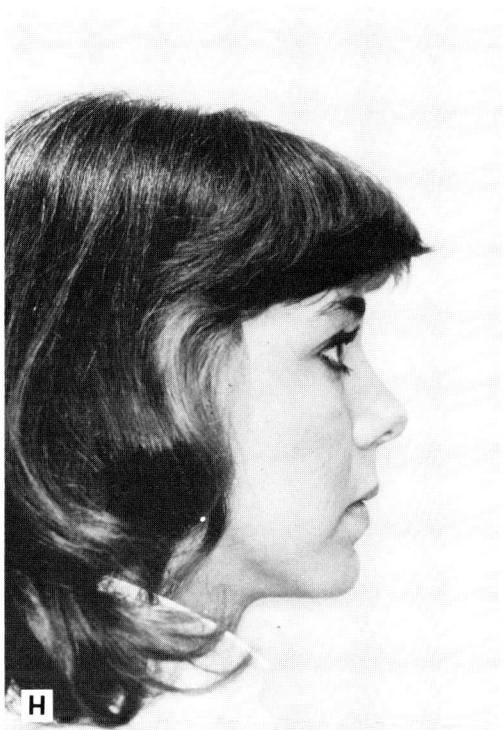

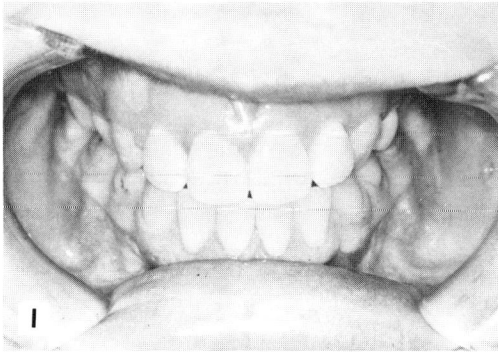

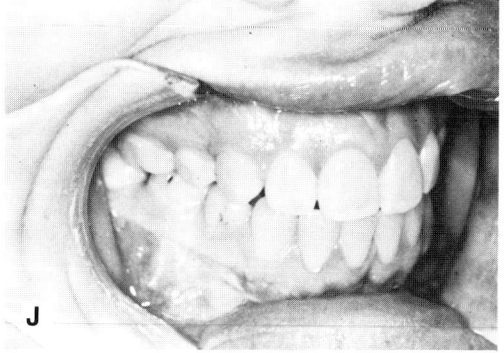

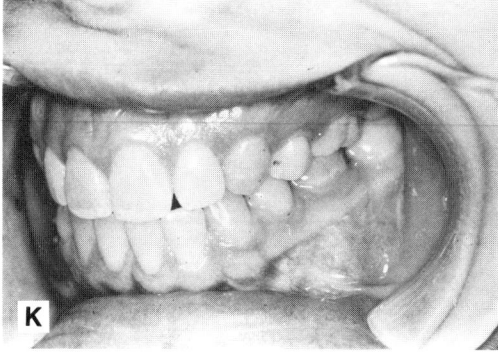

----- Presurgical 20.5 yrs.
——— 16 mo. Postsurgery 21.9 yrs.

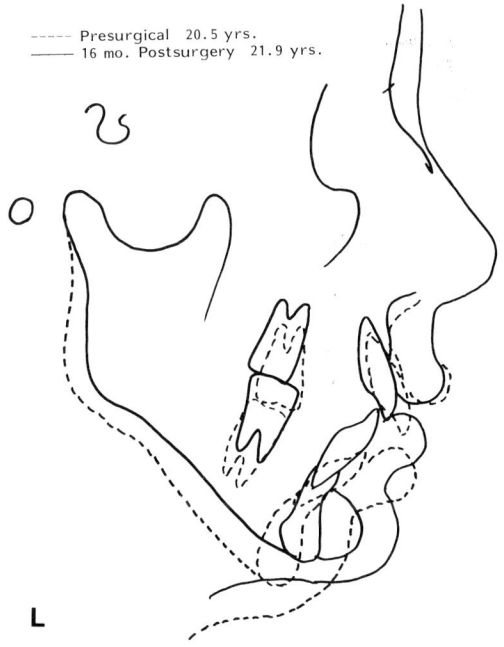

FIG. 22-30. *Continued. (G through K) Postoperative changes are noted. This patient was treated in the following manner: 1. Preoperative orthodontics to align and level the arches. 2. Superior repositioning of the maxilla. 3. Postoperative orthodontics to refine the occlusion. (L) Superimposition of the pre- and postoperative cephalometric radiographs demonstrates the changes achieved.*

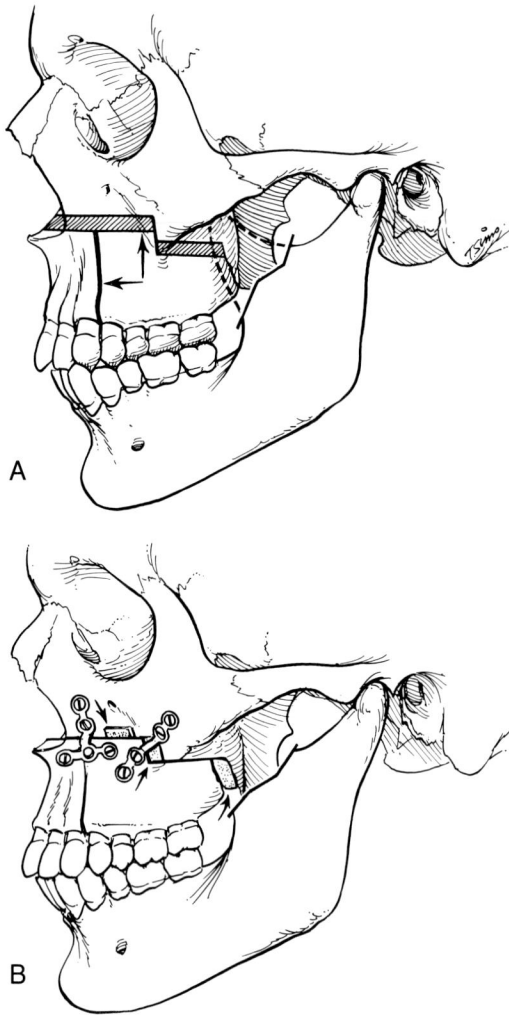

A

B

FIG. 22-31. (A) Vertical maxillary excess is usually corrected by removing a predetermined amount of bone above the maxillary teeth. (B) The dentoalveolus is then moved superiorly and stabilized with bone plates.

completing the correction of both jaws in one operation. Careful planning and accurate surgery are necessary to achieve optimal results.

Facial asymmetries, combined anteroposterior problems, vertical deformities, and/or transverse discrepancies frequently require double jaw surgery.

The occlusal plane angulation becomes a major factor that can be significantly altered with surgery. In extremely high occlusal plane angulation cases, the best aesthetic results are usually achieved by leveling the occlusal plane by moving the anterior maxilla upward and the posterior maxilla downward. Appropriate mandibular ramus surgery is then indicated to correct the mandibular deformity (Fig. 22-34). Patients with extremely low occlusal plane angulations may exhibit a prominent chin relative to the position of the dentoalveolus. They also tend to have short vertical facial heights and prominent mandibular angles. By increasing the occlusal plane level with double jaw surgery, not only can the occlusal problems be corrected, but the aesthetics can be significantly improved, creating increases in anterior vertical dimension and better balance between the chin, lips, and nose.

Temporomandibular Joint Problems and Orthognathic Surgery

Some patients exhibit problems of the temporomandibular joint as a result of their existing musculoskeletal deformities of the jaws or other insults such as trauma, bruxing and clenching, and stress. These patients must be evaluated carefully so that not only is there a complete diagnosis of the jaw deformity, but also a detailed diagnosis of the temporomandibular joint. Additional examinations, such as

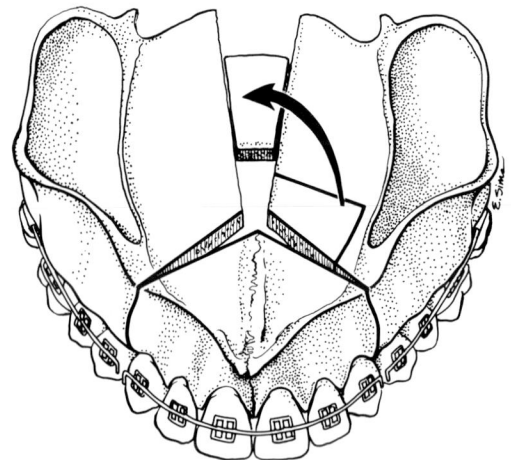

FIG. 22-32. Often the maxilla may be deficient in a transverse dimension, or occasionally it can be excessive in the transverse dimension. When a deficiency exists, a bone cut usually is done through the palate to expand it, and the midline area must be grafted with bone or synthetic bone.

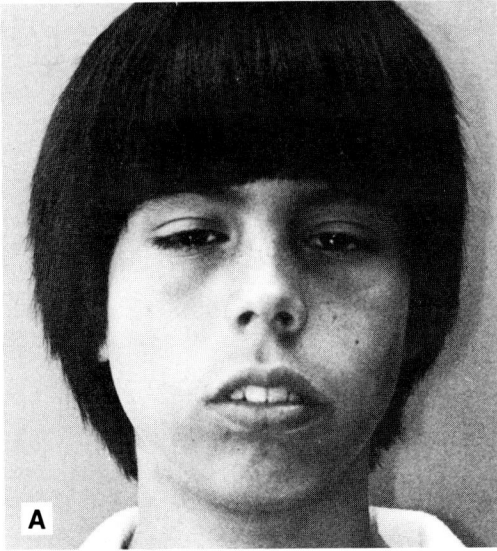

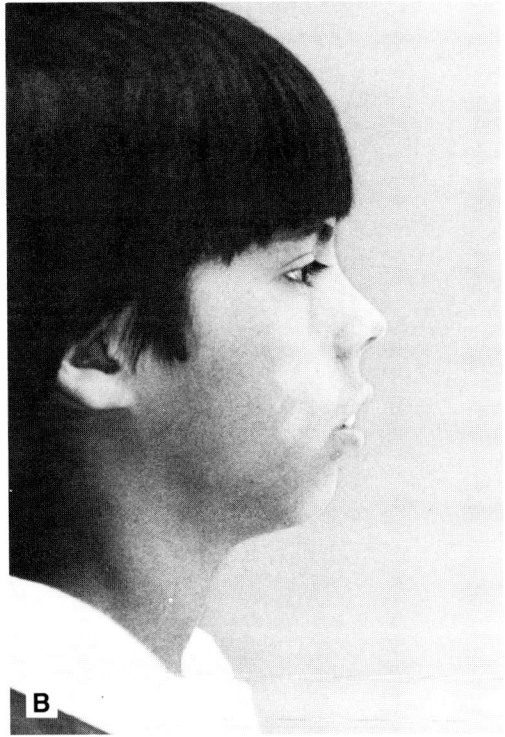

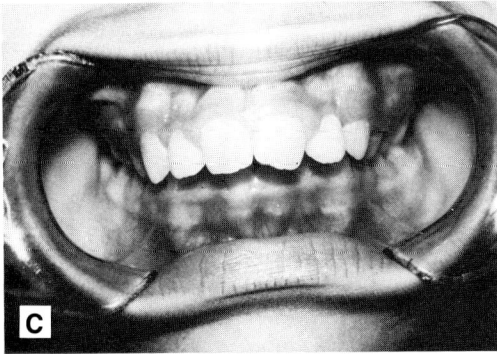

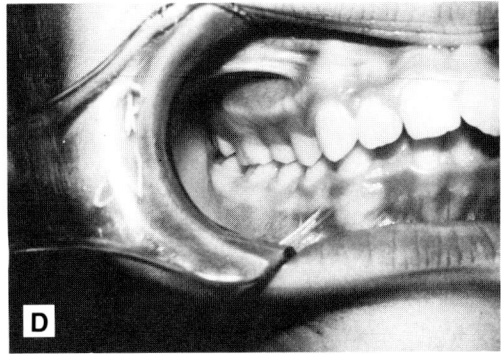

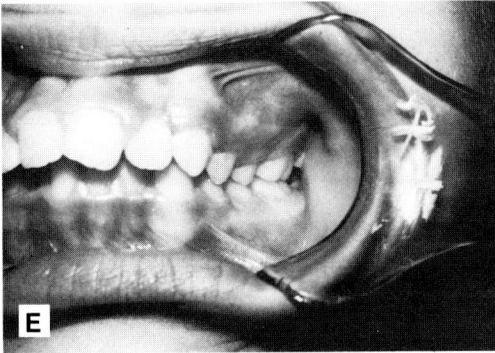

FIG. 22-33. (A and B) This 16-year-old man presents with vertical maxillary excess, A-P mandibular deficiency, and A-P microgenia. (C, D, and E) A Class II occlusion is present with crowding of the lower anterior teeth and overangulation of the upper anterior teeth. (F) Cephalometric analysis demonstrates vertical maxillary excess, A-P mandibular deficiency, microgenia, and overangulation of the maxillary incisors.

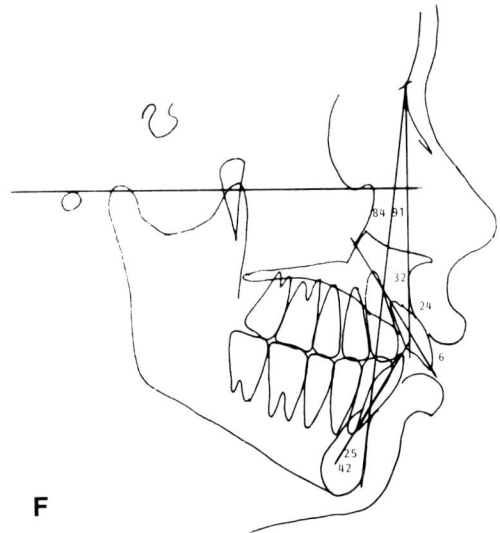

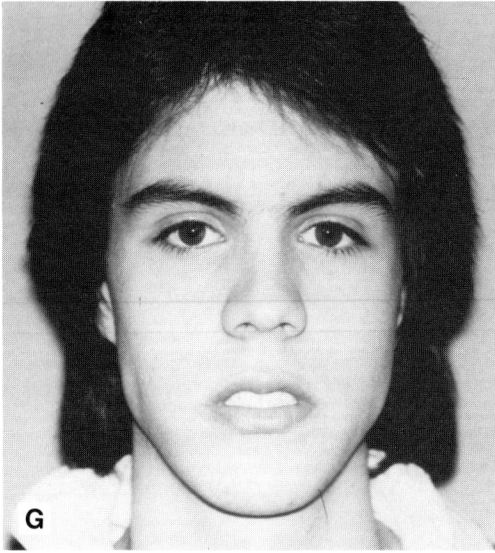

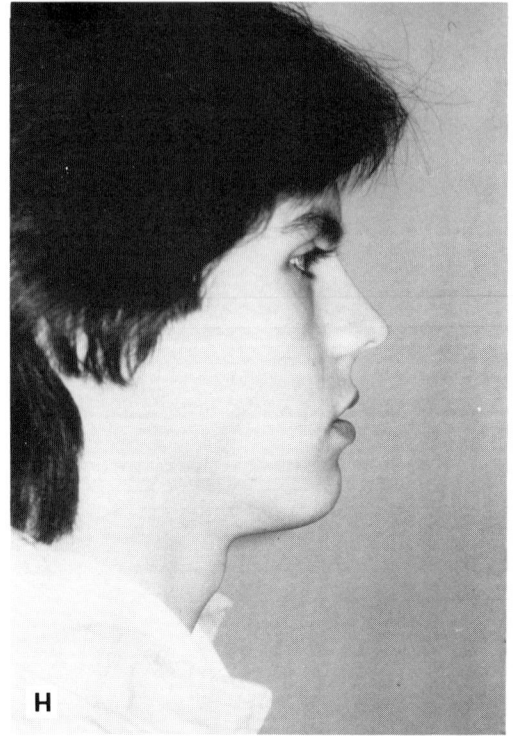

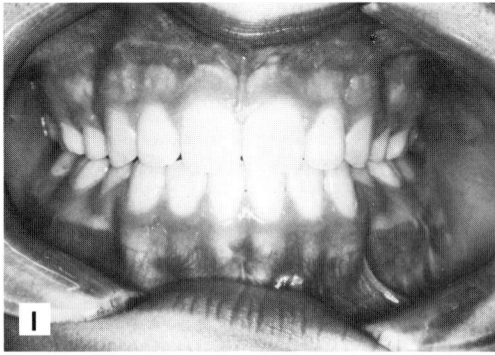

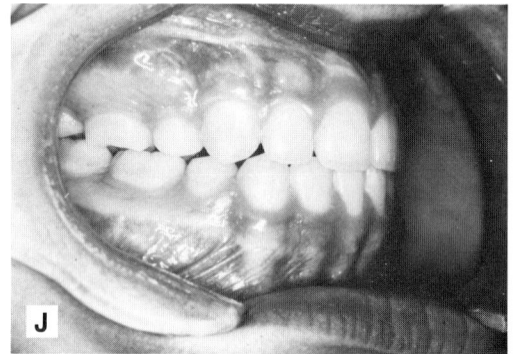

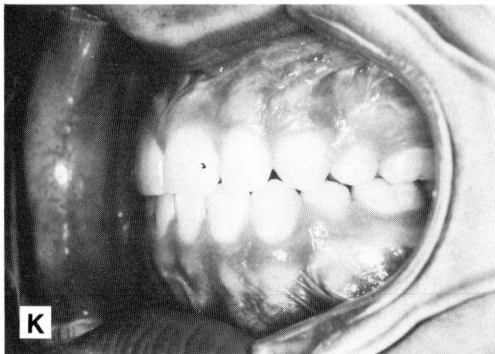

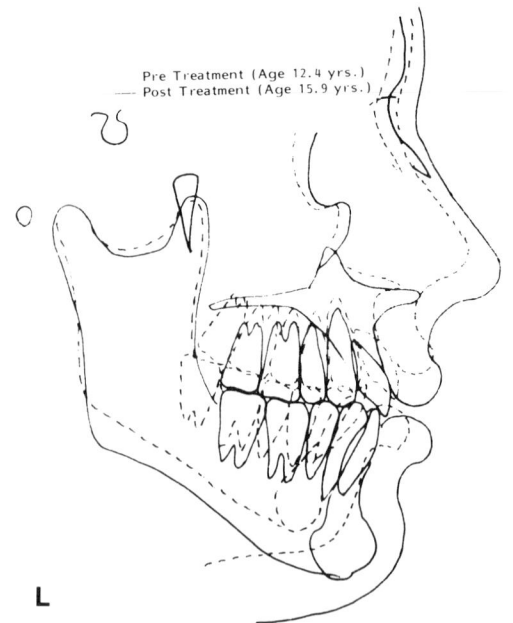

Fig. 22-33. *Continued. (G through K) Functional and aesthetic changes are observed after completion of treatment, which included: 1. Extracting all first bicuspids. 2. Preoperative orthodontics (aligning and leveling the arches, closing the lower extraction spaces). 3. Surgery—multiple maxillary ostectomies to move the maxilla upward and remove residual first bicuspid extraction spaces; mandibular advancement; augmentation genioplasty. 4. Postoperative orthodontics to finish and retain occlusion. (L) Superimposition of pre- and postoperative cephalometric tracings demonstrates overall results achieved.*

Pre Treatment (Age 12.4 yrs.)
Post Treatment (Age 15.9 yrs.)

L

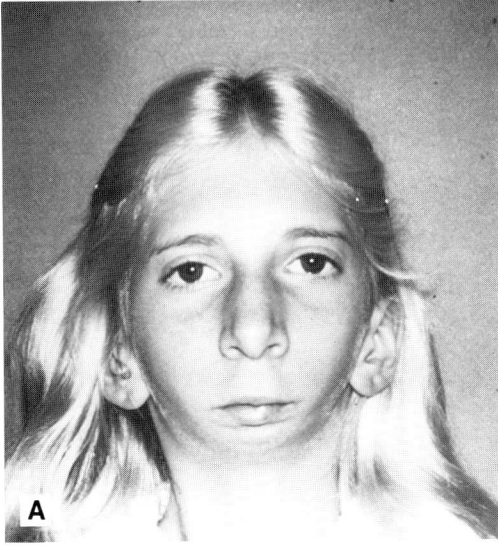

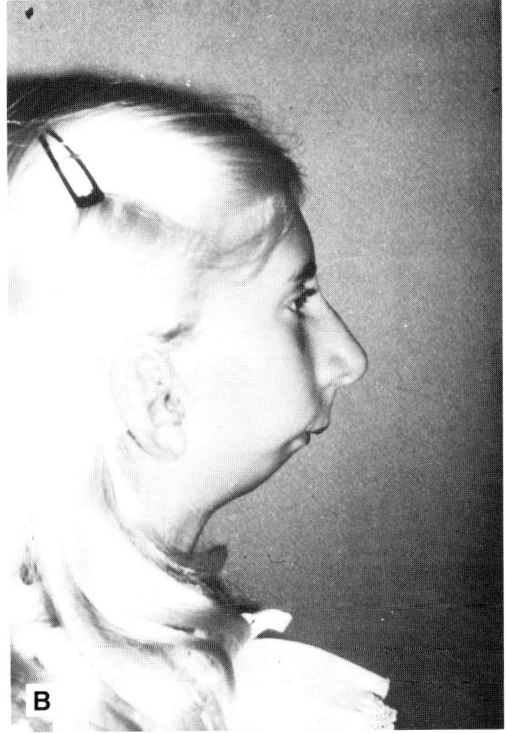

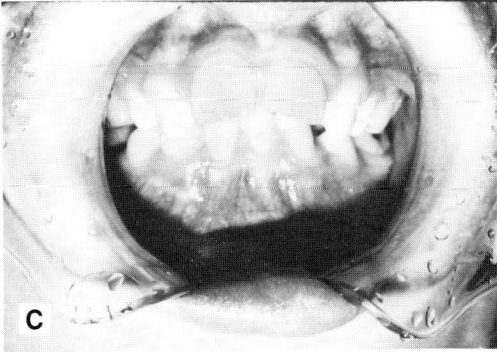

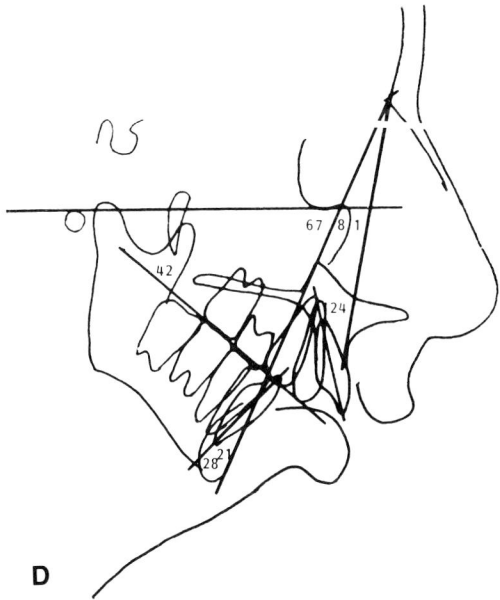

Fig. 22-34. *(A and B) This 12-year-old patient was diagnosed as having severe underdevelopment of the maxilla in a vertical direction, particularly posteriorly, and severe A-P mandibular deficiency. (C) A significant Class II malocclusion is noted. (D) Cephalometric analysis demonstrates severe vertical deficiency in the posterior maxilla, severe A-P deficiency in the mandible, and a severely overangulated occlusal plane.*

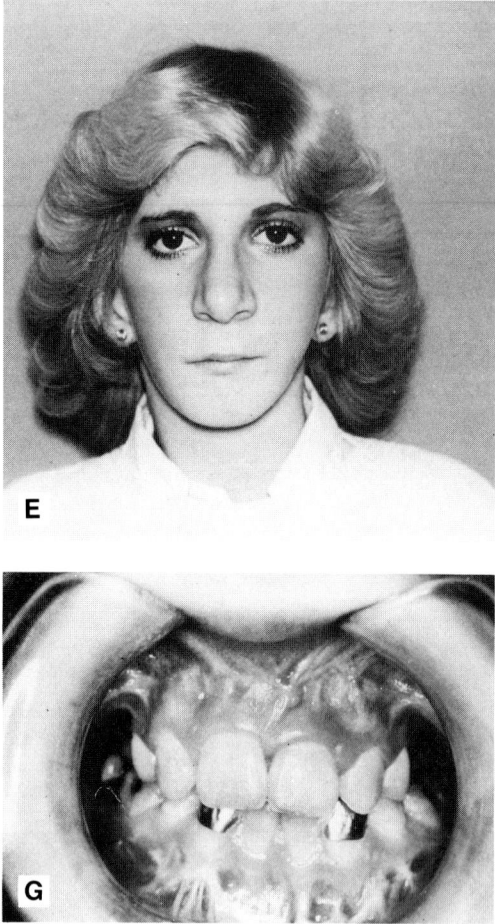

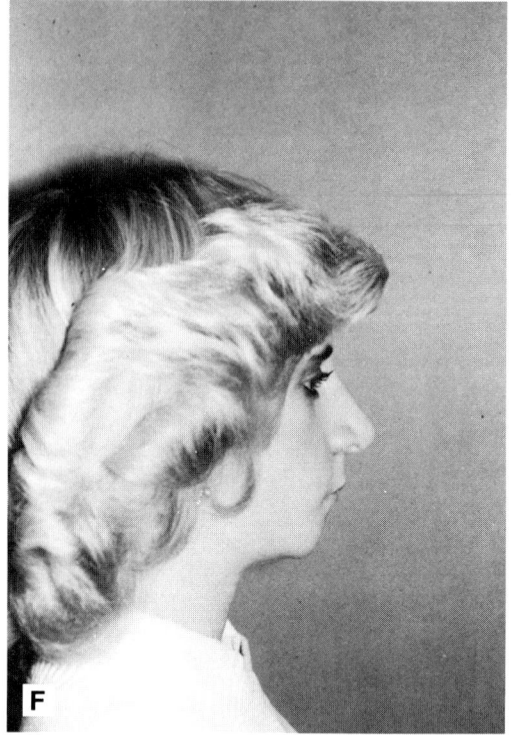

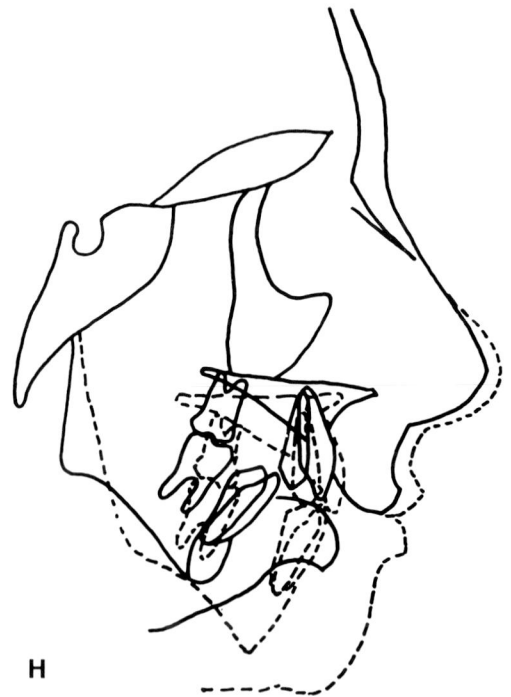

Fig. 22-34. *Continued. (E, F, and G) Postoperative results obtained for this patient. She was treated in the following manner: 1. Preoperative orthodontics to align and level the arches. 2. Surgery—maxillary osteotomies to downgraft the posterior maxilla; bilateral mandibular inverted "L" osteotomies (a modification of the vertical oblique osteotomy) to lengthen and advance the mandible; augmentation genioplasty. 3. Postoperative orthodontics to refine occlusion. (H) Superimposition of pre- and postoperative x-rays shows the tremendous changes functionally and aesthetically achieved for this patient.*

tomographic x-rays, transcranial x-rays, transpharyngeal x-rays, CT scans, magnetic resonance imaging (MRI), and arthrograms, may be required. Patients may demonstrate headaches and/or jaw and muscle pains that may very well be related to the jaw deformity or to the temporomandibular joint. If the jaw joints are relatively asymptomatic in regard to pain, then usually we proceed with the orthognathic surgery and monitor the temporomandibular joint long-term. However, if a patient has significant pain associated with the temporomandibular joint, conservative therapy is usually initiated first to see if it can resolve the problem. If not, surgical correction of the temporomandibular joint deformity may be indicated. Conditions such as articular disc dislocation with or without reduction, osteoarthritis, and rheumatoid arthritis may necessitate surgical intervention.

If surgical intervention is indicated, it can be managed in one of three ways. The first is to correct the temporomandibular joint problems and at a later operation correct the jaw deformity. The second approach is to correct the jaw deformities first and at a second operation, repair the temporomandibular joint problem. The third choice—and our primary method for managing these combined problems—is to correct the temporomandibular joint problem while the orthognathic surgery is being completed. In our experience this technique improves overall patient stability and comfort.

Other Craniofacial Deformities

Crouzon's and Apert's syndromes are developmental deformities affecting the facial structures. Because of premature closure of the cranial and middle face sutures, there is a severe lack of growth of the orbits, nasal, zygomatic, and maxillary bone components. Oftentimes the skull will be severely malshaped. Usually the mandible is the only normal bone in the entire head and face. The severe growth disturbance can cause significant functional and aesthetic deformities (Fig. 22-35A and B). Before surgery, these patients appear to have very prominent eyes, because they are protrusive beyond the orbital rims. They usually exhibit a skeletal Class III re-

lationship and a Class III malocclusion with posterior and anterior cross-bites (Fig. 22-35C, D, and E). Cephalometrically, the linear and angular measurements are unreliable because of the often severe distortion of the cranial base (Fig. 22-35F).

These types of deformities are corrected with orthodontics and the appropriate craniofacial surgery. Usually osteotomies are involved so that the nose, portions of the orbits, cheek bones, and maxilla can be separated from the cranial base structures and repositioned in an anterior direction. This allows the lateral, medial, and inferior orbital structures to be repositioned forward around the globe. These mobilized bones must be stabilized with either bone or hydroxyapatite grafting and preferably with bone plates. Sometimes the lower jaw also may require surgery to achieve the appropriate functional and aesthetic results (Fig. 22-35G through L). The earlier these problems are identified and managed, the less severe the deformity will be at a later time. Even with early correction, however, growth will still be disproportionate, with the mandible growing at a faster rate than the midfacial structures.

Hemifacial microsomia refers to the underdevelopment of the bony and soft tissue structures of half of the face (Fig. 22-36A through F). This condition can occur with varying degrees of severity and either unilaterally or bilaterally. These patients are often missing a portion of the mandible on the involved side including the condyle, ramus, and in more severe cases even a portion of the body of the mandible. They occasionally are missing the zygomatic arches and may have malformed ears. Patients are best managed at an early age with surgery designed to correct the aesthetic and functional deformity as well as to provide some growth potential by using a growth center transplant, such as a costochondral graft or a sternoclavicular graft. Not only are the bones severely deformed on the involved side, but deficiencies also exist in muscle, subcutaneous tissues, etc. These, likewise, are indicated to be reconstructed with such procedures as alloplastic augmentations to the mandible and maxilla, dermal grafts, and free vascularized grafts (Fig. 22-36, G through L). Orthodontic management in these patients is

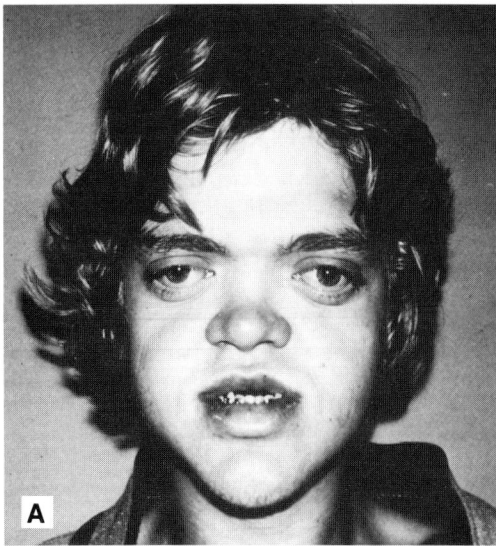

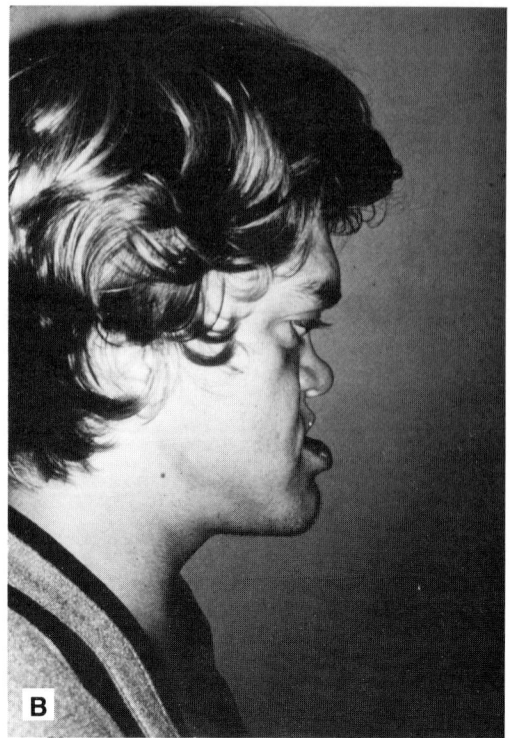

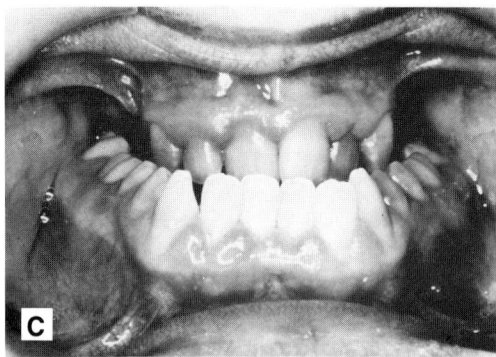

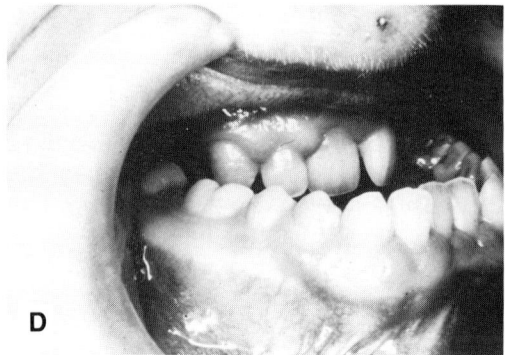

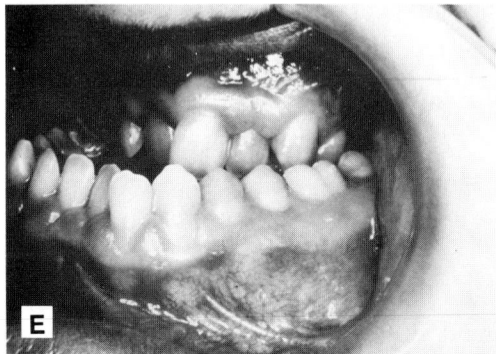

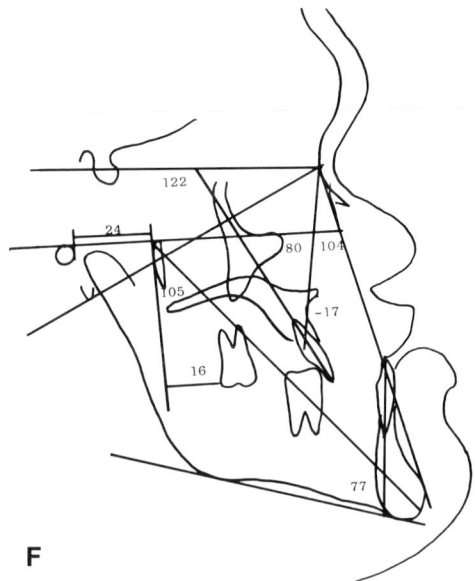

FIG. 22-35. (A and B) This 23-year-old man was diagnosed as having Crouzon's syndrome—severe underdevelopment of the nose, cheeks, and maxilla. In addition, he has overdevelopment of the lower jaw (mandibular prognathism). (C, D, and E) Severe Class III occlusion is seen as well as transverse maxillary deficiency. (F) Cephalometric tracings demonstrate severe facial deformity.

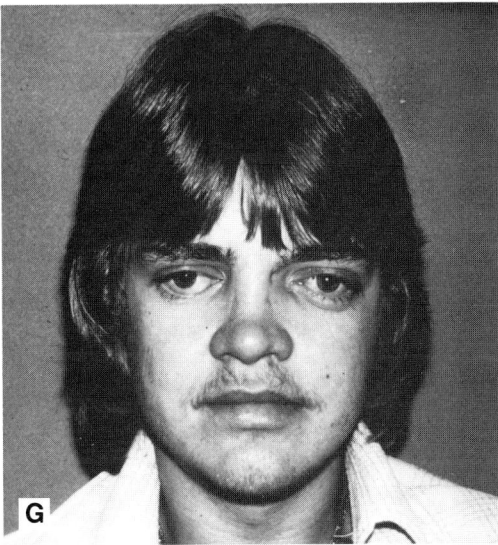

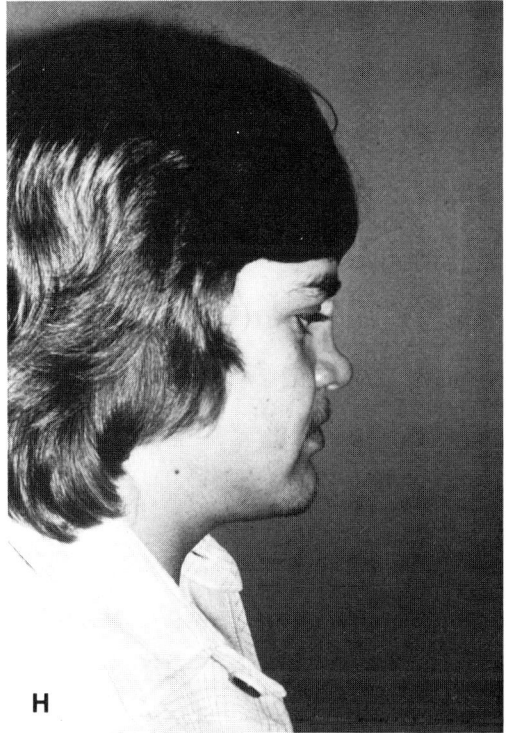

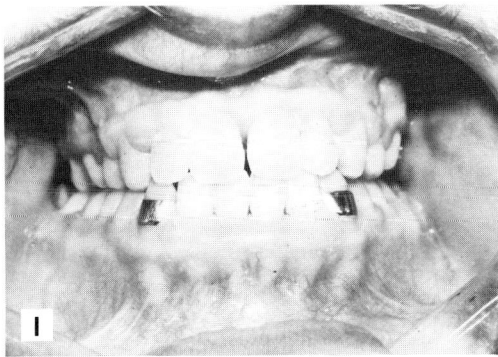

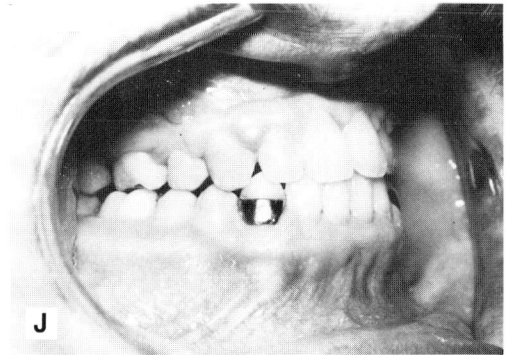

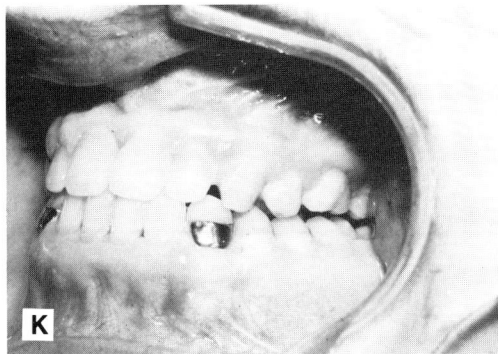

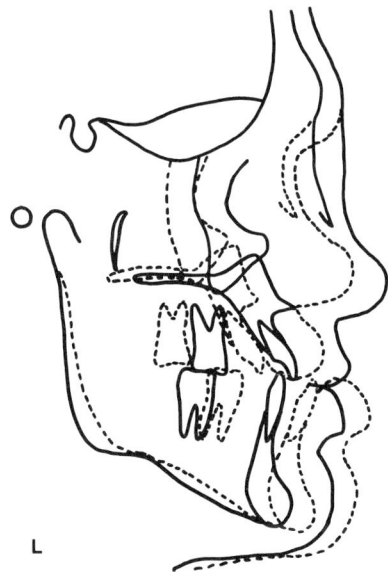

Fig. 22-35. *Continued. (G through K) Post-treatment photos demonstrate functional and aesthetic results achieved. The patient was treated in the following manner: 1. Extracting maxillary first bicuspids. 2. Preoperative orthodontics to align and level the arches. 3. Surgery—nasomalarmaxillary advancement (nose, cheeks, and upper jaw); mandibular setback. 4. Postoperative orthodontics to refine occlusion. (L) Superimposition of pre- and postoperative cephalometric tracings demonstrate the functional and aesthetic results obtained. (Orthodontics by Dr. Tom Wirick.)*

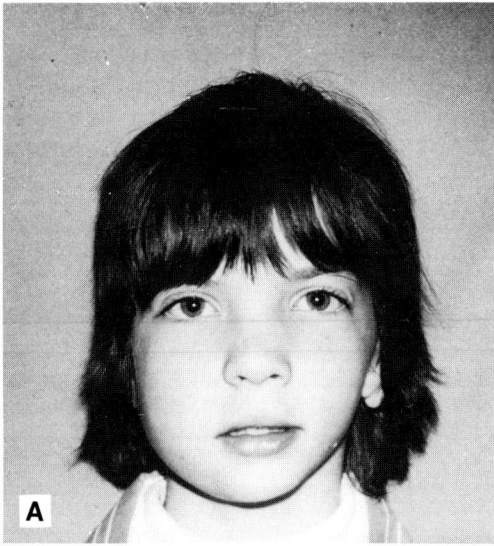

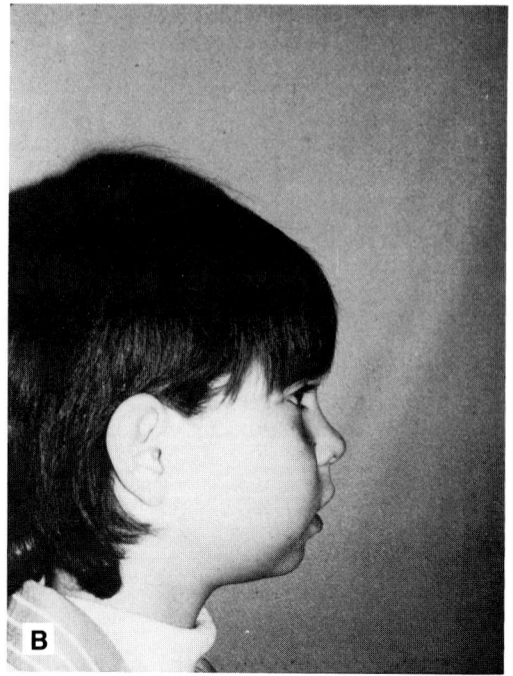

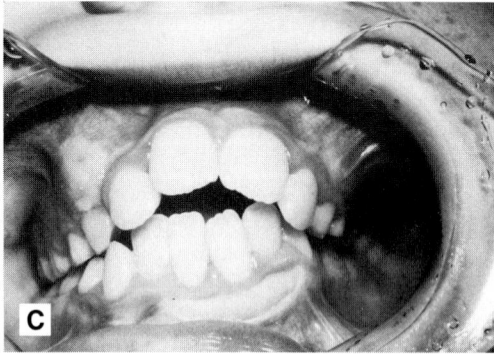

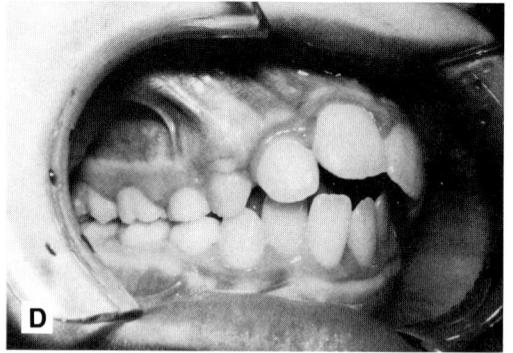

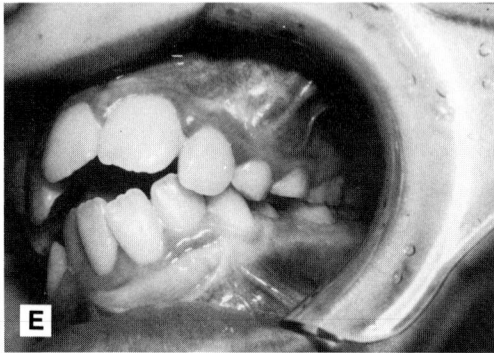

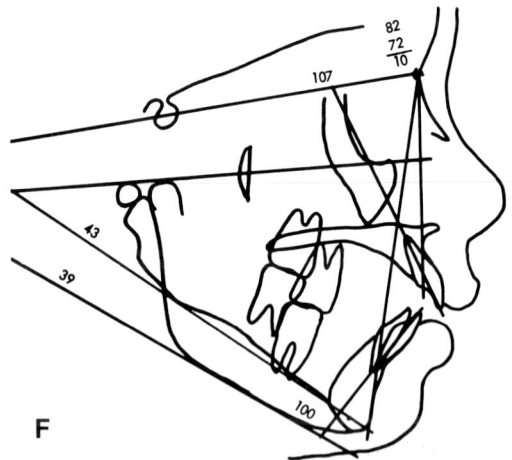

FIG. 22-36. (A and B) This 12-year-old female was diagnosed as having hemifacial microsomia with significant underdevelopment of the left side of the face vertically and anteroposteriorly. (C, D, and E) Demonstrate occlusion that is basically Class II and the tremendous cant in the occlusal plane secondary to vertical underdevelopment of the maxillary and mandibular dentoalveolus. (F) Cephalometric analysis confirms the diagnosis.

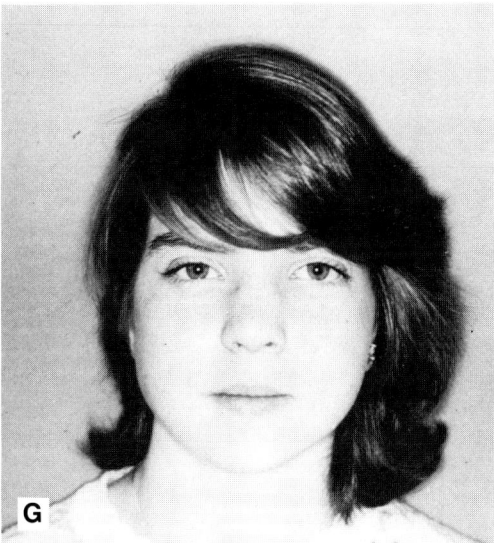

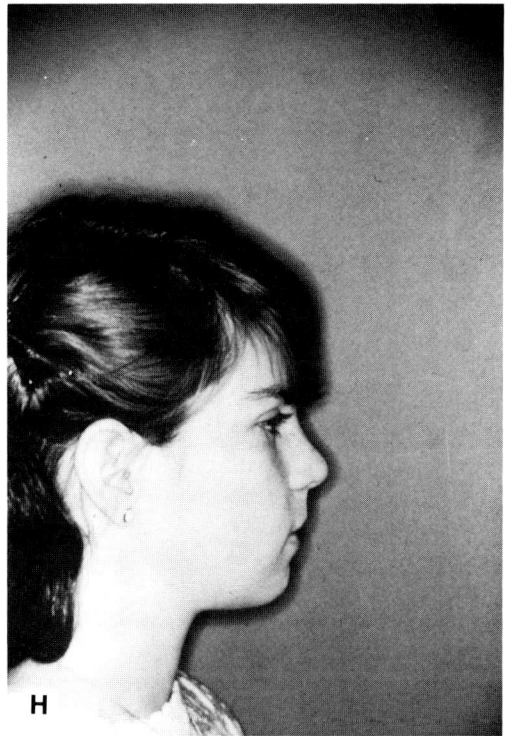

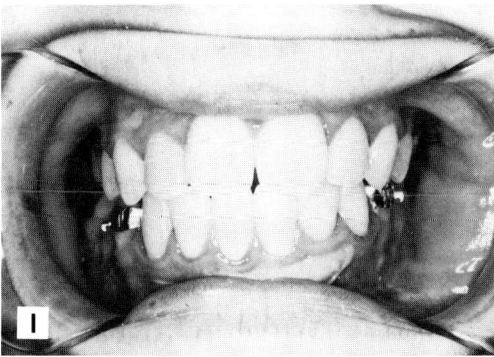

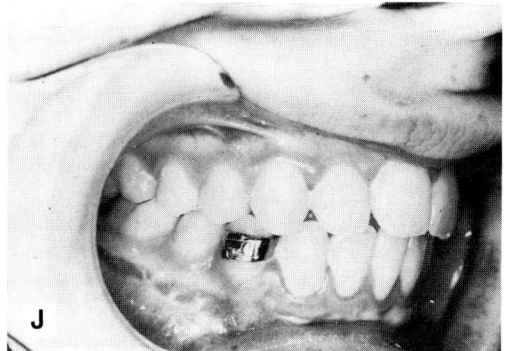

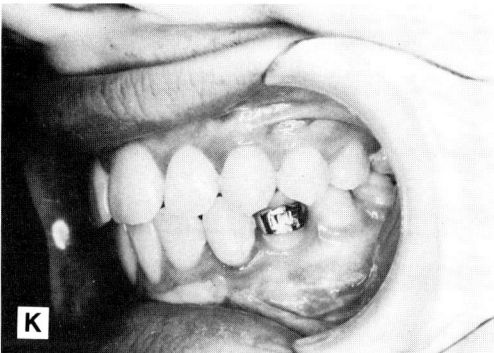

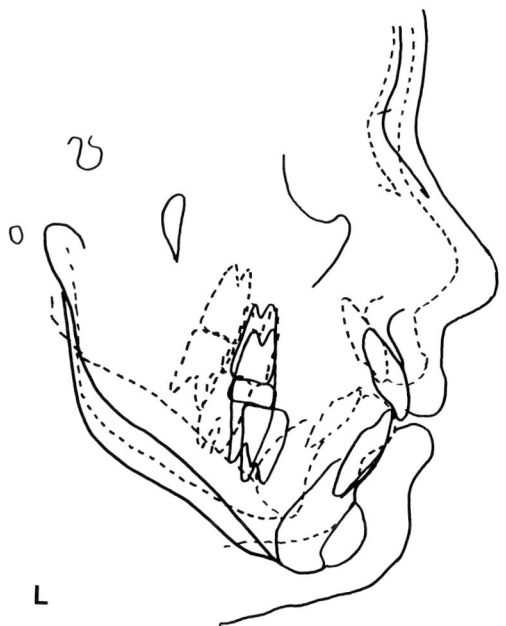

FIG. 22-36. *Continued. (G through K) The overall results achieved. Treatment consisted of: 1. Preoperative orthodontics to align and level maxillary and mandibular arch. 2. Surgery—Stage I— Mandibular ramus osteotomies to advance the mandible and open the bite significantly on the left side. 3. Orthodontics to extrude the maxillary teeth to level off the occlusal plane. 4. Surgery—Stage II— Alloplastic augmentation to the left mandible in the body and ramus area; alloplastic chin augmentation; dermal (fat) graft to left cheek. 5. Postoperative orthodontics to refine occlusion. (L) Postoperative cephalometric tracing demonstrates the establishment of good functional and aesthetic results. (Orthodontics by Dr. Leward Fish.)*

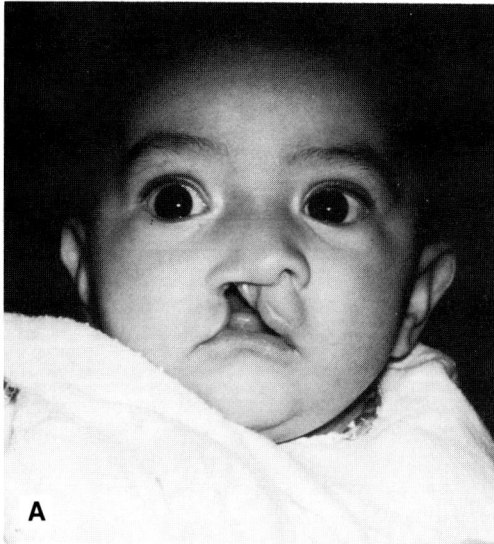

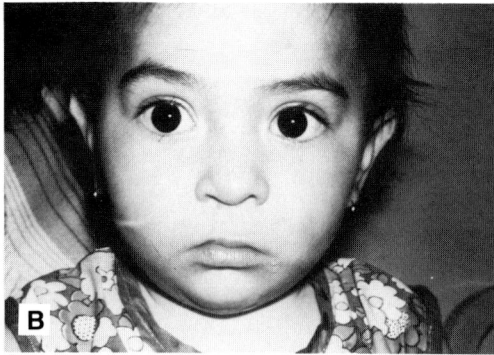

FIG. 22-37. (A) Unilateral cleft lip and palate. (B) Repair of the cleft lip.

deformities (Fig. 22-39A and B). These patients usually have alveolar clefts between the lateral and cuspid teeth (Fig. 22-39C, D, and E).

Frequently teeth are missing in this area, and occasionally extra teeth may be in the cleft area. The developing permanent cuspid teeth can erupt down into the cleft area, which could cause periodontal problems and subsequent loss of the tooth. Timing is crucial in placing bone in the alveolar grafts and closing a residual com-

usually lengthy, particularly if treatment is begun during the growth years.

Cleft lip and palate deformities develop because of lack of fusion or breakdown of the fusion processes of the upper lip and palate during the first six to nine weeks in utero. These deformities occur about one in every 750 live births. There is discontinuity in the lip, dentoalveolus, and/or palate (Fig. 22-37A) that can occur unilaterally or bilaterally. Repairs of the cleft lip are usually done at 10 weeks of age (Fig. 22-37B), and of the palate prior to the age of 2 years (Fig. 22-38). However, these repairs may cause growth problems of the maxilla later on. If these growth deficiencies occur, orthodontics and surgery may be necessary to correct the skeletal

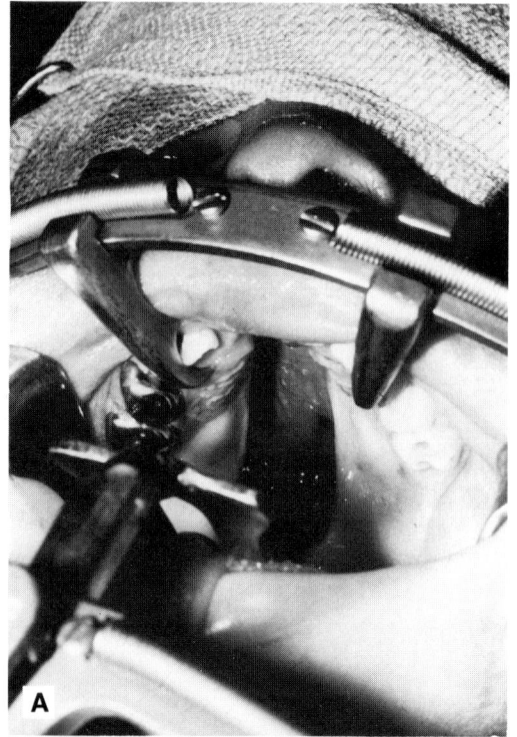

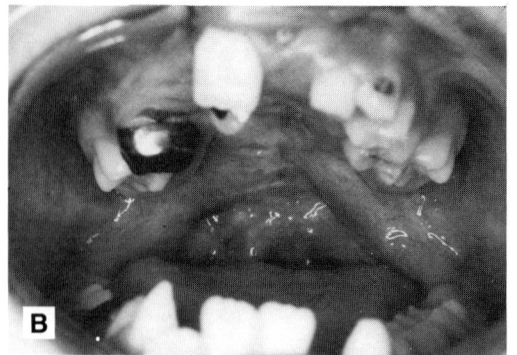

FIG. 22-38. (A) Cleft palate. (B) Repair of the cleft palate.

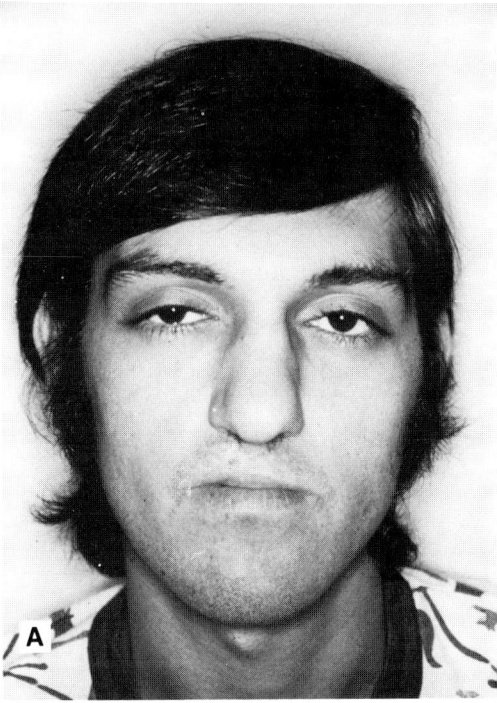

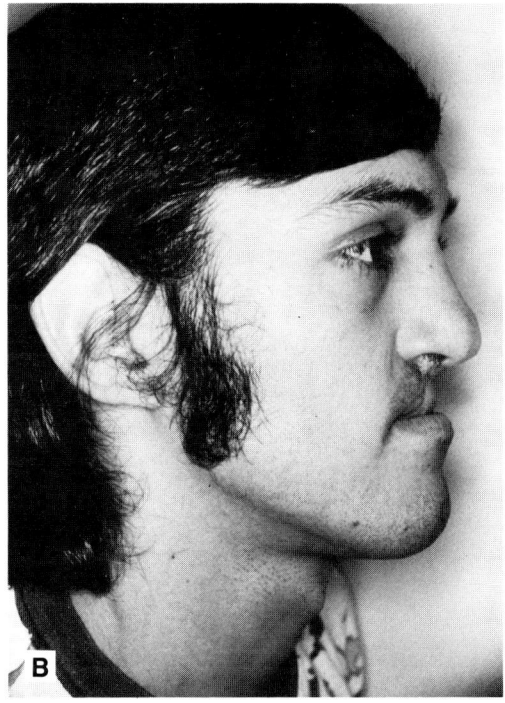

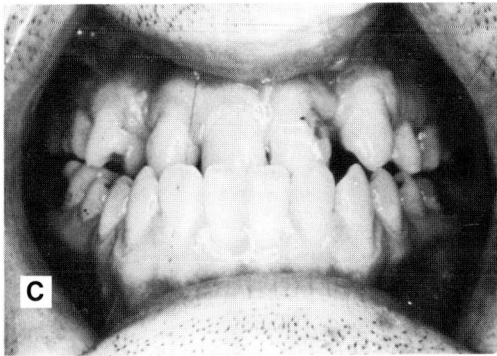

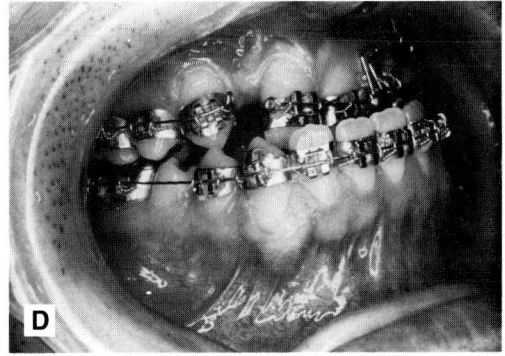

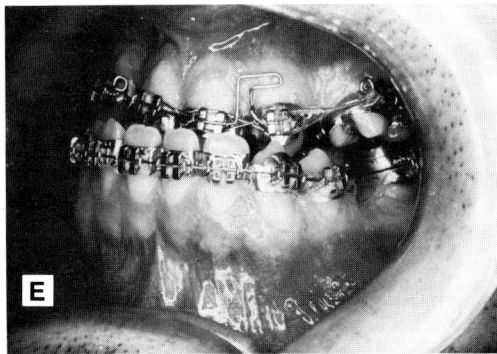

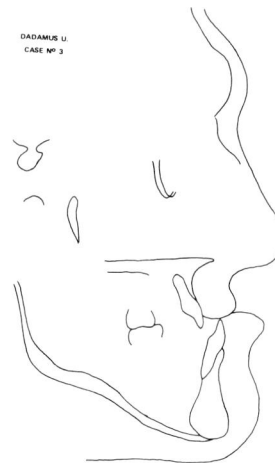

FIG. 22-39. (A and B) This 24-year-old man was born with a unilateral cleft lip and palate. They were repaired at a relatively early age, but A-P and vertical maxillary deficiencies remain. In addition, he has mandibular prognathism. (C, D, and E) The patient's Class III occlusal relationship. (F) Cephalometric analysis confirms the maxillary hypoplasia and mandibular prognathism.

469

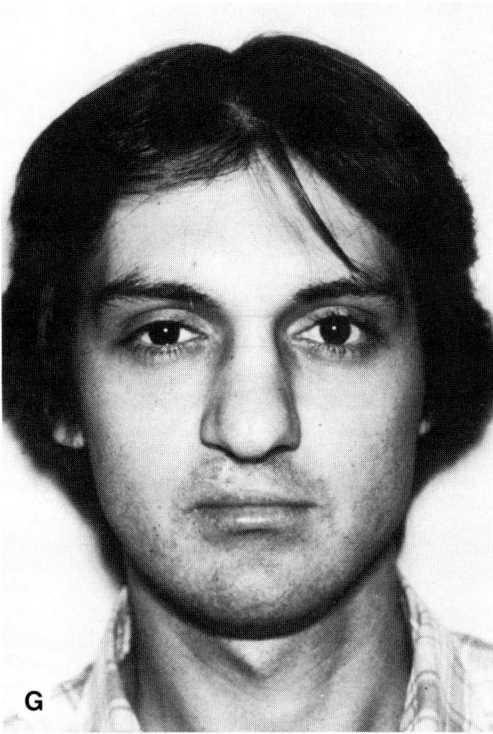

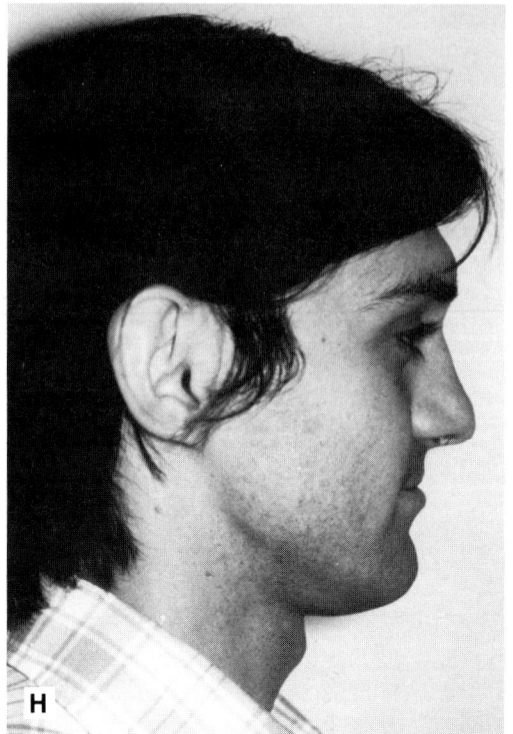

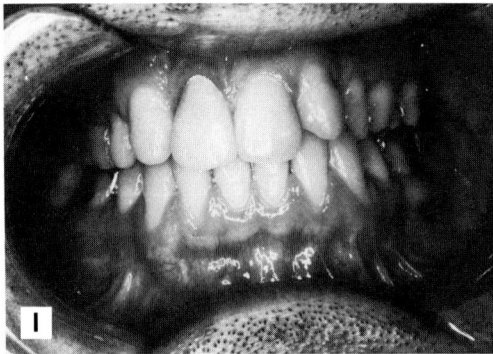

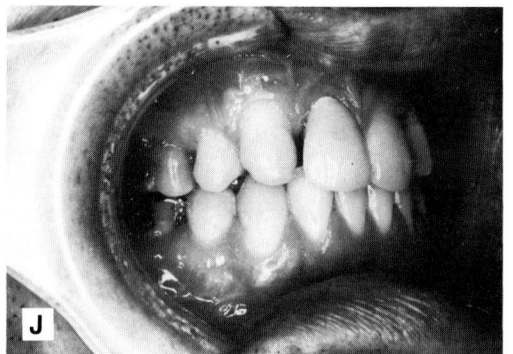

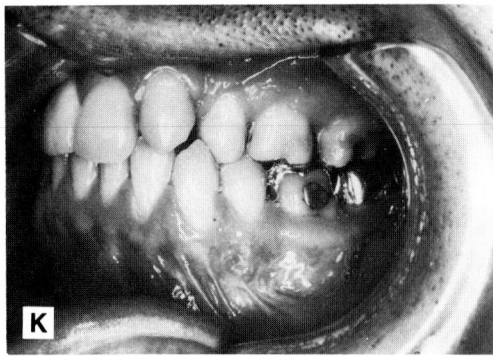

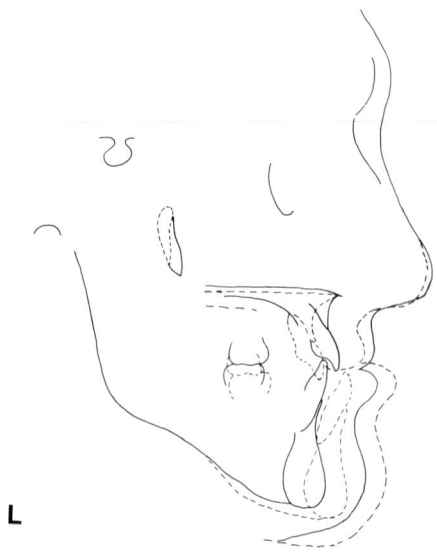

FIG. 22-39. *Continued. (G through K) Post-treatment results. Treatment included preoperative orthodontics to align and level the arches; multiple maxillary osteotomies to advance the maxilla; bone graft alveolar clefts; mandibular setback via bilateral mandibular body ostectomies (refer to Fig. 22-27); postoperative orthodontics to refine occlusion. (L) Superimposition of pre- and postoperative cephalometric x-rays demonstrates functional and aesthetic results.*

munication from the mouth into the nose in that area prior to eruption of the permanent cuspid. Placing a bone graft allows the cuspid teeth to erupt through the graft and into the oral cavity. Lower jaw surgery may also be necessary in these patients because of abnormal lower jaw growth or a deformity created in the lower jaw because of deficiency in upper jaw growth. Improved functional and aesthetic results can be achieved (Fig. 22-39G through L).

A myriad of craniofacial deformities can be corrected by orthognathic surgery. We have touched on a few of the more common types, but many combinations and existing problems are beyond the scope of this chapter. The field of orthognathic surgery continues to make significant advances. Surgical techniques and orthodontic mechanics improve, as do the technical skills of those performing them. Improvements in diagnostic equipment and the use of the computer will continue to improve diagnoses, treatment planning, and management for the correction of dentofacial deformities.

Orthognathic surgery to correct dentofacial deformities is a challenging and rewarding treatment area. To achieve optimal functional and aesthetic results, good training and cooperation of all health professionals participating in a patient's management are essential. It requires a team effort and rarely can problems be managed strictly by one health professional. Advances made in this area during the last 15 years have been remarkable, and future advances will continue to improve the quality of results and quality of life for patients undergoing this treatment.

References

1. Hullihen, S.P.: Case of elongation of underjaw and distortion of face and neck, caused by burn, successfully treated. Am. J. Dent. Surg., 9:157, 1849.
2. Angle, E.H.: Treatment of Malocclusion of the Teeth. Philadephia, The S.S. White Dental Manufacturing Company, 1907.
3. Cohn-Stock, G.: Die chirwigische Im-
mediatre-gulierung der Kiefer, speziell die chirwigische Behandlung der Prognathie. Vjschr Zahnheilk Berlin, 37:320, 1921.
4. Wassmund, M.: Frakturen und Luxationen des Gesichtsschadels. Berlin, 1927.
5. Hinds E.C., and Kent, J.N.: Surgical Treatment of Developmental Jaw Deformities. St. Louis, C.V. Mosby Co., 1972.
6. Epker B.N., and Wolford, L.M.: Dentofacial Deformities: Surgical-Orthodontic Correction. St. Louis, C.V. Mosby Co., 1980.
7. Bell, W.H., Proffit, W.R., and White, R.P.: Surgical Correction of Dentofacial Deformities. Philadelphia, W.B. Saunders Co., 1980.
8. Wolford, L.M., and Hilliard, F.W.: A practical method for diagnosis, treatment planning, and management of the surgical-orthodontic patient. Fort Worth, John Peter Smith Hospital, 1980.
9. Burstone C.J.: Lip posture and its significance in treatment planning. Am. J. Orthod., 53:268, 1967.
10. Spradley, F.L.: A study of normal anteroposterior contours of the soft tissue profile relative to an extra cranial vertical reference plane (thesis). Baylor College of Dentistry, 1980.
11. Scheideman, G.B., et al.: Cephalometric analysis of dentofacial normals. Am. J. Orthod., 78:404, 1980.
12. Ricketts, R.M.: Perspectives in the clinical application of cephalometrics. Angle Orthod., 51:115, 1981.
13. Tweed, C.H.: The diagnostic triangle in the control of treatment objectives. Am. J. Orthod., 55:651, 1969.
14. Ricketts, R.M.: Cephalometric analysis synthesis. Angle Orthod., 31:141, 1961.
15. Root, T.L., and Sagehorn, E.G.: Level Anchorage. Monrovia, CA, Unitek Corp., 1982.
16. Wolford, L.M., and Hilliard, F.W.: The surgical-orthodontic correction of vertical dentofacial deformities. J. Oral Surg., 39:883, 1981.
17. Bolton, W.A.: Disharmony in tooth size and its relation to the analysis and treatment of malocclusion. Angle Orthod., 28:113, 1958.
18. Wolford, L.M., Hilliard, F.W., and Dugan, D.J.: Surgical Treatment Objective: A Systematic Approach to the Prediction Tracing. St. Louis, C.V. Mosby Co., 1984.

CHAPTER 23

Cleft Lip and Palate

MICHAEL C. KINNEBREW

The secret of success is constancy to purpose.

Management of individuals born with cleft lip and palate seeks to habilitate these individuals into normally functioning and appearing children, adolescents, and adults. That these persons can ultimately take their places in society, without the encumbrance of real or perceived anatomic deformity, is due in significant part to contributions by the dental profession. Basic research and clinical practice, conducted under the auspices of dental schools and the National Institute of Dental Research and by individual practitioners, have added to present understanding of the underlying problems of the orofacial cleft.

Dentistry has participated synergistically with medicine and the allied health professions. General dentistry has been active, as have pediatric dentistry, orthodontia, prosthodontia, and oral and maxillofacial surgery, to name but a few. From medicine and the allied health professions have come other components of the treatment "team," including surgeons specializing in plastic surgery, otolaryngology, pediatric surgery and general surgery. Pediatricians, geneticists, and practitioners in special nursing, psychosocial services, and, of great importance, speech pathology and audiology have contributed their knowledge. Each role complements the others and provides its unique contribution within this orchestration of services offered by the "cleft palate team."

This chapter seeks to expand, for the dental student and practitioner, the background in craniofacial biology provided by dental education that is so readily modified toward management of the orofacial cleft. Existing knowledge is briefly reviewed, proceeding in a stepwise fashion through the salient points of embryology, pathologic anatomy and physiology, incidence, etiology, classification, and treatment. Historical perspectives and ongoing management controversies are also covered.

Embryology

Figure 23-1 illustrates the orderly sequence by which the facial structure is formed from the fusion of multiple embryonic processes. Failure of any process to fully form, or failure of neighboring processes to fuse, results in a facial cleft. The classically honored sequence is that the processes approach each other and "fuse," the intervening epithelium degenerates, and the neural crest-derived mesenchymal cores freely intermingle.[1,2] Histologic and morphologic differentiation then provides that the mesenchyme gives rise to such "mature" tissues as bone, muscle, blood vessels, and other connective tissues. Other specialized tissue, such as nerve tissue, develops simultaneously from the primordia of the processes. This schema is shown for the palate in Figure 23-2.

Formation of the lip and nose is essentially complete at 8 weeks in utero. Palatal fusion, proceeding from anterior to posterior, is completed at approximately 10 weeks. Development of the nasal septum and nasal chambers also occurs on either side. From that point facial growth and development continue according to the

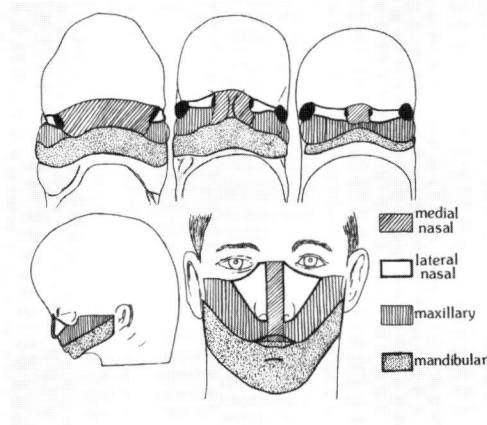

FIG. 23-1. *The sequence by which the adult face is formed from the union and subsequent interrelated growth of embryologic processes. (Adapted from Sicher and Tandler: Anatomie for Zahnartze, Berlin: Julius Springer, 1928)*

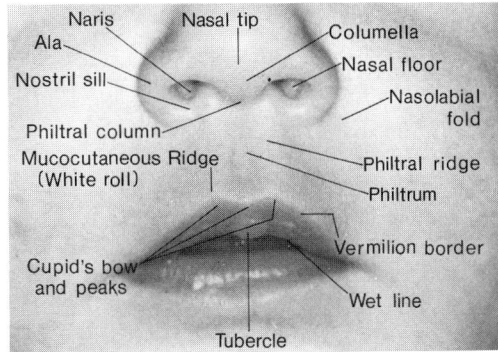

FIG. 23-3. *Tabulation of the component topographic points of the normal lip-nose complex in an infant.*

individual genetic code, with the ultimate expression of a "normal" face predicated first upon the genetic driving force, then upon anatomic and functional union of adjoining parts such that concordant growth will be achieved. These points are illustrated in the subsequent discussion of orofacial cleft anatomy.

Anatomy

Sound understanding of the abnormal morphology of the cleft situation arises from a grasp of normal anatomy. By way of review, let us first look at the normal external anatomy of the lip and nose (Fig. 23-3). At the same time, one must consider the underlying skeleton and the associated facial muscles supporting the visible soft tissue contours.

The mouth and nose are focal points toward which the facial muscles converge. Within the lip, the components of the or-

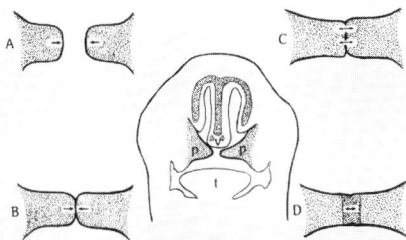

FIG. 23-2. *Formation of the palate (center) by the union of palatal shelves and vomer. A through D depict the apposition of embryologic processes, dissolution of the intervening epithelium, and intermingling of the primordial core. (From: Rampp, D.L., Pannbacker, M., and Kinnebrew, M.C.: Velopharyngeal Incompetency—A Practical Guide for Evaluation and Management. Tulsa, Modern Education Corp., 1984)*

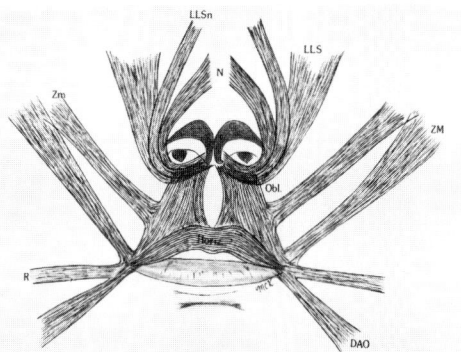

FIG. 23-4. *Facial muscles converging at the nose and oral stoma. Clockwise they include the nasalis (N); levator labii superioris (LLS), zygomaticus major (ZM), depressor angulae oris (DAO), risorsus (R), zygomaticus minor (Zm), and levator labii superioris alaeque nasi (LLSn). Within the lip are oblique and horizontal fibers; incisive fibers are not shown. (From: Rampp, D.L., Pannbacker, M., and Kinnebrew, M.C.: Velopharyngeal Incompetency—A Practical Guide for Evaluation and Management. Tulsa, Modern Education Corp., 1984)*

bicularis oris muscle—including the horizontal, oblique, and incisive fibers—intermingle further for normal animation (Fig. 23-4). By their association with the nasalis and levator labii superioris muscles, these muscles also serve a function of nasal respiration. In addition, the composite of muscles is thought to play a modulating role on growth of the facial skeleton, as will be seen in the review of cleft anatomy.[3]

The established orofacial cleft should be considered as both an absolute and relative tissue deficiency that is variably compounded by functional distortion. This statement of degree is well-supported by analysis of the unilateral complete cleft shown in Figure 23-5A. The overlying soft tissue distortion is readily seen and may be attributed to the abnormal muscular at-

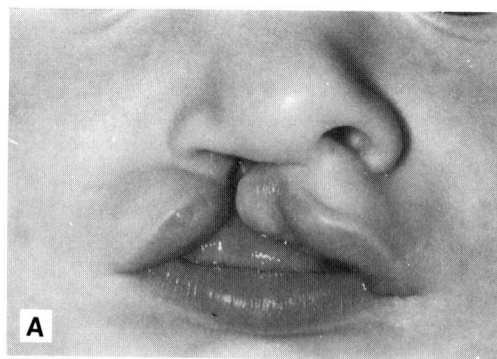

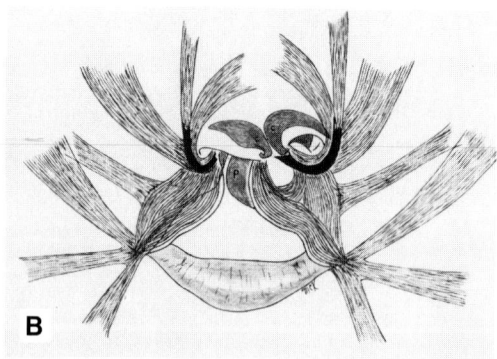

FIG. 23-5. (A) Topographic appearance of a unilateral complete cleft lip and palate in a newborn. (B) The distortion is further illustrated and amplified by the underlying muscular, cartilaginous, and bony abnormality. (From: Rampp, D.L., Pannbacker, M., and Kinnebrew, M.C.: Velopharyngeal Incompetency—A Practical Guide for Evaluation and Management. Tulsa, Modern Education Corp., 1984)

tachments and bony and cartilaginous distortion indicated in Figure 23-5B. Even if one were to assume that adequate mesenchyme was initially present, a lag in development of the involved region has occurred. The muscles, lacking functional continuity with their partners across the midline, have not pulled on one another to realize optimal growth.[4] Likewise, they have not pulled "normally" upon skin. Instead, they have pulled upon the margins of bone, cartilage, and skin to which they are attached, and with the lack of contralateral muscular antagonism, the net result is further distortion and widening of the cleft as the maxillary segments are distracted.

The complete bilateral cleft lip and palate presents a similar situation. Here the midline structures, the premaxillary segment, and associated prolabium (midline lip structure) are thrust forward on the protruding stalk of the nasal septum.[5] There is no bony continuity with the neighboring maxilla, and likewise no continuity of the muscles or skin. In the complete cleft, muscles are completely lacking in the prolabium; there has been no embryologic pathway for mesenchymal penetration and maturation.[6] The lateral muscle bundles have developed in relative isolation and are seen, as in the unilateral situation, to insert upon the lateral margins of the cleft. The result is a lag in anterior growth of the lateral maxillary segments as well as distraction of the segments (Fig. 23-6).

Following an anterior-to-posterior description of the cleft, one next envisions the cleft alveolus. The lateral incisor is commonly absent, and the remaining regional dental organs may be distorted.[7] The defect in the maxilla is merely a hole into which the overlying soft tissues may collapse, and through which the nasal and oral cavities are continuous. The hard palate is clefted with varying severity; a mere slit or a wide "U-shaped" deformity may be seen at the extremes.[8]

The soft palate (velum) is also affected with varying severity. Here, as in the lip cleft, abnormal muscular orientation occurs, with associated deficiency of bulk and function. Rather than discrete intermingling of the palatal and associated pharyngeal muscles across the midline, they are

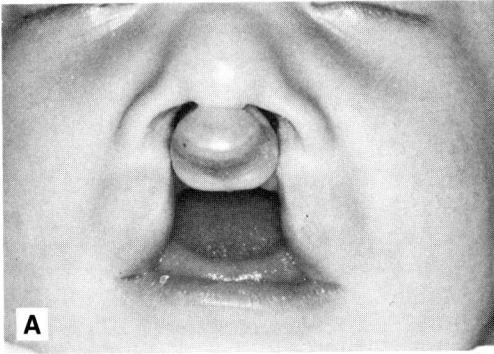

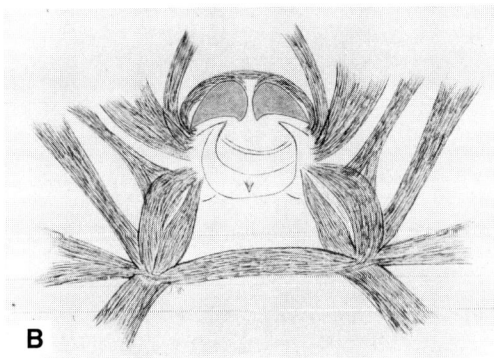

FIG. 23-6. (A) External features, and (B) musculoskeletal deformity of a bilateral cleft of the lip and primary palate. (From Rampp, D.L., Pannbacker, M., and Kinnebrew, M.C.: Velopharyngeal Incompetency—A Practical Guide for Evaluation and Management. Tulsa, Modern Education Corp., 1984)

speech with excessive nasal resonance and consonant distortion is present.[14] This is a function of the interrelated musculature of the soft palate and upper pharynx. While the velum is lifted and flexed and the pharynx constricted, the eustachian tubes are opened to allow equilibration of atmospheric and middle ear pressures, or "clearing" of the ears.[15,16,17] Without this latter activity, a chronic condition of negative middle ear pressure becomes established.

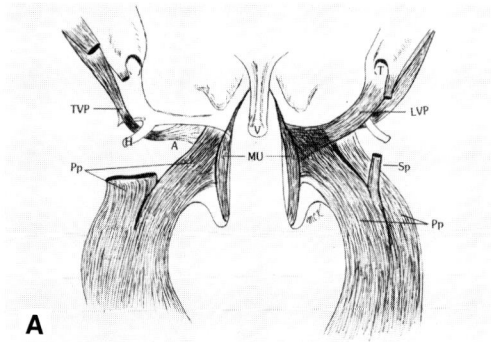

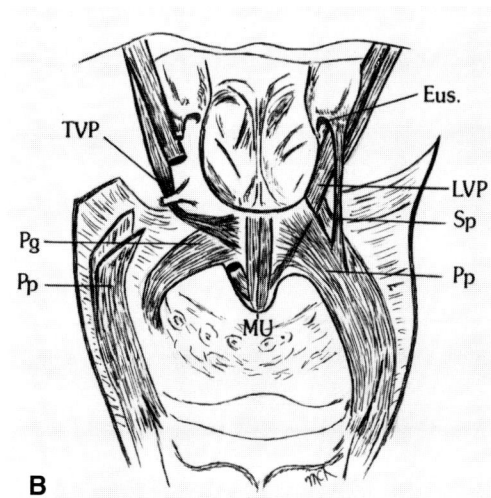

inserted confluently upon the hard palate and posterior nasal "hemi-spines" of either side.[9,10] This arrangement has deleterious implications for both normal speech and hearing.[11] The clefted velar anatomy, shown in Figure 23-7A, may be contrasted to the normal structure shown in Figure 23-7B.

Production of normal speech includes the important factor of velopharyngeal closure, or movement of the soft palate and posterior and lateral pharyngeal walls into apposition. This "velopharyngeal competency" provides that, during phonation of most consonants and some vowels, the major portion of exhaled air pressure is directed into the oropharynx and mouth by closure of the velopharyngeal portal[12,13] (Fig. 23-8). If closure is inadequate, leading to "velopharyngeal incompetency," the characteristic cleft palate

FIG. 23-7. (A) The structure of a bilateral cleft of the secondary palate, posterior view. Clockwise, one sees the vomer (V), eustachian tube opening (T), levator veli palatini (LVP), salpingopharyngeus (Sp), palatopharyngeus (Pp), musculus uvulae (MU), tensor aponeurosis (A), hamulus of pterygoid (H), and tensor veli palatine (TVP). (B) Normal muscular anatomy. (From: Rampp, D.L., Pannbacker, M., and Kinnebrew, M.C.: Velopharyngeal Incompetency—A Practical Guide for Evaluation and Management. Tulsa, Modern Education Corp., 1984)

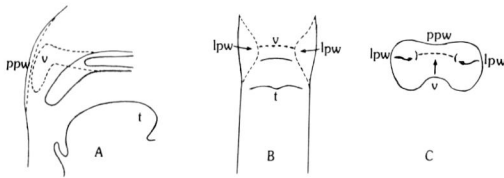

FIG. 23-8. *Velopharyngeal closure, seen from multiple views. (A) In lateral view broken lines depict elevation and flexion of the velum (V), with slight forward movement of the posterior pharyngeal wall. (B) Oral view shows velar lift and medial movement of the lateral pharyngeal walls (lpw). (C) Nasal view shows conjoint movement of all walls as the "large" portal closes competently to a slit. (From: Mason, R.M., and Grandstaff, H.: Evaluating the velopharyngeal mechanism in hypernasal speakers. Lang. Sp. Hear. Serv. Schools, 4:1, 1971)*

Effusion or "otitis media" follows, with the net result of commonly observed low frequency hearing loss.[18]

Figure 23-9 shows three situations of velar clefting, including a fully expressed cleft, a submucous cleft[19], and an occult submucous cleft.[20] The first two share a common muscular problem, as previously described. The occult submucous cleft, however, has only a portion of the muscular disorientation and is most properly termed a "microform," or minimally expressed cleft. All velar clefts have been associated with speech and audiologic problems, but these liabilities would expectedly be more prominent with the fully expressed defect. An individual with one of the submucous clefts may have little, if any, abnormality of speech or hearing. However, should recurrent middle ear infections lead to total removal of the adenoids, hypernasal (cleft palate) speech may result. The resultant speech defect is due to abrupt enlargement of the nasopharynx, in which the distance between the velum and posterior pharyngeal walls is increased by the removal of the adenoids. Without normal muscular contraction vectors, it is usually not possible for the velopharyngeal apparatus to adapt; therefore, normal speech is not regained as would be expected in the noncleft situation.[21]

Incidence and Prevalence

Clefts of the lip and palate occur with a rough frequency of 1 in every 800 live births, although considerable variation

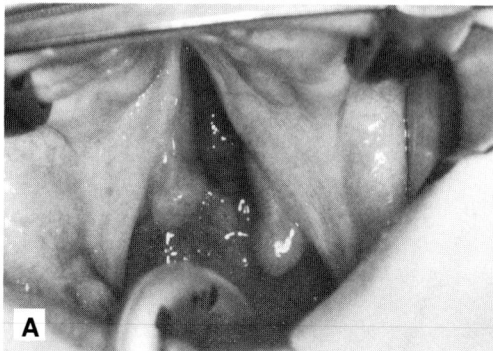

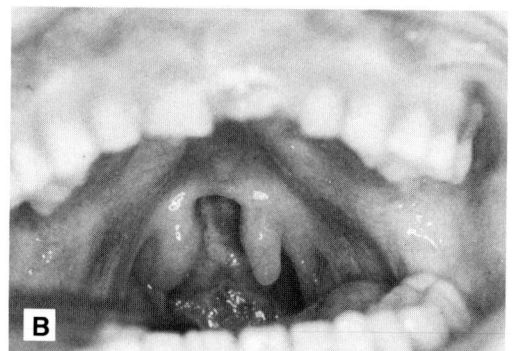

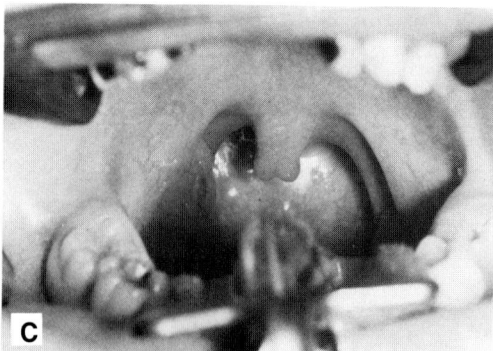

FIG. 23-9. *(A) An isolated cleft of the soft palate. (B) A submucous cleft palate, which features cleft anatomy with the exception of mucosal continuity. (C) The occult submucous cleft palate is seen with only minor physical markers of the preceding, fully expressed clefts. (From: Rampp, D.L., Pannbacker, M., and Kinnebrew, M.C.: Velopharyngeal Incompetency—A Practical Guide for Evaluation and Management. Tulsa, Modern Education Corp., 1984)*

exists in numerous studies from different populations. Cleft lip, with or without cleft palate, is more common in males, with a ratio of approximately 2:1 over females.[22] Cleft palate alone, however, is more common in females.

A slightly higher incidence occurs among Orientals and Caucasians, while incidence among blacks is somewhat lower. Multiple hypotheses, well supported and otherwise, ascribe cause and incidence to various sources; their number and bulk are well summarized in literature reviews.[23,24] For practical purposes, it is well to note that the incidence appears to be increasing in all groups. More importantly, irrespective of defined probability, the occurrence of any congenital anomaly impacts at 100 percent for the affected individual and family.

Whatever the active mechanisms, a genetic predisposition does appear to exist. A parent with a cleft lip may be told that a firstborn would have a 4 percent, or slightly greater than normal, chance of having a cleft. However, if the firstborn child has a cleft, the second child would face a 10 percent chance for orofacial clefting.[25]

Etiology

Most orofacial clefts are thought to follow a multifactorial mode of inheritance. This is to say that a genetic predisposition for clefting exists, but it is expressed only when other predisposing factors are present. For example, in the rapidly unfolding panorama of embryologic development, key nutrient provision or metabolic waste removal may not be adequate. This is the case with insufficient development of the placenta, or in maternal malnutrition. Teratogenic compounds ingested during the critical first trimester of pregnancy are also implicated. They include, among others, excessive or deficient concentrations of vitamin A, the administration of steroids, and alcohol.[26]

A number of named craniofacial syndromes may include cleft lip and palate.[27,28] This association hails back to the interrelated embryologic development of the face and brain, in which a sequence of induction and counterinduction between neural tissue, ectoderm, and mesoderm

takes place.[1] However, few syndromes are uniformly associated with clefting. Van der Woude's syndrome describes a variably penetrant, autosomally dominant condition that includes mucosal pits in the lower lip and complete or partial orofacial clefts (Fig. 23-10). Another, the Pierre Robin syndrome, includes mandibular micrognathia and a cleft of the secondary palate (Fig. 23-11).

Cleft palate development has been attributed to positional disturbances of the embryo during development of the face. For example, late unfolding of the cervical flexure during the "critical" period for fusion of the facial parts has been associated with isolated clefts of the secondary palate. The mandible is unable to migrate downward and forward because of its prolonged contact with the protruding "cardiac hump." The tongue, therefore, is maintained, by its association with the retruded mandible, within the space into which the

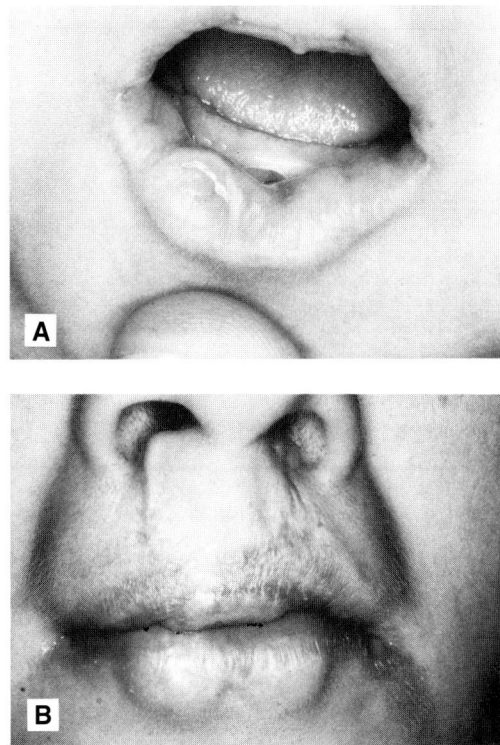

FIG. 23-10. (A) The lower lip pits of Van der Woude's syndrome, an autosomally dominant, genetic disorder that includes orofacial clefting. (B) Lower lip pits and repaired bilateral cleft lip in an older sibling.

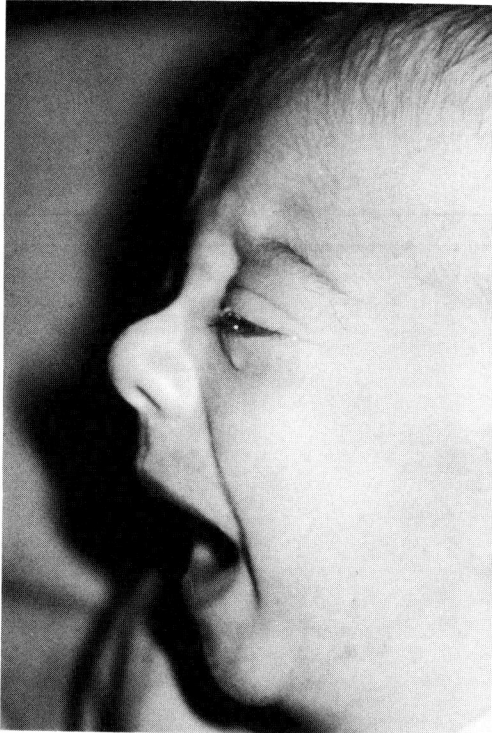

FIG. 23-11. *Pierre Robin Syndrome, which presents mandibular micrognathia, glossoptosis, and cleft palate. Note the facial convexity and mandibular retrusion in this crying patient.*

vertically oriented palatal shelves should rotate prior to fusion and completion of a continuous palate.[29] It has also been postulated that the embryonic processes can fuse and then separate to leave partial clefts, although this is poorly documented.[30] Incomplete fusion may also yield "microform" clefts, such as the occult submucous cleft palate.[31,32]

Classification

Classification of orofacial clefts is a simple matter that has been made painfully complex. Before continuing into the differing schemes of tabulation, let us say that most importantly one must succinctly and accurately express what he clinically observes.

Proceeding from anterior to posterior, the *lip* may be partially or completely clefted. The *palate* is divided into the *primary* and *secondary* palates. The *primary palate*, sometimes called the premaxillary segment, lies anterior to the incisive foramen

and normally gives rise to the four incisor teeth. The *secondary palate* includes all structures posterior to the incisive foramen, essentially the hard and soft palates.

As previously noted, clefts may include any or all of the fusion planes of the face. From these conditions arises the scheme of craniofacial clefting introduced by Tessier.[33] Focusing at the orofacial complex, clefts may be unilateral or bilateral, conditions that are identified simply by whether the clinician can see one or both sides of the nasal septum through the cleft. (Fig. 23-12).

A simple, graphic scheme of clefting, suggested independently by Kernahan, Elsahy, and Millard, is the "striped Y" diagram seen in Figure 23-13.[34,35,36] Historically, the classification of Veau,[4] that of Davis and Ritchie,[37] and that of the American Cleft Palate Association[38] deserve

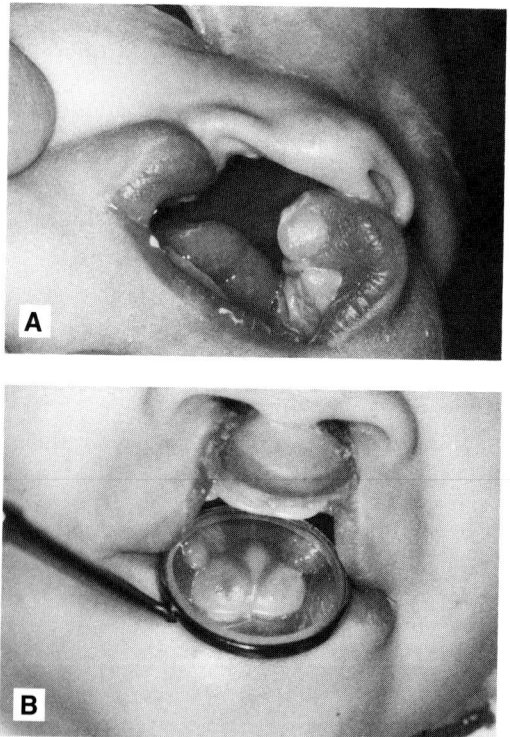

FIG. 23-12. *(A) Unilateral cleft, in which only one side of the nasal septum is visible. (B) Bilateral cleft of the primary palate. (From: Rampp, D.L., Pannbacker, M., and Kinnebrew, M.C.: Velopharyngeal Incompetency—A Practical Guide for Evaluation and Management. Tulsa, Modern Education Corp., 1984)*

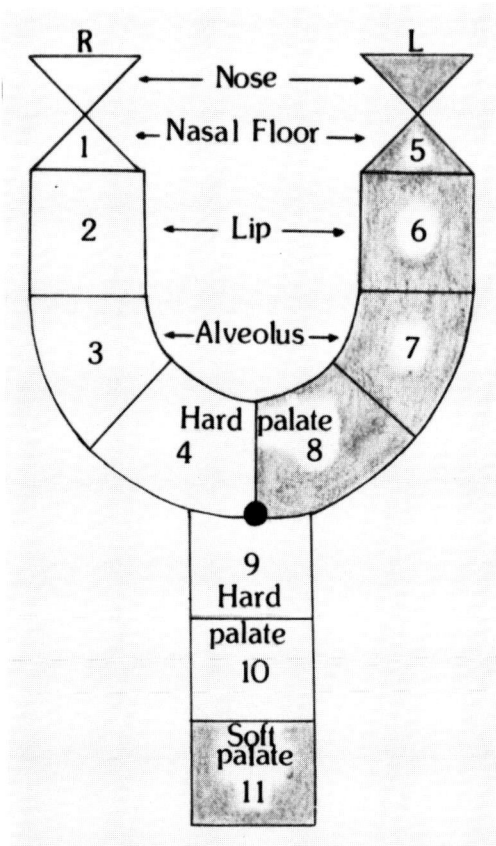

FIG. 23-13. *The "striped Y" scheme for cleft classification. Here, the darkened areas signify a unilateral cleft of the lip and primary palate, an intact "secondary" hard palate (behind the incisive foramen), and a velar cleft. (From: Rampp, D.L., Pannbacker, M., and Kinnebrew, M.C.: Velopharyngeal Incompetency—A Practical Guide for Evaluation and Management. Tulsa, Modern Education Corp., 1984)*

mention also, since they remain in common usage (Figs. 23-14 and 23-15).

To summarize, orofacial clefts may be complete or incomplete, unilateral or bilateral, "restricted" to the immediate region of the oral cavity, or miscellaneous. They may be blatantly obvious to the clinician, or subtle enough to escape the cursory clinical examination (Fig. 23-16). Additionally, different degrees of clefting may be present in the same patient as in an incomplete lip cleft with a partially or completely clefted secondary palate. The common orofacial clefts are listed in the following outline.

I. Complete—the cleft involves the lip, nasal floor, and primary and secondary palates

II. Incomplete
  A. Lip—partial lip clefting with the nasal floor variously intact—there may be a thick skin and vestigial muscular bridge or only a thin remnant of skin (Simonart's band)
  B. Palate
    1. primary—partial or complete alveolar clefts
    2. secondary—includes entire palate posterior to incisive foramen
      a. hard palate—rarely are clefts isolated here
      b. soft palate (velum)—complete or submucous
III. Unilateral
IV. Bilateral
V. Microform (lip, alveolus, palate)
VI. Miscellaneous facial clefts

Considerations in Treatment

The orofacial cleft presents a wide range of deformity. Its treatment raises some distinct needs and controversial issues. All revolve around the fact that normalcy must be restored in the growing child, and that multiple stages of treatment are required up to the endpoint, commonly the cessation of growth. Each stage may have its potential liabilities in further development, because of surgical scar and its deleterious effect on subsequent growth.[39,40] Potential psychologic scar to the patient's self-image,

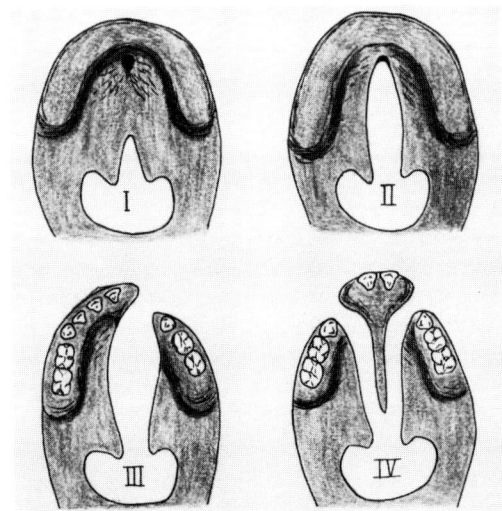

FIG. 23-14. *The Veau classification of clefting.*

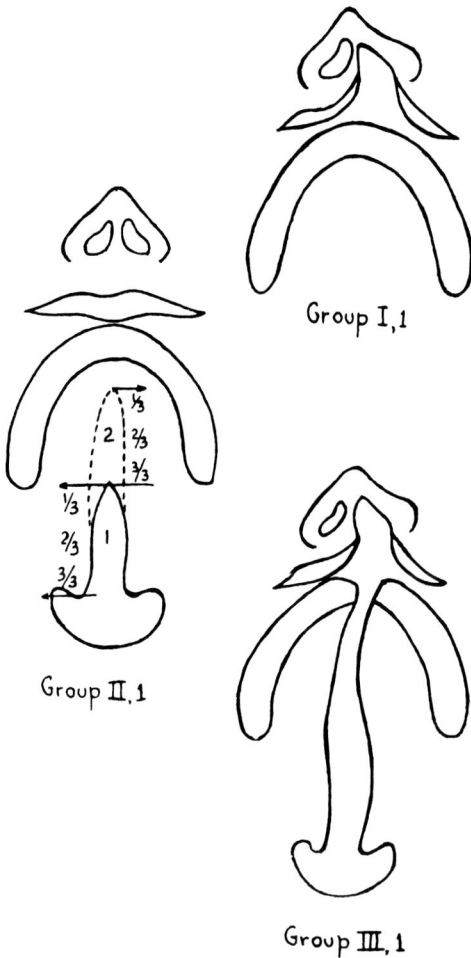

FIG. 23-15. *The classification of Davis and Ritchie.*

of the congenital anomaly in company with the individual characteristics that would have been expressed in the same, unaffected facial phenotype. However, some shared characteristics occur between differing cases, beyond generalities of anatomic classification. These similarities include the immediate needs posed by the birth of an affected infant, and the considerations of long-term treatment. Areas of consideration in the immediate treatment of a newborn with an orofacial cleft are discussed in the following paragraphs.

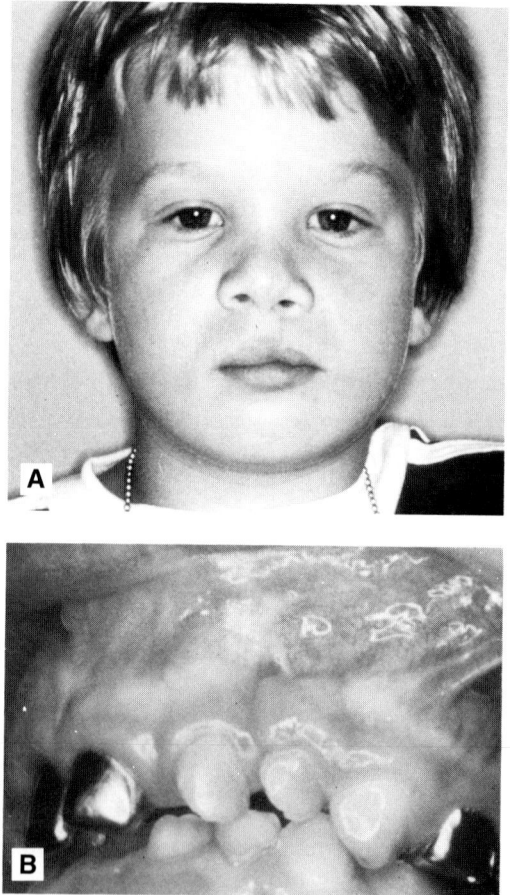

FIG. 23-16. *A "minimal" cleft lip or "congenital scar." (A) The vermilion is notched, lateral muscle bulging is present, and the alar base is depressed and lateralized, having "collapsed" into the underlying bony void. (B) The maxillary cleft is seen as a submucous declivity apical to the rotated lateral incisor. (From: Rampp, D.L., Pannbacker, M., and Kinnebrew, M.C.: Velopharyngeal Incompetency—A Practical Guide for Evaluation and Management. Tulsa, Modern Education Corp., 1984)*

caused by the deformity, and therefore decreased ability to cope with life's problems, may be a collateral problem. Herein lies the controversy. One would like to habilitate these individuals as early as possible in infancy, primarily to facilitate speech and hearing. However, by so doing one may significantly inhibit growth of the facial skeleton. Furthermore, lasting results may be elusory in the context of childhood and adolescent growth. This dilemma may be solved by compromise—a necessary prerequisite for those who wish to manage orofacial clefts.

Beyond flexibility, willingness to analyze individual problems and develop a "customized" treatment plan for each case is necessary because virtually all clefts are unique. They present the salient features

Airway

It is rarely necessary to resort to invasive means for airway provision. Appropriate positioning of the infant in the lateral or face-down posture usually is sufficient—not unlike during routine newborn care. When the situation is compounded by a small mandible and glossoptosis, however, upper airway obstruction of varying degree may indicate oxygen supplementation by a "hood," placement of a nasogastric tube to splint the tongue forward and out of contact with the pharyngeal walls,[41] sutures in the tongue for protraction, or a surgical procedure that sutures the tongue tip to the mandibular vestibule anteriorly.[42] With refractory airway obstruction, tracheostomy is another alternative.

Nutrition

An imaginative approach that obturates the open cleft has largely negated problems of nourishing the infant. Fabricated of acrylic upon casts of the cleft maxilla, these appliances also capably serve as orthopedic prostheses for guiding the growth and position of the segments, as will be discussed later. Before their use became widespread, a host of difficult nutritional schemes were used, including feedings through a nasogastric tube (gastric gavage), a host of specially prepared nipples, and alimentation through a surgically created gastric opening (gastrostomy).

Parental Attitudes

The importance of adequate counseling of the parents cannot be overemphasized. It is traumatic to have a pregnancy culminate with the birth of a deformed child, and in their confusion, anger, and often guilt, parents may embark on an ill-advised course of "emergency" surgical procedures to eradicate the problem. This approach holds only temporary solutions, however, and often introduces major compromise for the optimal habilitation of the child. Parents must be informed that (1) the ultimate habilitation of their child is commonly not completed until growth has ceased; (2) a rational approach to sequential therapy is the best course toward the best result; (3) beyond surgical intervention staged to his specific needs, the child needs little in the first 3 to 4 years other than nutrition, love, discipline, and emotional support.

Speech and Hearing

The bulk of current thinking about speech and hearing favors closure of the cleft as early as possible to facilitate normal speech acquisition.[43] However, speech production is not entirely a static phenomenon, and difficulties may arise if "heroic" reconstructive surgery is needed later to overcome any growth disturbances which premature invasive treatment introduces. This is to say that what has been gained for speech may in turn be lost, only to be regained by even greater surgical "heroism." This is further discussed later under "Secondary Procedures." With regard to hearing, it is not uncommon for ventilation tubes to be placed in the tympanic membranes to equilibrate middle ear and atmospheric pressures, and to remove thickened, "glue-like" secretions from the middle ear.[44] As previously noted, however, significant assistance to these interrelated, communicative faculties likely comes from anatomic reconstruction of the palatal muscles.

Growth Disturbance

At birth the cleft deformity is already 6 or 7 months old; a widespread, absolute, and relative tissue deficiency is further compounded by displacement of tissues; for example, a retruded maxilla on the clefted side. Considerable "catch-up" potential may be realized, however, if growth is not hampered by the scar of early surgery but instead is "directed" by orthopedic means.[45]

General Patient Tolerance

All needs of the infant considered, it is generally accepted that, if early repair is elected, the "rule of 10's" should be observed in staging in order to optimize conditions for the desired surgical result.[46] This rule states that the infant must be 10 weeks old, weigh 10 lbs., and register 10 g of hemoglobin per deciliter of whole blood. This interval has usually allowed the baby to overcome the early growth lag commonly seen in the cleft population.

"What's best for the child" is the best approach; consequently, support of an individualized, team-oriented treatment plan toward the discrete needs of the developing, future member of society should prevail. There are roughly equivalent landmarks regarding speech and growth. However, one needs to define these at the outset with the common goal of maximizing both. To that end, the following goals seem appropriate.

1. Achieve normal communicative faculties by school age.
2. Provide as near-normal appearance as possible from the sixth month on.
3. Commit no errors in early treatment that would seriously compromise the results at subsequent treatment stages, and at completion of growth.

Accordingly, a management scheme (such as that propounded by the cleft palate team at the University fo Zurich) holds attractive potential, especially if it is modified to the individual situation.[47] Following that lead, our present management philosophy is detailed below.

I. Birth to 6 months—maxillary orthopedics

A growth-guiding "orthopedic" obturator is fabricated and delivered in the first days of life. It also serves nutritive needs; the child is easily fed with a conventional nipple and a compressible bottle. The plate is adjusted selectively at intervals and refabricated as growth dictates. During the first 6 months of life, the segments of the

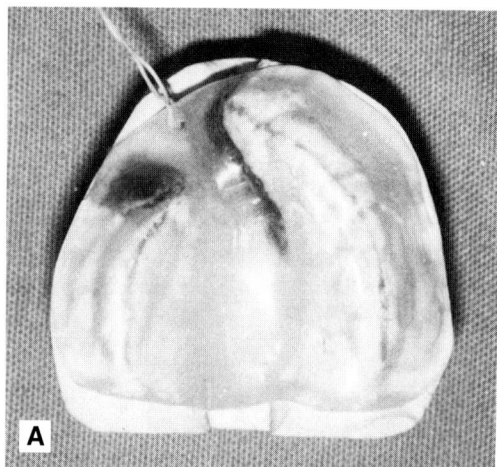

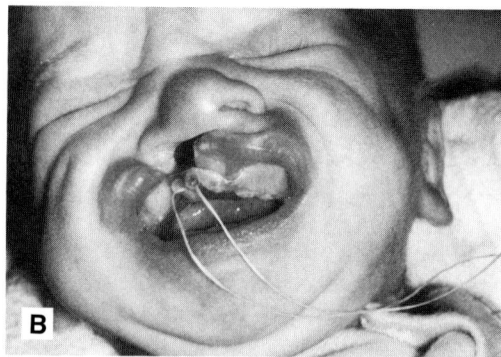

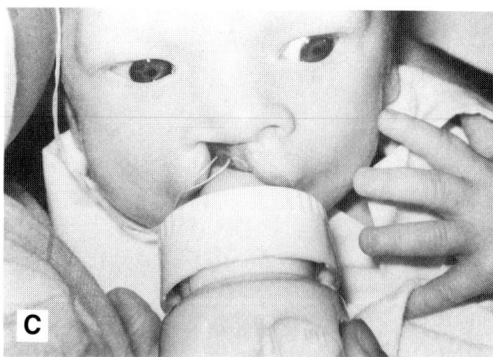

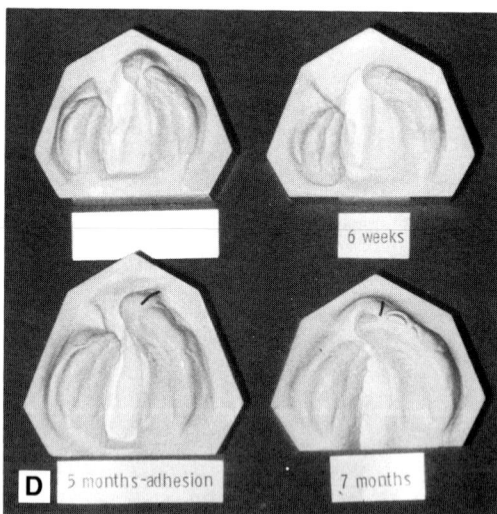

FIG. 23-17. *(A) The acrylic obturator, hollow ground in selected (darkened) areas to "direct" facial growth and align the maxillary segments. (B) Obturator in place. (C) Infant feeding with obturator, standard nipple, and compressible bottle. (D) Serial casts showing above and lower left, gradual control of maxillary segments. Lower right, after lip adhesion. (From: Rampp, D.L., Pannbacker, M., and Kinnebrew, M.C.: Velopharyngeal Incompetency—A Practical Guide for Evaluation and Management. Tulsa, Modern Education Corp., 1984)*

cleft maxilla grow anteriorly and are guided into proper alignment for a tension-free lip repair (Fig. 23-17).

II. 6 months of age—lip repair

At this age the child is beginning to formulate early speech, specifically the bilabial sounds *m* and *n*. For the first time, he *needs* a complete lip.

III. 6 to 12 months—soft palate repair

At the stage of babbling speech development, the soft palate is repaired. The closure features palatal lengthening and muscular union without violation of either the maxillary periosteum or its blood supply via the greater palatine arteries. The anterior palatal cleft is left open, but closes somewhat by spontaneous growth of the palatal shelves (Figs. 23-18 and 23-19). Importantly, no raw bony surfaces, and consequently minimal scar, are left to thwart subsequent maxillary growth.

IV. 12 months to 5 to 6 years—further obturation
V. 5 to 6 years—hard palate closure

Coinciding with eruption of the first permanent molars, the maxilla has attained approximately 80 percent of its ultimate transverse width.[48] At that time, closure of the remaining oral-nasal fistula, usually reduced to a mere slit, can be expeditiously achieved without much scar or threat to facial growth.

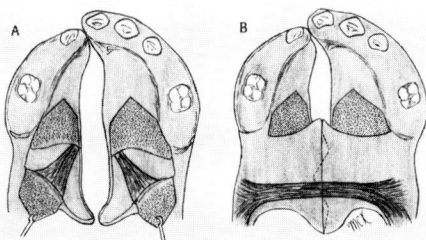

FIG. 23-19. *A residual anterior palatal oronasal communication after veloplasty and some spontaneous palatal closure (cleft of secondary palate).*

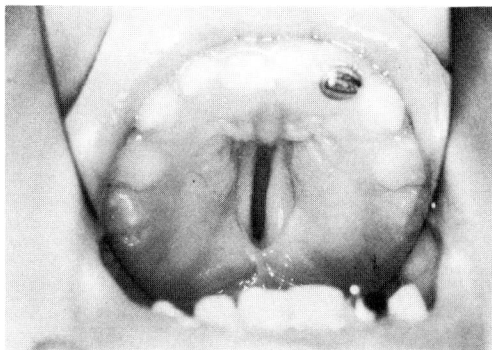

FIG. 23-18. *Two-staged palatal closure with initial veloplasty (A and B) which features lengthening, muscular dissection and "push-back," and minimal scarring. (Adapted from Perko, M.: Two-stage closure of cleft palate. J. Maxillofac. Surg., 7:76, 1979)*

The long-term benefits of this approach for facial growth, speech acquisition, and hearing are currently under considerable scrutiny. On the one hand, advocates for craniofacial growth have shown impressive results with later surgery and untrammeled growth which is "directed" by maxillary orthopedics.[49] From the opposite view, advocates for early surgery voice equal arguments that speech acquisition is better served with early complete closure, "before the first word."[50] Perhaps the best outcome from this debate is that of mutual awareness, such that future improvement will be sought through modification of the present techniques toward even greater support of the mutual goals. For the moment, it is appropriate to repeat that each case must be analyzed for its unique characteristics, and the optimal treatment must be derived with all components and individual needs firmly in mind. Individual treatment can then proceed by a variety of techniques, discussed in the following section.

Techniques for Repair

For simplicity, habilitative surgery for orofacial clefts may be divided into *primary procedures*, performed in the infant years, and *secondary procedures*, performed in childhood, adolescence, and occasionally in the adult years. The principles and the techniques are interchangeable between the two categories. In chronologic order, the *primary procedures* are discussed first, focusing upon lip and palatal repairs.

The *secondary procedures*, including palatal lengthening and pharyngoplasty for speech purposes, alveolar cleft grafts, surgical-orthodontic or orthognathic procedures upon the maxillofacial skeleton, and nose and lip revision, are then addressed.

Primary Procedures

LIP REPAIR (CHEILOPLASTY)

As might be expected, current approaches to primary lip repair represent a compendium of techniques. For in-depth coverage of the development of the procedures, the reader is referred to the writings of Still and Georgiade[51] or Millard.[36] For our purposes the more common, currently used repairs are discussed. They include the "Triangular,"[52] the "Quadrangular,"[53,54] and the "Rotation-Advancement" repairs.[55]

Triangular Repair. The major advantage of this repair is that a vertically short, "minor" side, lip segment can be lengthened to match the longer "major" side. Utilizing key landmarks such as the vertical length from the columellar base to the height of the cupid's bow on the major (noncleft) side, the lip is then marked and incised, and ultimately closed as shown in Figure 23-20A. Another advantage is capture of a normal-appearing cupid's bows and tubercle. Disadvantages include the placement of scars outside of the normal philtral ridge and a tendency for vertical height discrepancies that ensue as the minor side grows "longer" than its counterpart, which is thought to be in response to unbalanced muscle pull (Fig. 23-20B).[56]

Quadrangular Repair. Somewhat more complex in design, this repair (Fig. 23-21) seeks once again to establish equality of length and habilitation of the intrinsic lip components. While serving those goals, it also falls prey to unnatural scar lines and growth discrepancies.

Rotation-Advancement Repair. The popular use of this procedure testifies to its versatility and substantial reliability toward good results. Its advantages are that the incision lines ultimately place the cutaneous and mucosal scars in natural skin lines and that balanced reorientation of the labial muscular components is facilitated (Fig. 23-22). As mentioned above, some

surgeons avoid this technique, using a triangular design instead, when the minor, or "clefted," side is deemed to be vertically short. They argue that in such situations the rotation-advancement leads to excessive "notching" of the vermilion surface and mucocutaneous ridge. Indeed, this is a problem and represents the only real drawback to the rotation-advancement; the retraction is due primarily to scar contracture that would occur along any linear surface (here the philtral ridge). This is, however, an oversimplification. It fails to consider the effect of tension in the repaired lip which transpires as the mobilized lip portions scar back down to the

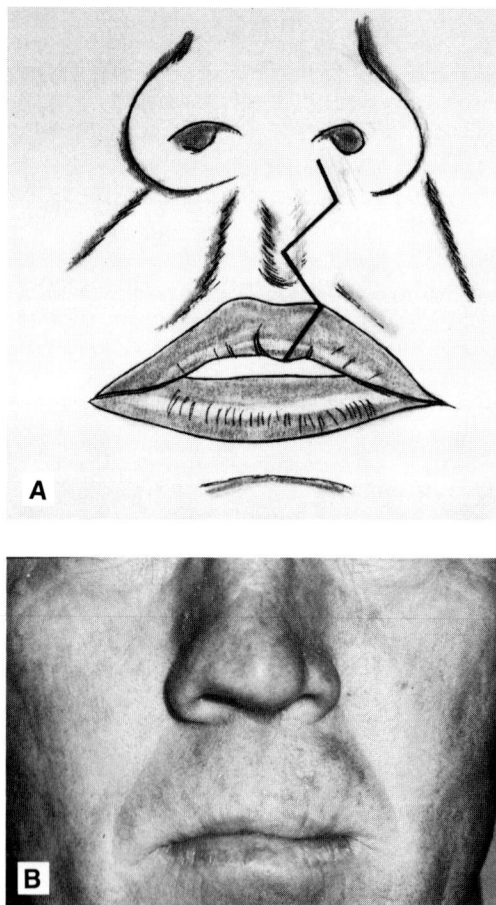

FIG. 23-20. *(A) Triangular repair. (B) Vertical height discrepancy as the lip (cleft) segment "outgrows" the medial, "major" portion. (Adapted from Tennison, C.W.: The repair of the unilateral cleft lip by stencil method. Plast. Reconstr. Surg., 9:118, 1952)*

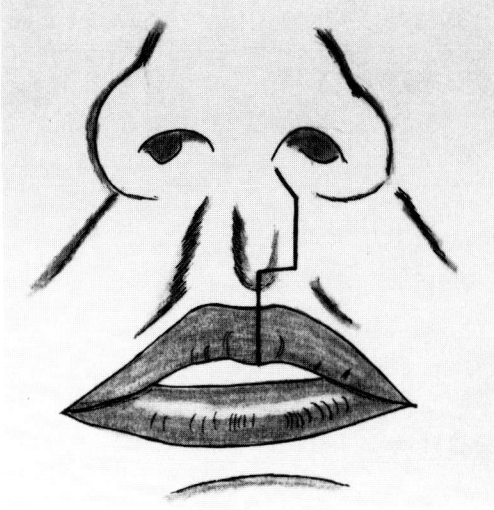

FIG. 23-21. *The quadrangular repair. (Adapted from Thomson, H.G.: Quadrilateral flap in the repair of unilateral cleft lip. In Cleft Lip and Palate: Surgical, Dental, and Speech Aspects. Edited by W.C. Grabb, S.W. Rosenstein, and K.Z. Bzoch. Boston, Little Brown, 1971)*

still-distracted bony maxillary segments and collapse into the underlying alveolar cleft (Fig. 23-23).

The skeletal and soft tissue discrepancies can be overcome by way of facilitating the best repair. These maneuvers include the previously discussed maxillary orthopedic alignment, and a simple, preliminary procedure known as the *lip adhesion*[57] (Fig. 23-24): The adhesion is performed at approximately 3 months, and tends to align the lip and maxillary segments by narrowing the cleft and to stimulate growth of the lip segments so that more tissue becomes available for the later, formal repair. Further, the rotation-advancement technique, even if notching develops, lends itself much more readily for secondary revision than the other approaches.

By way of summarizing the primary cheiloplastic techniques, it is wise to underscore this salient fact: *"Each individual patient demands an individualized approach if the best result is to be obtained."* Close scrutiny and planning indicate that elements of differing techniques can best suit the given task; for example, the so-called "triangular flap" technique that combines portions of the rotation-advancement and the triangu-

lar repair,[58] or the "wave-line" repair.[59] In passing, a second important axiom should be observed: *"Never assume that the goal of the moment is isolated; the final result will be realized only when growth is completed."*

The axioms of individualized treatment, in continuum, are also appropriate to the situation of the *bilateral cleft lip.* In dealing with the extremes of deformity that these present, and in view of the limitations that restricted blood supply imposes upon surgical intervention,[60] a number of named techniques have been devised. Among others, the Veau,[61] LeMesurier,[62] and Millard [63]designs remain in use. Each seeks to gain form, a task made difficult by the tissue deficiencies these clefts present. One problem is the diminutive mass of the nasal base (the columella), and the labial philtrum. The philtrum should have conspired with the lateral lip segments to form a mid lip portion and columella of "normal" length, as well as a labial sulcus. One repair, the LeMesurier, essentially devotes the prolabium to the columella to augment columellar length, relying upon transfer of lateral lip mass into the philtral area to complete the lip. Other repairs (Veau, Millard) retain the prolabium primarily in the philtral region, relying upon subsequent surgery to lengthen the columella.[64] All repairs face

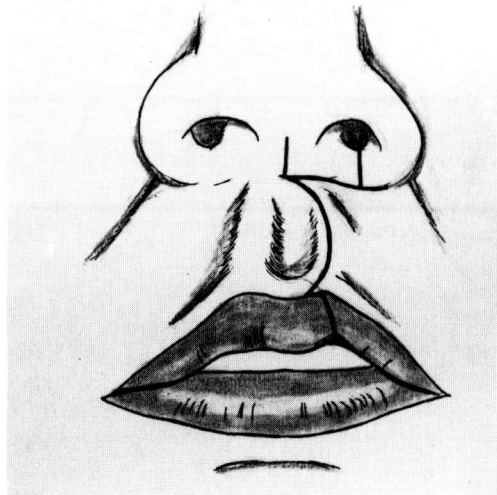

FIG. 23-22. *The rotation-advancement repair. (Adapted from Millard, D.R., Jr.: Extensions of rotation-advancement principle for wide unilateral cleft lip. Plast. Reconstr. Surg., 42:535, 1968)*

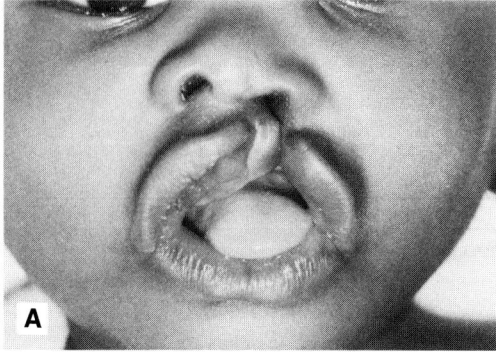

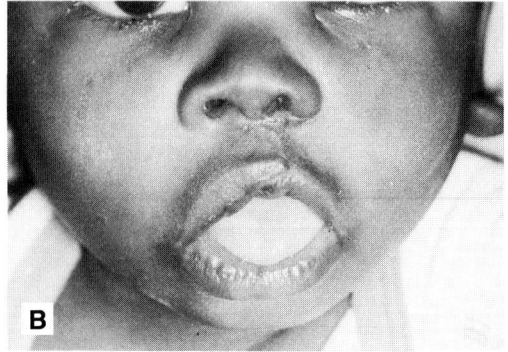

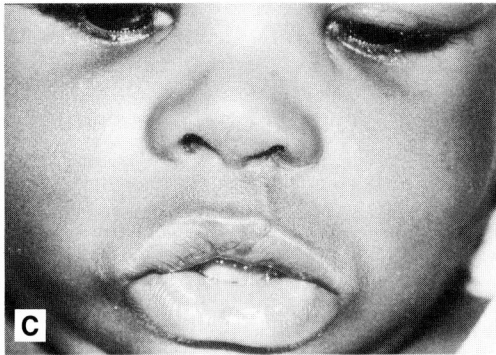

FIG. 23-23. *Illustrating relapse of lip repairs as soft tissues reattach to deficient underlying bony support. (A) Preoperative. (B) 3 months following rhinocheiloplasty by rotation-advancement technique. (C) 6 months postoperatively—note lateral migration of commissure and alar base.*

the challenge of establishing muscular continuity across the prolabium. This balanced muscle force achieves normal animation and is also necessary for a stable result; if the muscles are not joined, the prolabium is promptly widened and distorted by the action of isolated muscles pulling upon skin.

Figure 23-25 illustrates a bilateral cleft at presentation, its design for repair, and the results at 6 months. Further discussion of bilateral clefts appears under "Secondary Procedures."

PALATAL SURGERY

The differing philosophies of early, "one-stage" palatal closure versus delayed "two-stage" closure notwithstanding, the techniques for total and limited (velar) closure are now discussed. Since a foremost point in palatal surgery is proper reorientation of the musculature, this facet is discussed first in the context of soft palate repair, or "veloplasty."

Veloplasty (Staphylorraphy). Proper management of the palatal muscles is, again, thought to facilitate palatal growth, speech, and middle ear aeration. Let us

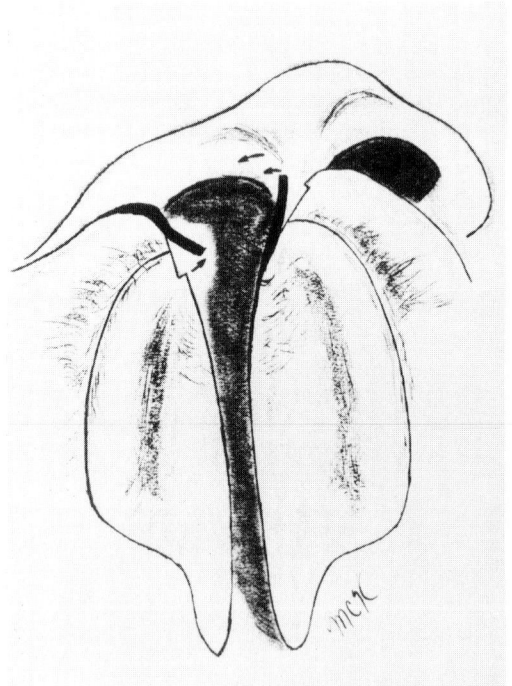

FIG. 23-24. *The lip adhesion, which achieves subtotal lip continuity to align bony segments prior to formal lip repair. (From: Rampp, D.L., Pannbacker, M., and Kinnebrew, M.C.: Velopharyngeal Incompetency—A Practical Guide for Evaluation and Management. Tulsa, Modern Education Corp., 1984)*

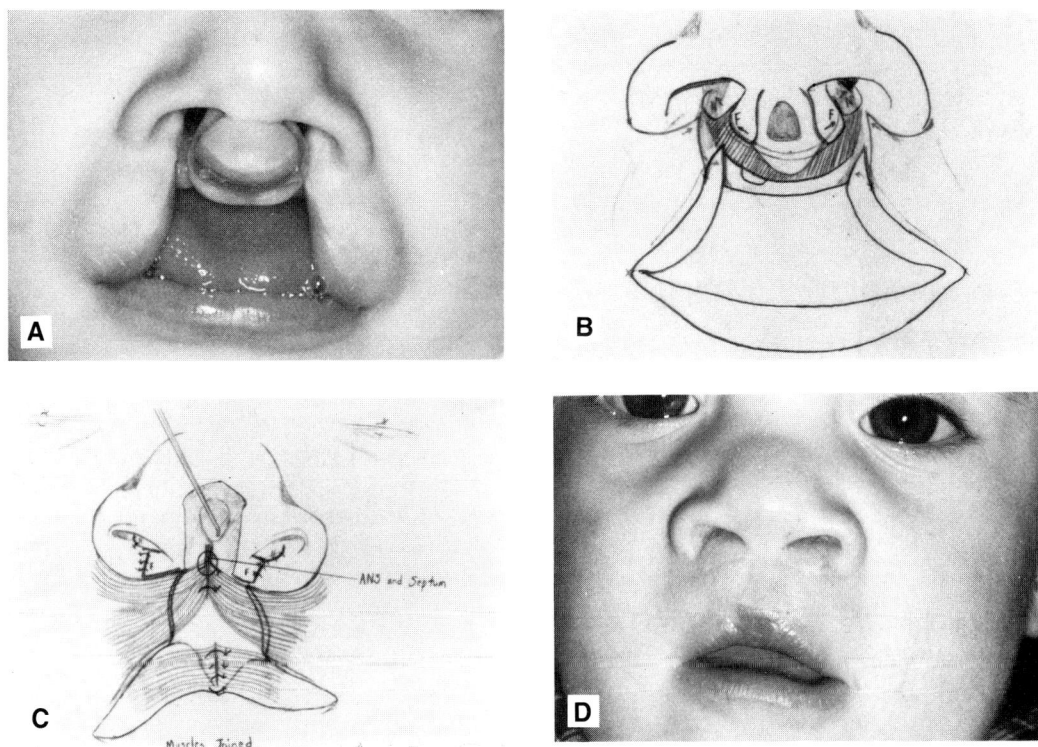

Fig. 23-25. *Bilateral cleft lip repair. (A) The previously seen bilateral cleft of the lip and primary palate; a lip adhesion was initially performed. (B) The reparative design. (C) Flaps "N" and "F" rotated into nasal floors and nostril sills, respectively, and muscular components joined. (D) Results at 6 months.*

consider the "Perko" veloplasty as a spring-board.[65] This technique differs from others in that the levator muscle group is specifically repositioned and joined posteriorly in the velum. This is in contrast to "edge-to-edge" closures, which leave the cleft muscle confluence attached to the hard palate (leaving a "submucous cleft" pattern). Lengthening is achieved by sliding split-thickness hard-palatal flaps posteriorly and by performing a "Z-plasty" on the nasal mucosa. The hard-palatal flaps split the glandular zone, leaving the periosteum and neurovascular bundle intact, deep to the dissection plane, and preserving epithelial remnants for rapid epithelial repopulation of the denuded area. The schema for this procedure is shown in Figure 23-18.

Even though long-term evaluation awaits the test of time, this approach is considered a laudable step in the right direction. However, this author's results raise the question that possibly more might be done with the muscles. If one considers the

normal muscular pattern, it seems reasonable that establishment of a palatopharyngeal ring would be appropriate, as would discrete reorientation of the levator and tensor veli palatini muscles across the midline. This has been done in a number of cases; when limited dissection of the contents of the palatopharyngeal muscle fold and sharp, transverse division of the nasal mucosa at the posterior border of the hard palate is performed. The "palatopharyngeus" muscles are then joined at the base of the uvula, somewhat more posteriorly than before, while the levator and tensor muscles are joined more anteriorly (Fig. 23-26).[66] The raw, triangular surface, formed on the nasal side with lengthening of the soft palate, is covered by a free graft of buccal mucosa to thwart scar contracture that otherwise would lead to loss of lengthening and also palatal motility.[67]

The resultant force vectors from this muscular placement yield a distinct "crease" of the uvular base, which indicates

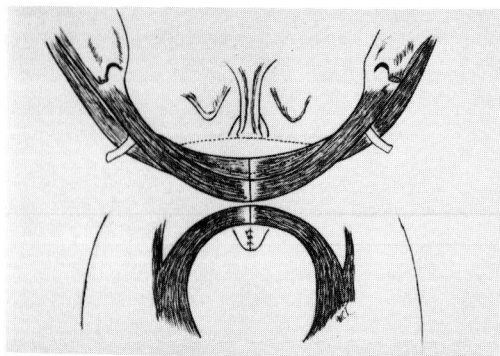

FIG. 23-26. *The muscular reorientation suggested for a more "functional" veloplasty. The palatopharyngeal ring is reconstituted at the base of the uvula, while the levator and tensor muscles are anastomosed more anteriorly. (From: Kinnebrew, M.C., et al.: The residual submucous cleft: A cause of persistent speech and hearing problems. Lang. Sp. Hear. Serv. Schools, 17:16, 1986)*

palatine canal, freeing its enclosed neurovascular bundle to allow velar lengthening. Once again it seems that it is possible to achieve the same goal with less surgical damage. Palatal closure and lengthening may be achieved by combining simple turnover flaps into the nasal floor with placement of a buccal mucosal graft on the oral surface, simultaneous to the veloplasty described previously.

For practical purposes, the discussion on primary procedures is completed. However, other procedures have been used historically in infancy, including pharyngeal flaps and alveolar cleft grafts. Both are discussed in terms of "secondary" procedures, in which they are more commonly used. The rationale for their use is evident, because the physiologic functions they serve in the secondary phase also apply in the primary phase.

up-and-back palatal pull (Fig. 23-27). This is in contradistinction to the mid-velar lift pattern of the more-limited muscular retrodisplacement. This palatal activity is believed advantageous for palatal growth and middle ear aeration.

Closure of the Secondary Palate (Uranoplasty). These approaches commonly involve full-thickness elevation of mucoperiosteal flaps from the hard palate, which are then transposed to the midline and posteriorly to provide oral closure. The nasal mucosal surface is obtained by turnover flaps hinged from the cleft margins. Figures 23-28 and 23-29 illustrate the Von Langenbeck[68] and Wardill-Kilner[69,70] approaches, respectively. The advantage of these procedures is that they can effect total functional closure of the cleft; the anatomic partitioning of oral and nasal cavities then segregates fluids within either passage and allows the impoundment of oral breath pressure for speaking. The disadvantages, most important to the small child, are that lifting the periosteum induces scar to an important bone-forming membrane and that transposition of the flaps leaves a raw bony defect in their wake. Healing by third-intention, with its obligatory heavy, nondistensible scar, leads to significant collapse of the maxilla. Further, these procedures often require fracturing of the posterior wall of the greater

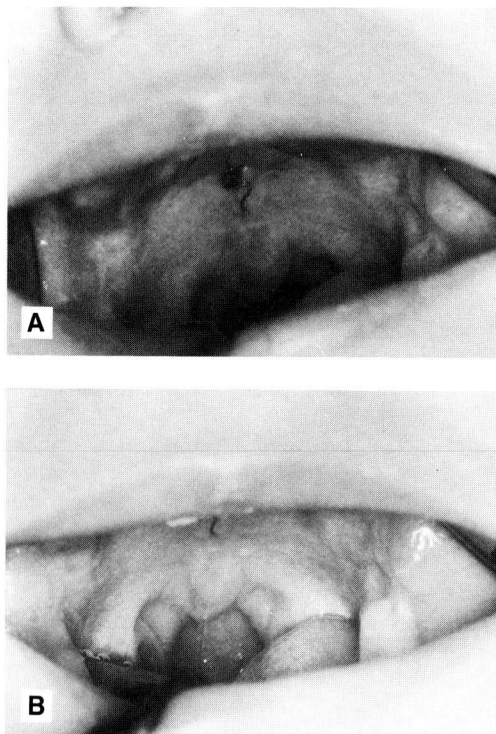

FIG. 23-27. *Palatal movement after the muscular dissection shown in Figure 23-26. (A) Repose (14 days postoperatively). (B) Elevation with subuvular crease and marked medial movement of lateral pharyngeal walls.*

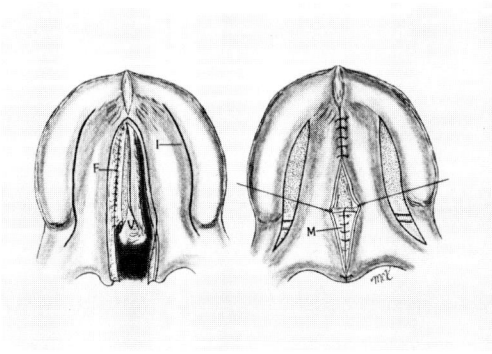

FIG. 23-28. *The Von Langenbeck palatal closure.*

Secondary Procedures

SECONDARY PALATAL AND
PHARYNGEAL REVISION FOR SPEECH
IMPROVEMENT
(PALATOPHARYNGOPLASTY)

A number of the best-laid plans for palatal management result in inadequate velopharyngeal closure. Consequently, it is often necessary to revise the velopharyngeal portal for more effective valving of expired air pressure. As stated by Morley,[71] the procedures fall roughly into two categories, those that *lengthen a short palate* or those that *provide baffles for or constrict the pharynx (or both)*. Even though we are speaking at this point of the preschool and

childhood years, these procedures may become necessary at any age as the velopharyngeal area increases in size. This may be a function of facial growth and involution of the adenoid tissues,[72] or it may follow maxillary advancement[73] or nasal revision.[74] This comprises another broad subject that can only be summarized here. For more in-depth discussion, the reader is referred to several published volumes on this specific subject.[14,71,74]

PALATAL LENGTHENING PROCEDURES

The Wardill-Kilner procedure, previously illustrated in Figure 23-29 under hard palate procedures, is merely a variant of the V-Y "pushback" attributed to Veau[4] (Fig. 23-30). Essentially full-thickness mucoperiosteal flaps are raised from the hard palate and displaced posteriorly, along with the soft palate, to decrease the size of the velopharyngeal portal. In that regard, these approaches are not unlike that described by Dorrance[75] (Fig. 23-31). As can be seen by the illustrations, these maneuvers should theoretically be sufficient. In practice, however, it is commonly necessary to provide lift to the palate as well, by adjustment of the intrinsic muscular vectors, by prosthetic means, or by suspension with a flap from the pharyngeal wall.[76] Additionally, it may be elected to augment or constrict the pharynx at a discrete level

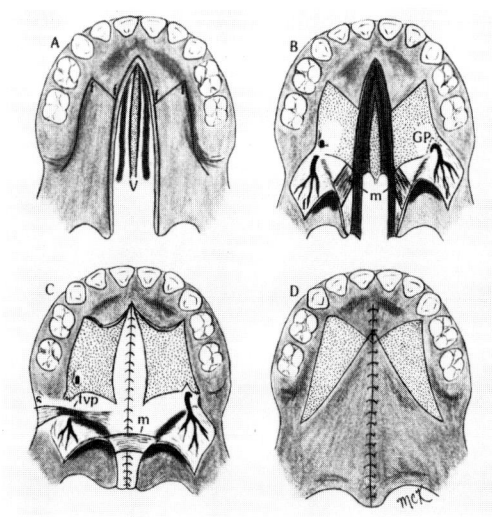

FIG. 23-29. *The Wardill-Kilner "four-flap" uranoplasty.*

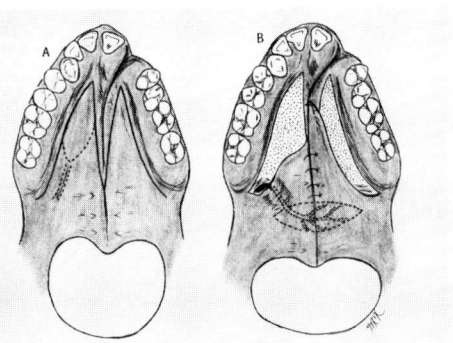

FIG. 23-30. *The "V-Y" palatal push-back. In the secondary repair shown here a mucoperiosteal island flap is mobilized on the greater palatine neurovascular bundle and turned onto the lengthened nasal surface of the velum. (From: Rampp, D.L., Pannbacker, M., and Kinnebrew, M.C.: Velopharyngeal Incompetency—A Practical Guide for Evaluation and Management. Tulsa, Modern Education Corp., 1984)*

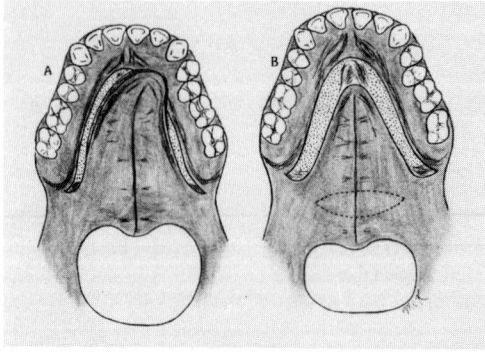

FIG. 23-31. *The Dorrance palatal pushback. The raw nasal surface is not covered (dotted ellipse) and poses a shortening predisposition through scarring. (Adapted from Dorrance, G.M.: Lengthening the soft palate in cleft palate operations. Ann. Surg., 82:208, 1965)*

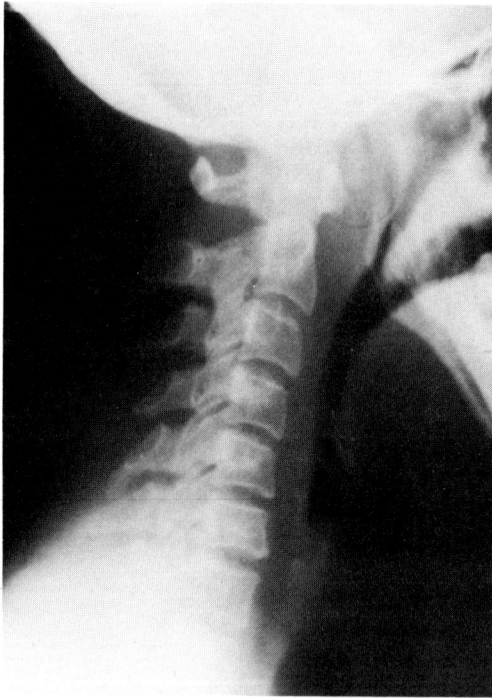

with the velum. This may be achieved by implants in the posterior pharyngeal wall,[77] or by transposition of the salpingopharyngeus muscles[78] or the palatopharyngeal folds and their overlying mucosa, respectively[79,80] (Figs. 23-32 through 23-34).

The *pharyngeal flaps* are used primarily as baffles or curtains that add to the air-diverting capability of the incompetent portal. As illustrated in Figure 23-35, they include the superiorly[81] or inferiorly based[82] pharyngeal flap. The superiorly based flap is more widely used because it lies at the more appropriate plane for velopharyngeal valving, even though it is technically more difficult. Both have potential strengths and weaknesses,[83] including inadequate valving, excessive closure that yields hyponasal vocal resonance along with compromised nasal respiration, and interference with facial growth.[84,85]

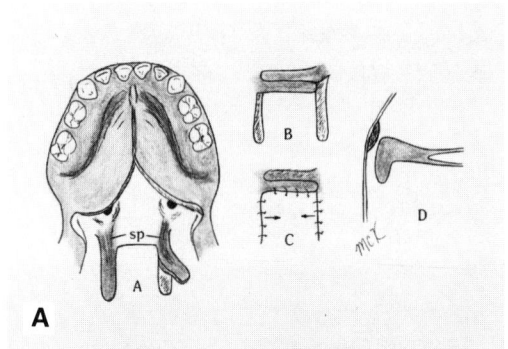

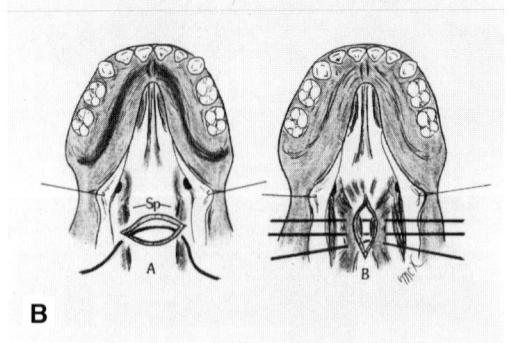

FIG. 23-32. *Augmentation of the posterior pharyngeal wall. A Proplast (Vitek Corp.) implant has been placed upon the prevertebral fascia at the level of velopharyngeal closure (circled). (From: Rampp, D.L., Pannbacker, M., and Kinnebrew, M.C.: Velopharyngeal Incompetency—A Practical Guide for Evaluation and Management. Tulsa, Modern Education Corp., 1984)*

FIG. 23-33. *Two modes of palatopharyngeal revision by manipulation of the salpingopharyngeus muscles. (A) Hyne's, (B) Wardill's pharyngoplasty.*

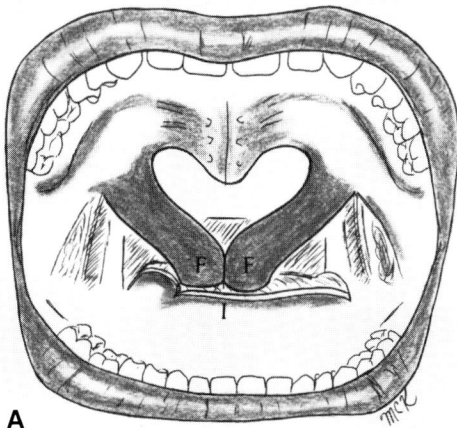

A

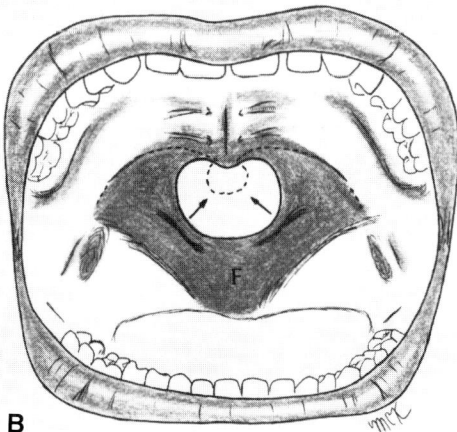

B

FIG. 23-34. *(A) Transposition of innervated palatopharyngeus muscles (the posterior tonsillar folds) onto the posterior pharyngeal wall by the orticochea procedure. (B) With healing, the resultant sphincter activity can then close the portal upon demand. (Adapted from Orticochea, M.: Construction of a dynamic muscle sphincter in cleft palates. Plast. Reconstr. Surg., 41:323, 1966)*

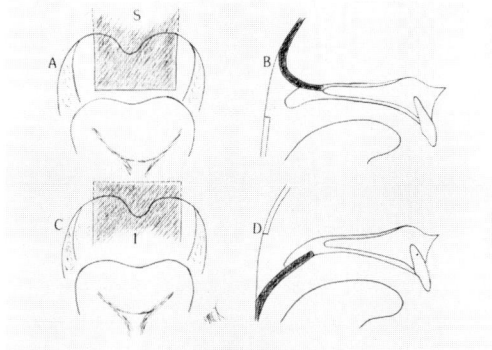

FIG. 23-35. *Composite of superiorly (above) and inferiorly (below) based pharyngeal flaps. (From: Rampp, D.L., Pannbacker, M., and Kinnebrew, M.C.: Velopharyngeal Incompetency—A Practical Guide for Evaluation and Management. Tulsa, Modern Education Corp., 1984)*

ALVEOLAR CLEFT GRAFTS

The goals of alveolar cleft grafting include provision of a continuous maxillary arch for orthodontic detailing of the permanent dentition, support for the overlying lip and nasal alar base,[86] and the closure of remaining fistulae between the oral and nasal cavities. In the past, the placement of bone grafts (of autogenous rib) at the time of primary lip repairs was widely practiced, and its modifications are convincingly advocated in some centers as a viable accompaniment to orthopedic alignment of the maxillary segments.[87] The practice has become controversial, however, because of reports of severe maxillary deformity developing in a number of patients so treated.[88] Other techniques of repair include the translocation of mucoperiosteal flaps from the neighboring maxilla,[89] closure and ablation with alloplasts,[90] or free transplantation of periosteum[91] to induce new bone formation in the cleft. For the most part, however, most techniques feature ablation of the bony defect with autogenous bone from the iliac crest, from the skull or rib, or with "banked" cadaveric bone.[92-94]

Grafting may be done in the late deciduous or mixed dentition stage (4 to 6 years) as a convenient additive to hard palate closure and "stabilization" of early orthopedic expansion of the maxilla, or it may be delayed. Not uncommonly, the behavior of the permanent dentition, specifically the cuspid tooth, dictates the age at which the graft is performed, assuming that further delay until the time of orthognathic maxillary surgery is not elected.

Figure 23-36A depicts the panographic appearance of an alveolar cleft at the mixed dentition stage. As is commonly seen, supernumerary teeth exist in the cleft itself and malpositioning of the other teeth at the cleft margin (age 8). Initially the su-

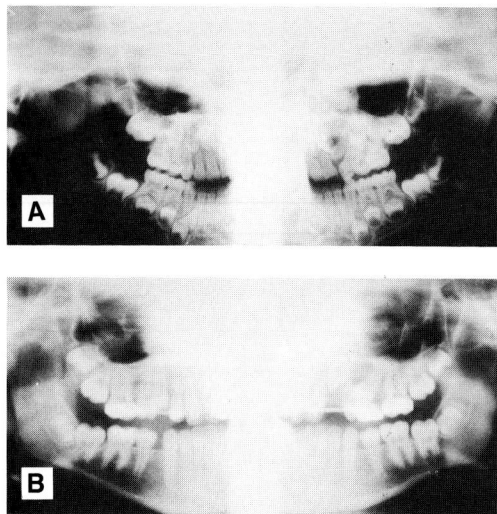

FIG. 23-36. *Panographic views of an alveolar cleft prior to and following bone grafting. (A) Initially, supernumerary teeth in the cleft were removed and the graft was performed. (B) Subsequently, the permanent canine is seen to be erupting normally through the graft.*

pernumerary teeth were removed, and the cleft was grafted approximately 3 months later. Figure 23-36B illustrates the sequence of canine eruption through the bone graft. In this case no orthodontic assistance was required for canine eruption, but at times it may be necessary.[95]

It is desirable that the graft be performed prior to eruption of the permanent canines into the cleft site, and that no other teeth be manipulated into the defect. If the canine is erupted and autogenous bone placed next to it, the risk of external resorption of the tooth, or ankylosis, becomes operative. If neighboring teeth have erupted through the cleft wall, considerable risk exists that a normal alveolar crest height will not be obtained with bone grafts; resorption of the graft bulk back to the preexisting crestal attachment level is commonly seen, leaving inadequate periodontal support.[96,97]

The alveolar cleft management technique is fairly standard, with major variation only in how the oral closure is performed. Initially, the cleft margins are incised to insure an adequate, tension-free eversion of flaps from the cleft wall into the nose. These are continuous above with

the lateral nasal wall mucoperiosteum and the nasal septal mucoperichondrium (Fig. 23-37). Watertight nasal closure to partition secretions is an absolute necessity for reliable "take" of the grafted bone. Following that, flaps are developed for oral coverage. These may include the advanced lateral maxillary wall flap[98] (Fig. 23-38), a trapezoidal flap from the lip[99] (Fig. 23-39), mobilized mucoperiosteal flaps on either side of the hard palate (Fig. 23-40), or in extreme cases musculomucosal flaps pedicled temporarily from the tongue[100] (Fig. 23-41). Clinical illustration of an alveolar cleft graft is shown in Figure 23-42.

Further nuances of detail are sometimes required in alveolar cleft grafting. The first hinges upon the need to transplant keratinized mucosa onto the ridge crest.[97] This maneuver provides an optimal host environment for "gingival" attachment to

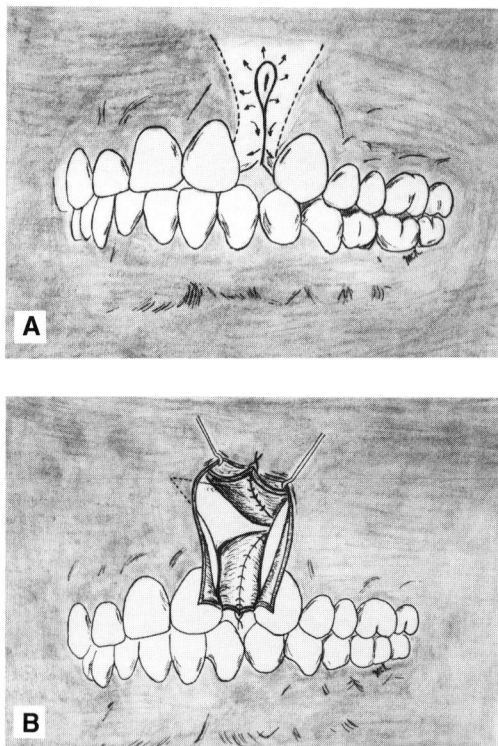

FIG. 23-37. *Alveolar cleft bone grafting. (A) Mucosal incisions outline the residual oral-nasal communication remaining from the congenital bony defect (broken lines). Arrows indicate the direction of flap elevation. (B) Flaps have been completed and sutured to provide nasal and palatal "floors."*

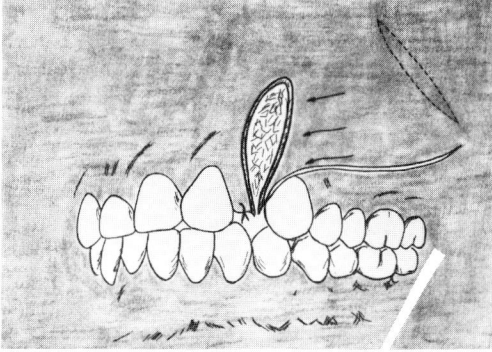

FIG. 23-38. *Lateral maxillary wall flap. Incision courses through and then superior to attached gingiva, with advancement (arrows) over the graft site and alveolar crest. Deep, periosteal relaxing incision is shown as broken line.*

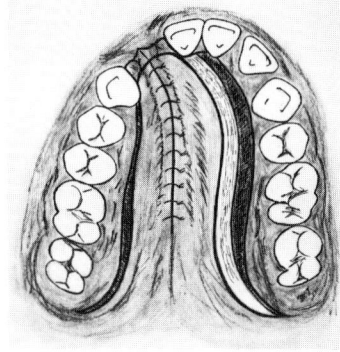

FIG. 23-40. *Mucoperiosteal, hard palatal flaps covering the cleft site. Beveled incisions at the alveolar slope minimize denuded bone and insure maintenance of the neurovascular bundle.*

erupting teeth. The second need is that of support for the overlying soft tissues; the pyriform rim of the nose and neighboring maxilla and zygoma may require, in addition to bone placed in cleft, simultaneous augmentation by onlay of cartilage or bone to increase their inadequate anterior projection (Figs. 23-43 and 23-44). This latter function may also be served by differentially moved maxillary segments when orthognathic surgery is necessitated to correct hypoplastic defects. A third important point is the remaining attachment of the nasalis muscle upon the wall of the alveolar cleft. It should be detached and secured across the cleft to the nasal septum.

The same protocols apply to bilateral alveolar clefts. However, the limitations of blood supply to the premaxillary segment

and the deficiency of covering tissue (mucosa) for the oral "side" of the cleft grafts introduce an extra degree of complexity. To maximize blood supply, it is important to preserve lip attachments, as "vascular pedicles," especially where repositioning osteotomy of the premaxillary segment is included.[101] For oral closure, it is sometimes necessary to rely upon lingual flaps.

ORTHOGNATHIC PROCEDURES

The evolution of combined surgical and orthodontic (orthognathic) reconstruction has provided a new vista for the orofacial

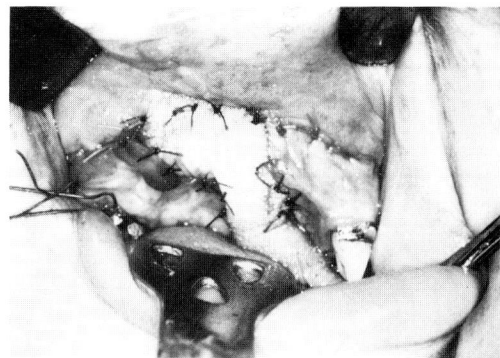

FIG. 23-41. *A lingual flap pedicled from the tongue sutured temporarily over a grafted alveolar cleft. It will be released and returned to the tongue after sufficient bony healing. (From: Kinnebrew, M.C. and Malloy, R.B.: Posteriorly based, lateral lingual flaps for alveolar cleft bone graft coverage. J. Oral Maxillofac. Surg., 41:555, 1983. Reprinted with permission from W.B. Saunders Co.)*

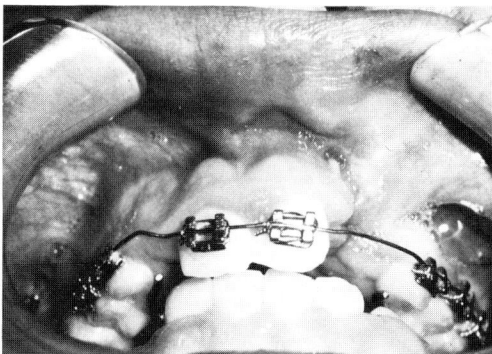

FIG. 23-39. *Trapezoidal lip flap in situ over a previously grafted cleft (viewer's right).*

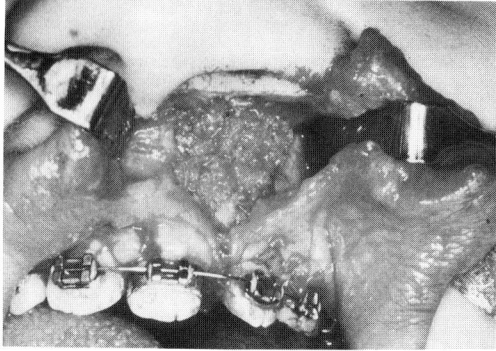

FIG. 23-42. *A grafted alveolar cleft prior to oral closure.*

FIG. 23-44. *(A) before and (B) after cartilage onlay of the lateral rim with cleft graft to restore alar base and check support. Mild residual edema is present.*

cleft patient. Commonly, the developmental years of these patients are attended by growth discrepancies in the individual parts of the facial skeleton, leading to varying degrees of malocclusion. When present, hypoplasia usually presents in the maxilla and midface, with maxillary constriction and a host of dental problems such as crowding, rotation, and abnormal angulation. Not uncommonly, the mandible appears prognathic, but in reality may be well-positioned relative to the cranium. Conversely, mandibular retrognathia may be present. The thrust of orthognathic surgery is to reposition the skeletal bases into functional harmony, complementing the orthodontic role of dental alignment and the prosthetic role of dental restoration. To that end, any of the orthognathic pro-

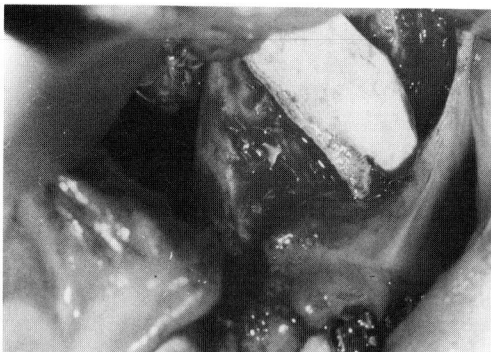

FIG. 23-43. *Onlaying the nasal pyriform rim simultaneous to bone grafting. Iliac crest cartilage is shown upon the lateral bony rim of the cleft; the nasal floor closure is also seen.*

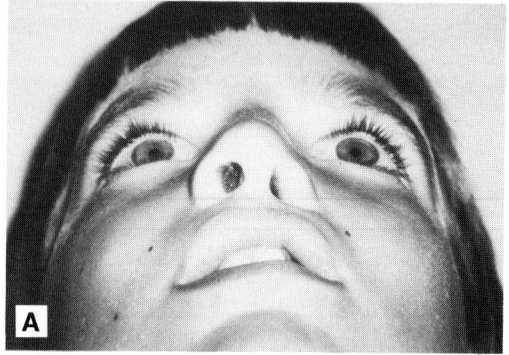

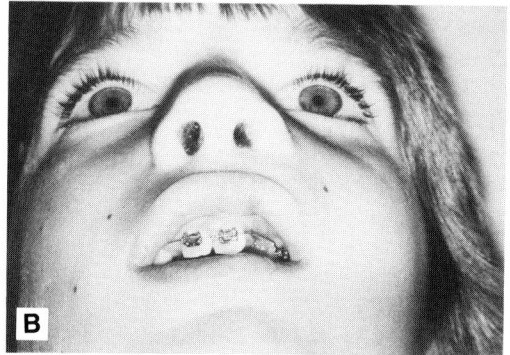

cedures (see Chapter 22) may be necessitated. The benefit to the dental picture should be obvious; an added dividend is that the soft tissues may be bolstered into proper contour by the bony movements. Selective design of the osteotomies intervenes discretely with the entire bony deformity at its multiple focal points, setting the stage for lasting revision and realignment of the soft tissues, specifically the lip and nose. When all is said and done, the "eyecatchers" that earlier invited close scrutiny of these patients are done away with; even though scars remain, they much less commonly draw a second look.

Not all cleft cases require jaw surgery. Indeed, a significant number may be managed primarily by orthodontic means with such surgical assistance as alveolar cleft bone grafts. It is important, however, that those cases requiring full-scale orthodontics and maxillofacial surgery be identified early and planned accordingly to avoid compromised results. For example, if max-

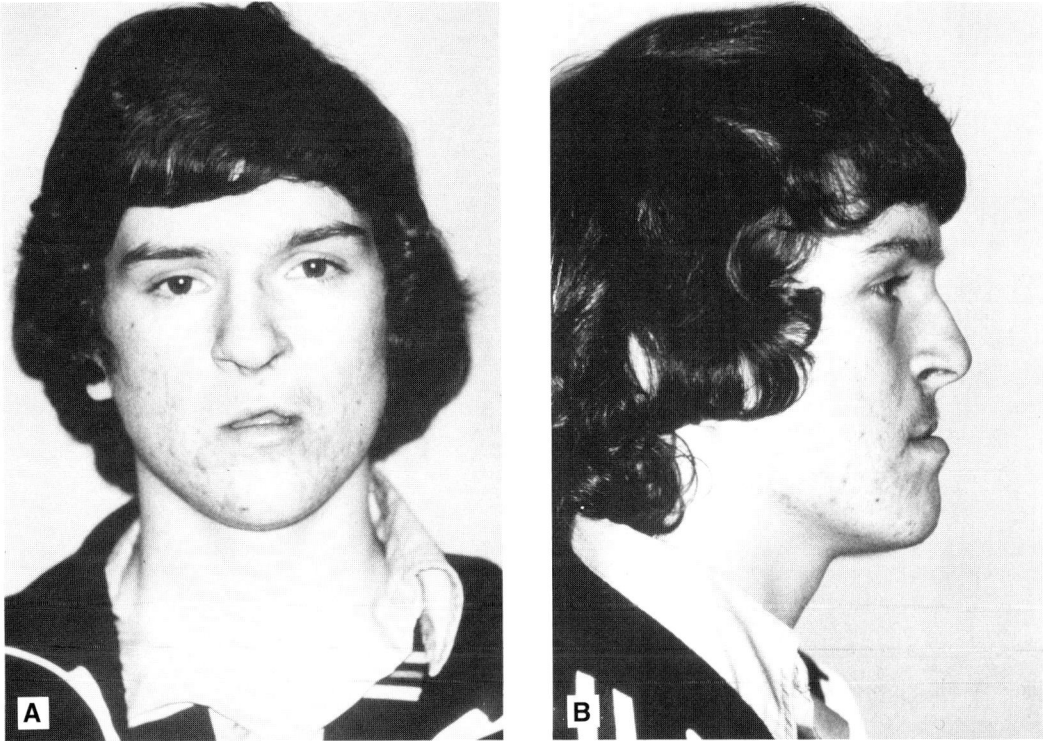

FIG. 23-45. *Frontal and lateral views of an adolescent with maxillary retrusion and lip-nose distortion residual to orofacial clefting. (From: Kinnebrew, M.C., and Kent, J.N.: Late definitive correction of the orofacial cleft: Report of a case. Am. J. Orthod., 84:104, 1983)*

illary constriction is present concomitantly with retrusion, it is considered favorable to limit major orthopedic expansion and to align the dentition in segments orthodontically, then surgically reposition the jaw in dentoalveolar segments.[40,98]

Let us consider, for illustration, the case of the boy depicted in Figure 23-45.[40] At age 14, obvious stigmata of cleft lip and palate are present and include midfacial hypoplasia, more marked at the maxillary plane, and lip and nose distortion. In addition to these problems, the speech exhibited excessive nasal resonance, or hypernasality, despite a previously performed inferiorly based pharyngeal flap. The occlusion is seen in Figure 23-46A. Treatment involved a sequence directed first to the dentition and skeletal balance, then the lip and nose; management of the incompetent velopharyngeal portal was deferred until later to allow complete involution of a significantly large adenoidal mass.

Over a 2-year period orthodontic forces aligned the dentition in the existing jaw segments. Selected extractions had been performed, including the removal of supernumerary teeth and the third molars. Minimal palatal expansion was sought orthopedically in lieu of later surgical expansion (Fig. 23-46B). Orthognathic surgery involved a LeFort I advancement osteotomy, in segments, with a simultaneous alveolar cleft bone graft to habilitate the occlusion (Fig. 23-47). Bone was transplanted from the iliac crest to the cleft and to the open interfaces created laterally and posteriorly by the maxillary movement. Fixation was obtained by multiple intraosseous wires that held the maxilla in its new position dictated by a prefabricated occlusal splint, and by maxillomandibular fixation. Permanent repositioning was obtained, as is demonstrated by the composite cephalometric tracings in Figure 23-48. Eighteen months following the or-

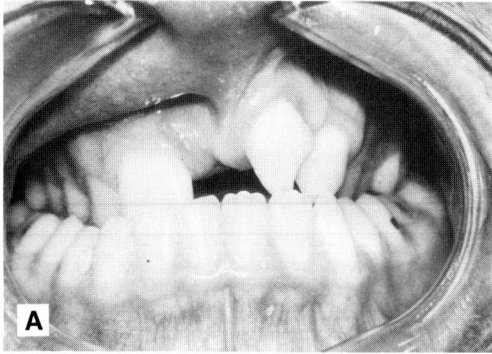

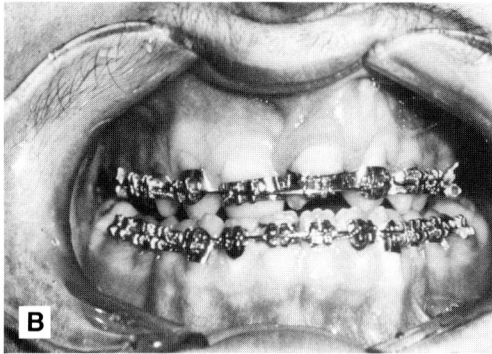

FIG. 23-46. (A) The pretreatment occlusion. (B) The intrasegmental orthodontic preparation for surgery.

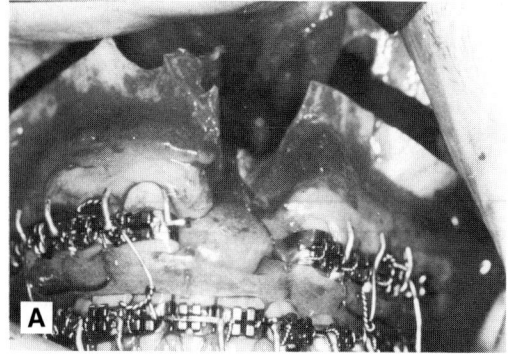

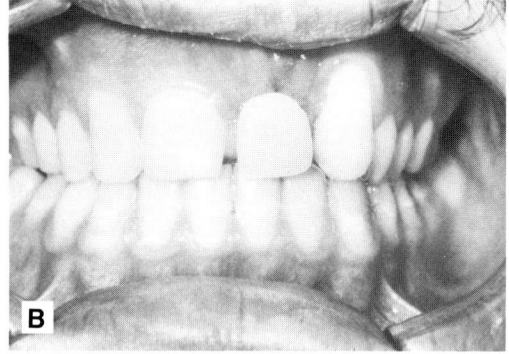

FIG. 23-47. (A) LeFort I (maxillary) osteotomy with simultaneous alveolar cleft graft. (B) Postosteotomy occlusion (temporary incisor prosthesis is present).

thognathic procedure, nose and lip revision was carried out, as discussed in the following paragraphs.

NOSE AND LIP REVISION
(RHINOCHEILOPLASTY)

Revisiting the congenital deformity of the nasal bones and cartilages, and the lip, it should come as no surprise that many of these focal deformities persist in the ensemble of secondary deformity. As well, there are added abnormalities subsequent to previous surgery, and scarring. These residua have been amplified by growth, as the small proportions of infancy attained adult dimensions. Returning to the previously discussed orthognathic case, these points will now be emphasized as the rhinocheiloplasty is detailed.

The clinical appearance of the lip and nose area is shown in Figure 23-49. Sketches of the deformity allowed tabulation from superior to inferior, as follows (Fig. 23-50A):

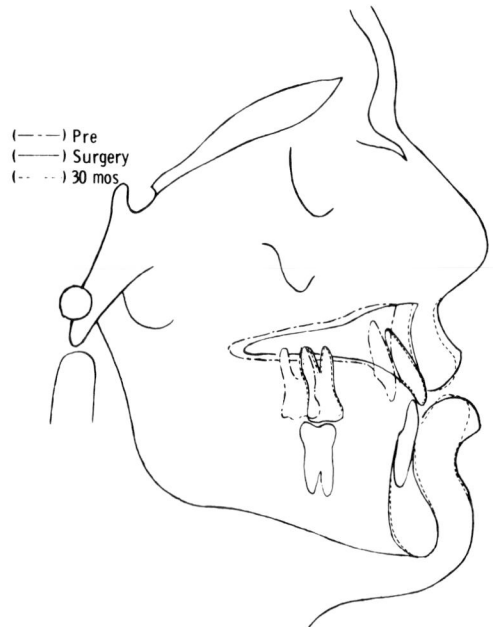

FIG. 23-48. Composite cephalometric tracings up to 30 months postoperatively, demonstrating marked stability.

CLEFT LIP AND PALATE • 497

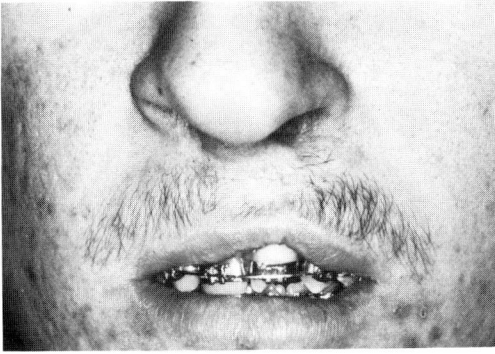

FIG. 23-49. *The clinical lip-nose deformity.*

The Nose
1. Deviation of the nose, including the bony bridge and cartilaginous septum, toward the "major" side (muscular pull)
2. Inferior rotation of the lower lateral (alar) cartilages, with greater distortion of the cleft or "minor" side such that the domes of these cartilages were poorly aligned
3. Lateral position of the minor side alar base
4. Left nasal sidewall in horizontal, rather than vertical angulation
5. Absence of a nostril sill across the cleft

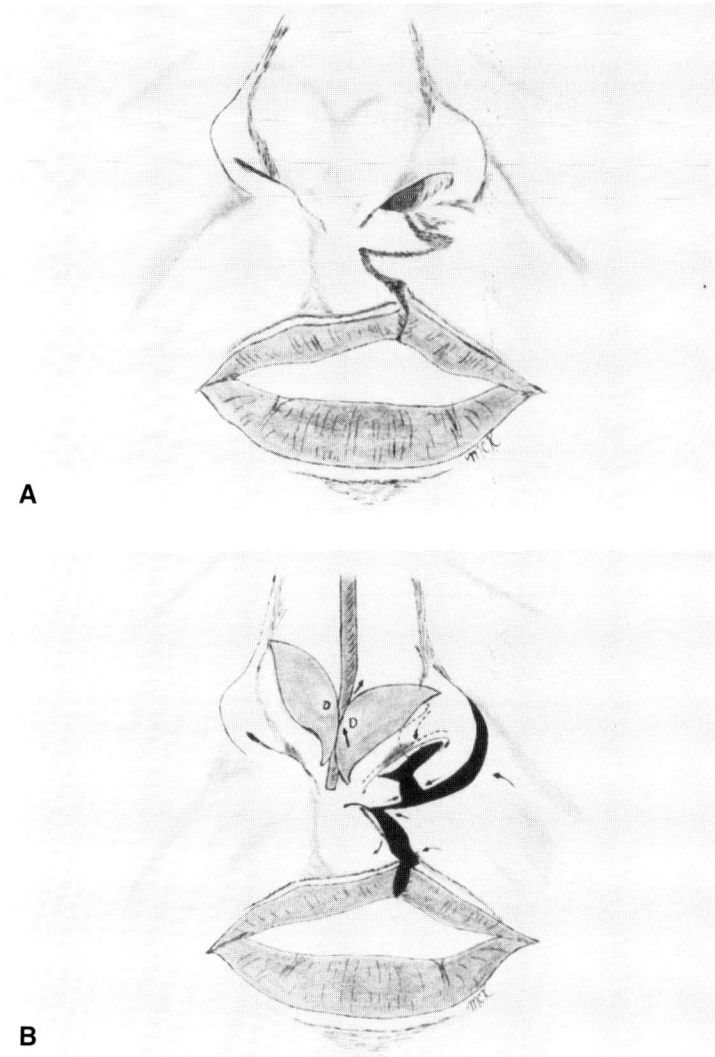

A

B

FIG. 23-50. *(A) Components of the lip-nose deformity. (B) Schema for the correction, as discussed in the text.*

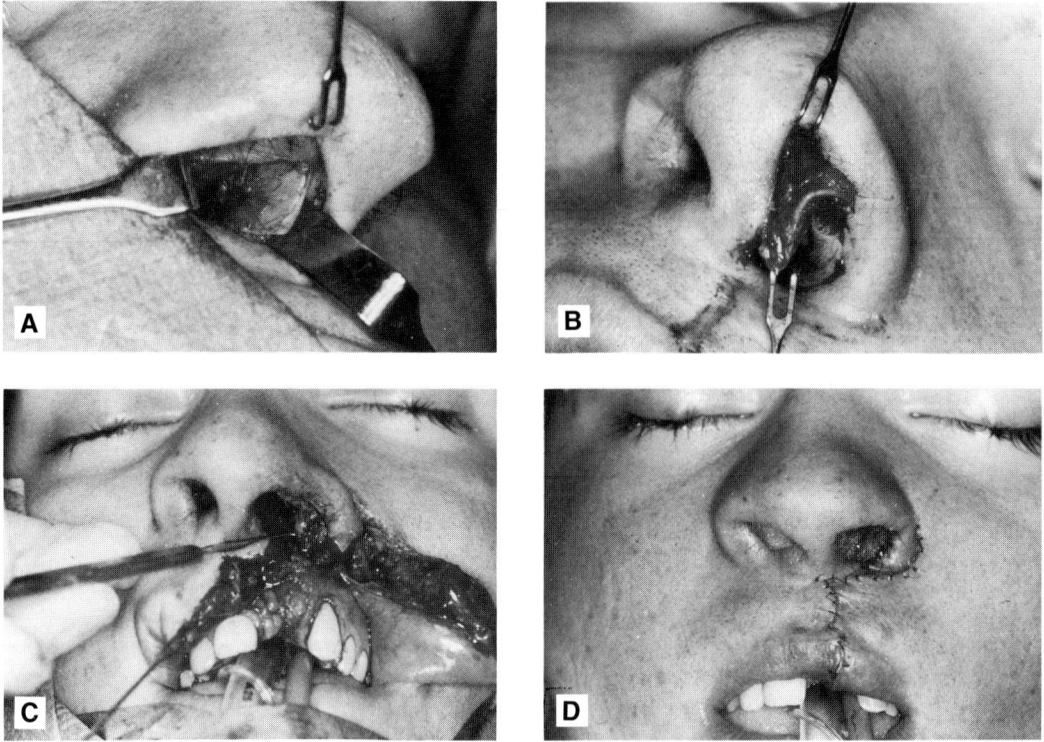

FIG. 23-51. *(A)Septoplasty by cartilaginous incisions for obliterating the memory of the deviated cartilage. (B) Dissecting the cleft-side alar cartilage for alignment of the domes. (C) Correcting the nasal sidewall and identifying the muscle components. (D) Routine closure.*

The Lip

1. Scarring residual to primary rotation-advancement repair
2. Superior retraction, or notching, of the labial contours, including the vermilion border
3. Discontinuity of the mucocutaneous ridge (white roll)
4. Muscular discontinuity and disorientation (bulges)
5. Lateral positioning of the labial commissure
6. Superior and lateral dislocation of the nasolabial fold

In summary, residua of the initial nasolabial deformity was accompanied by the residua of a rotation-advancement repair that had been either initially under-advanced or had relapsed laterally as the operated soft tissues reanchored themselves to their distorted bony base.

The surgical correction is schematized in Figure 23-50B, and clinically illustrated in Figure 23-51. It was elected not to intervene with the bony nasal bridge; instead straightening septoplasty was performed and the alar cartilages dissected and their domes aligned. The lip revision recreated the initial lines of the rotation-advancement, capitalizing on this pattern's allowance for scar resection and ease of revision. The orbicularis muscle components were dissected and securely anchored and the wound was closed in routine fashion. Pre-osteotomy and post-treatment photographs are shown in Figures 23-52 through 23-54. It can be seen, by comparison of the serial photographs, that the gross, eyecatching components of the secondary cleft deformity have been done away with; even though scarring and some distortions persist, they are minor and are not commonly scrutinized because attention is no longer invited to them.

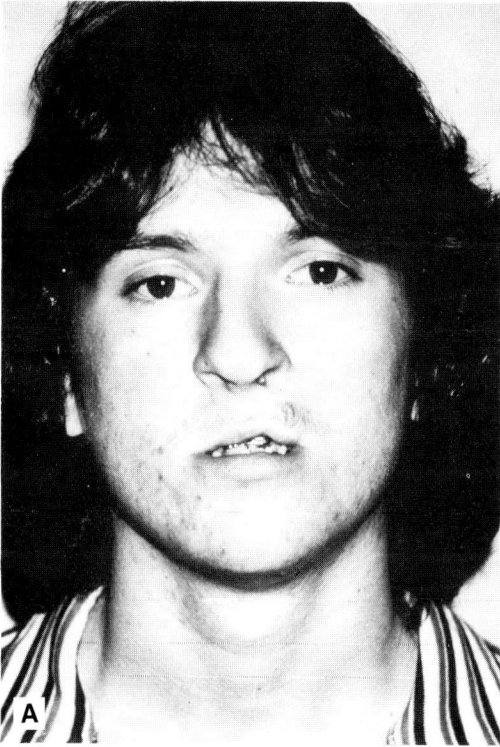

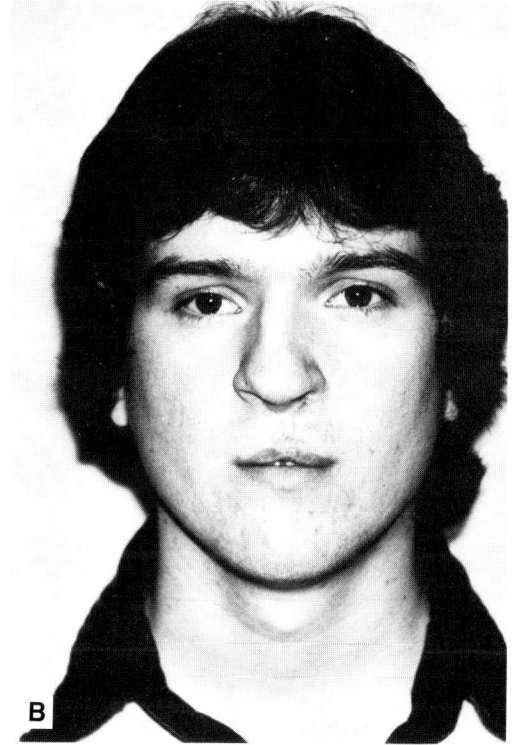

FIG. 23-52. *Frontal views. (A) Before osteotomy. (B) After completion of treatment.*

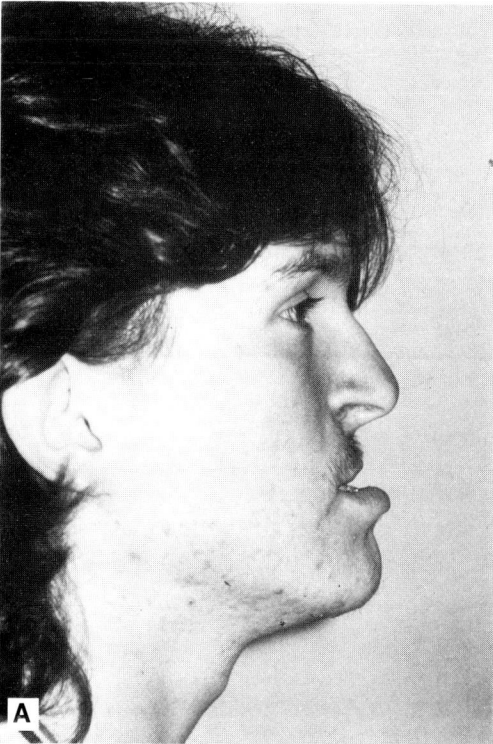

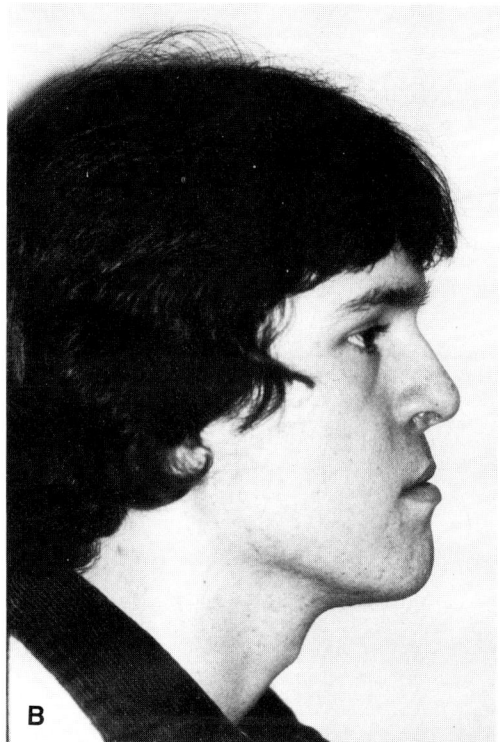

FIG. 23-53. *Lateral projections, before and after osteotomy.*

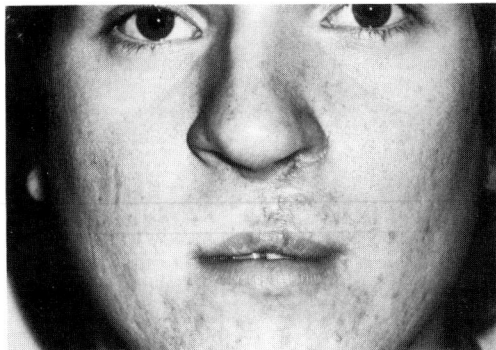

FIG. 23-54. *Labionasal anatomy is significantly improved, despite residual scarring.*

SIMULTANEOUS ORTHOGNATHIC SURGERY AND RHINOCHEILOPLASTY

At times it is elected to combine the soft-tissue aspects with simultaneously performed skeletal correction.[102,103] This abbreviated approach holds multiple advantages, from all viewpoints. For the patient,

the number of "finalizing" major operations is curtailed, after what is commonly a long series of surgical procedures. From the surgeon's view, this integrated approach allows one to "unravel" more of the deformity and take advantage of access and tissue availability to, in one procedure, redrape the soft tissues over a normalized skeleton. Additionally, the approach is significantly more cost-effective. Disadvantages include the degree of complexity and the length of the surgical procedures.

Figure 23-55 depicts a 28-year-old patient who desired further correction after multiple procedures of the lip, nose, maxilla, and palate. Analysis disclosed asymmetric midfacial hypoplasia, with the cleft side zygoma and maxilla lateralized and markedly retrusive (Fig. 23-56). An inadequately grafted alveolar cleft and an edentulous lateral incisor space were present. The midfacial midline was deviated toward the predominant muscles of the major

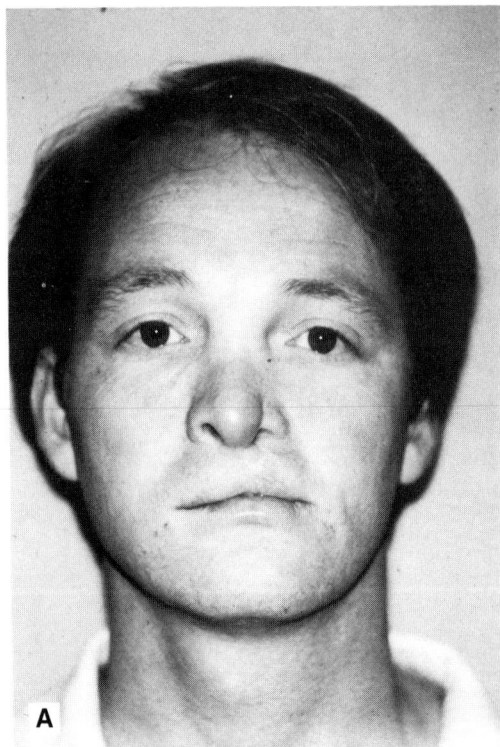

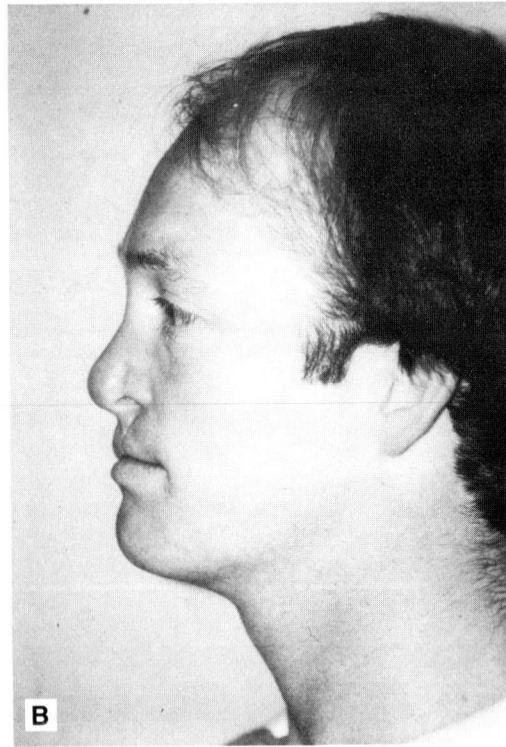

FIG. 23-55. *(A and B) Frontal and lateral views of a 28-year-old cleft patient with asymmetric midfacial retrusion, mandibular deviation, and labionasal distortion.*

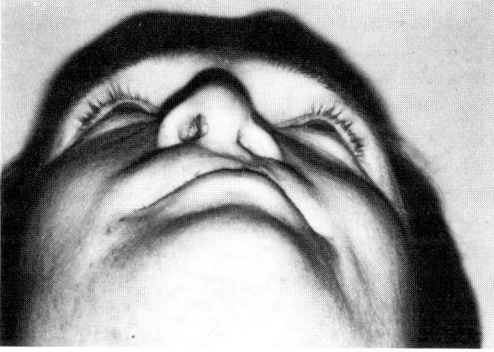

FIG. 23-56. *"Worm's eye" view of the degree of retrusion and the nasal collapse.*

side, and the "minor" lip segment was lateralized as well as superiorly retracted. In addition, residual displacement of lip skin into the nasal floor occurred as a carry over from the uncorrected congenital situation. Mandibular asymmetry was also present.

Utilizing a photocephalometric technique of treatment planning[104] (Fig. 23-57), it was elected to advance the midface differentially, by a LeFort III and LeFort I osteotomy on either side, to bring the zygomas into symmetry and correct the maxillary midline. The insufficient alveolar cleft graft was also to be augmented (Fig. 23-57D). The cleft-side cuspid tooth was advanced into the lateral incisor space, which movement also achieved normal support of the pyriform rim for the nasal alar base. The nasal revision included septoplasty, performed through the superior access of the alveolar cleft, onlay bone graft to the nasal dorsum, and cartilaginous tip reconstruction. The lip revision converted a previous straight-line repair, which was distorted, to a balanced rotation-advancement pattern (Fig. 23-58).

The midfacial and soft tissue surgery was performed as a first venture, through a facial degloving approach.[105,106] One month later the mandibular asymmetry was corrected by sagittal split osteotomy and genioplasty. At that time a previously planned, superiorly based pharyngeal flap was transferred to correct preexisting velopharyngeal incompetency that had been made worse by the maxillary advancement,

as the velum was pulled forward away from the posterior pharyngeal wall. As well, preexisting nasal occlusion, which had assisted the velopharyngeal closure in the reduction of nasal resonance, had been removed by the nasal revision. The patient's postoperative clinical photographs are shown in Figures 23-59 and 23-60, while the occlusion is shown in Figure 23-61.

REVISING THE BILATERAL CLEFT

Revisional rhinocheiloplasty in the bilateral cleft draws on techniques similar to those used for the unilateral cleft, not unlike the primary situation. Considerable variation in the secondary deformity is the rule here also, depending upon the initial severity, the procedures performed in infancy and childhood, and growth. The lip may be vertically long, as seen following the LeMesurier Repair, or it may be short and retracted, as in the straight-line closure. Commonly the nasal bridge and dorsum are wide, from muscular activity, and the nasal tip is depressed. It may be possible to perform the revision totally in the upper lip, but at times it is necessary to transfer unscarred, potentially dynamic tissue from the too full, ptotic lower lip to the tight, distorted upper lip as an "Abbe" flap.[107]

Figure 23-62 shows the nasal and labial morphology of an individual with a bilateral cleft; Figure 23-63 illustrates the clinical tabulation of the deformity and the proposed revision. The specifics of this case have been published previously, and consequently the interested reader is referred elsewhere for the surgical details.[108] The existing prolabium was shifted superiorly to lengthen the columella, the lip segments with their associated muscles were appropriately aligned, and tissue transfer from the lower to the upper lip was accomplished. Simultaneously, the nasal tip was stutted into greater projection. Post-treatment photographs (Figs. 23-64 and 23-65) demonstrate recaptured muscle balance and normal lip contours.

Conclusions

A broad overview of cleft lip and palate has been presented, seeking to condense the material of whole volumes into a single

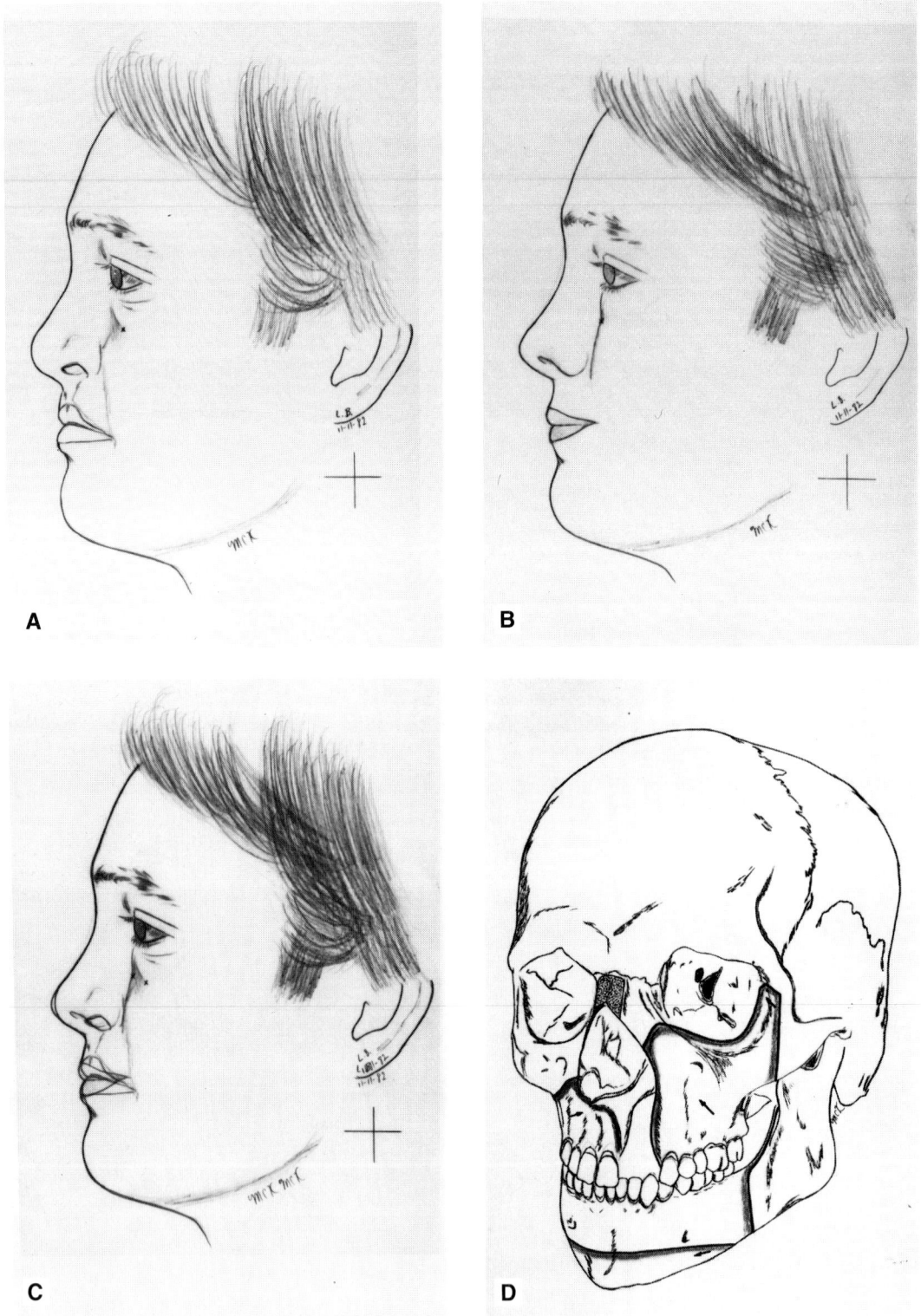

FIG. 23-57. (A) Photocephalometric treatment planning detailed in life-size tracings of the original feature. (B) Artistic depiction of what "could be." (C) Overlay of the two to ascertain and measure the degree of change. (D) The scheme of skeletal correction.

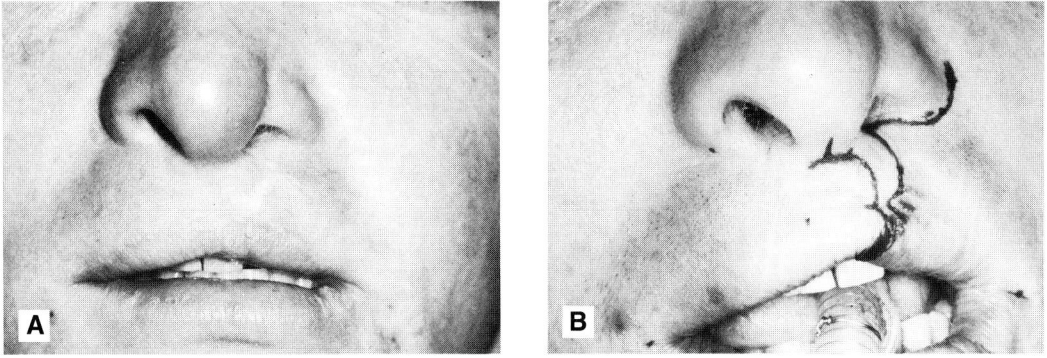

FIG. 23-58. *The existing lip scarring with (A) retraction (notching) and lateralization, and (B) its outline for correction.*

chapter. By no means should this chapter be considered a complete treatise, but instead a mere springboard and practical guide for the interested student. More in-depth coverage of the subject may be obtained from the following reference list.

The intended message of this chapter is that normalization of the orofacial cleft

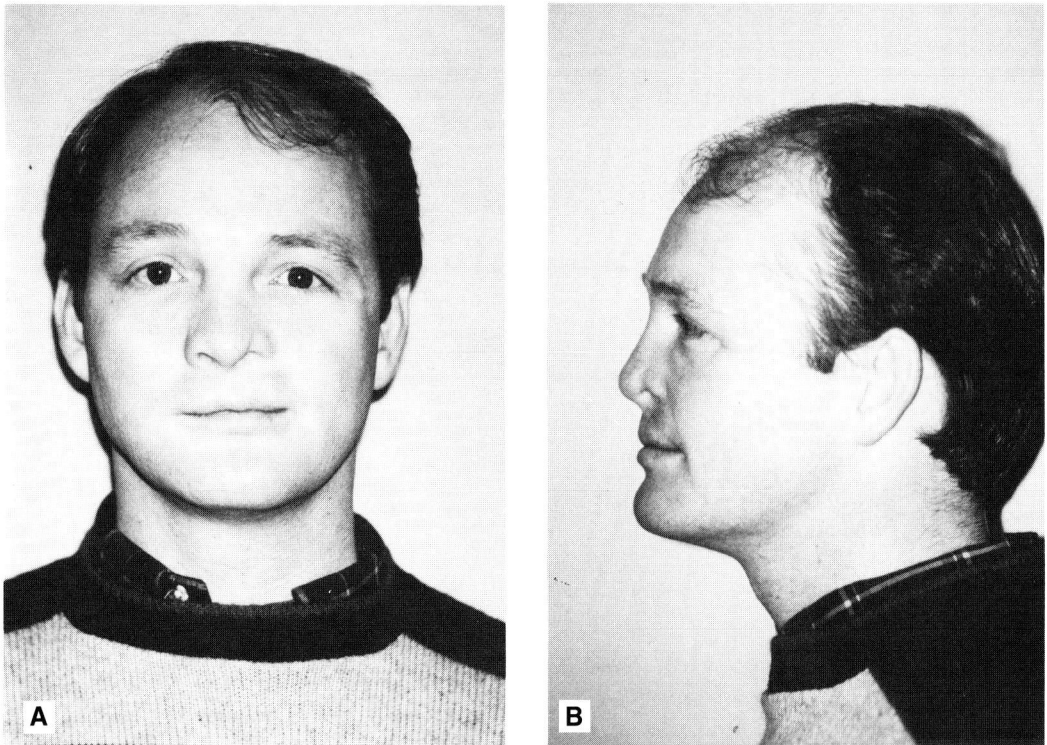

FIG. 23-59. *(A and B) Frontal and lateral projections, after treatment.*

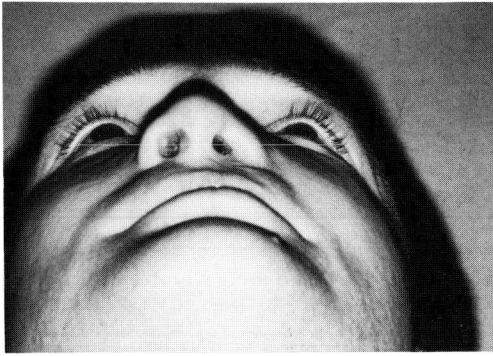

FIG. 23-60. *"Worm's eye" view, after treatment.*

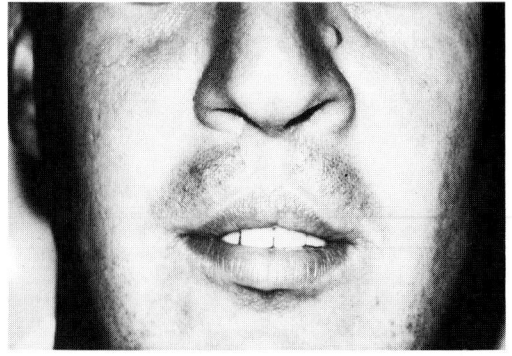

FIG. 23-62. *Lip-nose deformity secondary to bilateral cleft lip. (From: Kinnebrew, M.C.: Use of the Abbe flap in revision of the bilateral cleft lip-nose deformity. Oral Surg., 56:12, 1983)*

patient is substantially possible. Beginning with a basic understanding of the problems, continuing with a rational, common-sense approach to its treatment, and maintaining a genuine concern for the subject of one's efforts, *the patient,* much can be done. By the same token much remains to be done.

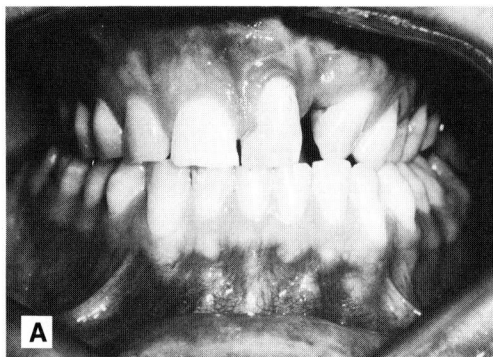

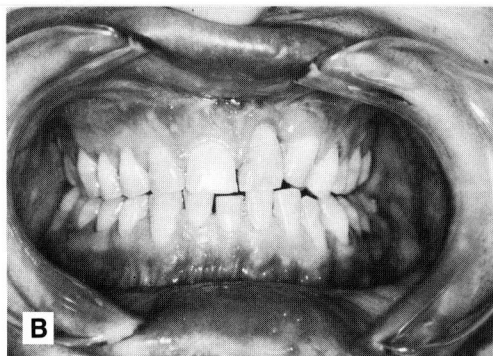

FIG. 23-63. *Photographic-sketch tabulation of (A) the irregular components, and (B) the scheme of correction.*

FIG. 23-61. *The occlusion, (A) before and (B) after surgery.*

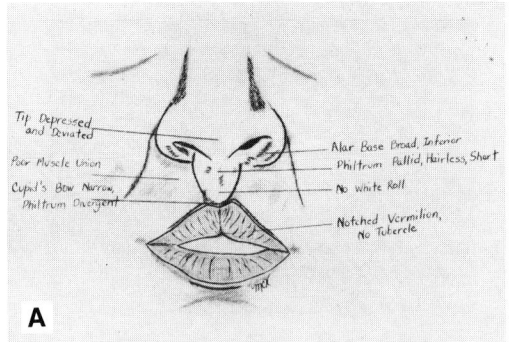

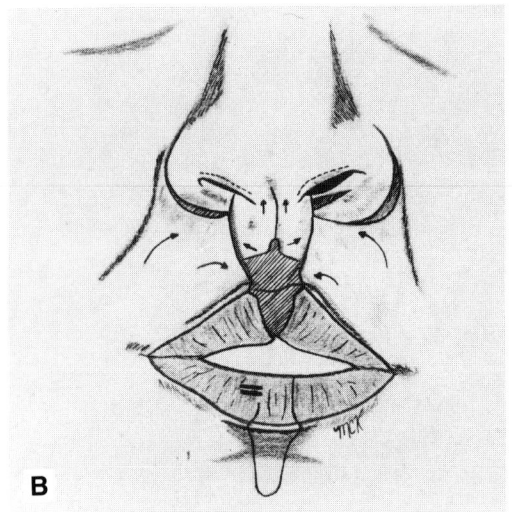

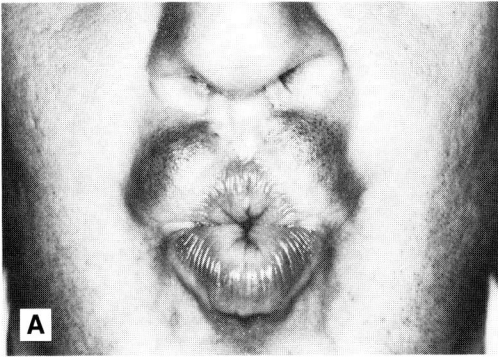

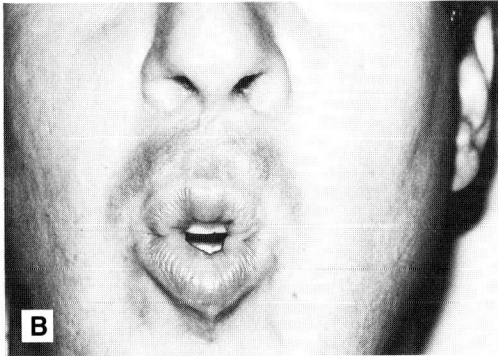

FIG. 23-64. *(A) The pursed-lip appearance prior to muscular reorientation, with lateral, discontinuous muscle bunching. (B) The post-operative muscular alignment is demonstrated.*

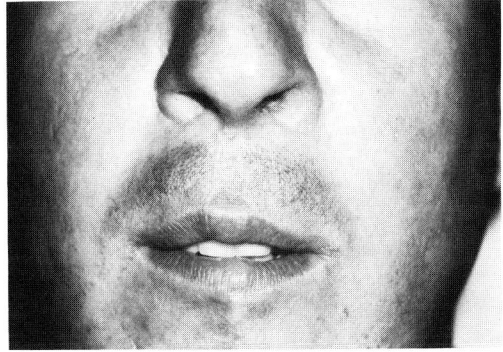

FIG. 23-65. *Habilitation of near normal labial structure following treatment.*

References

1. Patten, B.M.: Human Embryology. 3rd Ed. New York, McGraw-Hill Book Co., 1968.
2. Johnston, M.C.: Development of the face and oral cavity. *In* Orban's Oral Histology and Embryology, 8th Ed. Edited by S.N. Bhaskar. St. Louis, C.V. Mosby Co., 1976.
3. Delaire, J.: The potential role of facial muscles in monitoring maxillary growth and morphogenesis. *In* Muscle Adaptation in the Craniofacial Region. Monograph No. 8, Craniofacial Growth Series, Center for Growth and Development. Edited by D.S. Carlson and J.A. McNamara. Ann Arbor, University of Michigan, 1978.
4. Veau, V.: Division Palatine: Anatomie, Chirurgie, Phonetique. Paris, Masson, 1931.
5. Bishara, S.E., Olin, W.E., and Krause, C.J.: Cephalometric findings in two cases with unrepaired cleft lip and palate. Cleft Palate J., *15*:233, 1978.
6. Latham, R.A.: Development and structure of the premaxillary deformity in bilateral cleft lip and palate. Br. J. Plast. Surg., *26*:1, 1973.
7. Woolf, C.M.: Lateral incisor anomalies: Microforms of cleft lip and palate? Plast. Reconstr. Surg., *35*:543, 1965.
8. Bumstead, R.M.: A new method of achieving complete two-layer closure of a massive palatal cleft. Arch. Otolaryngol., *108*:147, 1982.
9. Kriens, O.B.: Anatomy of the velopharyngeal area and cleft palate. Clin. Plast. Surg., *2*:261, 1975.
10. Latham, R.A., Long, R.E., and Latham, E.A.: Cleft palate velopharyngeal musculature in a five-month-old infant: A three dimensional histological reconstruction. Cleft Palate J., *17*:1, 1980.
11. Morgan, R.F., Dellon, A.C., and Houpes, J.E.: Evaluation of the effect of levator retro-displacement upon conductive hearing loss in the cleft palate patient. Presented at the 39th Annual Session, American Cleft Palate Association, Denver, 1982.
12. Warren, D.W.: Velopharyngeal orifice size and upper pharyngeal pressure-flow patterns in normal speech. Plast. Reconstr. Surg., *33*:148, 1964.
13. Mason, R., and Grandstaff, H.: Evaluating the velopharyngeal mechanism in hypernasal speakers. Lang. Sp. Hear. Serv. Schools, *4*:1, 1971.
14. Rampp, D.L., Pannbacker, M., and Kinnebrew, M.C.: VPI: Velopharyngeal In-

competency - A Practical Guide for Evaluation and Management. Tulsa, Modern Education Corp., 1984.

15. Seif, S., and Dellon, A.L.: Anatomic relationship between the human levator and tensor veli palatini and the eustachian tube. Cleft Palate J., 15:329, 1978.

16. Bluestone, C.D.: Eustachian tube obstruction in the infant with cleft palate. Ann. Otol. Rhinol. Laryngol., 80:1,1971.

17. Cantekin, E.I., Doyle, N.J., and Bluestore, C.D.: Effect of levator veli palatini excision on eustachian tube function. Arch. Otolaryngol., 109:281, 1983.

18. Stool, S.E., and Randall, P.: Unexpected ear disease in infants with cleft palate. Cleft Palate J., 4:99, 1967.

19. Weatherly-White, R.C.A., et al.: Submucous cleft palate—its incidence, natural history, and indications for treatment. Plast. Reconstr. Surg., 49:304, 1972

20. Kaplan, E.N.: The occult submucous cleft palate. Cleft Palate J., 12:356, 1975.

21. Kinnebrew, M.C., and McTigue, D.: Submucous cleft palate: Review and two clinical reports. Ped. Dent., 6:252, 1984.

22. Stevenson, A.C., Johnson, H.A., Stewart, M.I.P., and Goldring, D.R.: Congenital malformations - a report of a study of consecutive births in 24 centres. Geneva, World Health Organization, 1966.

23. Zilberman, Y.: Observations on the dentition and face in clefts of the alveolar process. Cleft Palate J., 10:230, 1978.

24. Fraser, S.C.: Etiology of cleft lip and palate. In Cleft Lip and Palate - Surgical, Dental, and Speech Aspects. Edited by W.C. Grabb, S.W. Rosenstein, and K.R. Bzoch. Boston, Little Brown, 1971.

25. Lynch, H.T., and Kimberling, W.J.: Genetic counseling in cleft lip and cleft palate. Plast. Reconstr. Surg., 68:300, 1981.

26. Burdi, A.R.: Cleft lip and palate research. An updated state of the art. (I) Epidemiology, etiology, and pathogenesis of cleft lip and palate. Cleft Palate J., 14:261, 1977.

27. Gorlin, R.J., Pindborg, J.J., and Cohen, M.: Syndromes of the Head and Neck, 2nd Ed. St. Louis, C.V. Mosby Co., 1977.

28. Cohen, M.: Syndromes with cleft lip and palate. Cleft Palate J., 15:306, 1978.

29. Poswillo, D.: Mechanisms of congenital deformity. J. Dent. Res., 45:584, 1966.

30. Schubach, P.M.: Experimental induction of an incomplete hard-palate cleft in the rat. Oral Surg., 55:2, 1983.

31. Ross, R.B., and Johnston, M.C.: Cleft Lip and Palate. Baltimore, Williams and Wilkins, 1972.

32. Fraser, F.C.: Cleft lip and palate. Science, 158:1603, 1967.

33. Tessier, P.: Anatomical classification of facial, craniofacial and laterofacial clefts. J. Maxillofac. Surg., 4:69, 1976.

34. Kernahan, D.A., and Stark, R.B.: A new classification for cleft lip and palate. Plast. Reconstr. Surg., 22:435, 1958.

35. Elsahy, N., cited in Millard, D.R.: Cleft craft—the Evolution of Its Surgery, Vol. I. Boston, Little Brown, 1976.

36. Millard, D.R.: Cleft craft—the Evolution of Its Surgery, Vol. I. Boston, Little Brown, 1976.

37. Davis, J.S., and Ritchie, H.P.: Classification of congenital clefts of the lip and palate. JAMA, 2:1323, 1922.

38. Harkins, C.S., et al.: Report of the nomenclature committee: Proposed morphological classification of congenital cleft lip and palate. Cleft Palate Bull., 9:39, 1959.

39. Kremenak, C.R., and Searls, J.C.: Experimental manipulation of midfacial growth; a synthesis of five years of research at the Iowa Maxillofacial Growth Laboratory. J. Dent. Res., 50:1488, 1971.

40. Kinnebrew, M.C., and Kent, J.N.: Late definitive correction of the orofacial cleft: report of a case. Am. J. Orthod., 84:104, 1983.

41. McEvitt, W.G.: Treatment of respiratory obstruction in micrognathia by use of a nasogastric tube. Plast. Reconstr. Surg., 52:138, 1973.

42. Douglas, B.: The treatment of micrognathia associated with obstruction by a plastic procedure. Plast. Reconstr. Surg., 1:300, 1946.

43. Dorf, S.D., and Curtin, J.W.: Early cleft palate repair and speech outcome. Plast. Reconstr. Surg., 70:74, 1982.

44. Rood, S.: and Stool, S.: Current concepts of the etiology, diagnosis, and management of cleft palate otopathologic disease. Otolaryngol. Clin. N. Am., 14:865, 1981.

45. McNeil, C.K.: Orthodontic procedures in the treatment of congenital cleft palate. Dent. Rec., 70:126, 1950.

46. Wilhemsen, H.R., and Musgrave, R.H.: Complications of cleft lip surgery. Cleft Palate J., 3:223, 1963.

47. Hotz, M.M., and Gnoinski, W.: Comprehensive care of cleft lip and palate children at Zurich University: A preliminary report. Am. J. Orthodont., 70:481, 1976.

48. Bernstein, L.: The effect of timing of cleft palate operations on subsequent growth of the maxilla. Laryngoscope, 78:1510, 1968.

49. Gnoinski, W.N.: Early maxillary orthopedics as a supplement to conventional primary surgery in complete cleft lip and palate cases. J. Maxillofac. Surg., *10*:165, 1982.

50. Trost-Cardemone, J.: Effect of velopharyngeal inadequacy on speech. J. Childhood Commun. Dis., in press.

51. Still, J.M., and Georgiade, N.G.: Historical review of management of cleft lip and palate. *In* Symposium On Management of cleft Lip and Palate and Associated Deformities. Edited by N.G. Georgiade and R.F. Hagerty. St. Louis, C.V. Mosby Co., 1974.

52. Tennison, C.W.: The repair of the unilateral cleft lip by stencil method. Plast. Reconstr. Surg., *9*:118, 1952.

53. Skoog, T.: A design for the repair of unilateral cleft lips. Am. J. Surg., *95*:223, 1958.

54. Thomson, H.G.: Quadrilateral flap in the repair of unilateral cleft lip. *In* Cleft Lip and Palate, Surgical, Dental and Speech Aspects. Edited by W. C. Grabb, S.W. Rosenstein, and K.R. Bzoch. Boston, Little Brown, 1971.

55. Millard, D.R., Jr.: Extensions of rotation-advancement principle for wide unilateral cleft lip. Plast. Reconstr. Surg., *42*:535, 1968.

56. Kaplan, E.N.: Growth of the unilateral cleft lip. Cleft Palate J., *15*:203, 1978.

57. Meijer, R.: Lip adhesion and its effect on the maxillofacial complex in complete unilateral clefts of the lip and palate. Cleft Palate J., *15*:34, 1978.

58. Randall, P.: A triangular flap operation for the primary repair of unilateral clefts of the lip. Plast. Reconstr. Surg., *23*:331, 1959.

59. Holtje, W.J., and Ehmann, G.: Wave-line procedure in the repair of cleft lip. J. Maxillofac. Surg., *1*:198, 1973.

60. Frederiks, E.: Vascular patterns in normal and cleft primary and secondary palate in human embryos. Br. J. Plast. Surg., *25*:207, 1972.

61. Veau, V.: Operative treatment of complete double harelip. Am. J. Surg., *76*:143, 1922.

62. LeMesurier, A.B.: Hare Lips and Their Treatment. Baltimore, Williams and Wilkins, 1962.

63. Millard, D.R.: Closure of bilateral cleft and elongation of columella by two operations in infancy. Plast. Reconstr. Surg., *47*:324, 1971.

64. Ward, C.M.: An analysis, from photographs, of the results of four approaches to elongating the columella after repair of bilateral cleft lip. Plast. Reconstr. Surg., *64*:68, 1979.

65. Perko, M.: Two-stage closure of cleft palate. J. Maxillofac. Surg., *7*:76, 1979.

66. Kinnebrew, M.C., Pannbacker, M., and Rampp, D.C.: The residual submucous cleft: A cause of persistent speech and hearing problems. Lang. Sp. Hear. Serv. Schools, *17*:16, 1986.

67. Kaplan, E.N.: Soft palate repair by levator muscle reconstruction and a buccal mucosal flap. Plast. Reconstr. Surg., *56*:129, 1975.

68. Von Langenbeck, B.: Operation der angeboren totalen spaltung des harten gaumens nach eine neuen method. Deutsch. Klin., *12*:231, 1861.

69. Wardill, W.E.M.: The technique of operation for cleft palate. Br. J. Surg., *25*:117, 1937.

70. Kilner, T.P.: Cleft lip and palate repair technique. St. Thomas Hosp. Rep., *2*:127, 1937.

71. Morley, M.E.: Cleft Palate and Speech, 7th Ed. Edinburgh, Churchill Livingston, 1973.

72. Mason, R. and Warren, D.: Adenoid involution and developing hypernasality in cleft palate. J. Speech Hear Res., *45*:469, 1980.

73. Schendel, S.A., Oeschlager, M., and Wolford, L.M.: Velopharyngeal anatomy and maxillary advancement. J. Maxillofac. Surg., *7*:116, 1979.

74. Bzoch, K.R., ed.: Communicative Disorders Related to Cleft Lip and Palate, 2nd Ed. Boston, Little Brown, 1979.

75. Dorrance, G.M.: Lengthening the soft palate in cleft palate operations. Ann. Surg., *82*:208, 1965.

76. Mazaheri, M: Prosthodontic care. *In* Cleft Palate and Cleft Lip: A Team Approach to Clinical Management and Rehabilitation of the Patient. Edited by H.K. Cooper. Philadelphia, W.B. Saunders Co., 1979.

77. Wolford, L.M.: Proplast pharyngeal wall implants to correct VPI: Long term results. Presented at the 40th annual meeting of the American Cleft Palate Association, Indianapolis, 1983.

78. Hynes, W.: Pharyngoplasty by muscle transplantation. Br. J. Plast. Surg., *3*:128, 1950.

79. Orticochea, M.: Construction of a dynamic muscle sphincter in cleft palates. Plast. Reconstr. Surg., *41*:323, 1966.

80. Jackson, I.T., and Silverton, J.S.: Sphinc-

ter pharyngoplasty as a secondary procedure in cleft palates. Plast. Reconstr. Surg., *59*:518, 1977.

81. Owsley, J.Q.: The technique and complications of pharyngeal flap surgery. Plast. Reconstr. Surg., *35*:531, 1965.

82. Randall, P., Whitaker, L., Noone, R.B., and Jones, W.D.: The case for the inferiorly based pharyngeal flap. Cleft Palate J., *15*:263, 1978.

83. Whitaker, L.A., et al.: A prospective and randomized series comparing superiorly and inferiorly based pharyngeal flaps. Cleft Palate J., *9*:305, 1972.

84. Sphrinzten, R.J., et al.: A comprehensive study of pharyngeal flap surgery: Tailormade flaps. Cleft Palate J., *16*:46, 1979.

85. Subtelny, J.P., and Nieto, R.B.: A longitudinal study of maxillary growth following pharyngeal-flap surgery. Cleft Palate J., *15*:118, 1978.

86. Turvey, T.A., Vig, K., Moriarty, J., and Hoke, J.: Delayed bone grafting in the cleft maxilla and palate: A retrospective multidisciplinary analysis. Am. J. Orthod., *86*:244, 1984.

87. Rosenstein, S.W.: The case for early bone grafting in cleft lip and palate. Plast. Reconstr. surg., *70*:247, 1982.

88. Koberg, N., et al.: Present view on bone grafting in cleft palate. J. Maxillofac. Surg., *1*:185, 1973.

89. Sitzmann, F.: The alveolar flap for the repair of the cleft alveolus—related to the development of the upper jaw. J. Maxillofac. Surg., *7*:81, 1979.

90. Skoog, T.: The use of periosteum and surgicel for bone formation in congenital clefts of the maxilla. Scand. J. Plast. Surg. Reconstr. Surg., *1*:113, 1967.

91. Azzolini, A., Riberti, C., Roselli, D., and Standoli, L.: Tibial periosteal graft in repair of cleft lip and palate. Ann. Plast. Surg., *9*:105, 1982.

92. Kwon, H.J., et al.: The management of alveolar cleft defects. JADA, *102*:848, 1981.

93. Wolfe, S.A., and Berkowitz, S.: The use of cranial bone grafts in the closure of alveolar and anterior palatal clefts. Plast. Reconstr. Surg., *72*:659, 1983.

94. Boyne, P.J., and Sands, N.R.: Combined orthodontic-surgical management of residual palato-alveolar cleft defects. J. Oral Surg., *30*:87, 1972.

95. Hinrichs, J.E., et al.: Periodontal evaluation of canines erupted through alveolar cleft defects. J. Oral Maxillofac. Surg., *42*:717, 1984.

96. Eldeeb, M., et al.: Canine eruption into grafted bone in maxillary alveolar defects. Cleft Palate J., *19*:9, 1982.

97. Waite, D.E., and Kersten, R.: Residual alveolar and palatal clefts. *In* Surgical Correction of Dentofacial Deformities. Edited by W.J. Bell, W.R. Proffitt, and R.P. White. Philadelphia, W.B. Saunders Co., 1980.

98. Tideman, H., et al.: LeFort I advancement with segmental palatal osteotomies in patients with cleft palates. J. Oral Surg., *38*:196, 1980.

99. Epker, B.N., and Wolford, L.M.: Dentofacial Deformities, Surgical-Orthodontic Correction. St. Louis, C.V. Mosby Co., 1980.

100. Kinnebrew, M.C., and Malloy, R.B.: Posteriorly based, lateral lingual flaps for alveolar cleft bone graft coverage. J. Oral Maxillofac. Surg., *41*:555, 1983.

101. Westbrook, M.T., West, R.A., and McNeill, R.W.: Simultaneous maxillary advancement and closure of bilateral alveolar clefts and oronasal fistulas. J. Oral Maxillofac. Surg., *41*:257, 1983.

102. Schendel, S.A., and Delaire, J.: Functional musculoskeletal correction of secondary unilateral cleft lip deformities: Combined lip-nose correction and LeFort I osteotomy. J. Maxillofac. Surg., *9*:108, 1981.

103. Henderson, D., and Jackson, I.: Combined cleft lip revision, anterior fistula closure and maxillary osteotomy; a one-stage procedure. Br. J. Oral Surg., *13*:33, 1975.

104. Kinnebrew, M.C., Hoffman, D.R., and Carlton, D.M.: Projecting the soft-tissue outcome of surgical and orthodontic manipulation of the maxillofacial skeleton. Am. J. Orthod., *84*:508, 1983.

105. Egydi, D.: Degloving the nose. J. Maxillofac. Surg., *2*:101, 1974.

106. Kinnebrew, M.C., Zide, M.F., and Kent, J.N.: Modified LeFort II procedure for simultaneous correction of maxillary and nasal deformities. J. Oral Maxillofac. Surg., *41*:295, 1983.

107. Abbe, R.: A new plastic operation for the relief of deformity due to double harelip. Med. Rec., *53*:447, 1898.

108. Kinnebrew, M.C.: Use of the Abbe flap in revision of the bilateral cleft lip-nose deformity. Oral Surg., *56*:12, 1983.

CHAPTER 24 # Management of Chronic Craniofacial Pain

JAMES R. FRICTON

Pain is perfect misery, the worst of all evils. MILTON

Phenomena of Pain

Chronic pain is the most complicated of pain experiences and one of the most perplexing, frustrating, and feared problems in medicine and dentistry. Chronic pain costs our society an estimated 80 billion dollars annually in health services, medication, litigation, compensation and lost work.[1] Over 50 million individuals are either partially or totally disabled for days, weeks, months, or permanently because of chronic pain. Available data suggest that nearly one third of the population in the United States has persistent or recurrent chronic pain.[2] It is distressing that in this age of scientific and technological advances, millions suffer from chronic pain affecting their entire lives with serious physical and emotional disorders and little hope for relief. It is imperative that as clinicians in service to our community, we learn more about this societal problem. To do this, we must understand the multidimensional nature of the pain experience.

Patients often dread coming to the dentist for fear of pain, and dentists dread the patient who anxiously awaits pain or develops chronic pain. This fear creates significant adverse reactions from both patients and health professionals. These reactions can complicate the quality and enjoyment of clinical practice as well as the relationship with the patient. A clinician need not be reminded of the importance of under-

standing all the variables involved in pain and its prevention, diagnosis, and management. Pain experiences can vary from the brief sharpness of an easily forgotten pin prick to the throbbing agony of a chronic headache. This range in pain experiences demonstrates that pain is not a simple sensation but rather a complex physical, psychologic, and social experience. Aristotle described pain as a "Quale; a passion of the soul" rather than an ordinary sensory experience. Sternbach[3] defined it as a (1) personal and private sensation of hurt, (2) harmful stimulus that signals current or impending tissue damage, and (3) pattern of responses which operate to protect the organism from harm. Dorland's Medical Dictionary[4] defines it as a more or less localized sensation of discomfort, distress, or agony resulting from the stimulation of specialized nerve endings. Because no definition appears to fit the entire picture of the pain experience, it needs to be divided into three types of experiences: experimental pain, acute pain, and chronic pain. In addition, each type has four basic components: (1) the noxious or nociceptive stimulus, (2) the neurophysiologic pathway to the brain, (3) the person's cognitive perception, and (4) the emotional, behavioral, and social reactions to the pain. Understanding these experiences of pain and their components will facilitate control of them.

509

Experimental pain, as when we purposely pinch ourselves, stick ourselves with a needle, or perform a tooth pulp test is the simplest pain experience. Because of its nature, the noxious stimuli causes a localized sensation perceived as uncomfortable or painful and is self-limiting or can be terminated by ourselves. Thus, usually little, if any, anxiety or behavioral reaction to this type of pain occurs. If the locus of control in creating the noxious stimulation is taken away from the person experiencing the pain, the pain experience elicits a greater possibility for an emotional reaction. The degree of this reaction is generally related to anticipation of the pain and not to the sensation. As the stimulus strength and duration increases with a decrease in control, anticipation of pain and the emotional reaction become a greater part of the experience and can be far more important to the patient than the actual sensation felt. This is especially true of the pain and anxiety involved in dental phobic patients with a prolonged dreaded anticipation of a dental injection.

Acute pathologic pain as in an abscessed tooth or a broken leg has a greater possibility for adding a psychologic or behavioral reaction to the pain. The cause of this continuous pain is often unknown to the patient and, although the pain is eventually self limiting or treatable, it cannot be immediately terminated by the patient as with experimental pain. This can create reactions such as anxiety, verbal complaints, and partial disabilities that generally pass as the pain goes away.

Chronic pathologic pain, as seen in many pain clinics across the country, is a more complicated problem that includes experiences such as headaches, low back pain, facial pain, arm or leg pain, or abdominal pain that last many months to years. This pain can be very perplexing not only to the patient but to the physician or dentist managing it. A chronic pain condition has little apparent cause, is not self limiting, and often increases over time. It is difficult to terminate by both the physician and the patient and has no apparent function or purpose. These complicating factors create many psychosocial and behavioral reactions, such as persistent anxiety or depression, perceptual distortion of other sen-

sations, maladaptive behaviors such as verbalization of pain or clenching of teeth, and significant life-style disruptions.

This chapter reviews the characteristics and techniques of evaluation, diagnosis, and management of chronic craniofacial pain.

Chronic Pain Syndromes

A chronic pain syndrome is a pain problem that persists beyond a few months and has a network of interrelated psychosocial, behavioral, and somatic problems. Knowledge of these characteristics of chronic pain patients can help provide insight into the various factors that may complicate or perpetuate the pain. Because chronic pain appears to be permanent, patients may feel helpless, hopeless, and desperate in their inability to receive relief. They may become hypochondriacal, obsessed, and worried about any perceived symptom or sensation. Vegetative symptoms and overt depression may set in with sleep and appetite disturbances. Irritability and mood fluctuations are common. Loss of self-esteem, libido, and interest in life activities can add to their misery. Such behavior may erode personal relationships with family, friends, work associates, and health professionals.

Patients can focus all their energy on analyzing the pain problem and believe that it causes all their problems. They may visit one physician after another, desperately searching for a cure. They can become belligerent, hostile, and manipulative in seeking care. Many clinicians make gallant attempts with multiple drug regimens or multiple surgeries, but failure frustrates the clinician and adds to the patient's ongoing depression. Near the end of this progression, many chronic pain patients have multiple drug dependencies, high stress levels, loss of vocation, permanent disability, or involvement in litigation in addition to their pain problem.

Herein lies the importance of early recognition of the diagnosis and all contributing factors that may lead to a chronic pain syndrome. Comprehensive evaluation of a patient with chronic pain is critical. Rehabilitating the patient includes both the treatment of the physical diagnosis causing the pain as well as improving the contributing factors that perpetuate or result from the pain problem. Because this is often a complex, time-consuming, and difficult task, pain clinics with interdisciplinary teams have been developed to coordinate their care and provide a healthy environment for rehabilitation. Although recognition of persistent pain problems must be done at the primary care level, pain clinics may support the clinician in helping the patient improve long-term. Knowledge of evaluation techniques, differential diagnosis, and potential contributing factors help the clinician recognize these problems.

Evaluation for Craniofacial Pain

Understanding the patient with chronic pain depends on gathering as much information as possible about the patient and his experience. Such information can be gathered from history, physical examination, diagnostic studies, and other consultations. History of the problem often reveals information that points directly to a general diagnostic classification, if not to a specific diagnosis (Table 24-1). Physical examination of the patient should reinforce the clinician's perceptions about the patient and provide more information to support a definitive diagnosis (Table 24-2). Further diagnostic studies such as nerve blocks, pulp tests, radiographs, and psychometric testing can help rule out other disorders and provide information to complement the history and physical examination (Table 24-3). If doubt concerning the diagnosis persists or pathology not in your area of expertise exists, an appropriate consultation should be readily obtained to provide an additional perspective on the patient's status.

TABLE 24-1. *History*

Chief complaints
Associated symptoms
Characteristics of pain
Precipitating, aggravating, or alleviating factors
Onset and history of pain
Past and present medications, surgeries, and treatments
Personal history
Medical history
Review of systems

TABLE 24-2. *Physical examination for craniofacial pain*

General appearance
Mental status
Head and neck inspection
Cranial nerve function
Stomatognathic function
Myofascial palpation
Occlusal stability and function

TABLE 24-3. *Diagnostic studies for craniofacial pain*

Nerve blocks
  Peripheral nerve block
  Local infiltraton
  Epidural block
  Myofascial trigger point injection
  Sympathetic ganglion block
Radiographs
  TMJ arthrograms
  TMJ tomograms
  TMJ transcranials
  Sinus series
  Cervical series
  Computerized tomography (CT scan)
  Angiogram
Magnetic resonance imaging
Psychometric testing
Blood studies
Urinalysis
Radioisotope studies

History

The history should include the chief complaints and associated symptoms; character and severity of the pain; precipitating, aggravating, and alleviating factors; onset and history of pain; past and present medications; surgeries and other treatments; a personal history, medical history, and a review of systems.[5,6]

Establishing the patient's chief complaint includes listening carefully to the patient describe each type of pain or complaint present, including the locations, character, and severity of the symptoms. A chronic pain patient often has multiple pain complaints with different descriptions that may indicate several diagnoses involved in the pain problem. How the patient relates to the pain can also give important clues to the etiology. For example, patients with pain associated with a psychogenic conversion reaction frequently relate to the pain descriptively but indifferently as if it is another entity apart from them. The patient may have varying qualitative or quantitative descriptions for the pain to discern affective or sensory components of the pain or help in establishing a diagnosis.[7] For example, migraine headaches are typically described as throbbing, and a tension headache has a constant, steady quality like a dull pressure sensation. Pain may vary in timing during the day, week, or year. Cluster headaches occur in clusters of weeks and months, and the patient is pain free at other times.

Associated symptoms such as dizziness, numbness, blurred vision, or indigestion are seen frequently in patients with chronic pain. These symptoms may point to a specific diagnosis or an underlying structural disease, or they may be symptoms with unexplained etiology. Many of these symptoms can be benign and associated with a physical diagnosis such as myofascial pain, but some may uncover a serious structural disorder such as an intracranial neoplasm.

Precipitating, aggravating, alleviating factors also add clues to the origin of pain. Modifying factors such as stress, posture, weather, diet, heat, cold, and others are included. For example, precipitation of the pain associated with migraine headaches can occur with red wine, chocolate, cheese, and other foods.[8] Temporomandibular joint capsulitis is aggravated by chewing.

The onset and history of the problem includes learning about what events surrounded the initiation of the pain, how it has changed since onset, and various past evaluations and treatments. With acute pain, the history may be quite short, but with chronic pain the history may take an hour to obtain with many physicians, dentists, and other health professionals involved.

The effect of past medications, surgeries, and other treatments can provide insight into the pathologic process occurring as well as what approaches should be avoided in the future. For example, caffeine will alleviate a migraine or a caffeine withdrawal headache and not a muscular headache. Patients receiving physical therapy without relief of pain may be more prone to failure if a second trial of physical therapy is recommended. A personal history should include life facts and explore any factors involved in initiation and perpetuation of the problem or resulting from the problem. Collectively these are termed contributing factors. (The most common factors are discussed later in this chapter.) Life facts—including demographic information, race, marital status, or household situation, occupation, income, education, family physician, and family dentist—help in understanding the patient and his situation. If significant social and psychologic problems are elicited during personal history, it is wise to have the patient seek consultation with a psychotherapist to determine the extent of problems and if intervention is required.

A medical history may reveal some genetic predisposition to a particular problem like migraine headaches or some underlying serious illness that predisposes the patient to developing pain, such as lupus erythematosus. This history should include family history of similar or other illnesses, past surgeries, hospitalizations, and medications for other reasons, the last physical examination and results, a review of allergies and communicative illnesses such as hepatitis, diabetes, acquired immune deficiency syndrome, or venereal disease. It may also reveal the possibility for health care abuse by chronic pain patients. To supplement this knowledge, a review of all body systems includes asking about past or present problems related to the head and neck, skin, cardiovascular, respiratory, gastrointestinal, genitourinary, ear, nose and throat, neurologic, obstetric-gynecologic, musculoskeletal, and pyschiatric systems.

Physical Examination

A firm diagnosis may be established at any time from initial history to weeks of diagnostic tests or trials. By the time a clinician is familiar with the patient's problem through a thorough history, the diagnosis, diagnoses, or diagnostic group of most pain conditions should come into focus. The physical examination for pain may then be used to confirm thoughts about the history, to refine the diagnosis or diagnoses, or to indicate what further diagnostic tests, consultations, or trials are necessary to secure a diagnosis.

Physical examination for craniofacial pain varies depending on the location of pain and the apparent diagnosis. A physical examination may include inspection, palpation, percussion, auscultation, smell, and measurements to ascertain if pathology that involves the chief complaint is present.[6]

General inspection can reveal considerable information about the patient and any problems to the alert clinician. Slouching posture can point to depression. Rigidity in posture or clenching can show excess muscle tension in the neck, shoulders, or jaws and may be associated with myofascial pain. Asymmetry, swelling, weakness, loss of function, dysfunction, skin changes, and other signs may lead to finding a neoplastic or infectious process. Inspection of the skin may reveal scars of past surgeries, skin trophic changes of causalgia, and color changes of a local infection or systemic anemia. The patient's facial expression can reveal specific emotions, his relationship with the dentist or others in the room, or reactions to the specific questions asked.

Palpation is the process of using touch to examine the body for abnormalities. It can include finger palpation of the muscles for myofascial trigger points, the skin for hyperesthesia in causalgia, cold hands in migraine, lymph nodes for lymphadenopathy, joints for swelling and tenderness of arthritis, abdomen for organomegaly, and the rest of the head, face, neck, or body for size or consistency changes.

Percussion of teeth with the opposite end of a mirror can elicit problems with individual teeth. Also used for detecting normal densities of the body, percussion is performed by listening to the noise of striking the left finger lying flat on the body with a sharp blow by the middle finger of the right hand. These sounds reveal abnormalities in the lungs, liver, spleen, gallbladder, stomach, and urinary bladder.

Auscultation is the act of listening for normal body sounds through a stethoscope. The bruit of an arteriovenous fistula, murmurs of the heart and vessels, rales and friction rubs of lungs, crepitus in the joints, and bowel sounds in a scrotal hernia can be detected.

Smell is important in detecting abnormal odors in the breath, sputum, vomitus, feces, urine, or pus. Infections, diabetes, lung abscess, pancreas disturbances, gas gangrene, and many other illnesses have distinctive odors. A clinician managing chronic pain patients should use all senses and be aware of the possibility for a serious underlying disease causing persistent pain.

The examination can be divided into general appearance, mental status, head and neck inspection, cranial nerve function, stomatognathic function, and myofascial palpation. A general appearance assessment notes factors such as ambulation, general malaise, postural imbalances, and general motor function. Motor function of the body includes three systems: pyramidal or corticospinal, extrapyramidal, and cerebellar.[9] Lesions of the pyramidal system can cause paralysis, weakness, and spasticity of muscles plus hyperactive deep tendon reflexes. Lesions of the extrapyramidal system cause postural instability and diminished muscle tone and function. Lesions of the cerebellar system affect coordination of movements of the trunk and extremities on the contralateral side. Central or peripheral lesions of the nervous system can also be uncovered by detecting any sensory deficits in each nerve distribution including the cranial nerves. Symptoms of numbness or tingling can be verified by accurate two point discrimination testing, pin prick tests, and light touch tests. Disturbance of stereognosis or inability to recognize size and shape of objects reflects a parietal lobe lesion. Reflex testing of the deep tendon and superficial tendons can indicate upper or lower motor neuron disease as in compression neuropathy or multiple sclerosis.

A mental status examination reveals the patient's state of awareness, general appearance, behavior, mood, affect, language function, nonverbal function, and memory. Abnormalities in mental status may point to higher cortical lesions such as intracranial neoplasm, cerebral vascular accidents, hematomas, edema, or arteriovenous malformations within or causing traction on the cortex. Disturbances of cranial nerves result from a lesion of the cranial nerve nuclei, efferent or afferent pathways associated with cranial nerves. Disturbances of the senses of smell, sight, sound, balance, taste, and touch of the face reflect a disorder affecting the cranial nerves. For example, meningitis can cause double vision, multiple sclerosis can cause optic atrophy and diminished vision, and an acoustic neuroma can cause lack of sense of hearing. The motor function of the head and neck is mediated through the trigeminal (masticatory muscles), facial (facial expression), hypoglossal (tongue), and accessory (trapezius) cranial nerves. Paralysis, gross weakness, or spasticity of these muscles would dictate further evaluation of these nerves. Head and neck inspection includes examination of structure and function of the extracranial structures of the head and neck. Stomatognathic examination includes examination and measurement of the temporomandibular joint, function of the jaw, and occlusal stability and function (Table 24-4). This may often reveal temporomandibular joint pathology such as internal derangements or degenerative joint disease. Myofascial palpation is critical in the evaluation of myofascial pain. This examination consists of palpation of specific muscular trigger point sites

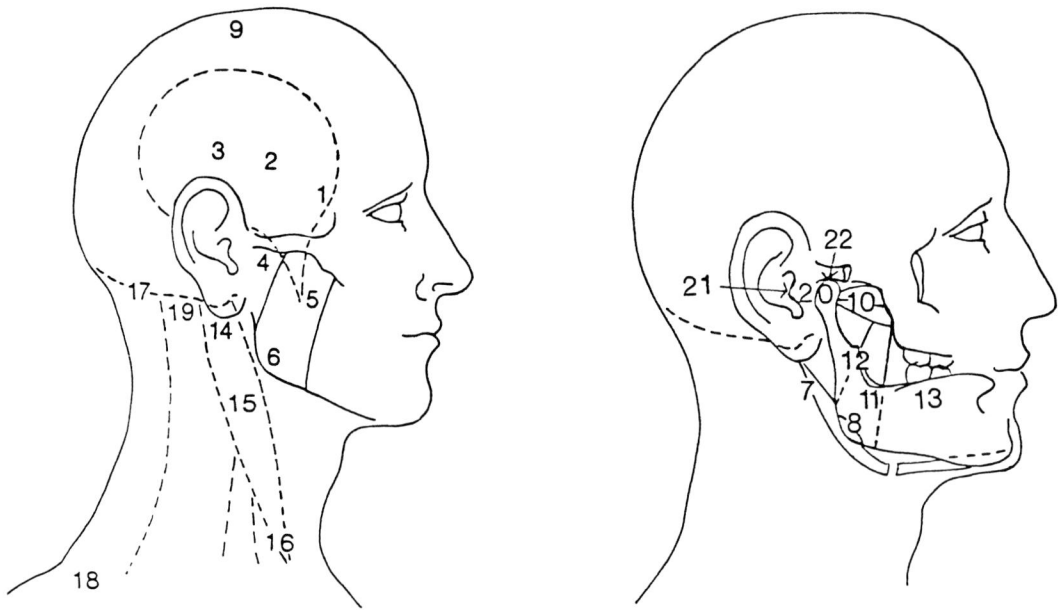

STRUCTURE

Muscle: Extraoral

1. Anterior Temporalis
2. Middle Temporalis
3. Posterior Temporalis
4. Deep Masseter
5. Anterior Masseter
6. Interior Masseter
7. Posterior Digastric
8. Medial Pterygoid
9. Vertex

Muscle: Intraoral

10. Lateral Pterygoid
11. Medial Pterygoid
12. Temporalis Insertion
13. Tongue

Muscle: Neck

14. Superior Sternocleidomastoid
15. Middle Sternocleidomastoid
16. Inferior Sternocleidomastoid
17. Insertion of Trapezius
18. Upper Trapezius
19. Splenius Capitis

TMJ

20. Lateral Capsule
21. Posterior Capsule
22. Superior Capsule

DESCRIPTION

Palpation is performed by first locating the distinct muscle band or part of joint and then palpating with the sensitive spade-like pad at the end of the distal phalanx of the index finger, using firm pressure (approximately 1 lb per square inch). The patient is asked "Does it hurt or is it just pressure?" The response is positive if palpation produces a clear reaction from patient, i.e: palpebral response, or if patient stated that the palpation "hurt" indicating that the site was clearly more tender than surrounding structures or contralateral structure. Any equivocal response by the patient would be scored as negative.

(From Fricton, J., and Schiffman, E.: Reliability of a craniomandibular index. J. Dent. Res., 65:1359, 1986.)

FIG. 24-1. *Description of palpation technique for head and neck muscles and temporomandibular joint.*

TABLE 24-4. *Stomatognathic examination*

Mandibular Movement (MM) (Normal Values in Parentheses)
Maximum Opening (incisor to incisor)
    ☐☐ mm (40-60)
Passive Stretch Opening (incisor to incisor)
    ☐☐ mm (42-62)
Restriction on Opening
Pain on Opening
Jerky Opening
"S" Deviation on Opening (≤ 2mm)
Lateral Deviation on Opening (≤ 2mm)
Protrusion—Pain
Protrusion—Limitation ☐ mm (≥ 7mm)
Right Laterotrusion—Pain
Right Laterotrusion—Limitation ☐ mm (≥ 7mm)
Left Laterotrusion—Pain
Left Laterotrusion—Limitation ☐ mm (≥ 7mm)
Clinically can lock open (subluxate, right or left)
Clinically can or is locked closed (right or left)
Rigidity of Jaw Upon Manipulation
TMJ Noise (TN)
Reciprocal Click ....
(Reciprocal Flim w/Mandibular Repositioning)
Reproducible Opening Click ....
Reproducible Laterotrusive Click Only ....
Reproducible Closing Click ....
Nonreproducible Opening or Closing Click ....
Crepitus—Fine ....
Crepitus—Coarse ....
Popping (audible) ....

for tenderness and alteration in the pain complaints (Fig. 24-1).

Differential Diagnosis of Craniofacial Pain

To simplify the process of obtaining a physical diagnosis, a working classification of craniofacial pain is essential.[10]

This classification method divides oral and craniofacial pain into eight groups, with each representing a different origin of pain. These origins of pain generally coincide with the type of tissue affected by the disorder. Each tissue type develops pain-producing pathology in a distinct manner, and the pain associated with it generally has unique characteristics and descriptions (Table 24-5). These characteristics can be used as initial information in arriving at a diagnosis, since the first thing a clinician asks a patient is "what are the symptoms?" The patient describes the qualities of his signs and symptoms and, in particular, describes the pain. The general description of the pain can lead a clinician to begin thinking toward ruling out any general

diagnostic group. Once the general diagnostic group is obtained, the specific diagnosis within that group can be deduced with added information from the history, examination, or diagnostic studies. This systematic approach helps the clinician simplify the diagnosis of complex chronic pain states, since frequent multiple diagnoses and psychologic symptoms can confuse the diagnostic process.

Different diagnoses can be elicited by closely listening to the patient's description of the various aspects of the pain experience and assessing if more than one experience and, potentially, more than one disorder is present. For example, a patient may complain of a constant dull ache in front of the ear and a periodic throbbing headache. Two patterns of pain are described and lead a clinician to consider ruling out a myofascial or rheumatic diagnosis for the ear pain and a vascular diagnosis for the throbbing pain. Knowledge of the general diagnostic group also helps to determine the appropriate somatic treatment. Different types of treatment are appropriate for different tissues affected, and thus, the diagnostic group is helpful. For example, physical and postural therapy is generally appropriate for all diagnoses within the myofascial group.

The eight diagnostic groups and their origins and characteristics are outlined in Table 24-6. It is important to be aware that the general symptom of each group has varying intensities and verbal descriptors adding to the difficulty in diagnosis. This general classification can help lead to the direction of an appropriate specific diagnosis, but obtaining all possible knowledge about the patient and the pain problem allows the clinician to exclude each diagnosis within each group until a definitive physical diagnosis is obtained. As the clinician obtains more knowledge about the patient and the problem, each general diagnostic group is ruled out with more confidence. Oral, facial, head, or neck pain resulting from diseases of extracranial structure or any intracranial pathology should be the first diagnostic groups ruled out. This includes lesions or pathology of the tooth pulp, periapical area, periodontium, eyes, ears, nose, throat, tongue, sinuses, and salivary glands. The general practitioner often rules out this diagnostic group, but scru-

TABLE 24-5. *General characteristics of each craniofacial pain diagnostic group*

	Diseases of Extracranial Structures	Diseases of Intracranial Structures	Migraine	Vascular Diseases Cluster	Arteritis
Basic Quality	Varies	Aching	Throbbing	Throbbing with ache	Throbbing with burning ache
Common Locations	Related to structure affected	Varies	Unilateral, frontal, temporal	Unilateral, periorbital Upper face	Area of artery Temples
Duration	Constant Varies	Varies	1–2 days	Minutes	Hrs.–days
Frequency	Intermittent Progressive	Progressive	Episodic	Clusters of days to wks. Remissions of mo. to yrs.	Persistent Progressive
Onset	All ages	All ages	Young, night	20–50 yrs., night	Over 50 years
Common Patient	None	None	Family history	Smoking, male	Polymyalgia rheumatica
Characteristic Signs/Symptoms	Sinus, periodontium, tooth pulp, eye, ear, nose, throat, salivary glands, lymph gland disorders	Seizures, loss of consciousness Loss of neurologic function Mental and emotional changes	Visual prodroma G.I. symptoms Hypersensitive to external stimuli Cold extremities	Lacrimation, rhinorrhea, perspiration, Horner's Syndrome, no prodroma, severe pain	Tender, swollen artery, fever, malaise, leads to blindness
Factors that Precipitate Pain	Inflammation, neoplasia, degeneration, obstruction, edema, compression	Hematoma, hemorrhage, abscess, neoplasm, angioma, aneurysm, edema	Dietary factors, tyramine, hypoglycemia, stress, alcohol, hypertension (D = 120)	Vasodilators Alcohol	Continuous
Factors that Aggravate Pain	Varies	Movement, straining	MAO inhibitors, stress, tension, estrogen imbalance	Stress, tension Vasodilators	Lying position Mastication
Factors that Alleviate Pain	Varies Reduction of cause	Reduction of cause	Hold head still Vasoconstrictors	Vasoconstrictors Walking around, Distractors	Upright position Pressure in artery
Key Diagnostic Determinants in Addition to Characteristics	Refer to specialists to rule out pathology	Arteriogram, EEG, MR scan, CT scan radiographs, not relieved with nerve block	Family history Relief with ergot	Family history, brought on with subcutaneous histamine or sublingual nitroglycerin	Biopsy of artery Elevated E.S.R.
Comment	Can display all types of pain	Should be ruled out first in all cases	Vasoconstriction and resultant vasodilation	Irritation of sphenopalatine ganglion Histamine release	Inflammation of vessel
Treatment	Specific treatment for underlying disease	Specific treatment for underlying disease Urgent	Ergotamine (abortive), stress reduction, biofeedback, Propranolol (prophylactic), Cyroheptamine (prophylactic children)	Similar to migraine	Prednisone 50 mg, alt. days for 2 wks. Urgent, check E.S.R.

TABLE 24-5. *Cont.*

	Myofascial Disorders	Rheumatic Disorders (Temporomandibular Joint)	Neuralgic Disorders Paroxysmal	Neuralgic Disorders Continuous	Causalgic	Psychogenic Disorders
Basic Quality	Steady ache	Steady ache	Sharp Shooting	Paresthesia	Burning	Descriptive
Common Locations	Head, neck, shoulders Pain can move	In ear Periauricular	Follows nerve distribution	Follows nerve distribution	Area of nerve Trauma	Unusual distribution
Duration	Constant	Constant	Seconds	Constant	Constant	Constant
Frequency	Fluctuates Nonprogressive	Fluctuates Nonprogressive	Intermittent	Fluctuates Nonprogressive	Fluctuates Nonprogressive	Continual
Onset	All ages	All ages	Usually older ages	After nerve damage	All ages	All ages
Common Patient	Female	None	None	Herpetic: Elderly	None	
Characteristic Signs/ Symptoms	Limitation of motion Occlusal disharmony Muscle tenderness Autonomic signs	Limitation of motion Crepitus, clicking, popping	Trigger area present, related to nerve affected	Herpetic: History of vesicular eruptions Dysesthesias	Hyperesthesia Eventual skin changes	Dull affect, indifferent toward pain, social and occupational incapacitation, life-threatening physical illness or emotional trauma
Factors that Precipitate Pain	Stress, tension, bruxism, clenching, trauma, sustained jaw opening, occlusal disharmony	Aging, repetitive microtrauma, macrotrauma	Touch or movement of trigger area	Touch, pressure, movement of area	Light touch	Psychologic trauma
Factors that Aggravate Pain	Strengthening exercise, immobility, cold weather, systemic disorders, stress	Movement, chewing Occlusal disharmony Yawning	Cold wind, activity Stress	Activity, stress, touch, movement of area	Movement, chewing, occlusal disharmony Yawning	Threatening situation Psychologic trauma
Factors that Alleviate Pain	Massage, heat, stretching exercise, relaxation	Rest, heat, cold Occlusal adjustment	Nerve block Avoid stimulating area	Nerve block	Relaxation Activity	Generally none reported
Key Diagnostic Determinants in Addition to Characteristics	Palpation of muscle trigger point and referral of pain Trigger point injection	Examination Radiograph	Nerve block	Pain distribution Nerve block	Stellate ganglion block	Rule out all other Dx first. Not relieved with nerve block Psychiatric history
Comment	Associated with TMJ disorders, muscle degeneration at site of muscle spindles with referral of pain to distant area	Frequently associated with myofascial pain of joint	Compression neuropathy	Damage to nerve due to herpes zoster virus or trauma	Hypersympathetic activity in area of trauma	Symbolic attempt to solve emotional turmoil
Treatment	Physiotherapy, occlusal therapy, acupuncture, trigger point injection stress, bruxism reduction, muscle relaxants	Stabilization splint and physiotherapy Occlusal rehabilitation Anti-inflammatory drugs, surgery	Carbamazepine Diphenylhydantoin, neurosurgery, acupuncture, hypnosis	Amitriptyline and anticonvulsants Steroid injection early in area for herpes, zoster, acupuncture and hypnosis	Stellate ganglion block Hypnosis	Guidance Situational therapy Psychotherapy

(From Fricton, J., and Kroening, R.: Practical differential diagnosis of chronic craniofacial pain. Oral Surg., 54:28, 1982.)

TABLE 24-6. *Diagnostic groups for craniofacial pain; origins and characteristics of pain*

Diagnostic Group	Origin of Pain	Basic Characteristic of Pain
Extracranial	Teeth and craniofacial organs	Varies
Intracranial	Brain and related structures	Varies
Vascular	Vascular system	Throbbing
Myofascial	Muscles and connective tissue	Steady ache or band
Rheumatic	Bones, ligaments	Periauricular ache
Neuralgic	Peripheral nervous system	Paresthesia along nerve
Causalgic	Autonomic nervous system	Burning hyperesthesia
Psychogenic	Mental functioning	Descriptive

tiny can lead to discovering a less obvious diagnosis such as a split or cracked tooth syndrome. After pain from extracranial structures is ruled out, intracranial disorders, which are of serious and immediate concern, should be carefully ruled out before progressing to the other diagnostic groups. If doubt exists in doing this, both the patient and the clinician can become more confident by obtaining appropriate consultation. Once done, the history, physical examination, and further diagnostic studies can lead the clinician to the correct diagnosis or diagnoses from the remaining groups. The specific diagnoses listed in each table are the most common disorders of each group. They do not make up a complete list.

Extracranial Group

Diseases of various head and neck organs and structures should be suspected first in any craniofacial pain condition (Table 24-7). The tooth pulp, periapical structures, periodontium, eyes, ears, nose, throat, tongue, sinuses, and salivary glands should be thoroughly evaluated with clinical, radiographic, or laboratory examination to rule out infectious, degenerative, edematous, neoplastic, or obstructive processes that may cause pain. Pain from this group varies from paroxysmal lancinating pain (as in pressure upon a nerve by tumor) to a throbbing of a tooth pulp and the dull ache of a sinus infection. Severity varies from excruciating in osteomyelitis to mild, as in periodontal disease. This group includes the tight, crushing, pressing pain from the sternum to the jaws that occurs during increased physical effort. This is

TABLE 24-7. *Diseases of extracranial structure*

Structures	Diseases
Tooth pulp	Infectious
Periapical structures	Degenerative
Periodontium	Edematous
Eye	Neoplastic
Ear	Obstructive
Nose	
Throat	
Sinuses	
Salivary glands	
Tongue	
Lymph glands	
Skin	

the pain of coronary artery disease. Glaucoma displays retrobulbar pain with a reduction in vision and visual haloes around lights.

Pain within the ear can be caused by a disease within the ear and related structures as in acoustic neuroma, otitis media, or mastoiditis, or can be referred from other structures such as the teeth, temporomandibular joint, tonsils, tongue, throat, trachea, or thyroid.[11,12]

Salivary gland disorders such as in Sjögrens syndrome can cause pain and tenderness usually associated with inflammation in the specific gland. In Sjögrens syndrome, parotitis is generally associated with diminished salivation, lacrimation, and a connective tissue disorder such as systemic lupus erythematosus or rheumatoid arthritis.[13]

Treatment of pain in this group consists of correcting or eliminating the cause of the pain. Some pain may persist after treatment since pain or disease may contribute to stress and tension and consequent development of myofascial pain.

Sinusitis is a common cause of a dull constant pain.[14] The location can vary from the maxilla and maxillary teeth as in maxillary sinusitis, upper orbit and frontal process in frontal sinusitis, between and behind the eyes from ethmoid sinusitis, and the junction of hard and soft palate, occiput and mastoid process in sphenoid sinusitis. Other characteristics include an elevated white blood count, stuffy nose, blood-tinged mucus, fever and malaise, postnasal drip, edema and inflamed turbinates, and radiographic or transillumination changes.

Intracranial Group

After all diseases of the extracranial structures are ruled out, it is critical to rule out intracranial pathology as the cause of pain (Table 24-8). Although this is a rare cause of pain in teeth, maxilla, and mandible, a neurologic or neurosurgical evaluation is critical to rule out space-occupying lesions such as tumors, hematomas, and arteriovenous malformations, if neurologic signs and symptoms suggest this. Intracranial causes of head and neck pain can be classified into two groups: those from traction of pain-sensitive structures and those from specific central nervous system syndromes.[15,16,17]

Pain-sensitive areas intracranially include venous sinuses, middle meningeal vessels, large arteries at the base of the brain, intracranial arteries, pia and dura mater, and cranial nerves. Pressure, trauma, spasm, contraction, and inflammation can cause pain within these structures and refer to all areas of the head, face, and neck. The quality can vary greatly between a generalized throbbing or aching to a more specific paroxysmal sharp pain. Associated with intracranial lesions can be many different neurologic signs or

deficits, such as: diminished reflexes, paresthesias, loss of hearing, tinnitus, visual disturbances, dizziness, inappropriate nausea and vomiting, ataxia, loss of corneal reflex, and weakness of facial or masticatory muscles. Patients may show variable concerns depending upon the acuteness of chronicity of the pain. These may be accompanied by gross personality changes or changes in levels of consciousness. If neurologic signs or deficits appear with a chronic craniofacial pain complaint, pain from intracranial sources must be ruled out.

A diagnosis is established through an appropriate neurologic examination of the head and neck, cranial nerves, motor, reflex, and sensory functions, and a mental status evaluation. Further explorations for diagnosis include EEG studies, radiograph skull series, computerized tomography scans, magnetic resonance imaging, arteriogram, lumbar puncture, brain scan, electromyography, diagnostic nerve blocks, and systemic disease laboratory investigations. Local anesthetic nerve blocks of the area of pain does not usually relieve pain from intracranial lesions. Head pain associated with space occupying lesions, such as tumor and edema, are described as deep, aching, steady, and dull. It is generally continuous and progressive and may be more intense in the morning. Coughing, straining, or sudden head motion aggravate the pain while aspirin, cold packs, and lying down alleviate it. If the lesion compresses a cranial nerve, a paroxysmal neuralgic complaint usually results. If the lesion is in the occipital area, a stiff aching neck and a tipping of the head toward the side of the lesion are evident. Treatment of these lesions, when appropriately diagnosed, requires neurosurgical intervention or appropriate medical treatment for that particular diagnosis.

Intracranial syndromes displaying chronic head and neck pain include benign and malignant lesions, meningitis, thalamic pain syndromes, and phantom pain syndromes.[8,16] Neurofibromatosis (Von Recklinghausen's Disease) is a genetic disorder characterized by pigmented skin lesions (café au lait spots), and multiple tumors of the spinal nerves, cranial nerves and skin. Clinical manifestations of pain

TABLE 24-8. *Disorders of intracranial structure*

Traction	Syndromes
Neoplastic	Neurofibromatosis
Aneurysmal	Meningitic
Abscess	Thalamic
Hematoma, hemorrhage	Phantom
Edema	
Angioma	

include headaches due to neurofibromata of cranial nerves producing increased cranial pressure. Numbness, paresthesias, and muscle weakness with involvement of the V, VII, VIII, and X cranial nerves are also associated with the syndrome. Diagnosis is made on clinical signs and symptoms and, in particular, the skin lesions. There are no somatic treatments other than tumor resection and palliative pain management.

Head pain from acute bacterial meningitis is related to the lowered pain thresholds of inflamed intracranial tissues. A throbbing pain at the base of the brain, it increases with each cardiac cycle and lowering of the head. The pain is usually accompanied by fever, vomiting, and stiff neck. Diagnosis is determined by lumbar puncture and cerebrospinal fluid analysis to determine if a pyogenic or viral meningitis exists. Appropriate medical treatment is directed by an accurate diagnosis for bacterial, fungal, or viral meningitis.

The thalamic syndrome is usually caused by a cerebral vascular accident that involves the vascular supply to the thalamus area in addition to the generalized cerebral apoplexy with distinct motor deficits, impairment of sensory perception, and disturbances in eye movements such as paralyzed upward gaze. Patients may complain of a protopathic burning pain with hyperalgesia and hyperpathia after the acute episode has resolved. It can occur on the entire ipsilateral side of the face or contralateral side of the trunk or limbs. Diagnosis is made on signs and symptoms as well as neuroradiologic studies.

Phantom pain, or central pain phenomenon, is a severe chronic pain associated with an amputated part of the body. It generally occurs with the extremities but can occur with different head and neck structures such as the nose or teeth. The pain may be similar to any pain before amputation or can resemble muscle pain or cramping. It is often alleviated with either cutaneous stimulation by rubbing or transcutaneous electrical nerve stimulation or by local anesthetic block. The pain is often aggravated with light touch to the stump or movement of it. Treatment generally has a poor prognosis but can include hypnosis, nerve blocks, transcutaneous electrical nerve stimulation, drugs, or acupuncture.

Vascular Group

The general symptom of vascular pain is a throbbing, pulsating pain (Table 24-9).

A *classic migraine headache* may begin as an ache but usually develops into a throbbing, pulsating, or beating nature as often described.[9,18,19] It is episodic and can last anywhere from several hours to days with short to long remissions. A visual prodromata or aura occurs 10 to 30 minutes prior to the onset of pain. These include blind spots (scotomata), zigzag patterns (teichopsia), flashing lights (photopsia), photophobia, dysesthesias, and other visual or auditory sensations. *Common migraine headache* is similar to classic migraine but proceeds into a headache without prodromata. Both types of migraines generally occur unilaterally in the frontal, temporal, or retrobulbar areas. Other symptoms include nausea, vomiting, diarrhea, hypersensitivity to noise, odors, and other stimuli, cold extremities, water retention, edema, and sweating. The usual onset of migraine occurs between the ages of 20 and 40, but can begin in childhood. Seventy percent of patients have a family history of migraine. Precipitating factors include stress and fatigue, foods rich in tyramine and nitrates, red wines and alcohol, histamines and vasodilators, thyroid diseases and estrogen imbalances. Once an attack occurs, a patient may hold his head rigid to prevent aggravation of the pain and develop myofascial and tension headaches in addition to the migraine. These are termed mixed headaches and both must be recognized and treated. If confusion exists about the diagnosis of migraine, .5 mg of ergotamine administered intramuscularly can be used to abort a migraine headache (but not other types).

Ergotamine (.5 mg I.M. for abortive therapy or 7 mg b. i. d. orally for prophylaxis), methysergide maleate (2 mg t. i. d.),

TABLE 24-9. *Vascular Disorders*

Migraine: Classic
Common
Complicated: Ophthalmoplegic/Hemiplegic
Cluster headache (ache with throbbing)
Cranial arteritis (ache with throbbing)
Toxic or metabolic vascular headache
Hypertensive headache
Carotidynia

and other migraine medications act to counter the rebound cranial vasodilation that occurs in migraine after the aura indicates vasoconstriction. The poorly understood vasoconstrictive phase occurs as a result of a variety of stimuli, including deposition of immune factors, ischemia, injury, activation of the Hageman factor, deposition of bacterial toxins, or muscular tension. This vasoconstriction begins a series of neurohumoral and vasohumoral reactions that result in a rebound vasodilation and resultant throbbing. Histamine, serotonin, SRS-A, prostaglandins, complement, and kinins have been implicated in this reaction. The more unusual and complicated forms of migraine include ophthalmoplegic and hemiplegic forms that develop distinct neurologic deficits outlasting the headache.[9,18,19] These may include transitory, partial or permanent monocular blindness, third nerve palsy, hemiparesis for days to weeks, hemisensory deficits, and occlusion of the retinal artery. These occur in less than 1 to 2 percent of migraine patients and usually have a strong family history. Hypertensive migraine can occur in hypertensive patients when their diastolic blood pressure rises above 120 mm of mercury. Usually it is worse upon arising and is reduced later in the day. Metabolic migraine occurs infrequently in some patients with fever, increased CO_2 retention, hypoglycemia, and toxic vascular substances. Toxic migraine can occur secondary to ingestion of excessive amounts of monosodium glutamate, alcohol, caffeine, nitrites, and carbon monoxide inhalation. Migraine-like head aches may also occur with caffeine withdrawal.

Cluster headaches differ from classic migraine headaches primarily in the pattern of occurrence and description of pain.[9,20] They occur in "clusters" of days to weeks with periods of remission of months to sometimes years. During a cluster period, headaches occur an average of six times in a day with a duration of 5 to 10 minutes. The pain is a continuous, intense ache with throbbing occurring with movements that increase blood flow to the head. The most common site is unilaterally around and behind the eye and in the maxilla, but can be in the temples and down into the jaws— rarely to the lower jaw and neck. It has been called a "lower half headache" be-

cause of its physical location. An aura is rarely associated with cluster headaches, but nasal stuffiness, lacrimation, rhinorrhea, conjunctivitis, perspiration, and Horner's syndrome are characteristic. Cluster headaches are found eight times more frequently in males than in females (and particularly in males who smoke). It is possible that chronic irritation of the sphenopalatine ganglion by smoke may cause autonomic instability, release of histamine and other substances, vasodilation, and pain. This is supported by the findings that intranasal stimulation of the sphenopalatine ganglia can mimic a cluster headache and nerve blocks of the ganglion will alleviate it. High histamine levels are also found with a headache. Thus, cluster headaches are also termed sphenopalatine ganglion neuralgia, histaminic headache, Horton's headache, Sluder's headache, and ciliary headache. Symptoms may resemble a cerebral vascular accident. Diagnosis is based on signs and symptoms as well as family history. Treatment is similar to migraine therapy, but prednisone (30 mg for 10 to 14 alternate days), lithium, and chlorpromazine (100-250 mg/day) have also been utilized.

Cranial arteritis resembles a migraine attack in that both have persistent throbbing qualities and last hours to days.[21,22] The difference lies with an additional quantitative burning ache in cranial arteritis, as well as additional signs and symptoms, including an elevated erythrocyte sedimentation rate (ESR), and the onset of pain occurring in patients over age 50. It is often seen with polymyalgia rheumatica. Since arteritis may be presented as a febrile disease, one is likely to see malaise, fatigue, anorexia, prostration, leukocytosis, or weight loss. Arterial inflammation can occur in any artery but generally affects the external carotid arteries such as the temporal artery and other major vessels of the upper aortic tree. The pain is frequently in the anatomic area of the artery, generally found unilaterally in the temples as in temporal arteritis or in and around the eye with ophthalmic arteritis. Pain can also radiate to the ear, zygoma, and occiput. Generalized scalp tenderness is also a common complaint. An examination of the artery reveals tenderness, a thickening enlargement, and lack of normal pulse. The pain increases with lowering of the head, palpation of the artery, mastication, and movements that create increased blood flow to that artery. Digital pressure with occlusion of the artery frequently alleviates the symptoms. Headache of similar origin can also be associated with periarteritis nodosa, connective tissue diseases, and hypersensitivity angiitis. Histologic examination of the artery reveals the elastic tissue to be frayed and giant cells are almost always found in the vessel walls. Anticapillary antibodies and immune deposits containing IgG are implicated in the inflammation. Definitive diagnosis should be established immediately as aggressive cases can lead to partial or complete blindness. Diagnosis is based on an elevated ESR above 45 mm/hr as well as arterial biopsy. Treatment includes emergency dosages of steriods (40-60 mg prednisone daily) and then with reduced ESR, a maintenance dose of 10-20 mg prednisone as clinically determined.

Carotidynia is characterized by throbbing pain overlying the carotid artery in the neck and submandibular area.[21] The pain is often associated with tenderness, swelling, and irritation of the carotid artery. It must be differentiated from superior laryngeal neuralgia by the lack of pain relief with a block of that nerve, absence of hoarseness, and absence of paralysis of the ipsilateral cricothyroid muscle on laryngoscopy. Treatment of it includes those medications found to be helpful for migraine if an arteritis has been ruled out.

Myofascial Group

The myofascial group consists of myofascial pain dysfunction syndrome (MPD), tension headaches, muscle contracture, recurrent muscle spasm, mixed tension/vascular headache, and muscular pain secondary to connective tissue diseases (Table 24-10). This group has a general pain description of continuous dull ache or band-like quality and is the most common cause of head and neck pain, although not generally the most severe.

Myofascial pain is also termed myofascitis, myofibrositis, fibrositis, and is included as part of the temporomandibular joint pain dysfunction syndrome.[23,24,25] The complexity of this syndrome make it difficult to diagnose and treat.

TABLE 24-10. *Myofascial disorders*

Myofascial pain (MPD) or TMJ pain dysfunction
Tension headache
Mixed tension/vascular
Contracture
Recurrent spasm
Secondary to connective tissue disease

It consists of a dull, steady ache perceived in a zone of reference that is referred to that area by trigger points within muscles distant from the area. The pain can be located in any structure of the head and neck with the most common areas being the vertex, frontal, temporal, temporomandibular joint, ear, occiput, and periorbital.

The trigger points are tender and firm nodular or rope-like areas located in the belly of skeletal musculature. Histologically, there is a high content of motor end plates, fatty deposits, lack of uniform striation, increase in mast cells and lactic acid accumulation, as well as increase in excitability of motor neurons within trigger areas termed a "local twitch response."[26] Clinically active trigger points display tenderness upon deep digital palpation with alteration of the pain complaints. Latent trigger points show tenderness with no alteration or referral of pain. Dermatographia of the skin over the muscle, weakness, and slight tightness of the muscle, as well as hyperactive stretch reflexes, are seen. Trigger points and related zones of reference are reproducible in most patients and display consistent patterns of referral. Extinction of the trigger points alleviates the referred pain, as well as other associated symptoms. The complexity of this syndrome lies in these numerous associated symptoms that can confuse the clinician and lead to misdiagnosis and mistreatment. These other symptoms include tinnitus, scratchiness, tearing, blurring of the eyes, ptosis, dysesthesias, dental hypersensitivity, increased salivation, nausea and vomiting, diminished hearing, coryza, dizziness, sweating and flushing of skin, edema, and asymmetry of jaws. This syndrome, often seen as an overlying diagnosis, is easily confused with other head and neck pain problems.

The pathophysiologic process originates with sustained muscle contraction or trauma. This may result from reactions to stress, poor postures, clenching, bruxism, systemic disorders, connective tissue disease, and other contributing factors. It is usually involved in vicious pain cycles beginning with muscle strain and continued by psychosocial stress, pathology, or trauma that results in trigger points with continued pain. This creates more stress and more muscle tension, and the self-perpetuating cycle continues.

Treatment lies in reducing the contributing factors as well as the trigger points. Stress reduction can be achieved with behavioral change and education; counseling, meditative techniques, biofeedback, self-hypnosis, or exercise. Alleviation of contributing factors such as occlusal disharmony, postural habits, bruxism, clenching, metabolic, or infectious processes is also important to prevent recurrence. Extinction of trigger points is accomplished through passive and active stretching of the musculature involved with prior application of a counter stimulant such as moist heat or vapocoolant spray (fluorimethane). Needling of the trigger point with injection of local anesthetic or normal saline, or acupuncture can reduce a trigger point. Also helpful is manipulation of the muscle through deep massage as in Rolfing and acupressure, ultrasonic massage, or transcutaneous electrical nerve stimulation. Progressive stretching exercises are an integral part of all therapy for myofascial disorders.

Tension headaches differ from myofascial pain in the quality of the pain.[27] They are often described as a tight band-like pain in muscles such as the temporalis, splenius capitis, or frontalis. Latent trigger points and muscle tenderness may be found. Electromyographic (EMG) levels of all the muscle may be high.

Management of this problem is similar to that of myofascial pain. Additionally, muscle relaxants (diazepam 5-10 mg t.i.d.) can be helpful for short periods while self-control techniques are learned by the patient.

Spasm of muscle occurs from the overstretching of previously weakened muscles, protective splinting, and subsequent acute muscle shortening. The muscle has gross limitation of movement and significant pain. Commonly termed a "charley horse," it can occur after sustained opening with dental work. A normal jaw opening of 40 to 50 mm may be reduced to 10 to 20 mm with contracture. If left untreated and shortened for several weeks, a decrease in pain with fibrous scarring or contracture occurs. Some "lock jaws" and organic torticollis result from contracture. Treatment of both spasm and contracture consists of gradual active stretching for 3 to 7 days with simultaneous application of counter stimulation with physical therapy modalities until restoration of original function is achieved.

Collagen diseases such as lupus erythematosus, scleroderma, and rheumatoid arthritis also cause myofascial type of pain.[13] Treatment is similar to that of myofascial pain and is coupled with treatment of the basic systemic disease.

Rheumatic Group

This group has a general characteristic of periauricular ache and involves intrinsic lesions of the temporomandibular joint, including traumatic derangement, capsulitis, and arthritis of various types (Table 24-11). Cervical spine disorders are also included in this group. It is possible to have several of these diagnoses affecting one joint. It is common to find myofascial pain associated with joint pathology and jaw dysfunction, thus the term myofascial pain dysfunction, or temporomandibular joint dysfunction syndrome, which often refers to both diagnoses.

Internal derangement of the temporomandibular joint may be clinically observed as clicking, popping, or locking of the joint upon opening or closing.[28,29,30] Attendant signs and symptoms may include preauricular ache, limitation of motion, fullness in the ear, locking of the jaw, hypermobility of the jaw, tinnitus, dizziness, and deviation of jaw upon opening or closing. Occlusal disharmony such as loss of posterior teeth, overclosure of jaws, and occlusal interferences in retruded and lateral movements may contribute to strain of the joint. Trauma to the joint resulting from accidents or the microtrauma of bruxism can also contribute to its development. Radiographic analysis of the joint by means of tomograms may reveal only a

TABLE 24-11. *Rheumatic—temporomandibular joint disorders*

TMJ capsulitis
TMJ derangement
TMJ arthritis: Polyarthritis
                Septic
                Traumatic
                Metabolic
                Rheumatoid
Cervical arthritis
Cervical ligament disorder
Disorder - secondary to rheumatic disease

mild posterior displacement of the condyle in the glenoid fossa, but arthrograms may reveal an anterior displacement of the articular disk. Functional analysis of the clicking joint reveals excessive caudal or posterior pressure on the disc, causing it to be extruded rapidly to the lateral or posterior direction upon opening and creating a clicking or popping noise or to be lodged anterior to the condyle creating locking. Treatment, depending on the specific nature of the derangement, may consist of surgical correction, redirecting the position of the condyle through mandibular repositioning with splints, and occlusal treatments or physiotherapy to recoordinate and rehabilitate the musculature.

Capsulitis, an inflammation of the pericapsular structures of the temporomandibular joint,[28,29] may present as a preauricular ache that is exacerbated with movement. It is usually associated with a structural disorder of the joint as a result of trauma. Diagnosis is confirmed by digital pressure posterior and lateral to the capsule with resultant tenderness of the capsule of the joint. It will be alleviated by infiltration of local anesthetic and aggravated by functions such as chewing or talking.

Arthritis of the temporomandibular joint can be divided into two general groups, osteoarthritis and rheumatoid arthritis.[28,29,31] Osteoarthritis includes postseptic, traumatic and metabolic arthritis, depending on the cause. Symptoms include a vague, dull ache in the preauricular area that is exacerbated by movement. The distinguishing clinical factor of arthritis is crepitus, grating, or cracking of the joint with active movement. Limitation in movement of the jaw may also occur. Radio-

graphic examination of the condyle reveals decreased joint space, subchondral sclerosis, cystic formation, surface erosions, osteophytes, or marginal lipping. The articular eminence may be flattened or eroded or may contain osteophytes. All laboratory findings are usually within normal limits.

Osteoarthritis may affect only the temporomandibular joint or involve many joints.[13,32] Degenerative osteoarthritis can affect most of the weight-bearing joints and includes Heberden's nodes of the terminal phalangeal joints. It usually affects females more than males and is progressive with age. Septic arthritis is related to degeneration of joints due to systemic infections that localize in a particular joint. Metabolic arthritis is related to degeneration of joints due to endocrine disturbances, such as hypothyroidism, acromegaly, and gout. Traumatic arthritis of the temporomandibular joint can occur unilaterally or bilaterally, and results from repetitive microtrauma from unusual occlusal forces or macrotrauma through accidents and injuries.

Treatment of osteoarthritis includes analgesics (aspirin or other nonsteroidal anti-inflammatory medication) for pain and the anti-inflammatory effects and physical therapy that includes rest, reduction of pressure on the joint, moist heat, or ultrasound. Reduction of the occlusal pressure on the joint can be accomplished via a maxillary or mandibular stabilization splint and through bruxism or clenching reduction. High intracapsular condylectomy or joint reconstruction with homografts or synthetic material is indicated for severe persistent symptoms that are transiently relieved by other methods.[31]

Symptoms of cervical osteoarthritis include crepitus on flexion, extension and rotation of the head, as well as dull to sharp pain on motion that may refer to the neck, shoulder, or occiput.[33] The delicacy of the cervical vertebrae and close proximity of the nerve roots to the joints of Luschka create a high incidence of degenerative joint problems in the cervical vertebrae, in particular, the C_4-C_5 and C_5-C_6 levels. Radiographic analysis may reveal osteophytic spurs at the joint spaces and osteophyte encroachment of the intervertebrae foramina. Whiplash injuries frequently precipitate a pain syndrome previously quiesent from underlying cervical osteoarthritis or inflamation and hypermobility of the vertebral ligaments. These ligaments may refer pain to the posterior neck, occiput, and center of the forehead.

Rheumatoid arthritis is an autoimmune systemic disorder that may resemble osteoarthritis in symptoms but occurs more often in young to middle-aged persons.[13] It affects smaller weight-bearing joints such as proximal phalangeal joints and includes the temporomandibular joint in 50 to 60 percent of cases. The symptoms decrease with function and spontaneous exacerbations and remissions can occur. Radiographic changes include gross deformities such as erosions, marginal proliferations, and flattening that are greater than occurs in osteoarthritis. This condition occasionally leads to open bite or ankylosis of the joints. Diagnosis is based on clinical characteristics, and elevated ESR, and a positive RA factor.

Treatment of the temporomandibular joint involvement is similar to the systemic disease itself, and includes analgesics and anti-inflammatory agents such as aspirin (4 g/day), indomethacin (25 mg t. i. d.), ibuprofen (400 mg q. i. d.), corticosterioids such as prednisone (10 mg daily), gold salts, and penicillamine. Physical therapy, occlusal treatment, and reduction of habits are other supportive measures. Surgical intervention is limited to severe cases with marked dysfunction.

Neuralgic Group

The general symptom of this group is a paresthesia-like pain along a distinct nerve distribution. Neuralgic pains fall into two main groups: those of a paroxysmal nature and those of a continuous nature (Table 24-12). Paroxysmal neuralgias include trigeminal neuralgia (tic douloureux), glossopharyngeal neuralgia, facial nerve neuralgia, occipital neuralgia, superior laryngeal neuralgia, nervus intermedius neuralgia, and Eagle's syndrome.[8,9,17,34,35] A paroxysmal lancinating sharp pain that follows a distinct unilateral course is common to all of these except the pains of facial nerve neuralgia. The pain is often described as electric-like, shooting, cutting, or stabbing. Attacks may last only a few seconds to minutes, with no discomfort in between attacks. They may occur intermit-

TABLE 24-12. *Neuralgic disorders*

Paroxysmal:	Trigeminal
	Occipital
	Glossopharyngeal
	Facial
	Nervus intermedius
	Superior laryngeal
	Eagle's syndrome
Continuous:	Postherpetic
	Post traumatic
	Postsurgical

tently, with days to months between a series of attacks. Patients may notice a vague prodromata of tingling as well as occasional ache after an attack. A trigger area on the skin or oral mucosa is located within the distribution of the nerve affected. Neural blockade of this area almost always relieves the pain for the duration of action of the local anesthetic. Should neural blockade not relieve the symptoms, either the diagnosis or the nerve block technique should be questioned.

With the exception of Eagle's syndrome, most paroxysmal neuralgias occur in elderly patients and are usually related to a neuropathic process secondary to compression of the nerve by aberrant arteries, tumors, bone, scar tissue, muscle or arteriovenous malformations.[36,37] Most lower the threshold of neuronal firing, and ordinary orofacial manuevers such as eating, teeth brushing, and swallowing precipitate an attack. They rarely occur in young people unless associated with a neuropathic process such as multiple sclerosis.

Each type of paroxysmal neuralgia has its own distinct characteristics. *Trigeminal neuralgia* usually affects one or at most two divisions of the nerve. Most common is the mandibular revision causing pain to shoot down the mandible into the teeth or tongue. Touching and washing the face, brushing teeth, cold wind against the face, shaving, biting, or talking sets off the trigger and results in pain. Patients go to extraordinary lengths to avoid stimulation of the trigger area. Occlusal and muscular dysfunction on the side of the pain may also be implicated. Maxillary, ophthalmic, or multiple division neuralgias are sequentially less common but occur within the same pattern in classical trigeminal distributions.

Glossopharyngeal neuralgia causes pain in the lateral posterior pharyngeal area, posterior of the tongue, down into the throat, the eustachian tube, the tonsillar area, and down the neck.[17] Eagle's syndrome has symptoms similar to those of glossopharyngeal neuralgia but with different etiology, and therefore, different precipitating factors.[38] The pain is related to a calcified elongation of the stylohyoid process that compresses the area of the glossopharyngeal nerve. Fast rotation of the head, swallowing, and pharyngeal motion in talking and chewing trigger a "sore throat," posterior tongue pain, or pharyngeal pain. The diagnosis is usually established he basis of radiographs, as well as intraoral finger palpation of the posterior pharyngeal area, location of the area of irritation, and the elongated stylohyoid process. Surgical resection of the stylohyoid process is indicated for definitive treatment.

Occipital neuralgia occurs in the distribution of the greater or lesser occipital nerves to the mastoid process and inferior to the infranuchal line.[39] Myofascial trigger points in the splenius capitis can exhibit similar patterns of pain referral.

Facial nerve neuralgia pain occurs in the preauricular and facial area and is usually associated with a sporadic convulsive tic that creates unilateral spasmodic contractions of facial muscles. The pain and spasm can be triggered by movement of the facial muscles.

Nervus intermedius, described as a lancinating "hot poker" in the ear, can occur anterior and posterior to, or on the pinna, in the auditory canal, and occasionally to the soft palate. The trigger area is usually in the external auditory canal. This neuralgia is also termed Ramsey Hunt Syndrome, geniculate ganglia neuralgia, or Wrisburg neuralgia.

Treatment of paroxysmal neuralgias generally consists of initial drug trials of carbamazepine (200 mg/day to 200 mg t. i. d.), diphenylhydantoin (200 mg t. i. d.), or chlorphenes (400 mg t. i. d.). Acupuncture, transcutaneous electrical nerve stimulation, and hypnosis have been used with some success. Also, percutaneous radiofrequency neuroablation and suboccipital or transtentorial cranial operations have a high success rate with severe cases.

Continuous neuralgias include postherpetic, posttraumatic, and postsurgical neuralgias. As with paroxysmal neuralgias, they follow the distribution of the cranial nerve involved, but differ in that they are continuous. Patients report altered sensations, dysesthesias, or pain in the distribution of the nerve that varies from tingling, numbness, and twitching to prickling or burning pain. The dysesthesias are generally discomforting to the patient because they are continuous and exacerbated by movement or touching of the area. As with paroxysmal neuralgias, local anesthetic blocks of the nerve eliminate all paresthesias except numbness. Peripheral degeneration or scarring of the nerve through trauma, surgery or viral infection is found by histopathologic examination.

Postherpetic neuralgia ("shingles") is usually a constant intense burning pain with hyperesthesia that occurs within days of a unilateral neural infection of a peripheral nerve or dorsal root ganglion with the herpes zoster virus.[34,35] Vesicular eruptions occur along the distribution of the nerve at the onset of the infection and pain develops as the infection continues. If treated early with local infiltration of corticosteriods, the chance of developing neuralgic discomfort is minimized. The longer the infection continues, the more difficult it is to manage the postherpetic pain. Postherpetic neuralgia most frequently affects the elderly and places a large emotional burden on them. It is common to see interruption of sleep, drug reliance, depression, and even suicidal ideation. The ophthalmic division of the trigeminal nerve is the most common head and neck nerve affected, although other divisions of the trigeminal nerve, as well as the auriculotemporal, occipital, and upper cervical nerves can be infected.

Treatment of the problem often includes a combination of tricyclic antidepressants (amitryptiline 75 mg/day) and with an anticonvulsant such as sodium valproate (250 mg t. i. d.), nerve blocks with local anesthetic and corticosteriods, acupuncture, or transcutaneous electrical nerve stimulation. Amelioration of the associated depression is as significant in therapy as reduction of the primary pain. Neurosurgical and cryoneuroablative techniques have also been reported as successful.

Post-traumatic and postsurgical neuralgias differ from postherpetic neuralgia in the history and quality of the pain.[40] Variations in paresthesias are perceived with both, but the pain has no intense burning quality. It is described more as a continuous tingling, numb, twitching, or prickly sensation. It results from damage to the nerve by trauma or surgery. The discomfort can be self-limiting, but total nerve regeneration is a slow inaccurate process and can result in permanent dysesthesias. Similar medicinal approaches to other neuralgias have been attempted with varying success. Acupuncture may also be successful with this condition.

Causalgic Group

Causalgia, sometimes termed reflex sympathetic dystrophy, is a pain syndrome with continual hypersympathetic activity.[41,42,43] Symptoms include a hot, burning sensation with associated cutaneous sensitivity to touch (hyperesthesia). It is a continuing progressive autonomic dysfunction that generally occurs after acute or chronic trauma to nerves supplying the area affected. Occasionally it is seen in the young with severe emotional problems. One may see vasomotor dysfunction with eventual trophic changes such as red, glossy dermal flushing. Causalgia is most commonly seen in the extremities but can be an underlying cause of atypical pain of the face or facial structures.

Osteoporosis, secondary to disuse, can be seen with it. The condition is related to an attempted aberrant regeneration of traumatized nerves with subsequent autonomic and sensory dysfunction. Definitive diagnosis and treatment of the condition can be accomplished through immediate reduction of pain and hyperesthesia with successful stellate ganglion nerve blocks with local anesthetic or stellate sympathectomy. Biofeedback and relaxation techniques also help reduce generalized sympathetic activity. Transcutaneous electrical stimulation, physical therapy, and acupuncture are helpful in providing relief and increasing function.

Psychogenic Group

The psychogenic group includes chronic pain resulting from conversion reaction, hypochondriasis, somatization, malinger-

TABLE 24-13. *Psychogenic pain disorders*

Conversion
Somatization
Malingerer
Münchausen's syndrome
Hypochondriacal reaction
Somatic delusion

ing, Münchausen's syndrome, and somatic delusion[44,45,46,47] (Table 24-13).

Many clinicians incorrectly use the term "psychogenic" to refer to patients who have a strong emotional component to the pain and who do not respond well to somatic treatments. It must be emphasized that most individuals with chronic pain have an emotional component such as depression that affects their perception of pain and behavioral reaction. Little therapeutic benefit exists in the pursuit of which came first, the depression or the pain. Pain is a psychophysiologic process that includes nociception via the peripheral and central nervous system as well as emotions and cognition via the higher cortical functions and limbic system. The definition of chronic pain implies that the patient has had the pain for a protracted period (approximately 6 months) and usually has received treatment that has resulted in failure. This situation creates both emotional strain for the patient and frustration for the clinician and leads to the premature label of "psychogenic pain." Most patients with chronic pain have a somatic diagnosis responsible for the pain.

Psychogenic pain should be reserved as a classification for those patients with two criteria. First, absolutely no organic neurologic or musculoskeletal findings should point to a somatic diagnosis after appropriate examinations, consultations, and diagnostic tests have been performed. Second, a definite psychosocial history should be present that would give evidence for a psychophysiologic process that somatizes emotional turmoil as pain. Myofascial pain is frequently overlooked as a somatic finding and mislabelled as psychogenic pain. A distinct difference exists between psychosomatic disorders, in which a physical disorder is caused by excess stress and tension and psychogenic pain, as described here. It is important to realize that whether or not the pain has an actual organic basis for the patient's complaint, it is still real to the patient and can be intense and as legitimate as any somatic pain.

Conversion reactions represent a successful subconscious symbolic attempt to solve emotional turmoil in the patient's life through development of a more valid somatic symptom such as pain. The quality of the pain can be related in descriptive affective terms such as; "lightning-like explosions," "heavy weight pressing on my head," "spike into my head," "rope choking my throat," "ugly pain," and others. Although patients describe the pain in elaborate terms, they may relate to it rather indifferently as another complaint that says "my life bothers me." Clinically, it is presented as a continuous unrelenting pain which is rarely affected by external somatic events. No muscular trigger points, autonomic signs, or other physical findings would contribute to the pain they describe. Patients can be of any age or sex. A history of the patient's complaint may reveal growing up with an ill parent or relative or prolonged childhood illness. Some patients are socially or occupationally incapacitated. Although true conversion reactions are rare, the close relationship between the face, head, and neck and personal identity, sexuality, and communicative skills are important in the development of conversion reactions in this area. Patients generally are under intense emotional stress in the past and present, have poor social relationships, but no major mental abnormalities. A conversion reaction can occur for a number of reasons. These may include handling of nonspecific stress, coping with a threatened uncontrollable rage, body symptoms reflecting inner conflict, anticipating a pending major life change situation, dealing with unchangeable life impasses, communicating with themselves and the world, a catastrophic life situation, manifestation of severe body image problem, expression of resentment for authority, temptation to rebel, or the need to inhibit self-inflicted sexual temptations. The patient subconsciously converts an apparently socially unacceptable psychologic illness to the socially acceptable physical complaint of pain which displaces emotional pain for somatic pain.

In contrast to the affective indifference to the complaint in conversion reactions, patients with a somatization reaction exhibit more elaboration of complaints about the subconscious pain. Patients outwardly display exaggerated agony, depression, and torment concerning the pain while dismissing any great emotional strife in their lives. They can be manipulative, belligerent, or demanding in their search for a physical cure to their pain. Psychologic events similar to patients with conversion reactions will contribute to the development of somatizing the events into a physical pain.

A malingerer is a patient that consciously exhibits and complains of pain with no physical origin for the purpose of secondary gain. The quality, frequency, and duration may be compatible with another diagnosis but have inconsistencies in response to nerve blocks or a treatment course. The pain is often patterned after an illness of a relative or social contact but invariably responds inappropriately to history, examinations, diagnostic studies, and treatment. The patient may actually have, or have had, an illness that gives rise to a self-limiting pain continued for secondary gain. The secondary gain that the patient achieves through his pain syndrome may range between psychologic and material motivations. These can include manipulation of intolerable family situations, assuring security and love in a relationship, maximizing litigation settlements, avoiding occupational tasks, and others. One differentiating factor between malingerer and conversion reaction is the lack of a serious subconscious emotional turmoil in malingering. Clinically they can present with similar characteristics. Münchausens' syndrome is a specific type of malingerer that shows up at a hospital with a major complaint but no apparent history.[48] After a few days of room and board, negative examinations, and diagnostic studies, the patient disappears only to turn up at another hospital often in a different city. The sequence may be repeated many times. Unsuspecting residents and veterans' hospitals lie prone to these individuals.

Hypochondriasis is a psychologic state in which much of the patient's attention and energy is focused on the body and its functioning. Patients usually have corresponding anxious obsession in viewing all bodily sensations and normal afferent impulses including normal minor pains as potentially threatening to their well being. This results in numerous complaints of pain and other symptoms that upon examination have no or a mild physical basis. This state can stem from a disturbed body image problem, numerous deaths or illnesses of close friends or relatives, general insecurity about one's health and life, as well as a fear of death.

Somatic delusions can occur in patients with psychiatric diagnoses such as psychosis or schizophrenia. They lose much rational thought and attachment to reality and display uncontrolled obsessions of pain or problems with their health. Psychiatric care or hospitalization is strongly indicated since the possibility of suicide is great.

Treatment of the psychogenic group of patients varies with the seriousness of the problem. Situational insight, supportive therapy, guidance, or counseling is occasionally sufficient to resolve the problem. In other cases, long-term outpatient psychotherapy, hypnotherapy, or medications such as antidepressants, antipsychotics, hypnotics, and tranquilizers help alleviate the pain. In serious cases with possible suicide, bodily injury to themselves or others, or aggressive behavior, inpatient psychiatric care is required.

Contributing Factors

Contributing factors are those that initiate, perpetuate, or result from a disorder and, thus, complicate management.[49] Because of their complicated interrelationship and lack of causal evidence, they are not referred to as etiologic factors. They can be categorized into biologic, behavioral, social, environmental, emotional, and cognitive (Table 24-14). Successful long-term management of chronic pain includes treating the physical diagnoses and reducing these contributing factors. Accomplishing one without the other can result in failure in symptom reduction or maintenance of that relief.

Biologic factors can be some of the most significant and include any factors related to the individual's mechanical or biologic constitution that would predispose them to developing chronic pain. This may include occlusal discrepancies,[50] unilateral short leg,[51] small hemipelvis,[52] past injuries,[53] and other coexisting medical problems.[26] It must be noted that occlusal discrepancies and other postural abnormalities may contribute to and result from abnormal muscle and joint function.[54]

Behavioral factors include any behavior or habit that is under a person's control and plays a role in perpetuating the disorder. Lifestyle habits and behaviors such as a nutrient deficient diet,[55] high caffeine intake in coffee or medications,[56] oral parafunctional habits[52,57] sleep disturbance,[58] and poor postural habits[59,60] may be involved in chronic problems. Parafunctional oral habits may include bruxism, clenching, deviated swallowing, fingernail biting, lip biting, object biting, gum chewing, protrusive and retrusive habits, tongue thrust habits, and mandibular opening habits with the facial or suprahyoid muscles. Each of these habits creates excessive muscle use and resultant muscle fatigue, and may perpetuate trigger points. Poor postural habits also perpetuate trigger points by using the muscle in a strained position. These positions such as an accentuated forward or lateral head position, shrugging the shoulders, or a tongue forced against the mandibular anteriors often result from habits such as poor pacing, chronic phone use, mouth breathing, poor work habits, sitting improperly in misfitting furniture, or carrying large objects (such as purses) on one side. Chronic immobility of muscles can also lead to myofascial trigger points by weakening a muscle and rendering it prone to strain with normal use.[25] This can occur with improper use of cervical collars or chronic inactivity and sedentary lifestyle.

Social factors include antecedent or consequential events that either affect an individual's perceptions and learned responses to pain or contribute to maladaptive behaviors. These events occur over a period of time and reinforce the behaviors of the patient that may in fact perpetuate the experience of pain and illness.[61,62] For example, a patient who is told or assumes he will receive more monetary compensation with more pain and treatments may neglect exercises to reduce pain until after the litigation is settled. Likewise, a patient

TABLE 24-14. *Contributing factors that may initiate, perpetuate, and result from (and thus complicate) chronic craniofacial pain*

Biologic	Environmental
Occlusal discrepancies	Weather changes
Developmental anomaly	Chemical ingestion
Short leg	Inhalants
Small hemipelvis	Chronic vibration
Skeletal malformations	Excess noise
Past injury	Improper lighting
Hormonal changes	
Other medical disorders	
Behavioral	**Cognitive**
Nutrient-deficient diet	Low understanding
Excess Caffine	Confusion
Parafunctional oral habits	Unrealistic expectations
Poor postural habits	Negative body image
Disturbed sleep	Low intelligence
Chronic inactivity	Low motivation
Pacing problems	
Immobility	
Social	**Emotional**
Chemical dependency	Irritability
Health care abuse	Anxiety
Excess pain verbalization	Anger
Disability	Depression
Litigation	Frustration
Avoidance of tasks	Fear
Social modeling	Guilt
Social dependencies	
Social Stressors	

who receives needed love and attention only when verbalizing pain will be less motivated to help decrease the pain.

Another set of social factors includes stressors that may be any novel or threatening situation or experiences that force a person to adapt. This can be seen in situations at home or work and may relate to financial difficulties, relationships, sexual problems, family conflicts, or recent losses or deaths.[63] Short-term stressors may be productive, but long-term stress may lead to maladaptive behaviors, cognitions, or emotions that can perpetuate or complicate a pain syndrome.[64]

Environmental factors include those stimuli in a person's physical environment that contribute to the pain problem and are not under direct control. Chronic exposure to chemicals such as lead, mercury, arsenic, and many toxins can lead to pain problems directly or indirectly. Excessive stimuli like chronic vibration, sounds, abnormal lighting, and excess use of video display terminals can contribute to headaches.

Emotional factors include any negative emotion that is sustained over time and affects the normal functioning of the individual. Although sustained negative emotions such as anxiety, anger, depression and frustration are very common among chronic pain patients, they do not directly cause pain, but, rather, may result from having persistent pain, make pain more difficult to tolerate, or prevent successful management.[65] Explaining emotional factors to the patient is a delicate process and should not be discussed as etiologic factors. The patient can better understand how these factors can result from persistent pain. Encouraging recognition and expression of feelings with artful listening frequently help alleviate any mild or transient emotional disturbances. Specific management of severe or prolonged emotional disturbances should proceed first if it becomes the primary problem, because it is often difficult for the patient to work on two problems simultaneously. The psychotherapy and counseling should be accomplished away from the clinic and, once alleviated, management of the pain can proceed again.

Cognitive factors often accompany emotional factors and include any dominant thought process that is counterproductive and related to the illness. Confusion and lack of understanding of the problem are common characteristics of chronic pain patients because of the long history of differing opinions from multiple sources about their problem. As a result of common assumptions they may have regarding medical care, patients may also be impatient or unrealistic about treatment and expect all the pain to go away or any reduction of pain to be immediate. These factors can greatly compromise treatment through poor physician-patient relationships and noncompliance. A thorough explanation of the problem, its contributing factors, and what to expect during treatment helps alleviate these factors.

References

1. Bonica, J.J., Liebeskind, J.D., and Albe-Fessard, D. (eds.): Advances in Pain Research and Therapy. Vol. 3. New York, Raven Press, 1973, pp. v-vii.
2. Bonica, J.J.: Preface. *In* New Approaches to Treatment of Chronic Pain. Edited by N.G. Lorenz. N.I.D.A. Research Monograph 36. Washington, U.S. Government Printing Office, 1981, pp. 1-11.
3. Sternbach, R.A.: Pain: A Psychophysiologic Analysis. New York, Academic Press, 1968.
4. Dorland's Illustrated Medical Dictionary. Philadelphia, W.B. Saunders Co., 1974.
5. Aranda, J.M.: The problem oriented medical records. JAMA, *229:*549, 1974.
6. DeGowin, E.L., and DeGowin, R.L.: Bedside Diagnostic Examination. London, Macmillan Co., 1978.
7. Melzack, R., and Torgeson, W.S.: On the language of pain. Anesthes., *34:*50, 1971.
8. Lance, J.W.: Mechanism and Management of Headache. Boston, Butterworth, 1978, pp. 84-103.
9. Diamond, S., and Dalessio, D.J.: The Practicing Physician's Approach to Headache. 2nd Ed. Baltimore, Williams & Wilkins Co., 1978, pp. 51-73.
10. Fricton J.R., and Kroening, R.: Practical differential diagnosis of chronic craniofacial pain. Oral Surg., *54*(6):628, 1982.
11. Payten, R.J.: Facial pain as the first symptom in acoustic neuroma. J. Laryngol. Otol., *86*(5):523, 1972.
12. Birt, D.: Headaches and head pains associated with diseases of the ear, nose, and throat. Med. Clin. North Am., *62:*523, 1978.
13. Arthritis Foundation: Primer on the rheumatic diseases. JAMA (Supplement), *5:*661, 1980.
14. Boles, R.: Paranasal sinuses and facial pain. *In* Facial Pain. 2nd Ed. Edited by C.C. Alling and P.E. Mahan. Philadelphia, Lea & Febiger, 1978, pp. 115-134.
15. Jannetta, P.J.: Treatment of trigeminal neuralgia by suboccipital and transtentorial cranial operations. Clin. Neurosurg., *24:* 538, 1977.
16. Macrae, D.: Intracranial causes of oral and facial pain. Dent. Clin. North Am., 529, 1959.
17. Walker, A.E.: Neuralgias of the glossopharyngeal, vagus, and intermedius nerves. *In* Pain. Edited by P.R. Knighton and P.R. Dumke. Boston, Little, Brown & Co., 1966, pp. 421-429.
18. Dalessio, D.J.: Classification and mechanism of migraine. Headache, *19:*114, 1979.
19. Friedman, A.P.: Migraine. Med. Clin. North Am., *62:*481, 1978.
20. Kudrow, L.: Cluster headache: Diagnosis and management. Headache, *19:*142, 1979.
21. Appenzeller, O: Headache in temporal arteritis and cerebral vascular disease. *In* Pathogenesis and Treatment of Headache. Edited by O. Appenzeller. New York, Spectrum Publications, 1976, pp. 115-130.
22. Troiano, M.F., and Gaston, G.W.: Carotid system arteritis: An overlooked and misdiagnosed syndrome. JADA, *91:*589, 1975.
23. Bell, W.E.: Orofacial Pains: Differential Diagnosis. 2nd Ed. Chicago, Year Book Medical Publishers, 1979, pp. 175-254, 322-334.
24. Travell, J.: Myofascial trigger points: A clinical view. *In* Pain Research and Therapy. Vol. 1. Edited by J.J. Bonica and D. Albe-Fessard. New York, Raven Press, 1976, pp. 919-926.
25. Travell, J., and Simons, D.: Myofascial Pain and Dysfunction: The Trigger Point Manual. Baltimore, Williams & Wilkins Co., 1983.
26. Simons, D.G.: Muscle pain syndromes (Parts I and II). Am. J. of Phys. Med., *54*(6):289, and *55*(1):15, 1975.

27. Kudrow, L.: Tension headache, scalp muscle contraction headache. *In* Pathogenesis and Treatment of Headache. Edited by O. Appenzeller. New York, Spectrum Publications, 1976, pp. 81-92.
28. Guralnick, W., Kaba, L.B., and Merrill, R.G.: Temporomandibular joint afflictions. N. Engl. J. Med., *299*:123, 1978.
29. Kreutziger, K.L., and Mahan, P.E.: Temporomandibular degenerative joint disease. Part I: Anatomy, pathophysiology and clinical description. Oral Surg., Oral Med., Oral Path., *40*:165, 1975.
30. Solberg, W., and Clark, G.: Temporomandibular Joint Problems: Biologic Diagnosis and Treatment. Chicago, Quintessence Publ. Co., 1980.
31. Poswillo, D.E.: Experimental investigation of the effects of intra-articular hydrocortisone and high condylectomy in the mandibular condyle. Oral Surg, Oral Med., Oral Path., *30*:161, 1970.
32. Christian, C.L.: Diseases of the joints. Part VII. *In* Cecil Textbook of Medicine. 15th Ed. Philadelphia, W.B. Saunders Co., 1979, pp. 186-193.
33. Edmeads, V.: Headaches and head pains associated with diseases of the cervical spine. Med. Clin. North Am., *62*:533, 1978.
34. Dalessio, D.J.: Wolff's Headache and Other Head Pain, 3rd Ed. New York, Oxford Univ. Press. 1972.
35. Poser, C.M.: Facial pain: Diagnostic dilemma, therapeutic challenge. Geriatrics, *30*:110, 1975.
36. Jannetta, P.J.: Arterial compression of the trigeminal nerve at the pons in patients with trigeminal neuralgia. J. Neurosurg., *26*:159, 1967.
37. Kerr, F.W.L.: Evidence for a peripheral etiology for trigeminal neuralgia. J. Neurosurg., *26*:168, 1967.
38. Massey, E.W., and Massey, J.: Elongated styloid process (Eagle's Syndrome) causing hemicrania. Headache, *19*:339, 1979.
39. Knox, D.L., and Mustonen, E.: Greater occipital neuralgia: An ocular pain syndrome with multiple etiologies. Trans. Am. Acad. Opthalmol. Otolaryngol., *79*:513, 1975.
40. Thompson, J.E.: The diagnosis and management of post-traumatic pain syndromes (causalgia): Aus. N.Z.J. Surg., *49*:299, 1979.
41. Bonica, J.J.: Management of intractable pain. *In* New Concepts in Pain. Edited by E.L. Way. Philadelphia, F.A. Davis Co., 1967, pp. 155-167.
42. Bonica, J.J.: The Management of Pain. Philadelphia, Lea & Febiger, 1953, pp. 785-824, 1263-1309.
43. Kozin, F., McCarty, D.J., Sims, J., et al.: The reflex sympathetic dystrophy syndrome (two parts) Am. J. Med., *60*:321, 1976.
44. Martin, M.: Psychogenic factors in headache. Med. Clin. North Am., *62*:559, 1978.
45. Maruta, T., and Swanson, D: Psychiatric consultation in the chronic pain patient. Mayo Clinic Proc., *52*:792, 1977.
46. Pilling, L.F.: Psychosomatic aspects of facial pain. *In* Facial Pain. 2nd Ed. Edited by C.C. Alling and P.E. Mahan. Philadelphia, Lea & Febiger, 1978, pp. 213-226.
47. Sternbach, R.A.: The Psychology of Pain. 1st Ed. New York, Raven Press, 1978.
48. Oldham, L.: Facial pain as a presentation in Von Munchausen's syndrome: Report of a case. Br. J. Oral Surg., *12*(1):86, 1974.
49. Fricton, J.R.: Behavioral and psychosocial factors in chronic craniofacial pain. Anesth. Progress, *32*:7, 1985.
50. Krogh-Poulsen, W.G., and Olsson, A.: Management of the occlusion of the teeth. *In* Facial Pain and Mandibular Dysfunction. Edited by L. Schwartz and C. Chayes. Philadelphia, W.B. Saunders Co., 1981.
51. Simons, D.G., and Travell, J.: Myofascial origins of low back pain Parts 1-3. Postgrad. Med., *73*:66, 1983.
52. Christensen, L.V.: Facial pain and internal pressure of masseter muscle in experimental bruxism in man. Arch. Oral Biol., *16*:1021, 1971.
53. Awad, E.A.: Interstitial myofibrositis: Hypothesis of the mechanism. Arch. Phys. Med. and Rehab., *54*:449, 1973.
54. Edmiston, G.F., and Laskin, D.M.: Changes in consistency of occlusal contact in myofascial pain-dysfunctional syndrome. J. Dent. Res., *57*:27, 1978.
55. Moldofsky, H., and Warsh, J.: Plasma tryptophan and musculoskeletal pain in nonarticular rheumatism ("fibrositis syndrome"). Pain, *5*:65, 1978.
56. White, B. C., et al.: Anxiety and muscle tension as consequences of caffeine withdrawal. Science, *209*:1547, 1980.
57. Rugh, J.D., and Solberg, W.K.: Psychological implications in temporomandibular pain and dysfunction. Oral Sci. Review, *7*:2, 1976.
58. Moldofsky, H., Scarisbrick, P. England, R., and Smythe, H.: Musculoskeletal symptoms and non-rem sleep disturbance in patients with "fibrositis syndrome" and healthy subjects. Psychosom. Med., *37*:341, 1975.
59. Kendall, H.O., Kendall, F.F., and Boynton, D.A.: Posture and Pain. New York, R.E. Krieger Publishing Co., 1970.

60. Kraus, H.: Muscle function and the temporomandibular joint. J. Prosth. Dent., *13:*950, 1963.
61. Fordyce, W.E.: Learning processes in pain. *In* The Psychology of Pain. Edited by R. Sternbach. New York, Raven Press, 1978, pp. 49-72.
62. Fordyce, W.E., and Steger, J.C.: Chronic pain. *In* Behavioral Medicine: Theory and Practice. Edited by O.F. Pomerleau and J.P. Brady. Baltimore, Williams & Wilkins Co., 1979, pp. 125-154.
63. Holmes, T.H., and Rahe, R.H.: The social readjustment rating scale. J. Psychosomatic Res., *11:*213, 1967.
64. Haber, J.D., Moss, R.A., Kuczmierczyr, A.R., and Garrett, J.C.: Assessment and treatment of stress in myofascial pain-dysfunction syndrome: A model for analysis. J. Oral Rehab., *10:*187, 1983.
65. Van Knorring, L.: The experience of pain in depressed patients. Neuropsychobiology, *1:*155, 1975.

CHAPTER 25

Oral Implants

ROBERT A. JAMES

Be not the first by whom the new is tried,
nor yet the last to lay the old aside.   ANON.

Considerable change has occurred in recent years in the field of oral implantology. This change has been brought about by numerous factors, including a better understanding of the biomaterials and the tissues that surround them. This increased knowledge, along with an ever increasing number of reports that describe long-term survival for various implant devices, has led to considerable change in the acceptance of oral implantology by the dental profession.

This chapter attempts to present a philosophy for implant therapy and to describe various devices available to the profession. The indications and contraindications for these implants are outlined. It must be recognized that in any new and developing field there is a divergence of opinions, and when this divergence is great, ignorance abounds. An attempt has been made to separate fact from opinion whenever the difference between them has been recognized.

One additional caution must be expressed. The great majority of devices available to the profession have been shown to be efficacious through the process of clinical usage rather than premarket testing. It is thus difficult to acquire specific information to indicate how effective such devices may be.

Permucosal devices are categorized generically in this chapter and grouped as endosteal, transosteal, and subperiosteal. Materials are discussed as they relate to individual devices.

While this is a text on oral and maxillofacial surgery, this chapter does not emphasize the surgical aspects. An attempt has been made to provide a basis for understanding the principles involved in implant and patient selection. Many clinicians are doing implants without adequate research and clinical background, and it is the authors' desire that this chapter will help enlarge the scope of understanding in this crucial area.

The Periimplant Tissues

It is important to understand the cellular responses of the host tissues to the various insults thrust upon them during the sequence of events that occurs while the implant is in place. This understanding affects implant selection, design, manufacture, handling, placement, and maintenance. It is concerned with the surgical wound incurred at placement and extends through healing, function, trauma, repair, necrosis, and finally, the surgical wound incurred during implant removal, and subsequent healing and repair. It is beyond the scope of this chapter to address thoroughly the topics of basic healing and repair. However, it attempts to cover those aspects that directly relate to, or are unique to, the tissues surrounding oral implants. The superficial or covering periimplant tissue and the pergingival defense mechanisms are described. This description is followed by a discussion of the deeper periimplant tissues and the support mechanisms involved.

Superficial Periimplant Tissue

At first it may seem preposterous that a dental implant can violate the integrity of the oral mucosa without disastrous results. On this issue the great majority of attacks have been directed against the practice of oral implantology. However, natural appendages of jaw bones penetrate the oral mucosa and function partly exposed to the outside environment. These appendages are the teeth, and they and their surrounding tissues are uniquely designed to allow for this penetration while maintaining the integrity of the mucosal barrier. Therefore, the similarities between the periimplant tissues and the periodontium must be noted.

The dental sulcular epithelium differs from the epithelial covering of attached and free gingiva in both appearance and function. It is not keratinized and resembles the mucosal covering more than the covering of gingival tissues exposed to direct masticatory function. It is more permeable to fluids and allows for the passage of certain cells, immunoglobulins, and various other items found in blood and interstitial fluids, from connective tissue and microvasculature to the oral cavity. At the base of the sulcus is the epithelial attachment, the tissue of most interest in our discussion because it forms the first line of defense where the tooth emerges from the deeper tissues. The "junctional epithelium" making up this attachment is very specialized, being found nowhere else in the body. It extends from the base of the sulcus a short distance apically and terminates abruptly where connective tissue fibers enter the cementum.

Along this junctional epithelium-tooth interface, and lying in contact with the tooth, is a basement lamina with ultramicroscopic plates called *hemidesmosomes*. Desmosomes are made up of a pair of these plates, one in each of two adjoining epithelial cells, and mark the site of intercellular adhesion and communication. A hemidesmosome (half a desmosome) may be found wherever an epithelial cell adjoins the surface of something other than another epithelial cell, such as at the basement membrane where epithelial tissue meets connective tissue; and apical to the gingival sulcus, where cells of the epithelial attachment form hemidesmosomes against the surface of the tooth by way of the basal lamina. This unique arrangement makes it possible for nearly inert biomaterials (implants) or less inert tissues (teeth) to penetrate the oral epithelium and maintain the integrity of this protective covering, a property not shared by epithelium covering the rest of the outside of the body. This factor has thus far prevented the successful long-term use of percutaneous implant devices for general medical and orthopedic applications in other parts of the body.

Evidence for an actual attachment was first demonstrated by Toto,[1] who used human and mouse gingiva and showed a Periodic Acid Schiff (PAS) positive material at the interfaces between the epithelial attachments to both dentin and enamel of teeth. This PAS positive material is indicative of a mucopolysaccharide cement. The first indication that an adherence of the epithelium to an implant could take place was presented by James and Kelln,[2] who demonstrated a similar PAS positive material at the interface between the posts of perforated metal plates made of surgical chrome-cobalt-molybdenum alloy (Surgical Vitallium, Howmedica) and junctional epithelium in dogs.

The dental cuticle is a thin layer of tissue that interfaces with the tooth and is believed to be involved in the original formation of the tooth. It is demonstrated histochemically as an orcin positive layer that is unique to the dental cuticle and lies adjacent to teeth. James and Kelln[3] also demonstrated an orcin positive extracellular material at the interface between the junctional epithelium and surgical chrome-cobalt-molybdenum implant posts. Thus, histochemically, the epithelial tissues interfacing with permucosal dental implant posts appear to react in a manner no different than when they interface with natural teeth.

Ponitz et al.[4] measured the crevicular fluid volume collected from around subperiosteal implant posts and natural teeth in man. He reported volumes similar in teeth and implants and an increase in volume when either had inflamed surrounding tissue. It has been well established that crevicular volume flow increases with gingival inflammation. Further indirect evidence of an epithelial attachment to the implant surface is found in the orientation of collagen fibers in the cervical region of the implant. James[5,5a] showed fibers in this area to extend from the crestal bone to the epithelium interfacing with the implant, thus orienting at a right angle to the implant surface. Since collagen fibers orient in the direction of tensile stress, this arrangement is consistent with adherence of the epithelium to the implant surface (Fig. 25-1).

Waerhaug[6] reported an interesting study in which he removed teeth, wrapped the roots with gold foil, and reimplanted them. Later he could recover the tissue and make histologic sections with the gold foil-epithelium interface intact. He showed cellular bridges between the gingival epithelial cells and the gold foil implant. These cellular bridges were similar in structure to the intercellular bridges (also called desmosomes prior to the development of the electron microscope and prior to their ultrastructural description). Stallard et al.,[7] using scanning electronmicroscopy, reported an in vitro study in which they placed glass and vitreous carbon in tissue culture and demonstrated epithelial cells adherent to both. Direct evidence for an attachment or adherence of epithelium to an implant was first reported by James and Schultz,[8] who showed hemidesmosomes with a basal lamina at the interface between epithelium and permucosal chrome-cobalt-molybdenum implants in monkeys.

Listgarten and Lai[9] demonstrated hemidesmosomes next to epoxy implants, Samida et al.[10] showed them next to carbon, again in monkeys (Fig. 25-2), Gould et al.[11] next to titanium in vitro, Ogiso et al.[12] next to hydroxyapatite implants in function, McKinney et al.[13] next to single crystal aluminum oxide implants, and Kavanagh et al.[14] next to titanium coated epon in rats. Swope and James,[15] in a longitudinal study, showed that hemidesmosomes are well developed next to the implant post within 48 hours after implantation of chrome-cobalt-molybdenum implants in monkeys. This study coincides nicely with the work of Taylor et al.,[16] who stripped away and then repositioned the epithelium to the teeth of monkeys and showed a hemidesmosomal reattachment within 48 hours.

Several studies have shown that dyes and bacteria fail to penetrate beyond the implant gingival sulcus. Hoppe[17] instilled dyes of various molecular size into gingival crevices surrounding subperiosteal implants in dogs and was unable to show diffusion beyond the deepest part of the sulcus. Pretreatment of the crevice with hyaluronidase failed to change the results. Gorhmann[18] performed similar studies around subperiosteal implants in dogs, using S^{35} labeled mycobacterium and staphylococci. His results were similar to

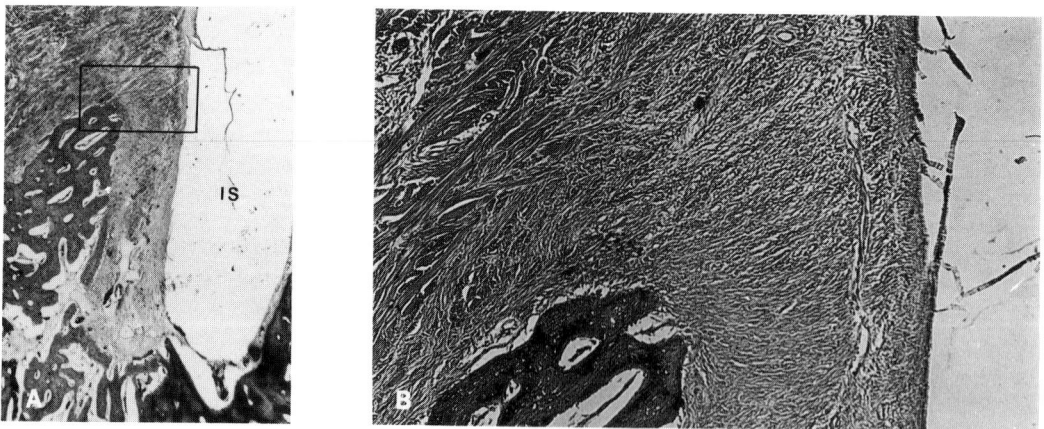

Fig. 25-1. (A) Photomicrograph of human autopsy periimplant tissue. Device was a stainless steel Ramus implant that had functioned in the mandible for three years. (B) Higher magnification of area outlined in (A). Horizontal crestal fibers can be seen extending from crestal bone on left to junctional epithelium on right. IS-Implant space. (From: James, R.A.: Histopathologic study of supporting tissues of an endosteal implant. Implantologist, 1:19, 1976)

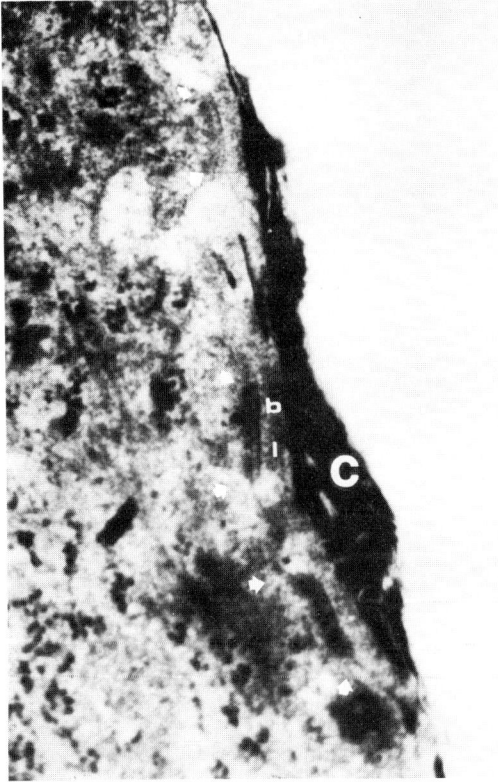

FIG. 25-2. *Transmission electron photomicrograph of monkey epithelial tissue interfacing with carbon fragments of a vitreous carbon implant. Note well defined hemidesmosomes (between arrows) and basal limina (bl). This intact interface was preserved when the carbon implant fragments (c) fractured away from the implant with the epithelium during an attempt to separate the implant from the tissue by means of thermal stress fracturing.*

implant's gingival sulcus (Fig. 25-3). It is widely accepted that bacteria play a key role in the etiology of periodontal disease. In light of the striking similarities between the periodontium and the periimplant tissues as outlined above, it seems reasonable to assume that bacteria play similar pathogenic roles in the disease process sometimes seen around dental implants. All the available evidence indicates the existence of active defense mechanisms that prevent the ingress of bacteria beyond the implant's gingival sulcus. These defense mechanisms attempt to protect the tissues from bacterial toxins that pose a threat.

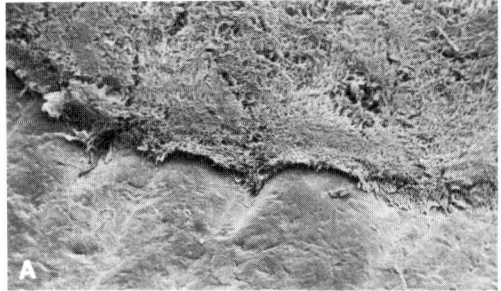

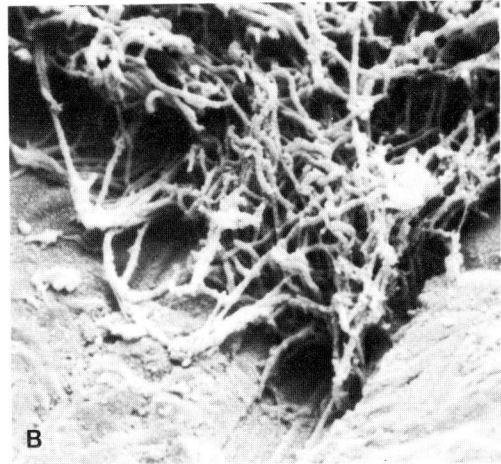

those of Hoppe. Schlegel et al.[19] worked with the tissues surrounding endosteal implants in dogs. They instilled phage-typed Staphylococcus aureus (which could not be confused with S. aureus endemic to the dog being studied) into each implant sulcus. This was immediately followed by feeding with pelleted dry food in order to exert masticatory pressure. After 5 minutes, venous blood was drawn and cultured. None of the cultures showed a growth of the test strain.

James and Kelln[3] showed a scanning electron photomicrograph of bacterial plaque adherent to an implant post that had functioned in a dog for 6 weeks. The plaque ended abruptly in the area of the

FIG. 25-3. *(A) Scanning electron photomicrograph of a highly polished surgical Vitallium implant post that had functioned in a dog for six weeks. Note bacterial plaque terminating along a definite front line in the area of the gingival sulcus. (B) Higher magnification of a polishing scratch. Note the opportunistic character of the plaque relative to its advancement into this fine surface scratch.*

Deep Periimplant Tissue

Frequently it is assumed that for an implant to function in healthy tissue, load transfer must occur by way of direct bone-implant interface. While such intimate relations have been documented on numerous occasions over the past several decades, some authors recently have claimed that the absence of such support represents pathology. Such claims are completely unfounded except for implants whose designs fail to provide adequate support by other means. Pathology from stress does not occur unless tissue is stressed beyond its physiologic limit. Thus far in the research conducted on tissue mechanics around dental implants, these physiologic limits have not been quantified. Failure to quantify, however, does not prevent us from benefitting from the concept.

The support:load ratio[11] refers to the amount of support the bone can provide for a given implant device as compared to the amount of load being placed upon it. The load can be measured, but until the elusive "physiologic limit" can be quantified, the support can only be guessed. One can attempt to overcome or perhaps sidestep this problem by referring instead to the "surface area:load ratio," which can be quantified. However, for this ratio to be useful, the condition of the interface must be known. Because the surface area does not vary and is a function of the configuration and surface texture of the implant, the support:load ratio of a given implant varies depending upon whether it is functioning with an implant/bone interface or an implant/connective tissue interface.

Thus, an implant in the form of a small screw with a nonporous surface will have a relatively low surface area/load ratio and can only function for extended periods of time with a direct bone interface. Relatively light loading can result in osteolytic activity and the development of a connective tissue interface. The "crown/root" ratio becomes critical; micromovement increases to macromovement and the connective tissue ligament becomes inflamed. It increases in size until the threads of the screw no longer can translate the load to the bone and the implant is lost. However, if the infrastructure of the implant is more complex, where occlusal forces can be translated over a larger area, either by increasing the size of the implant or by increasing the surface area by means of porosity or surface roughness, greater loading can occur before exceeding physiologic limits. If the design is further developed to allow for load transfer with either a bony or a connective tissue interface, long-term function without pathology can be extremely predictable.

With perforated metal plates (blades), physiologic forces can be transmitted to the bone through either a direct bony interface or a periimplant ligament. This periimplant ligament is made up of lamellar bone, Sharpey's fibers, and principal fiber systems.[5,5a,20]

Fibers resembling the gingival ligament can be observed in the pergingival area originating in part in the periimplant ligament (described later), in part from the palatal submucosa and buccal lamina propria, and in part from the bony crest. These fibers anastomose with circumferential fibers extending around the implant post in the free gingival area in a manner similar to circumferential fibers of the dental gingiva.[21] It would thus appear that this fiber system provides the architecture for the gingival crest noted as an elevation around the neck of pergingival implants.

Notwithstanding the dielectric forces involved, it is generally recognized that excessive pressure on the bone results in osteolysis, while tension is conducive to osteogenesis. Principal fiber systems have been observed passing apical to endosteal blade implants and extending as Sharpey's fibers into bundle bone buccal and lingual to the implant, thus forming a dynamic, functional, hammock-like suspensory ligament capable of transmitting the stress generated by occlusal and other forces directly to the bone from the implant (Fig. 25-4). This periimplant ligament can be observed to contain principal fiber systems resembling the alveolar crest, horizontal, oblique, and even apical fibers of the alveolar dental ligament (Fig. 25-5).

Subperiosteal implants have been shown to have similar but more complex suspensory ligaments. Early reports[22,23,24] described the collagen fiber system surrounding subperiosteal struts as running parallel to the implant surface. However, this does

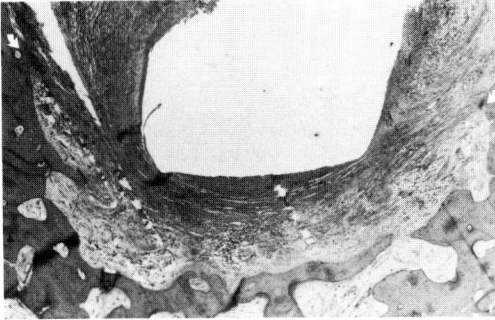

FIG. 25-4. *Photomicrograph of human autopsy periimplant tissue. Device was same implant as in figure 25-1, and this specimen was taken a few mm apical and distal to specimen shown there. Note suspensory ligament extending from lamellar bone on left, apical to the implant, and then to lamellar bone on right. (Arrows show supporting lamellar bone.) (From: James, R.A.: Histopathologic study of supporting tissues of an endosteal implant. Implantologist, 1:19, 1976)*

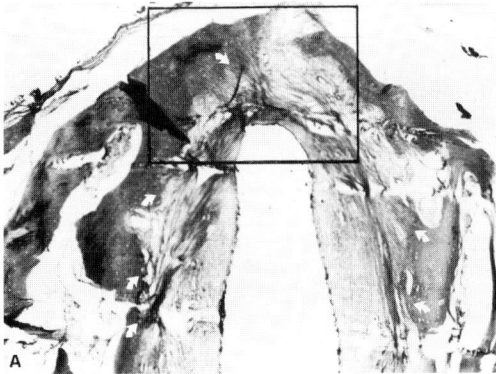

not explain satisfactorily how such a device absorbs occlusal forces effectively over such extensive periods of time. Careful examination of human and animal autopsy material reveals a subperiosteal implant suspensory ligament, similar in some respects to that seen in endosteal implants, and unique in other respects. The exact architecture of the ligament varies depending on the location of the strut, but is always determined by the external forces acting upon the implant and develops in a manner to translate those forces into tensile stress on the supporting bone.[25]

Struts crossing over the crestal ridge have no apparent means of support other than the underlying bone which, when subjected to pressure, resorbs under occlusal forces, thus allowing settling of the implant. This initial settling has long been observed. What has not been recognized is that only after the device has settled can a suspensory ligament be formed for such crestally located struts (Fig. 25-6).

On the other hand, the struts on the medial and lateral aspect of the mandible have potential for the development of the suspensory ligament without initial settling. Thus, the peripheral struts can provide the primary support for these devices. Failure to appreciate this critically important factor has led to designs that are generally underextended. Further, it has long

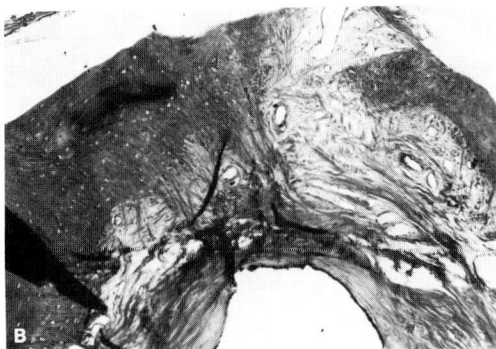

FIG. 25-5. *(A) Photomicrograph of human autopsy periimplant tissue. Device was a Vitallium Cranin Anchor implant which had functioned in the maxilla of a female patient for 2 1/2 years. Arrows indicate supporting bone. (B) Higher magnification of apical portion. Note apical fiber system with endochondral bone formation.*

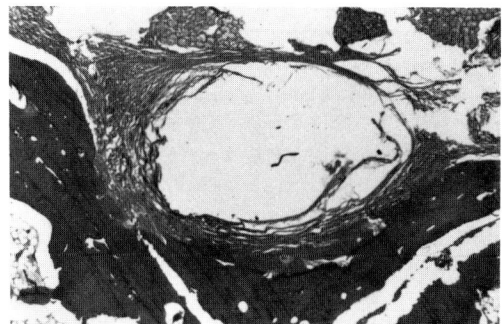

FIG. 25-6. *Photomicrograph of baboon autopsy periimplant tissue. Device was a subperiosteal implant which had functioned for one year. Note suspensory ligament which formed subsequent to the settling of the implant. Animal was partially dentulous and while implant was in full occlusion, the load was shared by natural dentition. Thus, the loads were less than if the animal had been totally endentulous.*

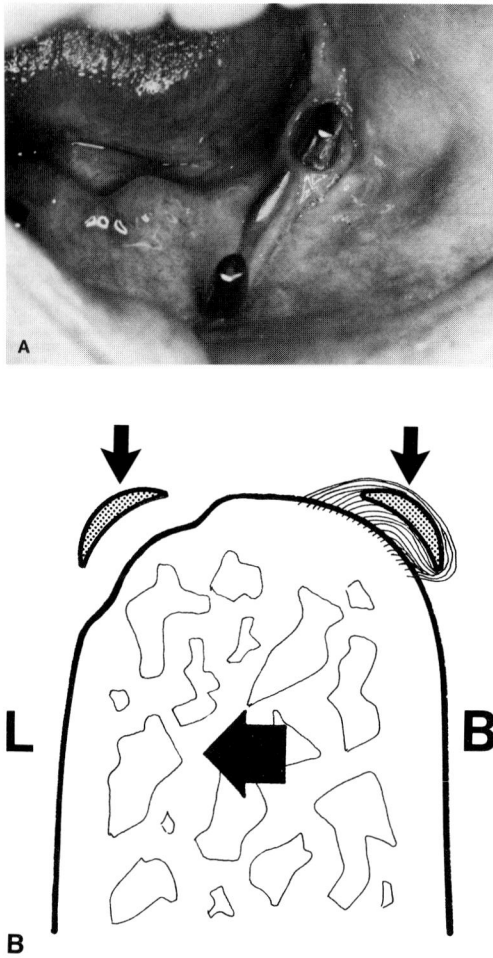

FIG. 25-7. (A) Dehiscent subperiosteal implant posterior lingual peripheral strut designed to cover the mylohyoid ridge when implant was placed 10 years earlier. (B) Graphic illustration showing architecture of ligament in the areas of the external oblique and mylohyoid ridges. Understanding the dynamics of the suspensory ligament offers explanation for this and other previously enigmatic problems. (L-lingual;B-buccal; large arrow indicates direction of medial deflection of mandible on opening; small arrows indicate direction of occlusal forces. See text.)

been observed that lingual posterior struts near the crest of the ridge develop early dehiscence. An understanding of the subperiosteal implant suspensory system offers explanation for these enigmatic problems.

When the mouth is opened a medial movement of the angle of the mandible occurs; thus, a posterior subperiosteal strut on the medial aspect of the mandible will cause bone resorption, etiologic to excessive pressure from the strut against the bone resulting from such movement. If the strut is near the crest, the resorption results in loss of the crest with resultant dehiscence (Fig 25-7). However, if the strut is several millimeters inferior to the crest, a suspensory ligament can be formed from the bone superior to the strut, and an eventual physiologic balance can be achieved (Fig. 25-8). This explains why we seldom see problems in the anterior lingual area, where the struts are more inferior on a medial surface and where the medial displacement is minimal. The connective tissue tends to be thicker in areas where pressure may be excessive. Such a response reduces pressure directly subajacent to struts and thereby decreases further resorption (Fig. 25-9).

Thus, it is apparent that the load-bearing capacity of struts of metal dental implants, whether endosteal or subperiosteal, is dependent upon medial and lateral bundle bone formation with resultant Sharpey's fibers that are continuous with principal fiber systems that form a sling or suspensory ligament around the strut. This mechanism forms from stress mediated from occlusal and other forces placed on the implant and provides a physiologic condition allowing for long-term function with healthy tissue.

Permucosal Endosteal Dental Implants

Historically, the permucosal endosteal implant is the oldest form of dental implant. Claims have been made of ancient Egyptian writings noting the use of dental implants, and there are reports of Mayan skulls unearthed with semiprecious stones carved to the shape of teeth embedded in the jawbones and having accretions of calculus.[26]

In the late 1800s several authors used endosteal devices for patient care. As early as 1913, Greenfield reported on one of his cases that had functioned for 5 years.[27]

Currently, the devices can be categorized as being either solid, porous, or vented cones or cylinders, with or without threads or fins; smooth or threaded pins; solid or perforated plates; or combinations or variations of any of the above. All of the hollow

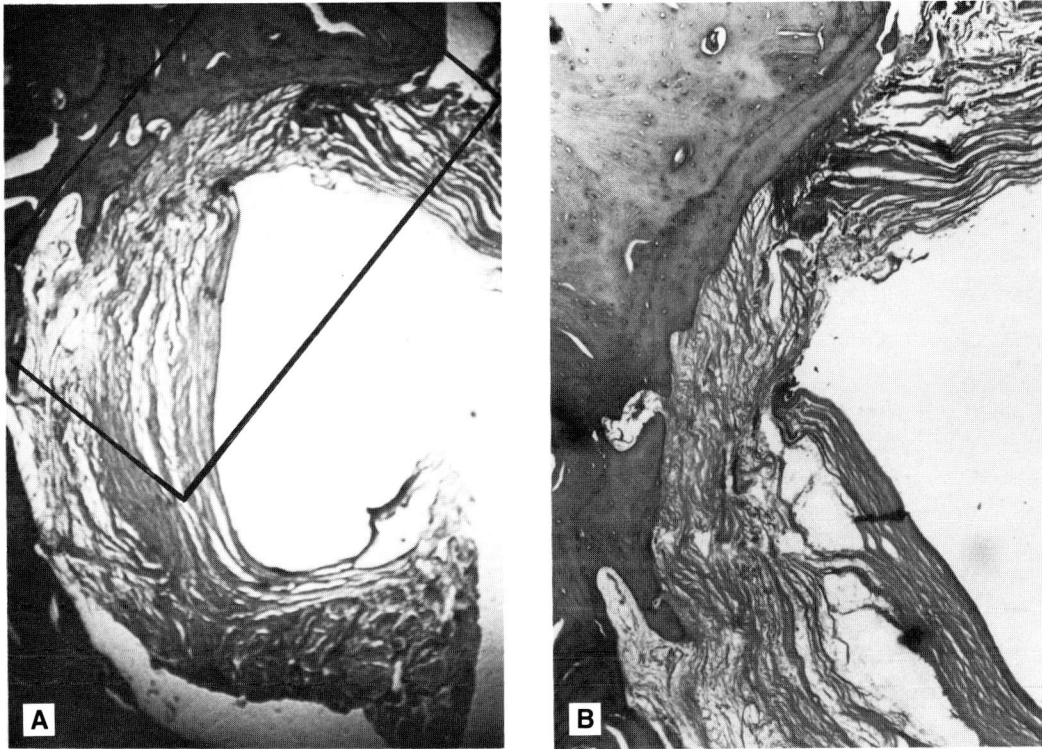

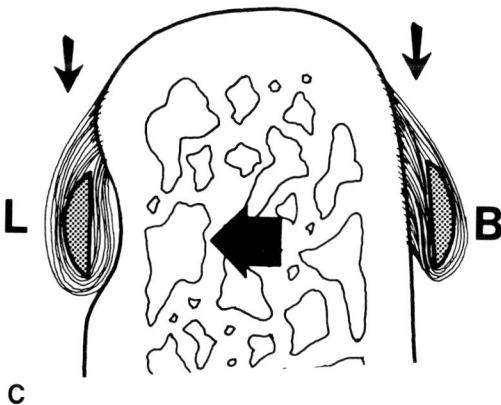

Fig. 25-8. *(A) Photomicrograph of human autopsy periimplant tissue. Device was a subperiosteal implant that had functioned for 11 years. Note the suspensory ligament which provides support from the lamellar bone coronal to this posterior lingual peripheral strut. (B) Higher magnification of area outlined in (A). (C) Graphic illustration showing architecture of ligament on posterior buccal and lingual struts placed on the lateral surface of the mandible. (Specimen courtesy of Dr. R. Bodine)*

cylinders and most of the plates are perforated. The perforations, called "vents," are provided to allow for the ingrowth of supporting bone. The surface may be smooth, textured, or porous, and may be coated with a different biomaterial. The most frequently used biomaterials in implant fabrication are titanium, titanium alloys, chrome-cobalt-molybdenum alloys, stainless steel, and nonmetals such as carbon, aluminum oxide, hydroxyapatite, and polymethylmethacrylate.

Thus, it is apparent that clinicians can choose from a broad array of commercial devices. This wide selection results in considerable confusion because most manufacturers portray their devices as being "best" and having universal application. What makes selection even more difficult is that, with few exceptions, the prognoses of these devices are unknown. For us to be confident of a favorable prognosis of any device, there are only two requirements. First, the device must have been in use for a reasonable length of time by a relatively large number of clinicians. Secondly, reports by independent clinicians must show at least 75 percent of the implants surviving for a minimum of 5 years.[28] With the

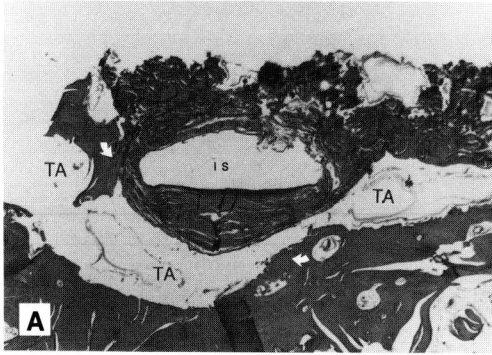

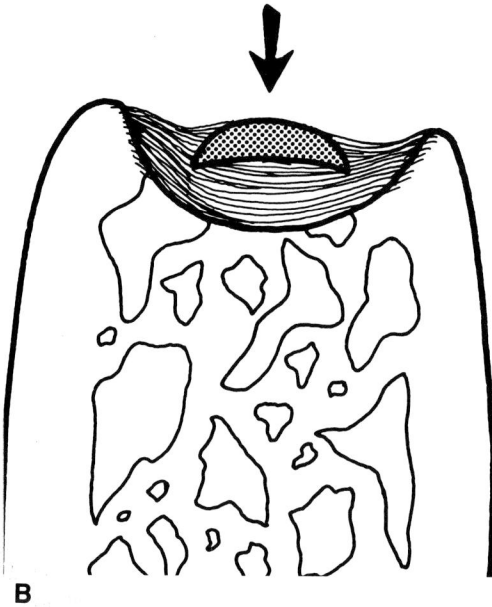

FIG. 25-9. *(A) Photomicrograph of human autopsy periimplant tissue. Device was a subperiosteal implant which had functioned for 12 years. Note thickening of suspensory ligament directly apical to strut where pressure would tend to be exerted on the bone. A similar thickening can be noted in Figure 25-8 medial to the strut where pressure results from the medial displacement of the mandible on opening (IS = Implant space, TA = Tear Artifact which resulted when implant was removed from the bone postmortem. Arrows point to areas of supporting lamella bone.) (B) Graphic illustration showing architecture of ligament which can only develop subsequent to implant settling. (Specimen courtesy of Dr. R. Bodine)*

adoption of these criteria, the options are greatly reduced and selection is simplified.

Examples of Currently Available Endosteal Implant Systems

The surgical placement of these systems is similar. All require low-speed drill prep-aration of the implant to avoid overheating the bone. Following placement of the implants, the tissue is sutured over them and they are left without loading for 3 to 6 months. The mandibular implants require 3 months integration time and the maxillary ones 4 to 6 months. A secondary phase is then required for placement of the abutments to be used in the restorative procedures.

Interpore IMZ Implant System. The Interpore IMZ Implant System was conceived in the early 1970s. It is composed of a pure titanium cylinder that is spray-coated with titanium plasma, thus increasing the surface area for bone interface. The design includes a stress-absorbing element to reduce the impact on surrounding bone structure and the residual dentition (Fig. 25-10). Indications include completely edentulous and partially edentulous maxilla and mandible. It may be used for retention of fixed as well as removable prostheses. The stress-absorbing element is replaceable each year. This encourages the patient's return for follow-up care.

Branemark Implant. The Branemark implant system consists of a pure titanium screw. It was developed in Sweden and has been in clinical use for over 20 years. The original research[29,30] related to a fixed prosthesis attached to 6 implants (fixtures) in the anterior portion of the maxilla or mandible (Fig. 25-11). Research data suggest over 80% success in the maxilla and over 90% success in the mandible. Recent studies on the use of these implants for restoration of partially edentulous cases show equivalent results.[31]

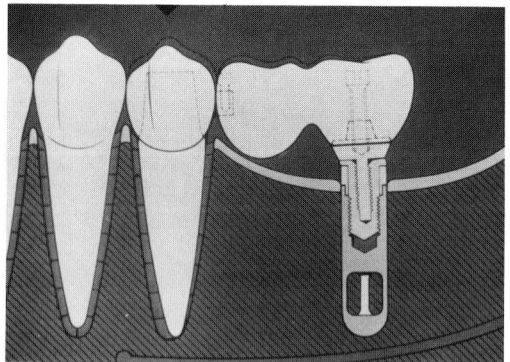

FIG. 25-10. *(A) IMZ implant device. (B) Schematic of IMZ implant. (Courtesy of Interpore Corporation)*

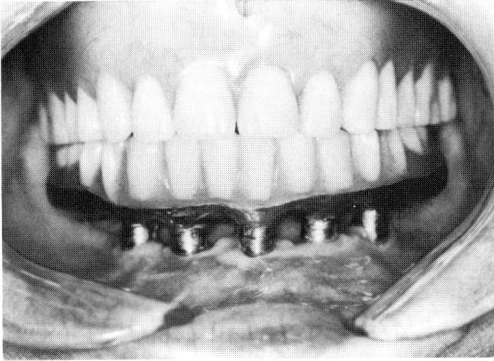

FIG. 25-11. *Five Branemark implants in place, with mandibular denture attached, 1 year after installation. The implants are exposed at the base of the denture to enhance periodontal care. (Courtesy of Dr. Donald G. Chiles)*

CoreVent Implant System. The CoreVent implant system was introduced in 1982 by Dr. Gerald Niznick.[32] This implant is made of a titanium alloy composed of 90% titanium, 6% aluminum, and 4% vanadium. It is reportedly 60% stronger than pure titanium (Core-Venture, Vol. 1, CoreVent Corp., 1986). The original design was a cylindrical hollow-vented implant with screw threads in the mid portion (Fig. 25-12). The system has been expanded to include a Screw-Vent (which looks very much like the Branemark design), a Sub-Vent (submergible Blade-Vent), and a Micro-Vent.

Basic Principles of Endosteal Implant Design

BACKGROUND AND DEFINITIONS

The principles of endosteal dental implant design are by no means new. They are based on two assumptions. The first assumption is that the primary etiology of pergingival periimplant pathology is related to the presence of bacterial plaque in the gingival sulcus surrounding the implant post. The second assumption is that, within limits, stress applied to the bone through functional loads placed upon an implant results in osteogenesis and bone maintenance, and that when loads are increased to exceed the physiologic limit, osteolysis will occur.

Careful application of the principles ensures the clinician the best possible prognosis for long-term function of the im-

plant. If one is to completely follow the principles at the present time, it will be necessary to custom design each device to most satisfactorily meet the needs of each patient. If it is decided that custom designing will not be employed, one must be alert to the compromises associated with the commercial devices chosen.

The principles are divided into two closely related categories. The first relates to the design of the post-cervix-crown complex, and is based on the assumption presented earlier: that chronic periimplant pathology originates in this area and that its etiology is related directly to bacterial plaque and their toxins. The second category involves the relationship between the bone and the load-bearing aspects of the implant, and recognizes that acute pathologic changes can occur when the bone and other supporting tissues are stressed beyond physiologic limits. Compromises in either of these categories will enhance pathologic changes in tissues associated with both.

Before proceeding further, certain definitions are in order:

Infrastructure—The portion of the implant that provides the load-bearing abilities of the implant.

Post—the portion of the implant that extends from the infrastructure to the cervix and must bear and transfer the total load to the infrastructure.

Cervix—the portion of the implant that forms the transition between the post and the crown.

Crown—the portion of the implant that interfaces with and provides retention for the intraoral prosthesis.

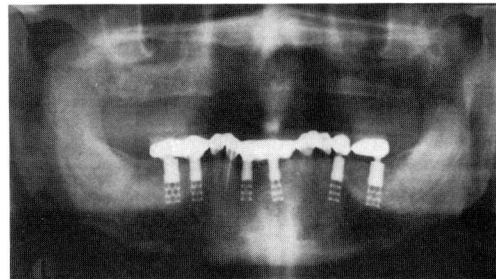

FIG. 25-12. *Radiograph of CoreVent implants in place, 2 years after installation. Hollow cylinder cores show good osseointegration. (Courtesy of Dr. Donald G. Chiles)*

CATEGORY I—THE POST-CERVIX-CROWN COMPLEX: THE ACHILLES' HEEL

Vertical bone loss around the post of all types of endosteal dental implants occurs frequently extending from the pergingival site. It is assumed to have an etiology tantamount to periodontal disease. Thus, the design of this post-cervix-crown complex is critical to the long-term maintenance of endosteal dental implant cases.

1. The Post Should Be As Long As Possible. Vertical bone loss around the post of endosteal implants is a consistent finding. The lesion extends from the pergingival site and spreads along the surface of the implant. If the infrastructure has a shoulder or other irregularity located near the pergingival site, when the lesion reaches and extends out along the irregularity it can be destructive to the covering crestal alveolar bone, and the eventual loss of the implant can result in considerable loss of alveolar bone. Once this lesion has extended apically into the interstices of the infrastructure, it can be extremely difficult or impossible to treat. It was learned from the use of the Chercheve[33] screw that, when the helical interstices of the implant infrastructure were implanted very deep in bone, the lesion could take several years to extend along the post from the pergingival site to the interstices. However, once the lesion reached the helix, the entire infrastructure became engulfed in granulation tissue over a matter of weeks or months, rendering the lesion unmanageable.

Using a long post has at least four advantages. First, it confines the pergingival lesion. The longer the post, the further isolated will be the complex configurations of the infrastructure from the pergingival site, the origin of most periimplant pathology. The pergingival lesion extends from the cervix, apically along the implant post. Once the lesion reaches the infrastructure, it can spread over a broad area and cause extensive damage, even while the infrastructure continues to provide support and function. This destructive lesion can progress asymptomatically until so much bony support has been lost that the critical support:load ratio is violated. Acute episodes generally do not occur until either the lesion has extended so far from the per-

gingival site that drainage from the lesion is hampered, or the support:load ratio becomes intolerable. If undetected or ignored until an acute episode occurs, so much damage may have taken place that subsequent implant or prosthetic management will be severely compromised.

Second, it controls the direction and location of the lesion, thus minimizing bone destruction. By having a long post, the lesion is directed apically and remains in the immediate vicinity of the post, destruction of the crestal bone is consequently minimized, and the original bone morphology is preserved.

Third, it provides a longer "fuse." Because the lesion becomes unmanageable when it reaches the interstices of the infrastructure, the post can be seen as a "fuse" along which the lesion must extend on its way to the infrastructure. A longer post provides a longer fuse, thus providing greater leeway for timing surgical intervention. It is highly desirable to intervene and treat the expanding lesion while still in this fuse stage, before it can do excessive damage. Such a lesion progresses slowly, and should be allowed to extend between one half to two thirds of the length of the post before initiating surgical intervention. This may take as little as 3 years, or up to 10 years or more before it reaches this critical point. Thus, one can plan and implement corrective surgery at a convenient time.

Finally, it simplifies the corrective surgery. It is highly desirable to intervene and correct a defect rather than to wait until damage is so severe that the entire implant must be removed and the crestal bone is irreversibly destroyed. When the lesion has been confined to only the post area, not only is the damage to bone confined, but its surgical management is greatly simplified. When the defect has extended to the interstices of the infrastructure, it becomes extremely difficult to remove all granulation tissue that has extended around them. When many of these appendages exist, corrective surgery often becomes impossible.

Surgical note: An incision is made parallel to and as near to the crest of the ridge as possible, extending anterior and posterior from the post approximately 1.5 cm. Full-thickness flaps are elevated buccally and lingually, and buccal relief incisions are extended only if necessary. Periodontal curettes are used to remove all granulation tissue from between the bony walls of the defect and the post. Following thorough debridement of the wound, the exposed post surface is cleaned mechanically with acrylic yarn that has been impregnated with sterile pumice. It is worked into the lesion and around the post with curettes. The yarn is removed and the wound is irrigated with copious amounts of sterile normal saline solution. A "prophyjet" can be helpful in cleaning, but precautions must be taken to maintain a sterile field. Next, yarn soaked in concentrated citric acid is worked into the wound, wrapped around the post, and left in position for approximately 5 minutes. The citric acid kills any remaining bacteria. Although some bone destruction will result, the action of the acid is self limiting and damage to the bone is minimal. After thorough irrigation with normal saline solution, a suitable graft material can be packed into the defect and the soft tissue flaps repositioned and sutured. The best graft material is autogenous bone harvested from any available source. A second choice is freeze-dried decalcified cortical powder reconstituted with whole autogenous blood. Packs and dressings are usually contraindicated.

2. The Post Should Be As Small As Possible, Consistent With The Strength Required. Few things can be more disconcerting than to have an implant fracture after it has served for a number of years with little or no evidence of pathology occurring. A cross-sectional area of 3 mm^2 is the minimum post size for surgical grade chromium cobalt-molybdenum alloys: although 4 mm^2 or 5 mm^2 is preferred, posts made of pure titanium require a minimum of 5 mm^2 or 6 mm^2 area for their cross-section because of the increased modulus of elasticity of titanium.

Although the post must have sufficient strength, it should be as small in cross-section as is consistent with the strength requirements necessary for the forces to be placed on it. As previously described, epithelium at the base of the periimplant sulcus is adherent to the implant post by the same hemidesmosomal adherent mechanism found at the base of the periodontal sulcus. This provides the seal necessary to impede the ingress of bacteria. The tooth, however, has the added advantage of having fibers extend directly into it immediately apical to the adherent epithelium, thus reinforcing and holding it in place. Without such fibers extending into the implant, the only protection this seal on an implant has is the elastic system of alternating circumferential bands of epithelium and connective tissue fibers. This viscoelastic system is subject to the same physical laws as any elastic material. The amount of deflection of such an elastic material increases logarithmically with the distance between supports. Thus, the deflection caused by the wedging action of objects like a popcorn husk or a toothbrush bristle has a much greater potential for mechanically tearing the adherent epithelium away from the implant if it is protected by a longer circumferential band of tissue as is present around a larger diameter post as opposed to the shorter circumferential band surrounding a small diameter post.

3. The Surface On The Postcervix Portion Should Be As Smooth As Possible. Because bacterial plaque plays such a prominent role in causing periimplant disease, and because the periimplant lesion originates at the pergingival site, it seems prudent that the cervical area be designed to facilitate the removal of bacterial plaque. This concept dictates that the coronal end of the post and the cervical region be as smooth as possible. Bacteria take advantage of any surface defect in their relentless efforts to multiply. Once entrenched in a surface irregularity, their mechanical removal is impaired (Fig. 25-3).

The American Society for Testing Metals specifies that stainless steel implants must have an electropolished surface throughout. Thus, all dental implants made from stainless steel have a highly polished cervical region. Kyocera's single-crystal aluminum oxide implants probably provide the best example of a smooth surface. Even scanning electron micrographs of 20,000 × magnification fail to show anything but a glassy smooth surface.

Numerous attempts to lure a fibrous attachment into the cervical region by providing a porous surface have met with failure. Once the bacteria begin to colonize in the porous surface, tissue breakdown rapidly ensues.

4. The Cervix Should Have A Morphology That Facilitates Bacterial Plaque Removal. All sharp angles in the cervical region should be eliminated. Corners must be rounded. A cross-section should be either circular or elliptic and, when viewed buccally or proximally, the transition from the post to the crown should curve gently, similar to that of a golf tee.

It is difficult to find a commercial product that adheres to this principle. The Cranin anchor had such a design, but is no longer commercially available. Almost all commercially available devices fall far short of fulfilling this requirement.

5. The Cervix-Crown Margin Should Be Supragingival. The periodontal compromises associated with subgingival margins have long been recognized, yet it seems difficult to find an implant patient who does not have subgingival margins on the implant retainers. There are only three justifications for the placement of subgingival margins: esthetics, caries, and retention. The most common endosteal implant location is in the lower posterior portion of the oral cavity. Certainly esthetics is of little concern here, no caries problem exists, and there are numerous methods of joining two metal parts without resorting to a long crown and cement. In other words, there is little justification for the widespread employment of subgingival margins on implant retainers.

6. No Mating Parts Of The Implant Should Join Subgingivally. Recently, there has been an increasing trend to develop multiple part endosteal implants with staged surgery.[32,34,35] The implant is placed initially in a totally submerged state and, after a suitable interval ranging from 2 to 6 months, it is surgically uncovered and a post is added. Such a regimen invariably leaves a compromised post and cervical region. It must be recognized that the sulcus continually extends apically and therefore eventually will encompass the joint where parts mate. Even with the highest level of sophistication in machining and in quality control aimed at improved fidelity in the mating parts, small spaces between them that can harbor anaerobic bacteria will exist. Thus, the potential has been achieved for establishing an endotoxin generator that discharges into the sulcus. With low fidelity between mating parts, pathologic changes can be detected early and are essentially untreatable.

There is no question about the improved tissue response around a totally implanted device but, once exposed, early gain is soon forfeited and the long-term maintenance of such devices is severely compromised. The important factor to remember is that this early gain comes from keeping the implant out of function and is achieved simply by keeping loads off the implant for a suitable period of time. Occasionally, it becomes necessary to place fixed or removable protective splints around the implant crown to protect it from muscular activity of the tongue during this healing period. However, this is much to be preferred, both in financial savings to the patient and in long-term prognosis, to the liabilities imposed by the subgingival or infrabony joining of parts.

Recent work by Akagawa et al.[36] supports this position. They implanted screw-shaped single crystal sapphire and titanium implants in dogs with some submerged and others exposed. In the dog, any device protruding into the oral cavity on the crest or the ridge will be in function even though it does not come into occlusal contact with an antagonist. Thus the variables were submerged implants vs. exposed and functioning implants. Their results showed a direct bony interface with all variables. While there was a more consistent and dense bony interface with the submerged implants, it must be remembered that the exposed implants were in function. No difference between the metal and nonmetal implants was noted.

In light of the evidence that hemidesmosomes have formed within 48 hours after implantation[15] (thus providing a protective seal), combined with the arguments cited in the preceding paragraphs, it is totally unnecessary to be burdened with all of the long-term compromises in the cervical area that are inherent with a submerged, multiple-part implant.

7. The Morphology Of The Cervix/ Crown Portion Of The Implant Must Be Harmonious With The Contours Of The

Dental Prosthesis And Must Facilitate Plaque Removal From Both The Implant And The Prosthesis. The contours of the implant and the crown must be harmonized to produce a total restoration that can be maintained as near plaque free as is possible. Overhanging margins, bulbous gingival contours, and closed embrasures are contraindicated on implant retainers for the same reasons that they are contraindicated on retainers cemented to teeth—the health of the soft tissue must be preserved through plaque elimination.

CATEGORY II—THE INFRASTRUCTURE

Support for dental implants can be achieved by means of a direct bone interface or a connective tissue suspensory ligament. Screw-shaped configurations appear to require a direct bone interface. When it is destroyed, loss of the implant follows shortly thereafter. Apparently there is no satisfactory mechanism whereby a connective tissue suspensory ligament can form around a screw-shaped device without having excessive shear forces develop to which such a ligament cannot adapt. Thus, it loses its loadbearing capabilities and as the mechanical interdigitations of the bone and implant are lost, the screw can no longer be retained. Fortunately, approximately 85 percent of the screw-shaped devices achieve a direct bone interface. Most other configurations can function either with a direct bony interface or with a connective tissue suspensory ligament. It seems reasonable to assume a direct bone interface is desirable. However, it is even more desirable to have an implant that can continue to function if such an interface does not develop or is subsequently lost.

Bone loss originating in the area of the infrastructure is directly related to overloading of the implant, rarely remains asymptomatic, and usually occurs early in treatment. This condition is best illustrated when an implant is loaded for the first time. Slight tenderness to heavy loads in which symptoms rapidly decrease with time is common. However, if the prosthesis is placed inadvertently in hyperocclusion, symptoms often rapidly increase and cause the patient severe distress within 48 hours. Location and correction of the occlusal prematurity invariably offers immediate relief, and symptoms will disappear within 24 hours. The three remaining principles apply to this vital loadbearing portion of the implant.

8. The Infrastructure Must Have Maximum Provisions For Loadbearing. It has been aptly demonstrated in perforated endosteal metal plates that a hammock-like suspensory ligament can form, extending through vents in and apical to the implant from the buccal and lingual bone. Thus the buccal and lingual bone provides the principal support for these devices when functioning in a ligament. To take best advantage of this system, two considerations are necessary. First, full advantage of all available bone must be taken. This means that the implant must extend in all directions to the full limit of available bone. Second, the implant must have ample provision for the maximum development of suspensory ligaments through extensive venting of the implant should the direct bone interface fail to occur or be subsequently lost. The Miter Titanalloy is an excellent example of this latter consideration.

9. Loadbearing Should Be Remote From The Pergingival Area. By keeping the infrastructure well isolated from the pergingival area, it is better protected from the pergingival lesion. (The rationale for this was covered under the topic of the long post.)

10. The Cross-Sectional Contour Of The Struts Should Approximate The Lines Of A Parabolic Curve, With No Macroscopic Concavities. The suspensory ligament discussed previously always follows a parabolic curve. If the struts are contoured to take advantage of this configuration, the epithelium that interfaces with an implant functioning in a suspensory ligament is discouraged from building up in multiple layers. Any surface concavity will be filled by excessive layers of epithelium and, even though the surface layer may adhere to the implant, multiple layers of epithelium located deep within connective tissue seems to be inviting unnecessary risk by providing a nidus for epithelial proliferation.

Transosteal Dental Implants

Transosteal implants are often referred to as orthopedic devices. They consist of transosteal pins or screws attached to a bony plate on the inferior border of the mandible. Transosteal implants are indicated when moderate to severe bone atrophy exists, or in cases of bone loss due to trauma.

A more common and better known device is the mandibular staple bone plate (Fig. 25-13). The implant is placed through an extraoral approach, seating the plate against the inferior border of the mandible in the symphysis region. Predrilled holes through the mandible permit the transosteal pins to penetrate into the oral cavity where the attachments connect to the denture to stabilize it. The prosthesis is tissue-supported.

Another transosteal implant, developed and used in The Netherlands with good success, is the transmandibular implant. The fixture is made of gold alloy with five individual bone screws and two transmandibular posts, all as separate units. This permits the path of insertion of each unit on an individual basis before attaching to the bone plate. Another advantage is that this unit permits vertical loading of the prosthesis, with increased patient satisfaction (Fig. 25-14). Like the mandibular staple, the transmandibular implant requires an extraoral approach.

Subperiosteal Dental Implants

The subperiosteal dental implant has been used for over 35 years to provide edentulous patients with improved function, comfort, and well-being (Fig. 25-15).

The subperiosteal implant concept, first proposed by Gustav Dahl in the early

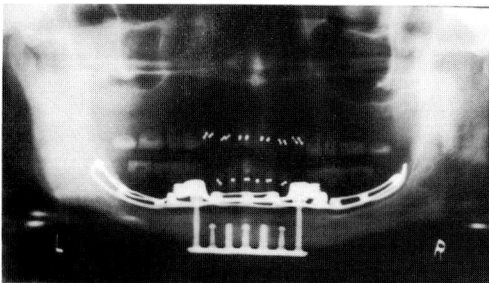

FIG. 25-14. *Composite radiograph of transosteal mandibular implant in place. Note the individual nature of each pin, permitting individual insertion with vertical loading ability.*

1940s, was introduced in the United States in 1949 by Gerskoff and Goldberg, who used intraoral radiographs to obtain bone contours of the mandible. Many of these early attempts resulted in premature failure probably, in part, because of the discrepancies in bone to implant proximity. Berman[37] suggested taking a direct bone impression as a first stage procedure and placing the implant at a second stage operation. By 1952 this practice had become

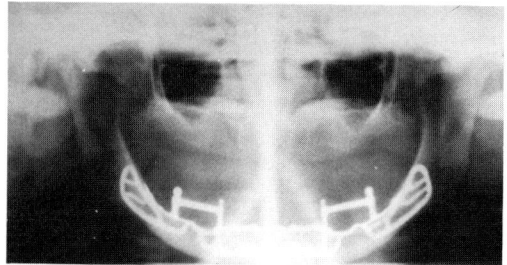

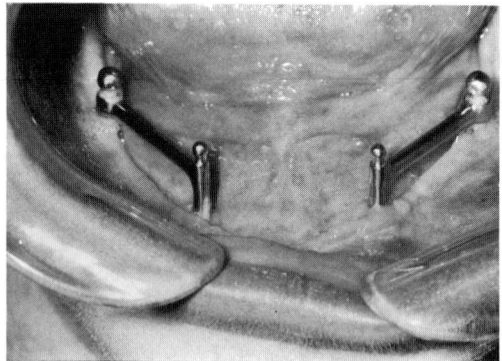

FIG. 25-15. *(A) Radiograph of subperiosteal implant placed in the usual 2-stage manner (2 years after insertion). (B) Intra-oral view of implant. Note cleanliness of superstructure and healthy quality of the gingivae.*

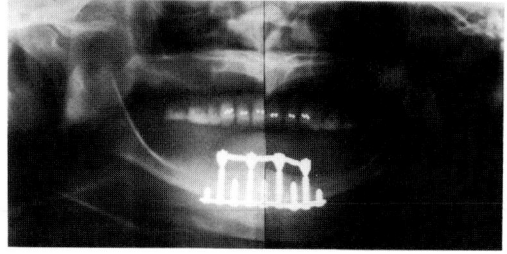

FIG. 25-13. *Radiograph of a transosteal mandibular staple bone plate. Note 7-pin appliance with stress-broken mandibular denture in place (7 years after installation). (Courtesy of Dr. Donald G. Chiles)*

the standard and continues to this date. Other early pioneers who worked with subperiosteal implants include Bodine,[38] Jermyne,[39] Lew,[40] and Cranin.[41]

In 1980, Harold P. Truitt at Loma Linda University School of Dentistry, developed a research program utilizing computerized tomography to produce a morphologic replication of the mandible. His original unpublished work consisted of comparing actual measurements to CT image measurements on dry skulls and subsequently cadavers. This work showed less than a 0.55 mm difference when using 18 separate anatomic landmarks, and was of sufficient accuracy to warrant proceeding to human subjects (Figs. 25-16, 25-17).

The advantage of such a technique is that it eliminates the second surgical procedure, the waiting time, and the further risk of infection in the two stage operation. The disadvantage of the CT imaging technique is that perfect replication of the bony tissue is not always possible and the casting may not fit accurately. In such instances small amounts of graft material may need to be added to fill in the minor discrepancies. Graft materials available are particulate bone marrow, freeze-dried human cancellous bone chips, and particulate hydroxyapatite.

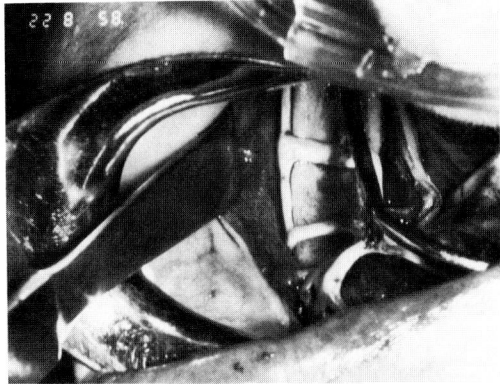

Fig. 25-17. *Body of mandible and seated implant made from a model obtained from a CT scan. Note excellent fit of the implant to the bone.*

Three-dimensional imaging is a rapidly expanding field. With new diagnostic techniques, new computer software, and continued research, accuracy will increase and this service will be more available.

Implant Disease and Management

Why are implants lost? With the exception of actual physical, mechanical, or structural failure of the device, all the etiologic factors are related to tissue pathology and fall into three categories: inadequate oral hygiene, adverse systemic conditions, and overloading or an inadequate support: load ratio.

Oral Hygiene

If the patient is not achieving adequate oral hygiene, what are the reasons? At least seven reasons can be given for why a patient may fail in this area. He may be unmotivated, uneducated, or have inadequate motor or psychomotor skills. An improperly designed implant, improper surface texture, improper implant placement, and an improperly executed prosthesis can affect oral hygiene. The responsibility for each of these situations lies, at least in part, with the treating dentist.

MOTIVATION AND EDUCATION

Although these matters may be listed separately, in practice they are too closely related to treat individually. If patients understand that poor oral hygiene can lead to early loss of their implants, they nearly always have the necessary incentive to be diligent in their efforts. It is rare to find an

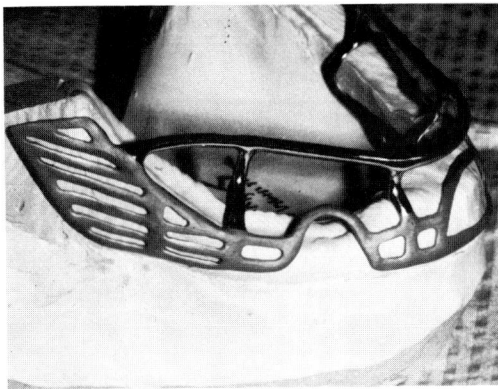

Fig. 25-16. *Current design of complete mandibular subperiosteal implant. Note extensive use of accessory struts on lateral aspect of the anterior ramus and body of the mandible. This area can allow for the early development of suspensory ligaments without a preceding settling. Note intraoral bar (Brookdale bar) which provides added strength for the appliance. (Model was generated from CT scan.)*

unmotivated implant patient. Once these patients have committed themselves to undergo surgery and have accepted its accompanying risks and discomforts, and once they have decided to embark on treatment involving considerable expense, time, inconvenience, and discomfort, with no guarantees of long-term implant survival, they are motivated. However, if they have not been educated and trained in the techniques necessary for plaque removal, motivation will not help. It will not eliminate poor oral hygiene. Patients must be provided with education and training, and dentists must educate their patients about the causes of periimplant disease.

MOTOR SKILLS

Some people do not have the motor or psychomotor skills necessary to maintain an adequate level of oral hygiene. Such persons generally have family members who are involved in the decision-making process leading to implantation and who can provide the necessary assistance, but only if they have been trained to do so. Even then, the implantologist must be responsible for training. It is not enough merely to tell people to brush and floss; they must have sufficient supervised, hands-on training to enable them to achieve their goal.

DESIGN AND SURFACE TEXTURE

The implant must be designed in such a manner, in both configuration and surface texture, to allow for the easy removal of bacterial plaque in the pergingival area.

PLACEMENT AND SUBSEQUENT PROSTHESIS

Even an implant designed for easy plaque removal can be surgically positioned in a way that frustrates hygienic efforts, and the morphology of the subsequent overlying prosthesis must harmonize with that of the implant so that the result may be maintained hygienically.

Systemic Conditions

As far as adverse systemic conditions are concerned, the implantologist has only limited control. Unsuitable candidates can be eliminated through proper medical screening. By capitalizing on the high level of motivation common to these patients, the treating dentist can often be instrumental in correcting existing conditions that adversely affect tissue response and bone maintenance. The patient is encouraged to establish life style changes that will promote health. The benefits thus accrued by the patient extend far beyond the immediate treatment of the edentulous or partially edentulous condition.

Support:Load Ratio

Unfortunately no significant data are available about what the proper support: load ratio might be. Suffice it to say that, in the design of our implants, it is reasonable to provide as much support as possible and to reduce loads on the implant to a minimum. Increased support can be achieved through direct implant bone interface as compared with that provided by a periimplant ligament. Thus, increasing the surface area through porosity or other forms of surface texturing may enhance the development and preservation of a bony interface. The risk of such texturing surfaces when a bacterial colony is established within such intersticies leaving it immune to all forms of therapy with the result of premature implant loss.[42,43] With this background in mind, the ten basic principles of endosteal dental implant design are presented.

Conclusions

Oral implantology offers reasonable options for the treatment of all stages of edentulousness. The subperiosteal implant provides a predictable solution for the totally edentulous atrophied arch and also can be employed in the partially edentulous atrophied arch. The Ramus Frame probably also offers a predictable result for the edentulous mandible that has adequate vertical height of bone in the region anterior to the mental foramina. The same can probably be said for the mandibular staple bone plate, however, the patient must continue to contend with a soft tissue-borne appliance. A number of root-shaped devices can be employed in the anterior region of the mandible, where there is sufficient height and width of bone. Several of these can be placed endosteally and splinted together to provide either a fixed prostheses which cantilevers posteriorly or provides support for a fixed removable combination.

Perforated metal plates can provide reliable support for fixed partial dentures in partially edentulous jaws where there is sufficient alveolar bone remaining.

Where sufficient facial-lingual width and vertical height of alveolar bone remains, the various root-shaped devices that can be used in the anterior mandible can also be used to replace individual teeth, either to stand alone or to provide support for a fixed prosthesis. These devices include conical and cylindrical shapes that may be solid, porous, or vented, with or without screw threads or fins. The surgeon should use caution with any of these tooth-shaped devices because with few exceptions, the prognosis is unknown, either because of their recent development, or because of the absence of reported survival studies by persons other than the developers who stand to profit from their sale.

References

1. Toto, P.D.: Mucopolysaccharides in the epithelial attachment. J. Dent. Res., *44*:451, 1965.
2. James, R.A. and Kelln, E.E.: A histopathological study of the nature of the epithelium surrounding implant posts, Parts I and II. Oral Implant., *3*:105, 1972 and *3*:137, 1973.
3. James, R.A., and Kelln, E.E.: A histopathological report on the nature of the epithelium and underlying connective tissue which surrounds oral implants. J. Biomed. Mater. Res. Symposium, No. 5 (Part 22), 373, 1974.
4. Ponitz, D.P., et al.: Passage of orally administered tetracycline into the gingival crevice around natural and around protruding subperiosteal implant abutments in man. Dent. Clin. North Am., *14*:125, 1970.
5. James, R.A.: Histopathologic study of supporting tissues of an endosteal implant. Implantologist, *1*:19, 1976.
5a. James, R.A.: The support system and the pergingival defense mechanism of oral implants. J. Oral Implant., *6*:270, 1976.
6. Waerhaug, J.: Observations on replanted tooth plated with gold foil; reaction to pure gold; mode of epithelial attachment to gold; expulsion of foreign bodies from pockets. Oral Surg., Oral Med., Oral Path., *9*:780, 1956.
7. Stallard, R.E., et al.: Vitreous carbon implants—and aid to alveolar bone maintenance. J. Oral Implantol., *VI(2)*:286, 1976.
8. James, R.A., and Schultz, R.L.: Hemidesmosomes and the adhesion of junctional epithelial cells to metal implants—A preliminary report. Oral Implant., *4*:294, 1974.
9. Listgarten, M.A., and Lai, C.H.: Ultrastructure of the intact interface between an endosseous epoxy resin dental implant and host tissue. J. Biol. Buccale, *3*:13, 1975.
10. Samida, M., et al.: The Effects of Surface Texture and Bacterial Plaque on the Tissues Surrounding Vitreous Carbon Implants. Proceedings, Third Annual Meeting of Society for Biomaterials. New Orleans, 1977.
11. Gould, T.R.L., et al.: The attachment mechanism of epithelial cells to titanium in vitro J. Periodont. Res., *16*:611, 1981.
12. Ogiso, M., et al.: Investigation of hydroxyapatite ceramic inplant under occlusal function. J. Dent. Res., *60A*:419, 1981.
13. McKinney, R.V., et al.: Clinical and histologic observations on the single crystal sapphire endosteal dental implant. Transactions of the 7th Annual Meeting of Society for Biomaterials, Troy, New York, May 28-31, 1981.
14. Kavanagh, et al.: A rodent model for the investigation of dental implants. J. Prosthet. Dent., *54*:252, 1985.
15. Swope, E.M. and James, R.A.: A longitudinal study of hemidesmosome formation at the dental implant-tissue interface. Oral Implantol., *9*:412, 1981.
16. Taylor, A.C., et al.: Reattachment of gingival epithelium to the tooth. J. Periodont., *43*:281, 1972.
17. Hoppe, V.W.: Tierexperimentelle untersuchungen uber den epithelansatz am implantatstift. DZZ, 14, 1959.
18. Gorhmann, A.: Untersuchungen uber die passage von 35-S-markierten mykobacterien und staphylokokken an perforationsstellen von gerustpfeilern. Inaugural dissertation, Kiel, 1969.
19. Schlegel, S., et al.: Experimental bacteremia to demonstrate the barrier function of epithelium and connective tissue surrounding oral endosseous implants. Internat. J. Oral Surg., *7*:569, 1978.
20. Jahn, E., et al.: Bindegewebige aufhangung bei blattimplantaten. Vorlaufige Mitteilung. Schweiz. Monatsschr. Zahnheilkd., *85*:1143, 1975.

21. Kaketa, T., et al.: Histopathological findings on endosseous implants in dogs (immediate implant method). Bull. Tokyo Dent. Coll., *10*:61, 1969.

22. Bodine, R.L., and Mohammed, C.I.: Histologic studies of a human mandible supporting an implant denture. J. Prosthet. Dent., *21*:203, 1969.

23. Bodine, R.L., and Mohammed, C.I.: Histologic studies of a human mandible supporting an implant denture, Part II. J. Prosthet. Dent., *26*:415, 1971.

24. Bodine, R.L., et al.: Long-term implant denture histology and comparison with previous reports. J. Prosthet. Dent., *35*:665, 1976.

25. James, R.A.: Host response to dental implant devices. *In* Biocompatability of Dental Materials, Vol. IV. Edited by D.F. Williams and D.C. Smith. Boca Raton, CRC Press, 1983.

26. Anjard, R.: Mayan dental wonders. Oral Implantol., *9*:423, 1981.

27. Greenfield, E.J.: Implantation of artificial crown and bridge abutments. Dental Cosmos, *15*:364, 1913.

28. Schnitman, P.A., and Schulman, L.B.: Dental implants: benefit and risk. An N.I.H. Harvard Consensus Development Conference, U.S. Dept of Health and Human Services, Publication No. 81:1531, 1980.

29. Hansson, B.O.: Success and failure of osseointegrated implants in the edentulous jaw. Swedish Dent. J., Suppl 1, 1977.

30. Branemark, P.I., et al.: Osseointegrated implants in the treatment of the edentulous jaw. Experience from a 10-year period. Scand. J. Plast. Reconstr. Surg., *11*:Suppl. 16, 1977.

31. Albrektsson, T., et al.: The long-term efficacy of currently used dental implants: A review and proposed criteria of success. International J. Oral & Maxillofacial Implants, *1*:11, 1986.

32. Niznick, G.A.: The Core-vent implant system. Implantologist, *3*:34, 1983/1984.

33. Chercheve, R.: Considerations d'actualite sur les implants dentaires et particulierement endo-osseus. Inform. Dent., 71, 1322, 1960.

34. Branemark, P.I.: Osseointegration and its experimental background. J. Prosth. Dent., *50*:399, 1983.

35. Roberts, E.: Rigid endosseous anchorage and tricalcium phosphate (TCP) coated implants. J. Calif. Dent. Assn., *12*(12):158, 1984.

36. Akagawa, Y., et al.: Initial bone-implant interfaces of submergible and supramergible endosseous single-crystal sapphire implants. J. Prosthet. Dent., *55*:96, 1986.

37. Berman, N.: Subperiosteal implant for full lower denture. Washington State Dental J., Dec. 5, 1950.

38. Bodine, R.L.: Canine experimentation with subperiosteal prosthodontic implants. J. Implant Dent., *2*:14, 1955.

39. Jermyne, A.C.: Ball-point balanced occlusion in the implant denture. J. Implant Dent., *2*:31, 1955.

40. Lew, I.: Progress in implant dentistry—an evaluation. JADA, 59:478, 1959.

41. Cranin, A.N.: Pharmacodynamics: pre- and post-operative care of the implant patient. J. Implant Dent., *3*:29, 1956.

42. Kent, J.N., and Homsy, C.A.: Pilot studies of a porous implant in dentistry and oral surgery. J. Oral Surg., *30*:608, 1972.

43. Schneider, et al.: Clinical evaluation of porous alumina ceramic dental implants. Oral Implant., 8:371, 1979.

Index

Numerals in *italics* indicate a figure, "t" following a page number indicates a table.